Minimally Invasive Surgical Techniques for Cancers of the Gastrointestinal Tract

Joseph Kim · Julio Garcia-Aguilar
Editors

Minimally Invasive Surgical Techniques for Cancers of the Gastrointestinal Tract

A Step-by-Step Approach

Second Edition

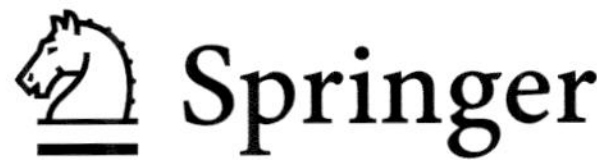

Editors
Joseph Kim
Department of Surgery
University of Kentucky
Lexington, KY
USA

Julio Garcia-Aguilar
Department of Surgery
Memorial Sloan-Kettering
Cancer Center
New York, NY
USA

Springer Science+Business Media New York
ISBN 978-3-030-18742-2   ISBN 978-3-030-18740-8   (eBook)
https://doi.org/10.1007/978-3-030-18740-8

This Springer imprint is published by the registered company Springer Nature Switzerland AG
The registered company address is: Gewerbestrasse 11, 6330 Cham, Switzerland

Preface

As we began our preparations for the second edition of this textbook, we were obliged to recognize the increasing implementation of laparoscopic and robotic surgical techniques for routine and advanced cancer operations of the gastrointestinal tract. We recruited authors that are experts in their respective fields to provide details on the surgical procedures while providing experienced insight to avoid technical errors. Similar to our first edition, the second edition of our textbook provides different approaches for various organs of the gastrointestinal tract. We are confident that surgeons at all levels of training will derive benefit from this work.

For the second edition, we recruited two assistant editors who have performed numerous robotic procedures for upper (Dr. George Georgakis) and lower (Dr. Garrett Friedman) cancers of the gastrointestinal tract. We owe them a debt of gratitude for their tireless work in support of completing the second edition. We were also fortunate to have Ms. Miranda Lin as an editorial assistant, without whose help, this textbook would not have been completed. She is the glue that binds this book together.

As always, we thank the support of our family members: Elsa in the Garcia-Aguilar family and Sarah, Anderson, and Lauren in the Kim family for their patience and understanding as we committed our efforts to organize a textbook that will benefit both early learners and advanced practitioners of gastrointestinal surgery.

Lexington, KY, USA
New York, NY, USA

Joseph Kim
Julio Garcia-Aguilar

Contents

Contributors

Warqaa M. Akram Brody School of Medicine at East Carolina University, Greenville, NC, USA

Amr Al-Abbas University of Pittsburgh Medical Center, Pittsburgh, PA, USA

Matthew Albert Department of Colorectal Surgery, Center for Colon & Rectal Surgery, Florida Hospital, Orlando, FL, USA

Ciro Andolfi Department of Surgery, The University of Chicago Pritzker School of Medicine, Chicago, IL, USA

Brian Badgwell The University of Texas MD Anderson Cancer Center, Houston, TX, USA

Nicholas Baker Department of Cardiothoracic Surgery, University of Pittsburgh Medical Center, UPMC Presbyterian-Shadyside, Pittsburgh, PA, USA

Sudeep Banerjee Department of Surgery, University of California, Los Angeles, Los Angeles, CA, USA

Department of Surgery, University of California, San Diego, San Diego, CA, USA

Felix Berlth Department of Surgery, Division of Gastrointestinal Surgery, Seoul National University Hospital, Seoul, Republic of Korea

Department of General, Visceral and Cancer Surgery, University Hospital of Cologne, Cologne, Germany

Matthew T. Brady Department of Surgery, Division of Colon and Rectal Surgery, University of California, Irvine Medical Center, Orange, CA, USA

Peter A. Cataldo Department of Surgery, University of Vermont Medical Center, Burlington, VT, USA

George J. Chang Department of Surgical Oncology, The University of Texas MD Anderson Cancer Center, Houston, TX, USA

Edward Cho Hepatobiliary Surgery, Methodist Richardson Medical Center, Richardson, TX, USA

Robert K. Cleary Department of Surgery, St Joseph Mercy Hospital Ann Arbor, Ann Arbor, MI, USA

Natalie Coburn Sunnybrook Health Science Centre, Toronto, ON, Canada

Marc Dakermandji Department of Colorectal Surgery, Center for Colon & Rectal Surgery, Florida Hospital, Orlando, FL, USA

F. Borja de Lacy Gastrointestinal Surgery Department, Hospital Clinic, University of Barcelona, Barcelona, Spain

Wolfgang B. Gaertner Division of Colon and Rectal Surgery, Department of Surgery, University of Minnesota, Minneapolis, MN, USA

Julio Garcia-Aguilar Department of Surgery, Memorial Sloan Kettering Cancer Center, New York, NY, USA

Georgios V. Georgakis Department of Surgery, Stony Brook University Hospital, Stony Brook, NY, USA

Jose L. Guerrero-Ramirez General Surgery, Hospital Universitary Virgen del Rocío, Sevilla, Spain

Naoki Hiki Department of Upper Gastrointestinal Surgery, Kitasato University School of Medicine, Kanagawa, Japan

Kelsi Hirai Department of Surgery, Stony Brook University Hospital, Stony Brook, NY, USA

Melissa E. Hogg University of Pittsburgh Medical Center, Pittsburgh, PA, USA

Santiago Horgan Department of Surgery, Center for the Future of Surgery, University of California, San Diego, San Diego, CA, USA

Christina N. Jenkins Loma Linda University Medical Center, Loma Linda, CA, USA

D. Rohan Jeyarajah Hepatopancreaticobiliary Surgery, Methodist Richardson Medical Center, Richardson, TX, USA

Rosa Jimenez-Rodriguez Department of Surgery Colorectal Service, Memorial Sloan Kettering Cancer Center, New York, NY, USA

Craig S. Johnson Oklahoma Surgical Hospital, Tulsa, OK, USA

Margaret W. Johnson The University of Texas, Austin, TX, USA

Chang Hyun Kang Department of Thoracic and Cardiovascular Surgery, Seoul National University Hospital, Seoul, Republic of Korea

Kaitlyn J. Kelly Department of Surgery, Center for the Future of Surgery, University of California, San Diego, San Diego, CA, USA

Jae Kim Division of Thoracic Surgery, Department of Surgery, City of Hope Comprehensive Cancer Center, Duarte, CA, USA

Joseph Kim Department of Surgery, University of Kentucky, Lexington, KY, USA

Young Tae Kim Department of Thoracic and Cardiovascular Surgery, Seoul National University Hospital, Seoul, Republic of Korea

Yuko Kitagawa Department of Surgery, Keio University School of Medicine, Tokyo, Japan

Laz Klein Department of General Surgery, University of Toronto, Toronto, ON, Canada

John R. Konen Department of Surgery, University of Vermont Medical Center, Burlington, VT, USA

Tsuyoshi Konishi Department of Gastroenterological Surgery, Colorectal Division, Cancer Institute Hospital of the Japanese Foundation for Cancer Research, Tokyo, Japan

Antonio M. Lacy Gastrointestinal Surgery Department, Hospital Clinic, University of Barcelona, Barcelona, Spain

Jenny Lam Department of Surgery, Center for the Future of Surgery, University of California, San Diego, San Diego, CA, USA

David W. Larson Mayo Clinic, Colon and Rectal Surgery, Rochester, MN, USA

Jin-Tung Liang Department of Surgery, National Taiwan University Hospital, Taipei City, Taiwan

Amy L. Lightner Cleveland Clinic, Colorectal Surgery, Cleveland, OH, USA

Miranda Lin Department of Surgery, University of Kentucky, Lexington, KY, USA

James Luketich Division of Thoracic and Foregut Surgery, UPMC Presbyterian, Pittsburgh, PA, USA

Songphol Malakorn Department of Colorectal Surgery, Faculty of Medicine, Chulalongkorn University, Bangkok, Thailand

Department of Surgical Oncology, The University of Texas MD Anderson Cancer Center, Houston, TX, USA

Shaila Merchant Department of Surgery, Division of General Surgery and Surgical Oncology, Queen's University, Kingston, ON, Canada

Sumana Narayanan Department of Surgical Oncology, Roswell Park Comprehensive Cancer Center, Buffalo, NY, USA

Timothy E. Newhook The University of Texas MD Anderson Cancer Center, Houston, TX, USA

Steven J. Nurkin Department of Surgical Oncology, Roswell Park Comprehensive Cancer Center, Buffalo, NY, USA

Houssam Osman HPB Surgery, Methodist Richardson Medical Center, Richardson, TX, USA

Spyridon Pagkratis HPB Surgery, Methodist Richardson Medical Center, Richardson, TX, USA

C. Palanivelu Gem Hospital and Research Centre, Coimbatore, India

Vanessa Palter St. Michael's Hospital, Toronto, ON, Canada

Emmanouil P. Pappou Department of Surgery, Memorial Sloan Kettering Cancer Center, New York, NY, USA

Alessio Pigazzi Department of Surgery, Division of Colon and Rectal Surgery, University of California, Irvine Medical Center, Orange, CA, USA

Owen Pyke Department of Surgery, Stony Brook University Hospital, Stony Brook, NY, USA

Felipe Quezada-Diaz Department of Surgery Colorectal Service, Memorial Sloan Kettering Cancer Center, New York, NY, USA

Elizabeth R. Raskin Loma Linda University Medical Center, Loma Linda, CA, USA

Dan Raz Division of Thoracic Surgery, Department of Surgery, City of Hope Comprehensive Cancer Center, Duarte, CA, USA

Maria Luisa Reyes-Diaz General Surgery, Hospital Universitary Virgen del Rocío, Sevilla, Spain

Tarik Sammour Department of Surgical Oncology, The University of Texas MD Anderson Cancer Center, Houston, TX, USA

Colorectal Unit, Department of Surgery, Royal Adelaide Hospital, University of Adelaide, Adelaide, SA, Australia

Inderpal Sarkaria Shadyside Medical, Pittsburgh, PA, USA

Palanisamy Senthilnathan Gem Hospital and Research Centre, Coimbatore, India

Jason K. Sicklick Department of Surgery, University of California, San Diego, San Diego, CA, USA

Jesse Joshua Smith Department of Surgery Colorectal Service, Memorial Sloan Kettering Cancer Center, New York, NY, USA

S. Srivatsan Gurumurthy Gem Hospital and Research Centre, Coimbatore, India

Hiroya Takeuchi Department of Surgery, Hamamatsu University School of Medicine, Shizuoka, Japan

Julia H. Terhune Department of Surgical Oncology, Roswell Park Comprehensive Cancer Center, Buffalo, NY, USA

Hannah Thompson Department of Surgery, Stony Brook University Hospital, Stony Brook, NY, USA

Catherine Tsai Department of Surgery, Center for the Future of Surgery, University of California, San Diego, San Diego, CA, USA

Konstantin Umanskiy Department of Surgery, The University of Chicago Pritzker School of Medicine, Chicago, IL, USA

Patrick Varley University of Pittsburgh Medical Center, Pittsburgh, PA, USA

Han-Kwang Yang Department of Surgery, Division of Gastrointestinal Surgery, Seoul National University Hospital, Seoul, Republic of Korea

Part I

UGI

Nicholas Baker, Inderpal Sarkaria, and James Luketich

Historical Perspective

Open approaches to esophagectomy have historically been associated with elevated morbidity and mortality. A 10-year review of the Veterans Affairs' population demonstrated 50% morbidity and 10% mortality [1]. In the 1990s, the growing confidence in laparoscopic surgical techniques and instrumentation led to the introduction of various minimally invasive approaches to esophageal resection. Early minimally invasive resection techniques often hybridized more traditional open techniques with newer less invasive approaches. Collard was the first to describe a thoracoscopic technique for esophageal dissection, and DePaula was the first to describe the first entirely laparoscopic transhiatal esophagec-

tomy in 1995. In the following year, Luketich and associates at the University of Pittsburgh began performing totally minimally invasive esophagectomy (MIE) via a McKeown approach and later published one of the first, large series with zero mortality in their first 77 patients [2].

Indications

Indications for MIE are the same as standard open esophagectomy, including end-stage achalasia, failed antireflux surgery, intractable esophageal stricture, high-grade Barrett's esophagus not amenable to ablative or endoscopic techniques, and esophageal cancer. A thorough history of previous interventions to the chest and abdomen, including endoscopic management and pre-and postoperative symptoms in failed benign esophageal surgery, is mandatory. Chemoradiotherapy history, staging, and location of tumor are also necessary in order to appropriately plan the surgical approach.

There are multiple minimally invasive techniques described throughout the literature. In our experience, Ivor Lewis esophagectomy is the surgery of choice for standard esophageal cancer resections of the gastroesophageal (GE) junction and low mid-esophageal tumors, benign strictures, and failed antireflux surgery. McKeown (three-hole) esophagectomy is indicated for high mid-esophageal tumors, extensive high-grade

Electronic supplementary material The online version of this chapter (https://doi.org/10.1007/978-3-030-18740-8_1) contains supplementary material, which is available to authorized users.

N. Baker
Department of Cardiothoracic Surgery, University of Pittsburgh Medical Center, UPMC Presbyterian-Shadyside, Pittsburgh, PA, USA

I. Sarkaria (✉)
Shadyside Medical, Pittsburgh, PA, USA
e-mail: sarkariais@upmc.edu

J. Luketich
Division of Thoracic and Foregut Surgery, UPMC Presbyterian, Pittsburgh, PA, USA

© Springer Nature Switzerland AG 2020
J. Kim, J. Garcia-Aguilar (eds.), *Minimally Invasive Surgical Techniques for Cancers of the Gastrointestinal Tract*, https://doi.org/10.1007/978-3-030-18740-8_1

dysplasia, or end-stage achalasia. Overall, the goal is an R0 resection for malignancy and complete resection of diseased esophagus in benign cases.

Preoperative Considerations

Anesthesia preoperative planning should focus on the need for accurate hemodynamic monitoring, adequate intravenous access, and lung isolation. Invasive arterial line placement is necessary for accurate blood pressure monitoring as perfusion pressure to the conduit is top priority to prevent postoperative complications. Most cases require central venous catheterization to ensure adequate intravenous access throughout the case. Double lumen endotracheal tube is needed for the thoracic portion of the case and is typically placed at the beginning of the operation.

Positioning planning will include a well-padded foot board for steep reverse Trendelenburg position. The patient should also be positioned on the right lateral aspect of the surgical table to allow room for the liver retractor.

Surgical Technique for MIE

Video 1.1

Endoscopy

Before beginning the operation, endoscopy is used to confirm the pathology of the esophagus and distance from the incisors. The decision on approach may be altered at this time based on the findings. Ivor Lewis esophagectomy would begin with laparoscopy, whereas McKeown esophagectomy would begin with right video-assisted thoracic surgery (VATS). Bronchoscopy is also performed to confirm the absence of airway involvement and confirm normal airway before dissection begins.

Laparoscopy

The xiphoid process and the umbilicus are identified, and a ruler is used to measure 15 cm distal to the xiphoid with marks at 5 cm and 10 cm. At the 10-cm mark, the right paramedian 10-mm port is placed 2 cm to the right of the midline via a Hasson cut-down technique. The right paramedian port is the primary working hand of the surgeon. The abdomen is insufflated to 12–15 mm Hg, and the patient is placed in steep reverse Trendelenburg position. Next, under direct visualization with a 10-mm 30° laparoscopic camera, the remaining ports are placed. The camera port is placed one hand-breadth to the patient's left from the right paramedian port. Two subcostal 5-mm ports are placed, and a right lateral subcostal port is placed just inferior to the 12th rib and is used for the liver retractor. Finally, a right lower quadrant 12-mm port is placed at approximately at one-third the distance from the anterior superior iliac spine to the umbilicus (Fig. 1.1). This port will be used later for placement of the jejunostomy tube and retraction for gastric conduit creation.

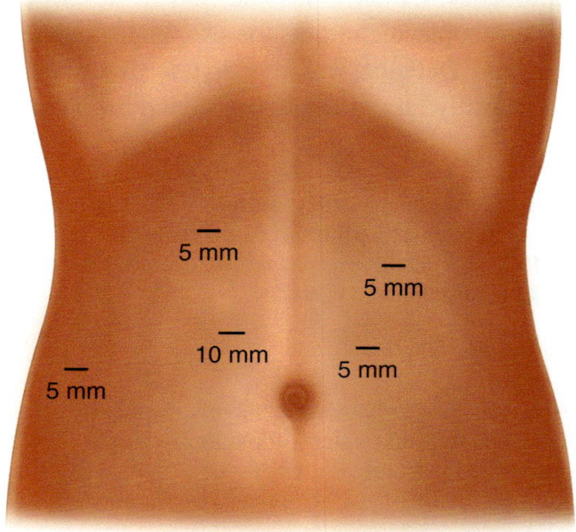

Fig. 1.1 Port placement for laparoscopic procedures. (© Heart, Lung, and Esophageal Surgery Institute University of Pittsburgh Medical Center)

Abdominal Dissection

After all ports are placed, detailed diagnostic laparoscopy is performed to rule out metastasis in malignant cases and evaluate aberrant anatomy. A self-retaining liver retractor is positioned to elevate the left lobe of the liver to expose the hiatus. Next, the dissection begins with incising the gastrohepatic ligament. With the hiatus completely exposed, dissection continues up the right crus anteriorly and down the left crus. Circumferential exposure of the crus helps to gain access into the chest, and mediastinal dissection is carried out between the bilateral pleural, the pericardium, and the spine/aorta. This can be carried up to the inferior pulmonary veins to help with the thoracic dissection but only needs to be enough to place the specimen into this space at the end of the abdominal portion of the procedure.

The left gastric pedicle is approached to identify the base, and lymph node tissues are dissected from the base toward the specimen to remove all nodal tissue associated with the celiac axis. The dissection is carried out laterally on top of the splenic artery and pancreas over to the splenic hilum. All the lymph node tissues are again pushed up toward the specimen, and using an endovascular stapling device, the left gastric artery is taken at its base.

Next, using a "no touch" technique, the short gastric arteries are divided and the left gastroepiploic artery is identified. The omental arteries are now identified and divided leaving a couple of centimeters of tissue on the lateral aspect of the right gastroepiploic artery to ensure it is not damaged. An omental flap can be created at this step using approximately two to three of these omental branches creating a 3–4-cm-wide omental flap to be used later to buttress the anastomosis. We routinely do this on induction cases where radiation is used. Complete mobilization of the entire gastroepiploic artery is necessary for full mobility (Fig. 1.2). A Kocher maneuver is performed, and retrogastric and duodenal attachments are incised as well to help with mobilization. At this step, the pylorus should reach to above the caudate lobe of the liver. This indicates adequate mobilization. After full mobilization of the stomach, the three remaining portions of the abdomen include conduit formation, pyloroplasty, and jejunostomy tube placement.

Laparoscopic Pyloroplasty

A Heineke-Mikulicz pyloroplasty is performed laparoscopically with an endoscopic suturing device (Endo Stitch 2.0, Medtronic) with 2-0

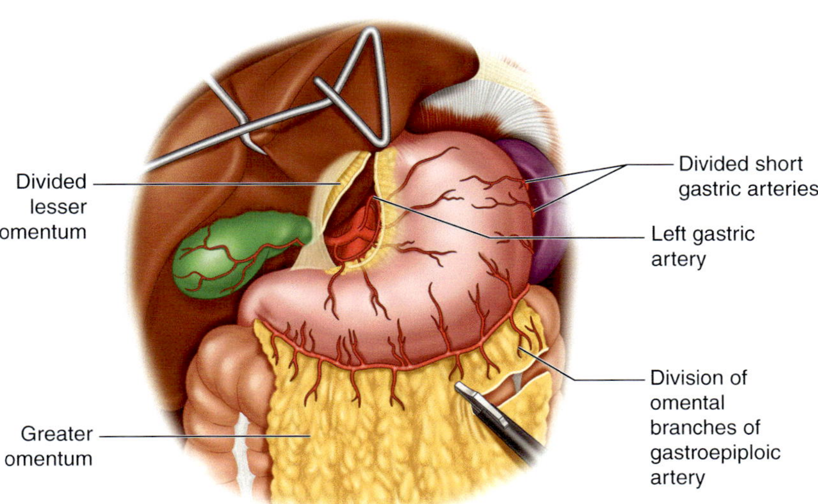

Fig. 1.2 Mobilization of gastroepiploic arcade. (© Heart, Lung, and Esophageal Surgery Institute University of Pittsburgh Medical Center)

sutures placed at the most superior and inferior aspect of the pylorus. The pylorus is incised using ultrasonic shears (Harmonic Scalpel, Ethicon Inc.) in the midline horizontally with care to ensure complete full thickness incision. The pylorus is then closed in a vertical fashion with the Endo Stitch incorporating mucosa with each suture (Fig. 1.3). Routinely, omentum is placed over the pyloroplasty prior to completing the abdominal portion of the procedure.

Laparoscopic Jejunostomy Tube

The patient is placed back in level supine position and the insufflation of the abdomen is reduced to 8–10 mm Hg. The omentum is retracted cephalad and the ligament of Treitz is identified. Approximately 40 cm distal to the ligament of Treitz, a portion of mobile jejunum is chosen and tacked to the anterior abdominal wall. Using a 12-Fr needle jejunostomy kit, a needle is passed into the jejunum and a wire is

passed. Serial dilators are passed in a Seldinger technique until the introducer is passed. Next the jejunostomy tube is inserted into the jejunum. Two 2-0 Witzel sutures are placed around the J-tube, and then a purse-string suture is placed around the jejunostomy tube tacking it to the anterior abdominal wall. One single interrupted 2-0 suture is placed approximately 2 cm distal to the feeding tube as an anti-torsion suture (Fig. 1.4).

Creation of Gastric Conduit

The gastric conduit is formed by retracting the fundus of the stomach into the left upper quadrant as far as possible, and the antrum is retracted toward the patient's right foot. The surgeon gently retracts the gastric conduit. The stapler is passed though the right paramedian port. This begins with a 2.5-mm endovascular staple to divide the lesser curve vessels. These steps should form the desired diameter of the tube. We prefer

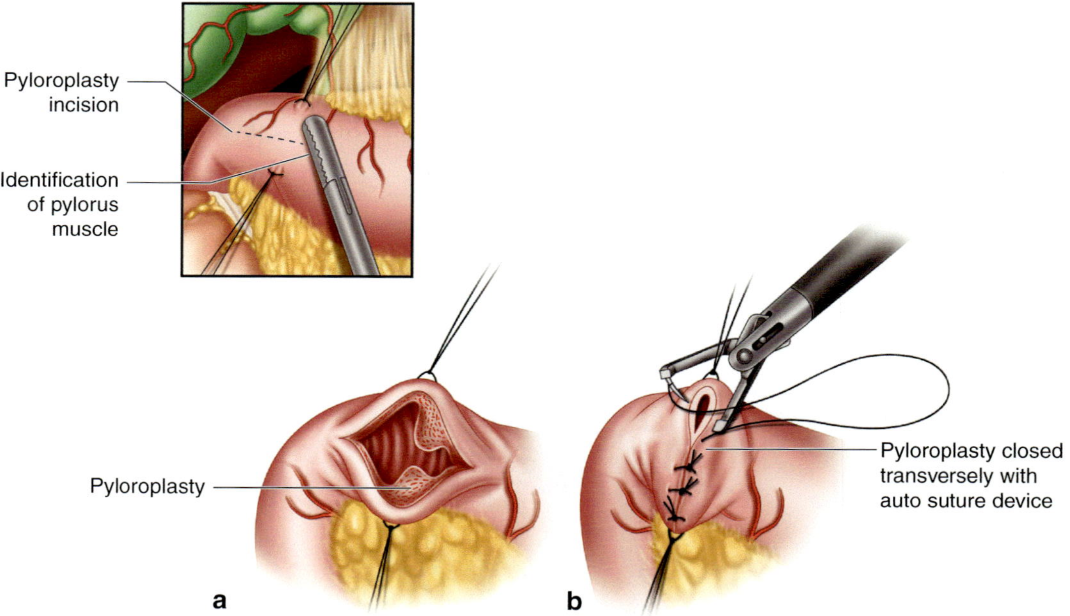

Fig. 1.3 Laparoscopic pyloroplasty is performed by (**a**) creating a longitudinal incision across the pylorus. (**b**) An Endo Stitch is used to close the pyloroplasty with a transverse incision

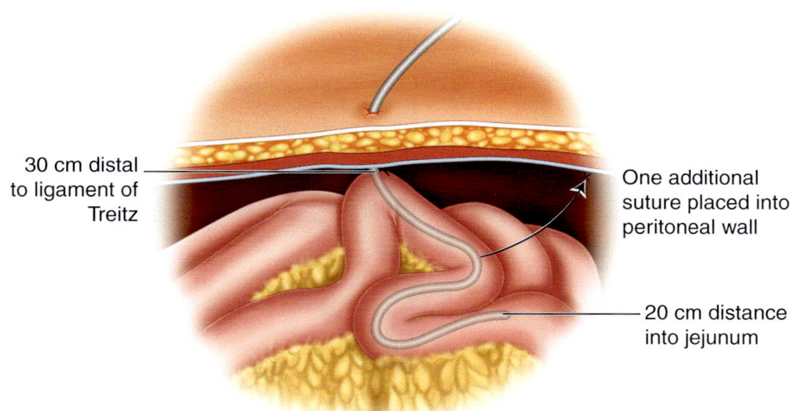

Fig. 1.4 Laparoscopic jejunostomy tube is placed approximately 30 cm distal to the ligament of Treitz. One additional suture is placed distal to the catheter insertion to prevent torsion of the jejunal limb. (© Heart, Lung, and Esophageal Surgery Institute University of Pittsburgh Medical Center)

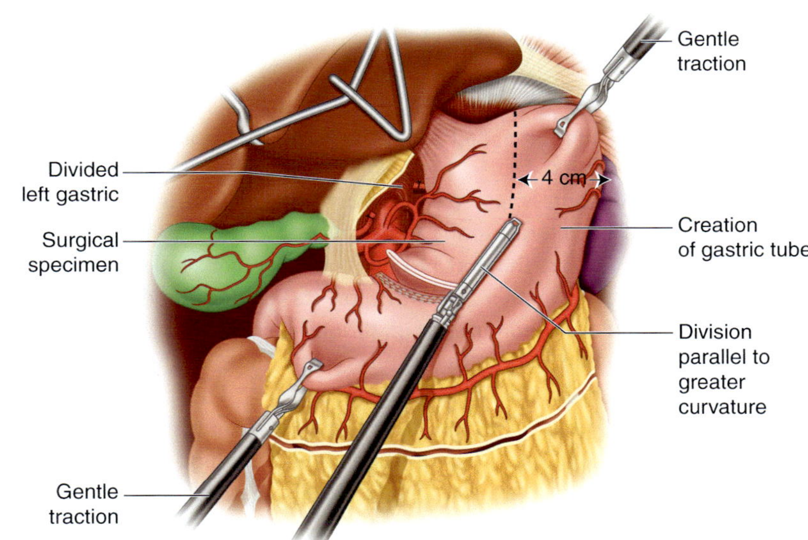

Fig. 1.5 Creation of the gastric conduit with a linear stapler. The assistant provides gentle traction and counter-traction of the stomach. (© Heart, Lung, and Esophageal Surgery Institute University of Pittsburgh Medical Center)

a 3–4-cm-wide gastric tube (Fig. 1.5). Gastric staple loads usually begin with a 5-mm endovascular staple load and subsequently progress to 4 mm. The staple line should parallel the greater curve in the desired width to ensure not spiraling the conduit. After the conduit has been fully created, the specimen is placed into the hiatus and the conduit is sutured to the specimen maintaining proper orientation with the specimen staple line sewn and attached from the lesser curve to the greater curve of the conduit (Fig. 1.6).

Thoracoscopy

A nasogastric tube (NGT) is placed at this time, and double-lumen endotracheal tube is placed if not already done. The patient is placed in a left lateral decubitus position, and with the double-lumen tube confirmed in appropriate position, the right lung should be isolated immediately to provide adequate time for decompression. The operating table is flexed to move the iliac crest away from the costal margin and

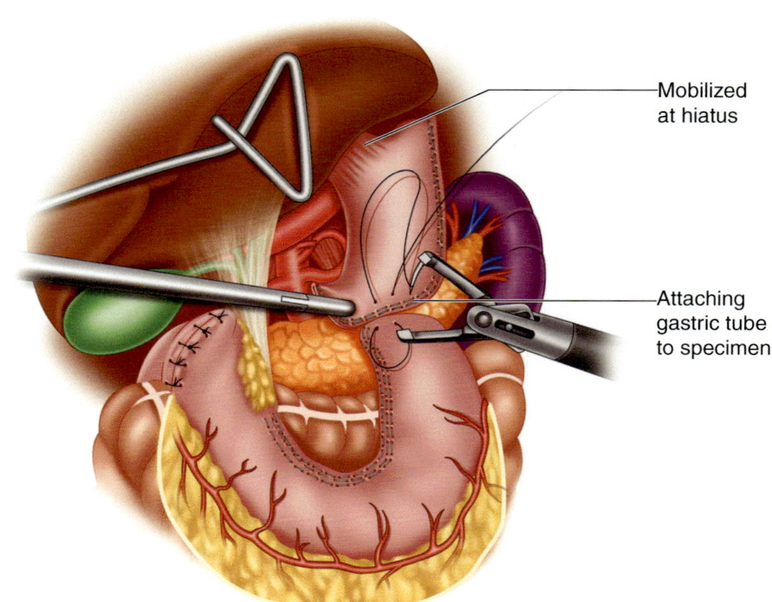

Fig. 1.6 Attachment of the specimen to the gastric conduit with the Endo Stitch and maintaining proper orientation. (© Heart, Lung, and Esophageal Surgery Institute University of Pittsburgh Medical Center)

expand the intercostal spaces, and the position of the right scapula is marked.

A 10-mm camera port is inserted in the eighth intercostal space just anterior to the mid-axillary line. This typically places the port just above the costophrenic recess. Another 10-mm port is placed in the scapular tip line in the eighth intercostal space. This is the surgeon's working port. Next a 5-mm port is placed at the scapula tip, and 5-mm port is placed in the sixth intercostal space at the anterior axillary line. The fifth and final 10-mm port is placed in the fourth intercostal space anterior axillary line, and a fan retractor is passed through this port to retract the lung. A full-length Endo Stitch is placed in the central tendon of the diaphragm and retracted through the costophrenic recess via an Endo-close device (Medtronic) and is secured to the outside of the chest wall to retract the diaphragm inferiorly, allowing full visualization of the distal esophagus and hiatus.

The chest dissection begins with taking the inferior pulmonary ligament down and identifying the pericardium. This usually connects with the hiatal dissection that was carried out in the abdomen. The dissection is carried up the pericardium to level 7 lymph nodes and the right bronchus intermedius. This is a critical dissection point, and care must be taken not to injure the posterior membrane of the airway. The anterior dissection is continued up the mediastinum to the azygos vein that is taken with a 2.5-mm endovascular staple load. The dissection above the azygos vein should be carried out directly on the esophageal wall, and this can be carried safely up to the level of the thoracic inlet and beyond if needed.

The posterior dissection is performed in a similar fashion, but clips are deployed in an attempt to prevent thoracic duct injury. This is carried up to the thoracic inlet as well. The last remaining plane is the deep plane along the left pleural and aorta. After all the periesophageal tissue, esophagus, and level 7 lymph nodes have been successfully mobilized up to the thoracic inlet, the conduit is delivered into the mediastinum with care to ensure appropriate orientation with the staple line facing toward the operators.

The access incision is created for passage of the end-to-end anastomosis stapler (EEA) and removal of the specimen. This is one rib space above the surgeon's working port and is <4 cm in length. A wound protector (Applied Medical) is placed to protect the wound from spillage and tumor implants. The specimen is incised above the level of the azygos vein and passed out of the chest via the access incision.

Assessment of the proximal esophagus is then performed and the decision on which EEA stapler to use is made. Most commonly, a 28-mm EEA stapler is used, and the esophagus can be dilated with a Foley catheter if needed. The anvil is passed into the chest and placed into the proximal end of the esophagus. Two purse-string 2-0 sutures are placed around the anvil with each stitch ensuring incorporation of mucosa (Fig. 1.7). The conduit is completely delivered into the chest and the stapler is passed into the chest. It is placed into the conduit in a "sock over foot" type fashion (Fig. 1.8). After the stapler is inserted, it is progressed up to the anvil, and an assessment of length is again made. The staple line should be facing the operator and the spike can be brought out of the conduit in line with the gastroepiploic artery. The stapler is locked and fired (Fig. 1.9a, b). The rings of the stapler must be examined to confirm they are complete. The excess conduit is resected with a 3.5-mm endovascular stapler, and this is the final gastric margin (Fig. 1.10).

Lastly the omental flap should be placed around the anastomosis making sure there is flap between the airway and the anastomosis. A 10-mm flat Jackson-Pratt drain is placed posterior to the conduit with the tip adjacent to the anastomosis. The chest is irrigated with copious antibiotic solution. One 28-Fr chest tube is placed in an apicoposterior position. After wound closure, the patient is placed back in a supine position and the oropharynx is irrigated and suctioned. The double lumen tube is exchanged for a single lumen tube and repeat bronchoscopy is carried out to inspect and clear the airway. The final reconstruction is depicted in Fig. 1.11.

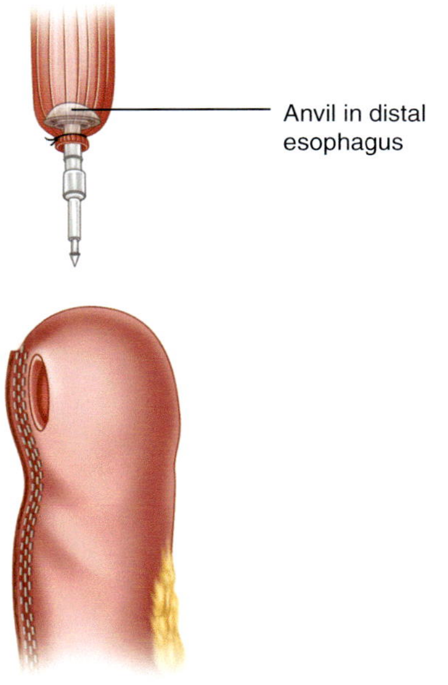

Fig. 1.7 The anvil has been placed in the esophagus. (© Heart, Lung, and Esophageal Surgery Institute University of Pittsburgh Medical Center)

Fig. 1.8 Insertion of the EEA stapler into the conduit in a "sock over foot" fashion. (© Heart, Lung, and Esophageal Surgery Institute University of Pittsburgh Medical Center)

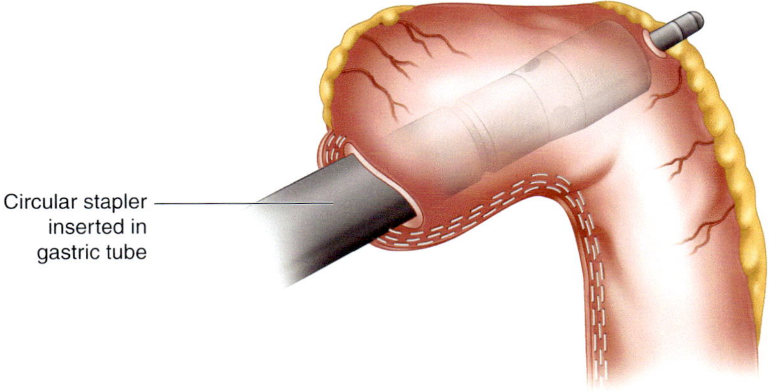

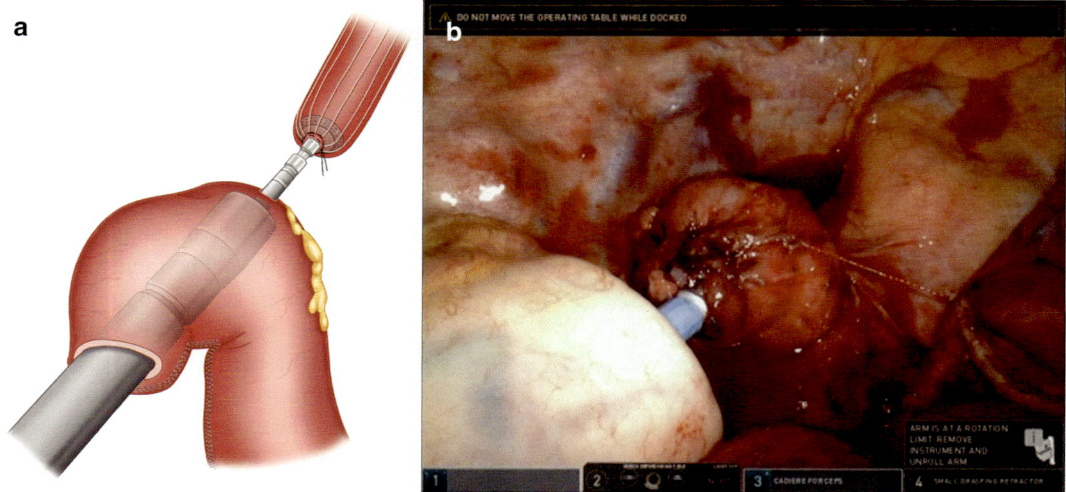

Fig. 1.9 (**a**) Illustration of the alignment of the EEA stapler pin/trocar with the anvil. (**b**) Intraoperative image of the stapler alignment. (© Heart, Lung, and Esophageal Surgery Institute University of Pittsburgh Medical Center)

Fig. 1.10 Resection of proximal gastric conduit with a linear stapler. (© Heart, Lung, and Esophageal Surgery Institute University of Pittsburgh Medical Center)

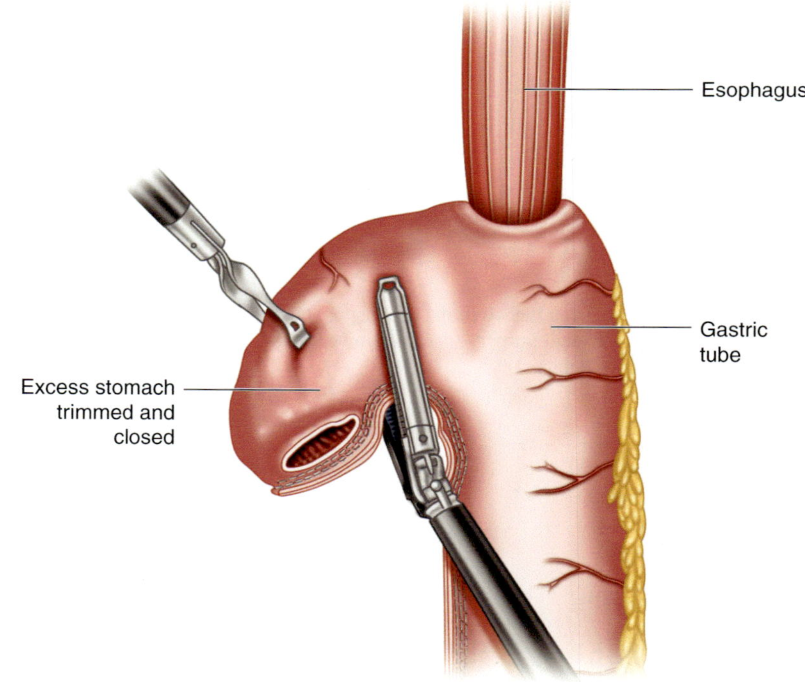

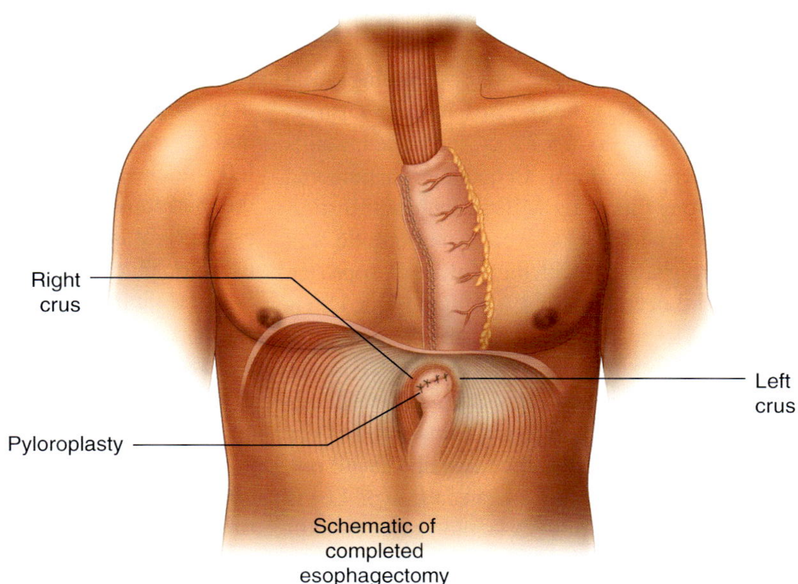

Fig. 1.11 The finished reconstruction with the gastric conduit in the chest and the pyloroplasty near the hiatus. (© Heart, Lung, and Esophageal Surgery Institute University of Pittsburgh Medical Center)

Postoperative Care and Complications

Thoracic Complications

Bleeding and transfusion requirements were less with the minimally invasive approach, but it is important to note that even small amounts of bleeding can obscure the operative field, making progress difficult and requiring conversion to an open procedure. Hence, the aorto-esophageal vessels must be identified and clipped and bleeding from the azygos vein and peribronchial arteries avoided. Injury to the posterior membranes of the bronchus and trachea must be carefully avoided, especially during mediastinal lymph node dissection. Cautery, auto-sonic, or harmonic scalpel use in close proximity to the posterior membranous airway can lead to tissue damage resulting in an air leak, local ischemia, and subsequent development of a tracheogastric conduit fistula.

The thoracic duct is at risk for subtle injuries leading to the development of a chylothorax. Early in our experience with our initial 77 patients undergoing MIE, we noted 3 patients with delayed chylothorax, leading us to become more cautious in this area and transitioning to the liberal use of metal clips on thoracic duct

branches. Vocal cord paralysis from injury to the recurrent laryngeal nerve is minimized by dividing the vagus nerve just above the azygos vein and dissecting this away from the esophagus. We generally do not perform a lymph node dissection above this level in an effort to avoid injury to the recurrent laryngeal nerves and the lack of definitive evidence that lymph node clearance in the upper chest is essential for gastroesophageal junction tumors.

Abdominal Complications

Disruption of the main gastroepiploic arcade can be devastating to the viability of the gastric conduit. Likewise, one must be certain that there is adequate room at the hiatus for the conduit to lie without strangulation. In our series, there was an incidence of gastric tip necrosis of 3.2%. Delayed hiatal herniation of abdominal viscera is also a possibility if the gastric conduit is not properly tacked to the hiatus. Kent et al. reported approximately 2% incidence of diaphragmatic hernias and 2% risk of redundant gastric conduit leading to delayed gastric emptying, reflux, and obstruction. Eighty-five percent of patients with such anatomical complications benefited from reoperative revisional surgery [3].

Other Major Complications

Cardiopulmonary complications, including atrial fibrillation (2.9%), Acute Respiratory Distress Syndrome (ARDS) (5.7%), and pneumonitis (3.8%), were the most frequently encountered complications following MIE in the multi-institution E2202 trial [4]. Our overall anastomotic leak rate requiring surgery with the McKeown approach was 5% and decreased to 4% with the Ivor Lewis approach. The reported leak rate for the open procedure is approximately 9.1%. Other MIE series demonstrate similar leak rates. Moderate strictures at the gastroesophageal cervical anastomosis are common and generally can be managed with one or two outpatient dilations. Using the Ivor Lewis approach and a 28-mm EEA stapler, strictures still occur but generally are less clinically important and respond favorably to dilations.

Robot-Assisted Minimally Invasive Esophagectomy

Robot-assisted minimally invasive esophagectomy (RAMIE) approach is largely adapted from our MIE approach as described earlier. There are several selected differences that we will expand on below.

RAMIE Preoperative Planning

The robotic platform uses four arms with two operating consoles with the operating surgeon and trainee at the controls and an assistant at the bedside. The tower is to the patient's right and the robotic cart is to the left of the patient. Bedside positioning is similar to MIE except the left arm may be tucked to avoid collision.

RAMIE Surgical Technique

Setup for the abdominal portion of RAMIE involves docking the robotic cart (Da Vinci Surgical Robot) and arms directly over the mid-line of the patient with the patient in steep reverse Trendelenburg position (Fig. 1.12). The camera port is placed in the midline just above the umbilicus. A 5-mm left lateral subcostal port is placed and is used for an atraumatic grasper. An 8-mm left midclavicular port is placed and is used for the harmonic scalpel (Ethicon). An additional 5-mm right lateral subcostal port is placed and is used for placement of the liver retractor, and an 8-mm right midclavicular port is used for a bipolar atraumatic grasper. An additional 12-mm assistant port is placed by triangulating between the umbilicus and the right midclavicular port and is used for suction by the assistant as well as jejunostomy tube placement. It is important to maintain a minimal distance of 9–10 mm between robotic ports to minimize collisions (Fig. 1.13).

The thoracic portion of the case setup begins with placement of the camera port in the eighth intercostal space in the mid to posterior axillary line under direct video guidance (Fig. 1.14). Carbon dioxide insufflation at 8 mm Hg is used for better visualization. A 5-mm robotic port is placed in the third intercostal space in the mid to posterior axillary line, and an 8-mm robotic port is placed in the fifth intercostal space. An additional 8-mm port is placed laterally in approximately the eighth or ninth interspace. A 12-mm assistant port is placed under direct vision at the diaphragmatic insertion midway between the camera port and the lateral 8-mm robotic port (Fig. 1.13). The robot is docked to the ports, and the robotic camera is placed within the chest at a 30° downward orientation.

RAMIE operative components are the same as MIE. RAMIE allows the surgeon to perform all exposures without the need for an assistant, allowing the surgeon to be in complete control. The camera offers better visualization with three-dimensional optics. Wristed instruments offer greater precision while suturing. Potential disadvantages of the RAMIE approach include reduced versatility in large operative fields such as the thorax with a large area between the hiatus and the inlet. This can lead to multiple collisions and decreased range of motion. Also, the robot has to be undocked to change positions of the operative

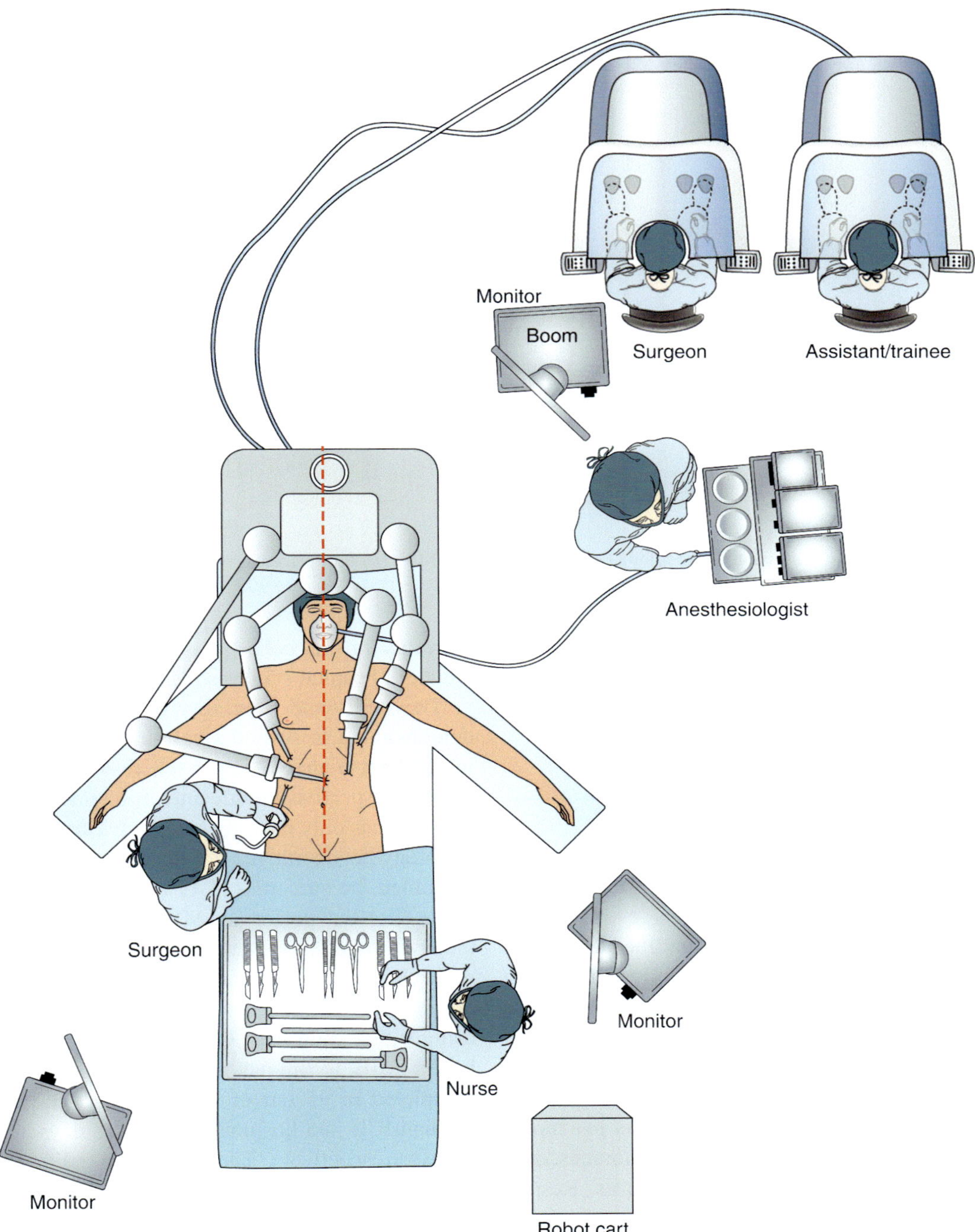

Fig. 1.12 Robotic setup for the abdominal steps of RAMIE

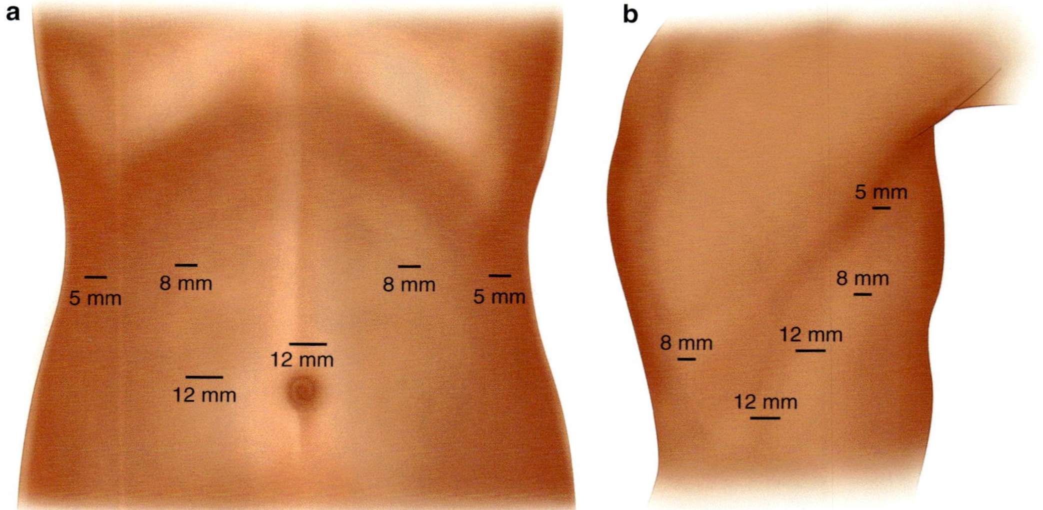

Fig. 1.13 (**a**) Port placement for abdominal steps of robotic RAMIE. (**b**) Port placement for thoracic steps of robotic AMIE

table. These disadvantages have been somewhat reduced with newer technologies such as Da Vinci Xi with an integrated operating room table (Intuitive Surgical Inc.).

Conclusions

Our institutional approach at the University of Pittsburgh Medical Center has evolved over time, initially developed as a modified McKeown (three-hole) technique with a cervical anastomosis, and transitioned to a primarily Ivor Lewis approach with intrathoracic anastomosis. In an initial series of 222 patients, 8 initial cases were performed as laparoscopic transhiatal operations, with quick adaptation thereafter to a modified McKeown approach with thoracoscopic mobilization and cervical anastomosis. Results from this early experience yielded a median hospital stay of 7 days and an operative mortality of 1.4%, which is equivalent or better to the majority of open series. An anastomotic leak rate of 11.7% and stage-specific survival were similar to open series. In a follow-up institutional series of 1011 patients undergoing elective MIE, including 530 patients operated via the currently preferred Ivor Lewis MIE approach, operative

mortality in this cohort was 0.9% and median length of hospital stay was 8 days [2].

The safety and feasibility of MIE has been demonstrated in several single-institution studies and meta-analyses, yet the results from a large, prospective, multicenter trial investigating MIE has only recently emerged. The eastern oncology cooperative group study (E2202) examined the outcomes of 17 credentialed sites in the USA that performed MIE on patients with biopsy-proven high-grade dysplasia or esophageal cancer of the mid-esophagus or distal esophagus. Esophagectomy was performed using either modified McKeown MIE or Ivor Lewis MIE technique. Protocol surgery was completed in 95 out of 104 patients (91.3%). Median ICU and hospital stay were 2 days and 9 days, respectively. The 30-day mortality for patients who underwent MIE was 2.1%. Adverse events included anastomotic leak (8.6%), acute respiratory distress syndrome (5.7%), and atrial fibrillation (2.9%). At a median follow-up of 35.8 months, the estimated 3-year overall survival was 58.4%. Locoregional recurrence occurred in only seven patients (6.7%). This trial demonstrated that MIE is safe and feasible and has low perioperative morbidity and mortality and good oncologic results and suggests that

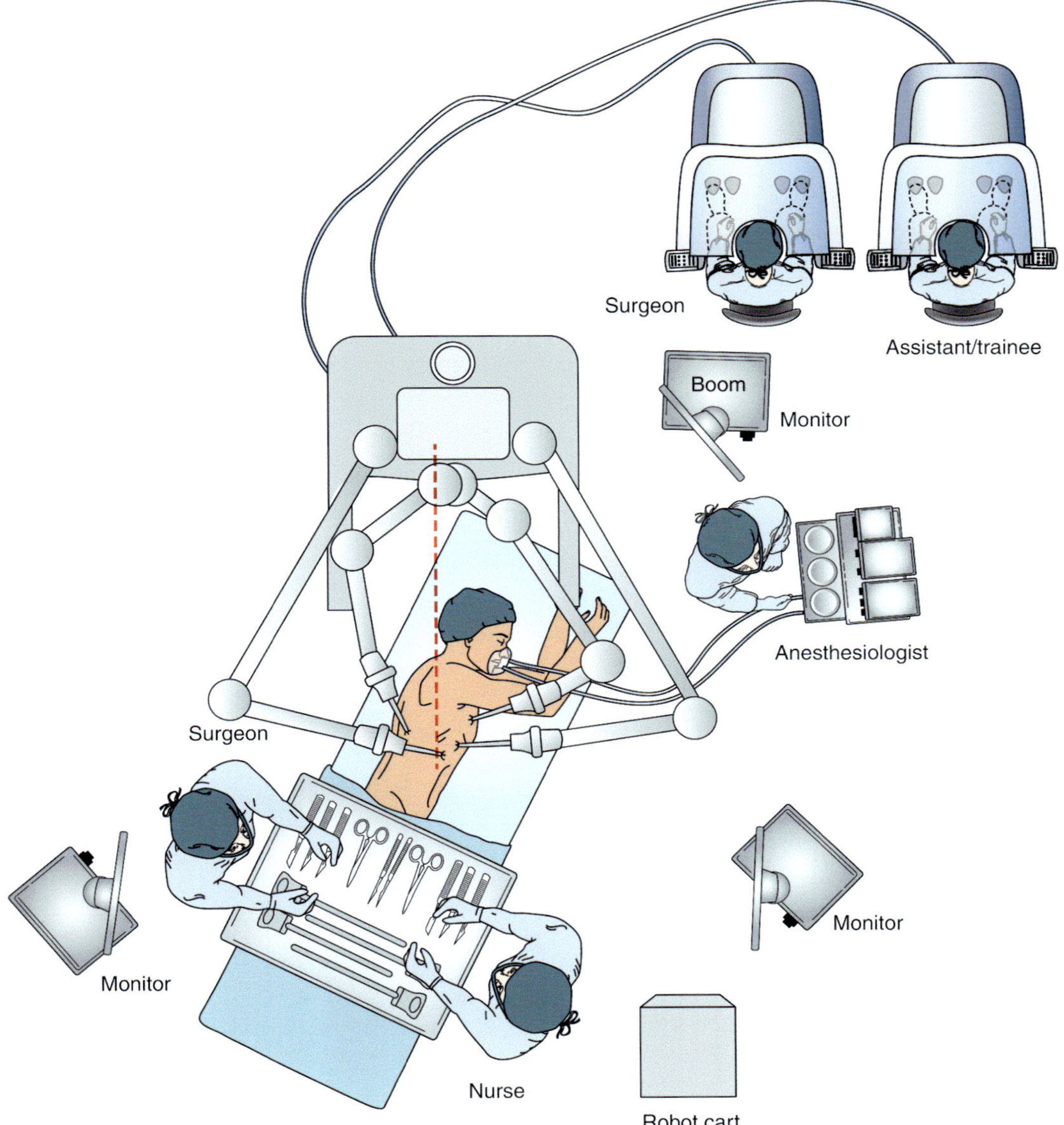

Fig. 1.14 Robotic setup for the thoracic steps of RAMIE

MIE can be adopted by other centers with appropriate expertise in open esophagectomy and minimally invasive surgery [4].

References

1. Bailey SH, et al. Outcomes after esophagectomy: a ten-year prospective cohort. Ann Thorac Surg. 2003;75(1):217; discussion 222.

2. Luketich JD, Pennathur A, Awais O, et al. Outcomes after minimally invasive esophagectomy: review of over 1000 patients. Ann Surg. 2012;256(1):95–103.

3. Kent MS, Luketich JD, Tsai W, Churilla P, Federle M, et al. Revisional surgery after esophagectomy: an analysis of 43 patients. Ann Thorac Surg. 2008;86: 975–83.

4. Luketich JD, Pennathur A, Franchetti Y, et al. Minimally invasive esophagectomy: results of a prospective phase II multicenter trial-the eastern cooperative oncology group (E2202) study. Ann Surg. 2015;261(4):702–7.

Jae Kim and Dan Raz

General Approach

We perform minimally invasive Ivor Lewis esophagectomy through a combined laparoscopic/robotic approach. The abdominal portion of the operation is typically performed laparoscopically without the robot, and the thoracic portion is performed robotically. We have observed limited advantage to using the robot for the gastric mobilization; and additional ports are required for robotic mobilization. In the abdomen, there is also the disadvantage of having to undock the robot for any adjustment in table positioning, unless an integrated operating room table is used. In the chest, there is less need to adjust table or patient positions during the course of the procedure. The robotic wristed instrumentation enables the circumferential esophageal mobilization to be performed with greater ease [1]. Likewise, suturing the esophageal purse string for the esophagogastric anastomosis is also facilitated by the robot.

Electronic supplementary material The online version of this chapter (https://doi.org/10.1007/978-3-030-18740-8_2) contains supplementary material, which is available to authorized users.

J. Kim (✉) · D. Raz
Division of Thoracic Surgery, Department of Surgery,
City of Hope Comprehensive Cancer Center,
Duarte, CA, USA
e-mail: jaekim@coh.org

Laparoscopic Mobilization of Gastric Conduit

Positioning and Preoperative Esophagoscopy

The patient is positioned on the operating room table with the right arm tucked and a foot board well-secured on the bottom of the feet. Before preparing the patient, the table should be placed in steep reverse Trendelenburg to test bed positioning. Esophagogastroduodenoscopy (EGD) should be performed intraoperatively prior to prepping the patient. It is important to assess the length of the tumor and Barrett's disease and to inspect the stomach for ulcerations or other lesions. Excessive insufflation should be avoided. During endoscopy, we inject botulinum toxin (200 units) into the pylorus and balloon dilate the pylorus. We do not perform pyloroplasty or pyloromyotomy and instead favor endoscopic botulinum toxin injection and pyloric dilatation. Alternatively, botulinum toxin can be injected into the pylorus during the laparoscopic procedure using a 25-gauge needle. A nasogastric tube (NGT) is then placed following endoscopy.

Surgical Technique

Port Placement

The surgeon stands on the patient's right side with the assistant standing on the patient's left side

© Springer Nature Switzerland AG 2020
J. Kim, J. Garcia-Aguilar (eds.), *Minimally Invasive Surgical Techniques for Cancers of the Gastrointestinal Tract*, https://doi.org/10.1007/978-3-030-18740-8_2

(Fig. 2.1). A 12-mm port is placed two-thirds of the distance between the xiphoid process and umbilicus to the right of the midline. Later, the linear stapler will be inserted through this port to create the gastric conduit. We use a 5-mm 30° laparoscope to allow the camera to be used in multiple ports. The peritoneum and omentum are inspected for carcinomatosis and the liver is inspected for metastases. A 5-mm port is placed to the left of the midline in the same line to mirror the other port. The patient is then placed in reverse Trendelenburg position. A 5-mm port is placed along the costal margin in the right mid-clavicular line and another 5-mm port is placed in the left mid-clavicular line (Fig. 2.2). A 5-mm port is placed laterally on the right and close to the costal margin. A 5-mm liver retractor is then inserted, and the left lobe of the liver is retracted to expose the esophageal hiatus.

Fig. 2.1 Operating room setup for laparoscopic steps

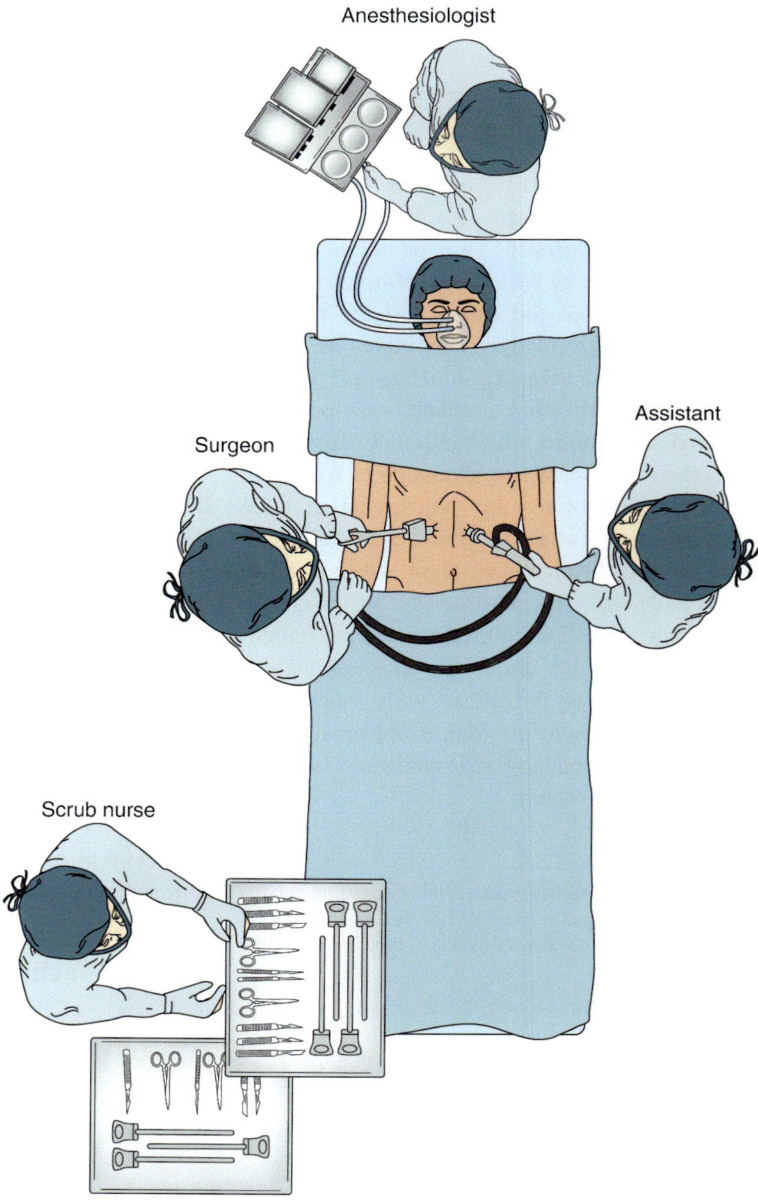

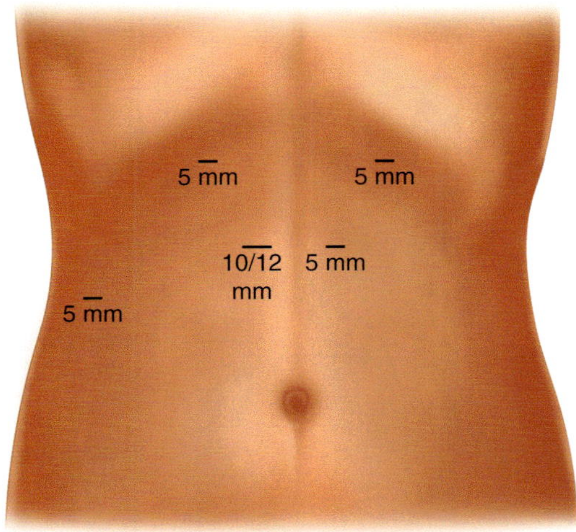

Fig. 2.2 Port placement for laparoscopic steps

Gastric Mobilization

The dissection is started at the hiatus. The right crus is exposed using an energy device and blunt dissection. The LigaSure (Covidien) and Harmonic Scalpel (Ethicon) are both adequate instruments for this step. We typically remove the peritoneal lining around the crus, but do not routinely excise muscle fibers unless the tumor is directly adherent. The dissection from the right crus is followed anteriorly and over to the left crus. If there is a hiatal hernia, it is helpful to reduce the sac and completely separate the sac from the crura. For patients who do not have a hiatal hernia or only a small hernia, we divide some of the right crural fibers to enlarge the hiatus so that it will easily accommodate the size of the gastric conduit. It is important not to divide the fibers of the left crus to avoid development of a paraesophageal hernia.

Next, the right gastroepiploic artery is visually identified. The stomach is separated from the omentum and mesocolon by retracting the omentum caudally near the point of transection and dividing the omentum using an energy device away from the gastroepiploic artery (Video 2.1 Robotic Ivor Lewis Esophagectomy). We avoid trauma to the gastric conduit by mini-mizing grasping of the stomach itself. We usually harvest an omental flap by leaving a pedicled portion of the omentum attached to the conduit perfused by two to three branches of the gastroepiploic vessels—any more vessels would be too bulky. This "tongue" of omentum is dissected directly off the colon. Then, the dissection continues parallel to the gastroepiploic artery until the short gastric vessels are identified. All short gastric arteries are then serially transected using a vessel-sealing device, and the stomach is completely mobilized free from the spleen and left crus. Additional attachments to the mesocolon are then divided. To prevent paraesophageal hernia and to allow maximum mobility of the gastric conduit, the gastrocolic ligament as well as adhesions between the posterior stomach and mesocolon are completely divided. Extreme caution must be taken in the vicinity of the takeoff of the right gastroepiploic artery from the gastroduodenal artery to avoid accidental injury of either artery. The lesser sac is then dissected, freeing the stomach from the pancreas. While the assistant retracts the gastric conduit anteriorly, the left gastric artery pedicle is dissected from the celiac axis. Nodal tissue is carefully dissected and swept towards the stomach (Fig. 2.3). Once this step is completed, the left gastric artery pedicle is transected using a vascular stapler cartridge or between clips.

Before the gastric conduit is created, we check to ensure that the stomach is circumferentially free, and that the pylorus easily reaches the hiatus. A Kocher maneuver is not necessary for an Ivor Lewis esophagectomy, but can be easily performed laparoscopically. The posterior gastroesophageal junction is then dissected, and the mediastinal esophagus is circumferentially dissected as cephalad as safely possible. It is easy to enter one or both pleural cavities during the mediastinal dissection, so it is best to wait until the latter part of the laparoscopic procedure to perform this dissection. A pleural defect can be a nuisance during laparoscopy and impair the surgeon's ability to insufflate the abdomen adequately.

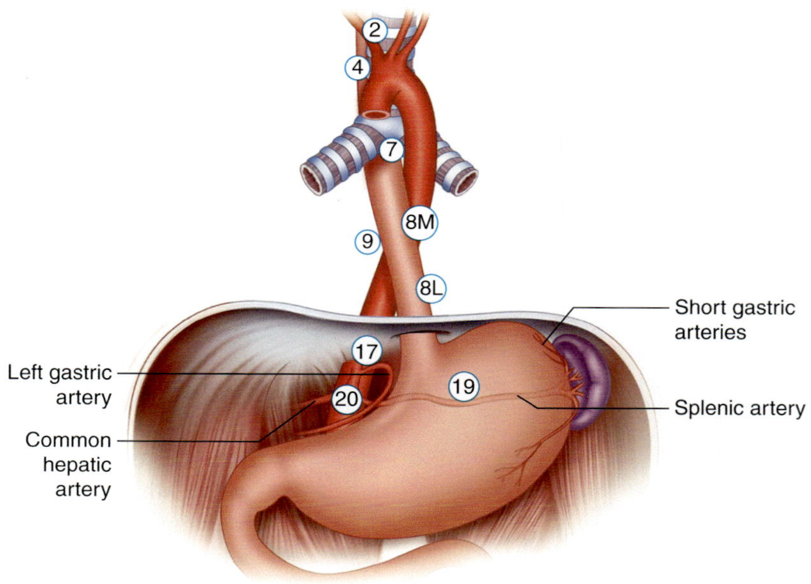

Fig. 2.3 Key lymph node stations for Ivor Lewis esophagogastrectomy

Creating the Gastric Conduit

The NGT is then pulled back into the pharynx. A point on the lesser curvature of the stomach between the right and left gastric arteries is identified just proximal to the incisura. Collateral vessels overlying this point are divided. Medium/thick tissue staple cartridges are then used to create the conduit, firing multiple stapler loads up until a point on the gastric fundus. We do not oversew the staple line. Ideally, the gastric conduit is no smaller than 4 cm in width. The gastric conduit is then sewn back to the specimen with a single mattress stitch. Alternatively, the last 2 cm of the stomach can be left undivided while creating the gastric conduit and can be later divided within the chest. We leave a quarter inch Penrose drain around the GE junction, secured by a suture, to facilitate retrieval of the gastric conduit and dissection within the chest.

Feeding Jejunostomy

Finally, the feeding jejunostomy is placed. A loop of jejunum approximately 30 cm distal to the ligament of Treitz is identified and the proximal bowel is tacked to the anterior abdominal wall near the site of the proposed jejunostomy using 2-0 silk suture. We insert a jejunostomy catheter using a modified Seldinger technique and a peel away catheter kit. An additional stitch is placed on the opposite side of the first stitch to secure the jejunum to the abdominal wall in a Stamm fashion. One additional stitch is placed 2–3 cm distally, tacking the jejunum to the anterior abdominal wall to prevent twisting of the jejunum around the jejunostomy insertion site.

Closure

The fascia of the 12-mm port is closed with a figure-of-eight 0-vicryl suture. All the skin incisions are then closed, and sterile dressings are applied. If the left pleural cavity is entered during the mediastinal dissection, a 19-Fr round Blake drain may be placed through one of the abdominal ports in the left pleural space to prevent accumulation of an effusion postoperatively.

Thoracic Procedure

The following narrative describes the robotic esophagectomy technique with the Xi version of the intuitive robot platform. The Si version is nearly identical with the exception of using a 12-mm camera port and a 5-mm posterior retraction port rather than the 8-mm ports of the Xi system. Also, the Si robot is docked over the patient's right shoulder rather than from an anterior approach as described below for the Xi robot.

Esophageal Mobilization

After the abdominal incisions are closed, the patient is placed in the left lateral decubitus position. After single lung ventilation has been established, an 8-mm port is initially introduced in the anterior axillary line, at approximately the seventh intercostal space. The chest is insufflated to 8-mm Hg pressure with a low flow rate to prevent hypotension. An 8-mm port is placed approximately 1 cm posterior to the posterior axillary line at the level of the major fissure to be used for the robotic camera. This is typically in the same interspace as the first port. Another 8-mm robotic port is placed one-hand breadth posterior to the camera port in the same intercostal space. Another 8-mm robotic port is placed one intercostal space caudally, just lateral to the transverse process. A 12-mm assistant port is placed in the tenth intercostal space, just above the insertion of the diaphragm (Fig. 2.4). The robot may be docked from the patient's anterior side, roughly perpendicular with the table (Fig. 2.5).

We begin with a 30° down-viewing scope. With the aid of insufflation, additional retraction on the diaphragm is rarely necessary. The inferior pulmonary ligament is divided and any lymph nodes at that station should be removed. A thoracic grasper placed through the most posterior port is used to retract the lung anteriorly, exposing the esophagus. We divide the azygous vein with a vascular staple cartridge. The mediastinal pleura overlying the esophagus is then opened

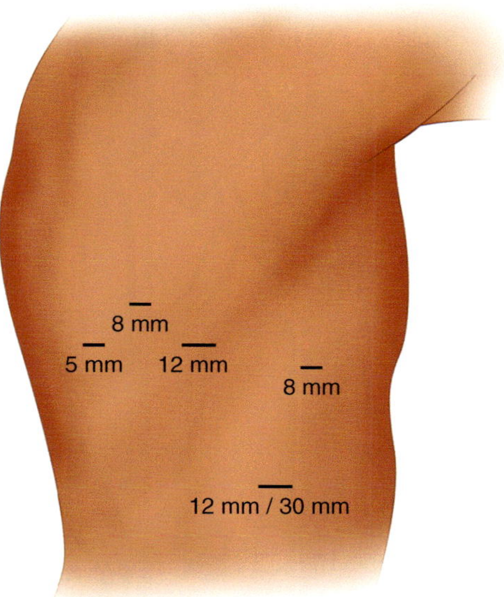

Fig. 2.4 Trocar placement for robotic and thoracoscopic dissection and anastomosis

anteriorly and posteriorly, allowing a layer of mediastinal pleura to stay attached to the esophagus. The esophagus is mobilized circumferentially using the robotic harmonic scalpel or vessel sealer to ligate small perforating vessels from the aorta. This is typically performed using the energy device in robotic arm 4 and a Cadiere forceps in robotic arm 2. The borders of the dissection are the pericardium anteriorly, the aorta and spine posteriorly, and the edges of the mediastinal pleura laterally. All tissues within these borders should be mobilized and removed en bloc with the esophagus. The network of lymphatics overlying the aorta should be removed en bloc as well. Using the Cadiere forceps to grasp the Penrose drain and providing traction on the esophagus greatly facilitate this part of the dissection (Fig. 2.6a, b). For our standard Ivor Lewis operation, the esophagus is mobilized from just above the azygous vein to the diaphragmatic hiatus. Above the level of the aortic arch, use of electrocautery should be minimized, as the left recurrent laryngeal nerve is at risk for injury.

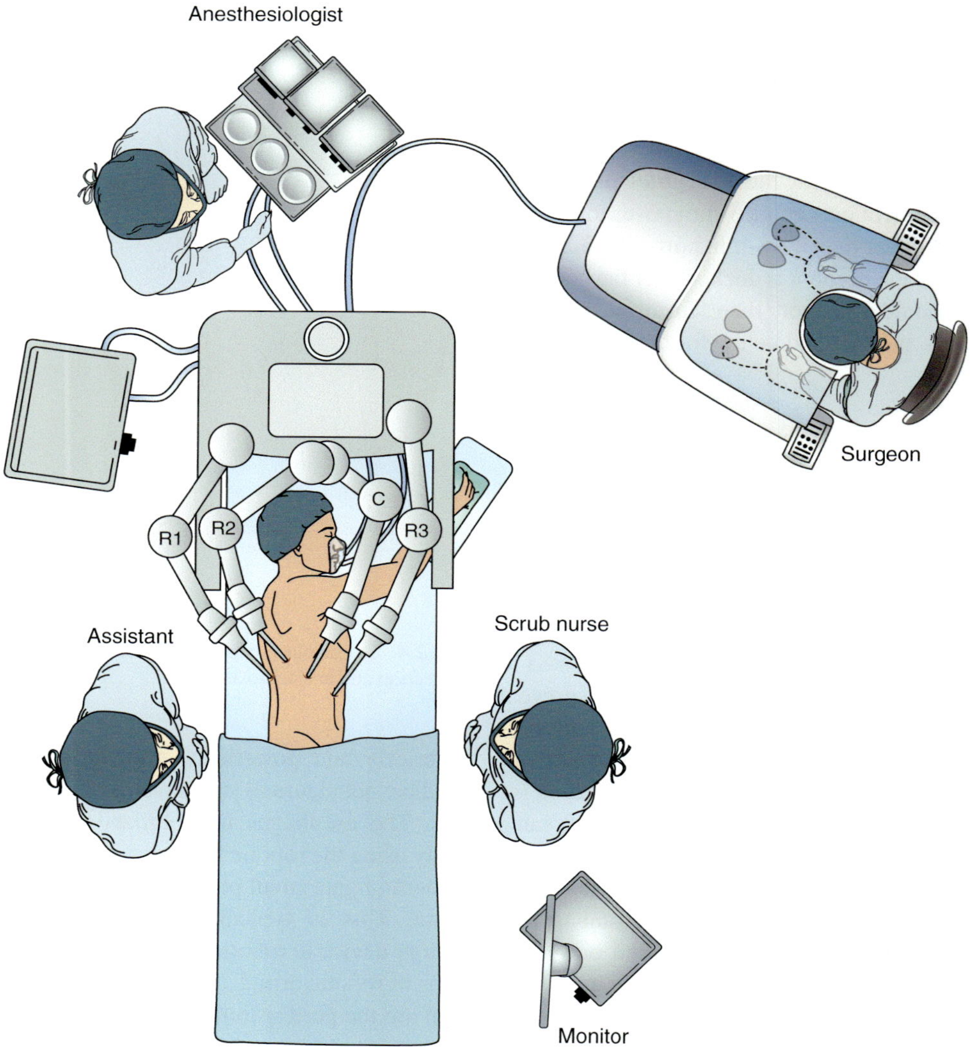

Fig. 2.5 Operative positioning for robotic dissection and esophagogastric anastomosis

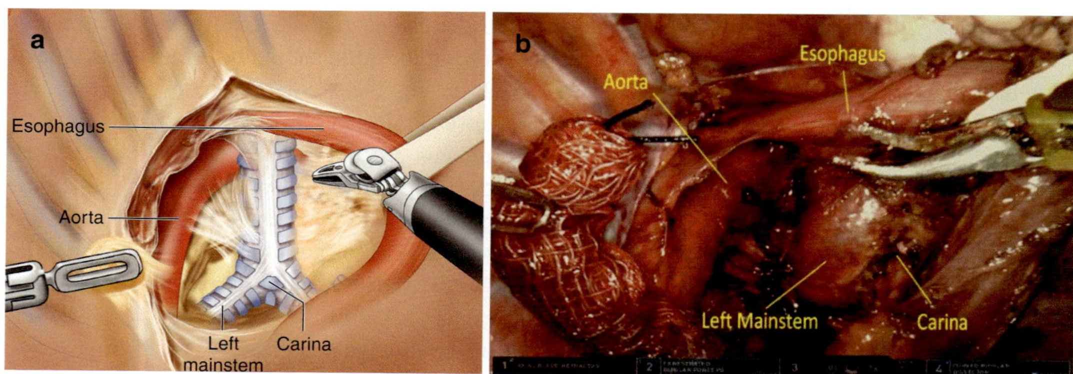

Fig. 2.6 (**a**) Illustration showing lateral retraction of a Penrose drain encircling the esophagus. (**b**) Intraoperative image showing retraction of the esophagus

The subcarinal lymph node station should be completely excised. To facilitate exposure, we typically divide the bronchial branches of the vagus nerve and the main bronchial artery to the level of the right mainstem bronchus. The thoracic duct is easily ligated using the robot to ligate all the tissue between the azygous vein and the aorta at the level of the diaphragmatic hiatus (i.e., mass ligation) using a 0-silk tie.

Anastomosis

After the mobilization is complete, the gastric conduit is gently pulled into the chest along with the omental flap. The esophagus is divided sharply at the level of the azygous vein. If the conduit has not yet been divided completely from the specimen, it is done so at this point using a linear stapler. Otherwise, the suture attaching the conduit to the proximal stomach and specimen is cut. The

assistant port is enlarged to accommodate the specimen and an extra-small wound protector is placed. Frozen section is obtained on the proximal and distal margins. The proximal esophagus is sized using a Foley catheter balloon to gauge the appropriate-sized stapler. The anvil of an EEA stapler is placed through the assistant port and then placed into the proximal esophagus. Using a robotic needle driver in robotic arm 4, a double purse string suture using 2-0 absorbable suture is placed around the anvil. A zero-degree camera usually provides a better image for this step of the operation. After confirming the absence of cancer at the margins, the robot is undocked.

The remainder of the operation is performed using a 5-mm 30° camera placed through the anterior port. A gastrotomy is made in the proximal conduit by opening up the lesser curve staple line. The stapler is placed through the gastrotomy and the spike is brought out in a well-perfused portion of the greater curve (Fig. 2.7). The anastomosis

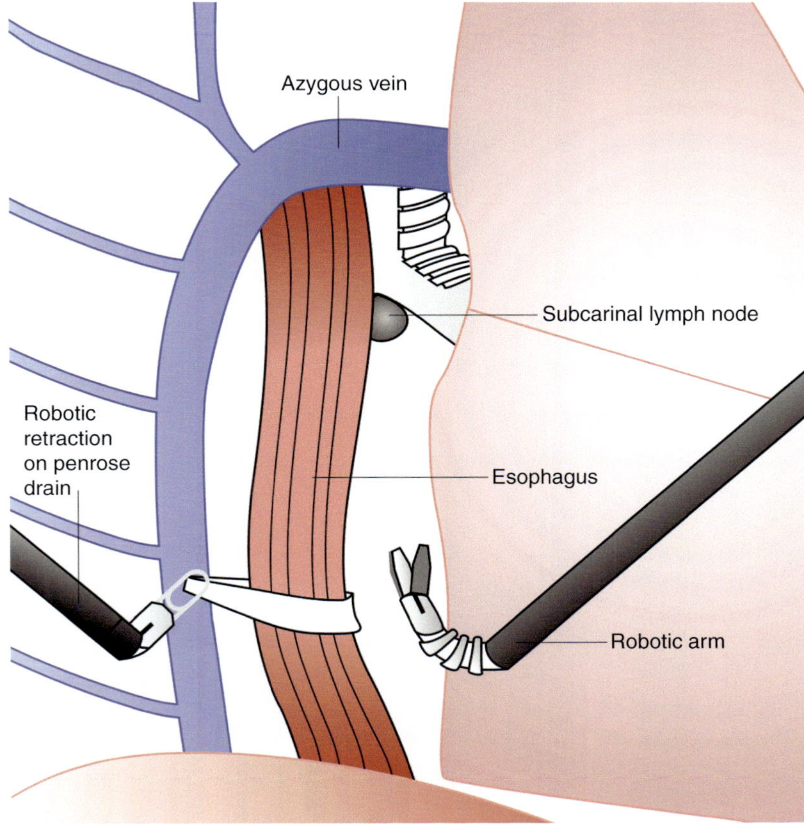

Fig. 2.7 Illustration showing a circular stapler inserted through the staple line into the gastric conduit. The spike is attached to the anvil in the distal end of the esophagus

should be made at the lowest point possible on the greater curve that will not create tension. Creating the anastomosis too high (i.e., too proximal) on the conduit can result in a redundant conduit within the chest, allowing the conduit to take on a sigmoid shape above the diaphragm and impeding conduit emptying. Also, the lower on the conduit (i.e., more distal), the better the blood supply. After firing the stapler, the donuts are inspected for completeness. The NGT is advanced beyond the anastomosis. The linear stapler is then used to close the gastrotomy and remove the excess portion of conduit that lies proximal to the anastomosis. We routinely perform a repeat endoscopy at this point to inspect the anastomosis and test for leak by insufflating endoscopically while submerging the anastomosis under irrigation. This is a very safe maneuver and poses virtually no risk to the anastomosis if performed by an experienced endoscopist. The omental flap is placed between the anastomosis and the posterior wall of the trachea and secured to the pleura with sutures.

Closure

A 24-Fr chest tube and 19-Fr Blake drain are placed in the posterior mediastinum. Local anesthetic is infiltrated into the intercostal spaces. The lung is reinflated and the remaining port sites are closed with absorbable sutures.

Reference

1. Sarkaria IS, Rizk NP. Robotic-assisted minimally invasive esophagectomy: the Ivor Lewis approach. Thorac Surg Clin. 2014;24(2):211–22. https://doi.org/10.1016/j.thor-surg.2014.02.010. vii

Robotic Three-Field Esophagectomy

Chang Hyun Kang and Young Tae Kim

Introduction

Minimally invasive esophagectomy (MIE) has become a popular option for the treatment of esophageal cancer. MIE reportedly decreases postoperative complications [1–5], and its long-term survival is comparable to open esophagectomy [3–6]. Robot-assisted minimally invasive esophagectomy (RAMIE) has been recently introduced as an alternative option for MIE. The robotic system enables more meticulous dissection of tissues and gentle handling of organs. Several studies reported early and long-term results of RAMIE, and the outcomes were comparable to other surgical modalities [7–9]. However, the techniques of RAMIE are diverse because of the heterogeneous patient population and different levels of experience in RAMIE. In this chapter we will present the three-hole RAMIE technique, which can be applied to esophageal squamous cell carcinoma located mostly in the upper to mid-thoracic esophagus. In our institute, the abdominal procedure in RAMIE has been performed robotically rather than by a laparoscopic technique. The detailed technical features will be discussed.

Advantages of Robotic Esophageal Surgery

RAMIE has several advantages over conventional thoracoscopic and laparoscopic MIE. Because RAMIE enables well-controlled fine motion during the operation, it facilitates meticulous dissection of tissue with less traumatic manipulation of organs. These advantages can be especially helpful during dissection of lymph nodes along the recurrent laryngeal nerve (RLN). Dissection along the RLN is a critical and important procedure in mid- and upper thoracic esophageal cancers. The RLN lymph node is the site of most frequent lymph node metastasis and is more closely related to survival than any other lymph node station [10, 11]. So, it has been considered that RLN dissection is critical for predicting prognosis and preventing locoregional recurrence. Robotic technology enables the performance of this critical step more easily. Radical and extensive dissection along the RLN can be possible by robotic upper mediastinal dissection [12] and could reduce the rate of vocal cord palsy [13]. These features of RAMIE may

Electronic supplementary material The online version of this chapter (https://doi.org/10.1007/978-3-030-18740-8_3) contains supplementary material, which is available to authorized users.

C. H. Kang · Y. T. Kim (✉)
Department of Thoracic and Cardiovascular Surgery, Seoul National University Hospital, Seoul, Republic of Korea
e-mail: chkang@snu.ac.kr; ytkim@snu.ac.kr

© Springer Nature Switzerland AG 2020
J. Kim, J. Garcia-Aguilar (eds.), *Minimally Invasive Surgical Techniques for Cancers of the Gastrointestinal Tract*, https://doi.org/10.1007/978-3-030-18740-8_3

lead to reduction of locoregional recurrence and improved overall survival in these patients.

The next important advantage with robotic esophagectomy is gentle manipulation of organs. This is an important advantage when operating on the trachea and stomach. Excessive tracheal retraction during esophagectomy or lymphadenectomy may result in insufficient ventilation or tracheal injury. Very close coordination between the operator and assistant surgeon is required during tracheal retraction in thoracoscopic MIE. However, in RAMIE, the force and extent of tracheal retraction can be controlled by the surgeon and better visualization can be easily achieved without the help of assistant surgeons. Therefore, airway injury during esophagectomy or lymphadenectomy can be minimized. The robotic approach also has advantages in stomach mobilization. Careful handling of the stomach, as in open surgery, is possible using robotic surgery. Excessive traction and traumatic manipulation can jeopardize the submucosal vascular network and decrease blood flow in the graft, which is an important cause of poor healing of the anastomosis with subsequent leakage. Using the robotic technique, the gastric graft can be manipulated gently and less traumatically, which helps to reduce graft-related complications.

The final advantage of robotic surgery is its flexibility in technically challenging situations, which can be frequent during MIE. These situations are the main cause for open conversion. Examples include extranodal metastatic LNs, anatomical variation, adhesion to critical organs (trachea or descending aorta), and extreme left-sided esophagus. The robotic technique can overcome these challenging conditions. The approach enables fine dissection and access to difficult areas. In our series of RAMIE, only two cases of thoracic conversion were necessary. In both cases, the cause was secondary to diffuse severe pleural adhesions. We did not experience any thoracotomy conversion after docking the robot or any conversion during robotic abdominal procedures. This low incidence of conversion is indicative of the high performance of the robotic system in difficult surgical situations.

Indications of RAMIE

RAMIE has been performed in our institute since 2008. In the early period of its use, RAMIE was performed sporadically for highly selected patients. However, the indications of RAMIE were expanded gradually from patients with low-risk early esophageal cancer to patients at high risk with advanced esophageal cancer. RAMIE has become the most commonly performed surgical procedure for esophageal cancer in our institute. Currently, there are several contraindications for RAMIE, which depend on the condition of the patients and the progression of esophageal cancer. The contraindications of thoracic robotic esophagectomy are severe pleural adhesions, previous major chest surgery, large-size esophageal cancer that is not reduced after neoadjuvant treatment, suspicion for airway invasion, intolerance to one lung ventilation, and salvage esophagectomy after definitive chemoradiation therapy. Contraindications of abdominal robotic procedures are previous history of peritonitis, previous major abdominal surgery, abdominal lymph node metastasis, and suspicion for invasion to adjacent organs. Hybrid RAMIE that comprises robotic esophagectomy combined with open laparotomy can be performed when the abdominal situation is not favorable for robotic surgery. However, if the thoracic situation is not favorable for robotic surgery, then we usually do not perform robotic surgery at all. We think that avoiding thoracotomy is the most important component of MIE, rather than avoiding laparotomy.

Position of Patient, Port Placement, and Robotic Setup

In the thoracic procedure, patients are in the left lateral decubitus position with a slight tilt in the anterior direction (Fig. 3.1). In the early period of robotic surgery, we used the prone position during the thoracic procedure. However, we changed to the decubitus position because of the difficulties in airway management during anesthesia and pleural adhesiolysis with whole pleural adhesion.

With experience in RAMIE, we now know that the decubitus position is not inferior to the prone position for esophagectomy.

We prefer the four-arm technique during the thoracic and abdominal procedures and usually use four ports during the thoracic procedure (Fig. 3.2). A camera port is made in the seventh intercostal space just below the scapular tip. The level of the camera port is very important because an optimal surgical view cannot be obtained when the location is too high or too low. The vertebral body and lung parenchyma in high- and low-position camera locations, respectively, can hinder visualization of the esophagus and peri-

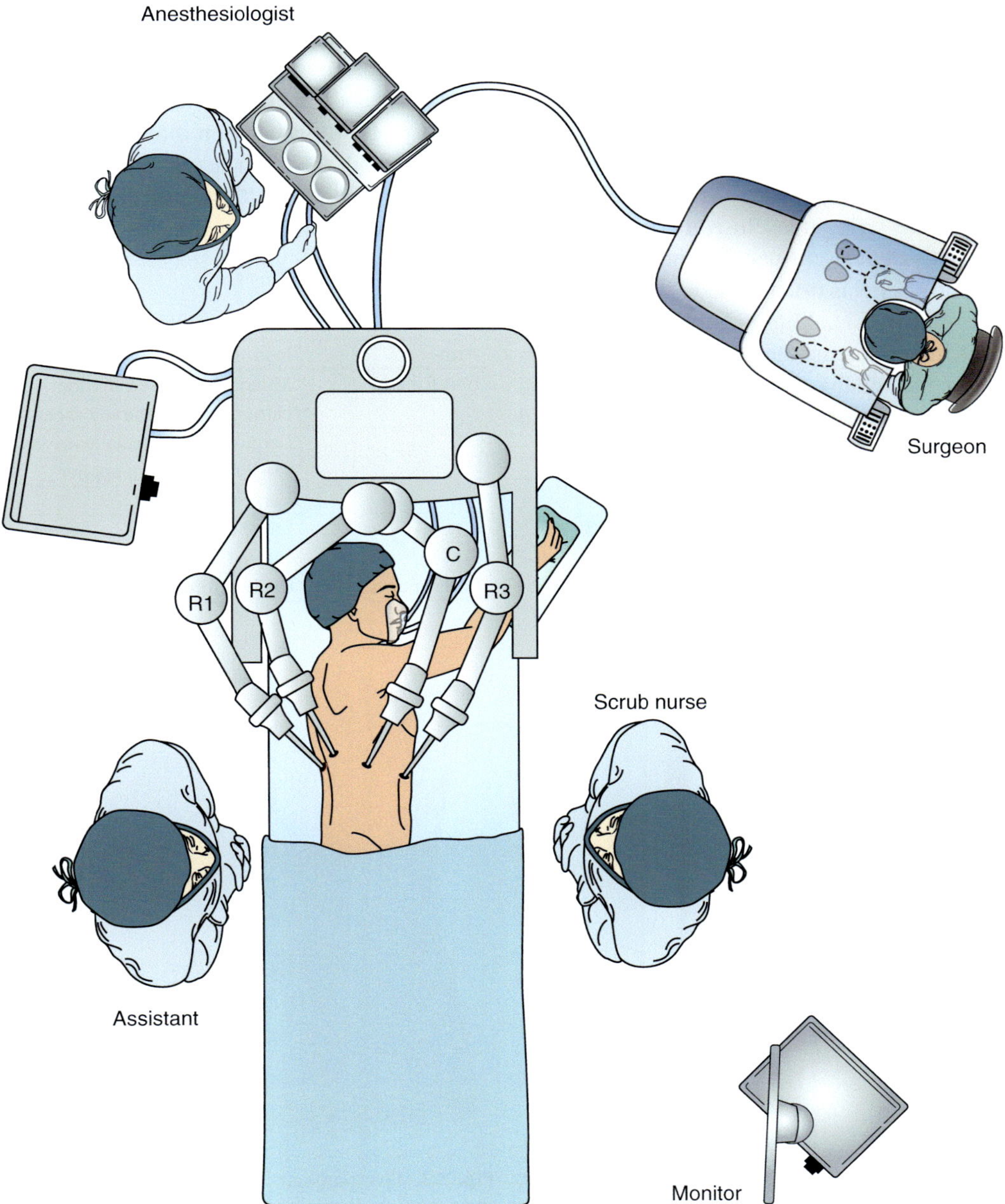

Fig. 3.1 The position of the robot and patient during robotic esophagectomy

esophageal structures. Other ports are usually made to maintain distances >8.5 cm between the arms. Arm 3 port is placed in the third intercostal space of the axillary fossa. The location of this arm should be checked after docking because it can compress the right arm of the patient. Arm 3 is usually used for retraction of structures, so a Cadiere grasper is usually used in this arm. Arm 1 port is made in the fifth intercostal space in the posterior axillary line. This port can be used for the robot but can also be used by an assistant surgeon. Therefore, we make a 4-cm sized port and use a single incision silastic port (Glove port, NELIS Co., South Korea). Arm 2 port is made in the tenth intercostal space on the back of the patient. This arm is exclusively used for the robotic dissecting grasper. Robotic scissors or harmonic scalpel is usually used as the dissection device (Table 3.1). Minimizing clashing of the arms is important and the surgeon should always consider the relative positions of each arm and use the arms properly in each surgical procedure.

In the abdominal robotic procedure, we always place five ports. Four are robotic ports and the remaining port is an assistant port. The camera port is 2 cm in size and made just lateral to the umbilicus. The glove port used for the thoracic procedure can also be inserted in this port. We place a feeding jejunostomy catheter through this port after finishing the robotic procedure. Other ports are placed as depicted in Fig. 3.3. We also use the four-arm technique in the abdominal procedure; most of the robotic arms used in thoracic procedure can be used in the abdominal procedure.

We prefer to use carbon dioxide (CO_2) insufflation in both the thoracic and abdominal procedures. We reduce the CO_2 pressure below 5–8 mm Hg to minimize hemodynamic instability during

Table 3.1 Robotic ports and instruments used in RAMIE

Arms	Instruments
Port for arm 1	Monopolar curved scissors
	Harmonic ACE curved shears
	Large suture cut needle driver
	Medium-large clip applier
	Large clip applier
	Small clip applier
Port for arm 2	Curved bipolar dissector
Port for arm 3	Cadiere forceps

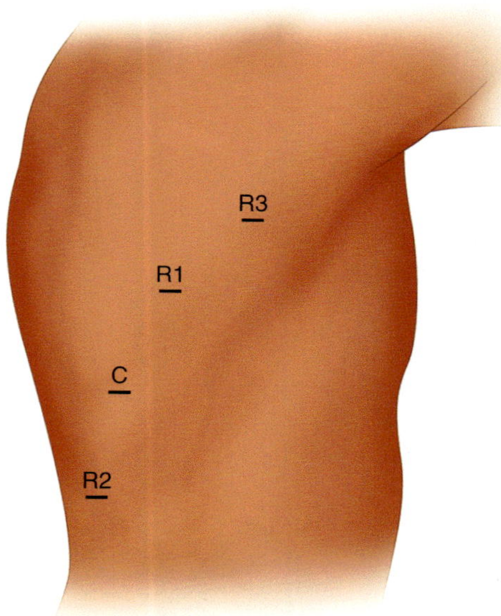

Fig. 3.2 Four ports are made for the robotic thoracic procedure. A silastic port can be applied using a small utility incision. The utility incision can be used by robotic arm #1 or by the assistant surgeon

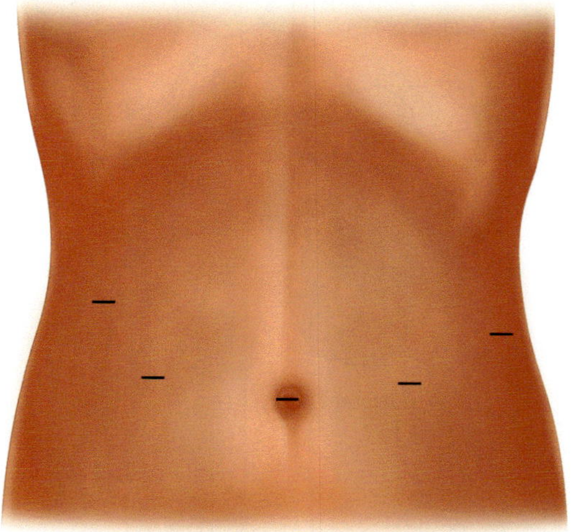

Fig. 3.3 Five ports are made in the robotic abdominal procedure. A silastic port used in the thoracic procedure can be also used in the periumbilical port. However, the assistant surgeon uses a different port

the thoracic procedure. Both bipolar and monopolar electrocoagulation are used during surgery with dissectors in arm 2 connected to bipolar coagulation and scissors in arm 1 to monopolar coagulation.

Surgical Techniques (Video 3.1)

Thoracic Procedure

We start the esophagectomy from the level of the azygous vein. After dividing the azygous vein and the right bronchial artery, we open the mediastinal pleura along the vagus nerve and dissect the lymph nodes in the right upper mediastinum. Then we dissect peri-eosphageal tissue downside along the azygous vein and thoracic duct to the level of the diaphragmatic hiatus. Lastly, we finish by dissecting the subcarinal area and the left paratracheal area. The order of dissection can be dependent on the surgeon's preference.

After dividing the azygos vein, the right bronchial artery can be divided by robotic hemoclips from the origin of aorta. The right main bronchus and vagus nerve can be visualized at this point, and dissection can be performed along the vagus nerve. The distal vagus nerve can be cut just distal to the right pulmonary branch of the vagus nerve. Dissection can proceed to the upper mediastinum along the vagus nerve. The right RLN can be identified at the junctional point between the right subclavian artery and the vagus nerve. Lymph nodes along the right RLN (station 2R in American Joint Committee on Cancer [AJCC] [14], 106recR in Japanese Esophageal Society [JES] mapping [15]) can be dissected from this point. The dissection can be performed up to the level of the inferior thyroidal artery. A portion of cervical paraesophageal lymph nodes can be removed at this area (1R in AJCC, 101R in the JES). Complete removal of lymph nodes and perilymphatic tissue along the right RLN is possible. Figure 3.4 demonstrates lymph node dissection view around right RLN.

Mid- to lower thoracic esophageal dissection is relatively easy compared to upper mediastinal

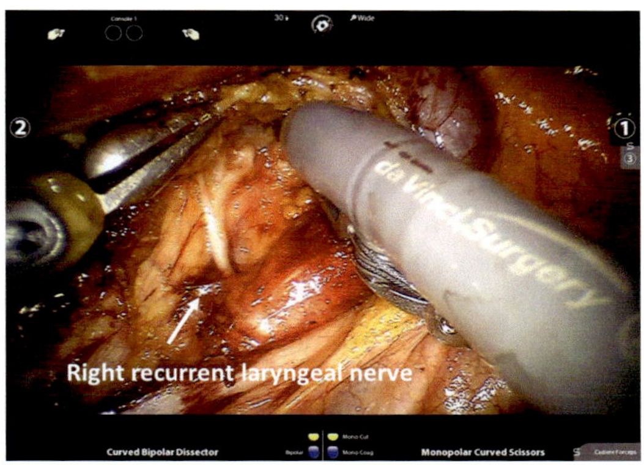

Fig. 3.4 Robotic view during dissection of lymph nodes in the right upper mediastinum along the right recurrent laryngeal nerve

dissection. Mediastinal pleura can be exposed by sharp dissection with scissors. In other areas, the harmonic scalpel is usually sufficient for dissection. Paraesophageal lymph nodes (8M and 8L in the AJCC map, 108 and 110 in the JES map) are usually dissected in an en bloc fashion with the esophagus. Complete removal of the whole thoracic duct is a routine procedure in our institute, and the thoracic duct is divided just above the diaphragmatic hiatus. The contralateral lung, left pulmonary vein, and left main bronchus should be entirely exposed, and lymph nodes in the left mediastinal side should be completely removed. Anterior para-aortic lymph nodes (112aoA in the JES map) can be removed by converting the camera angle to 30° upside. Dissection can be performed to the level of the hiatus and supradiaphragmatic LNs can be removed (15 in the AJCC map, 111 in the JES map). Along the left main bronchus, the left vagus nerve can be identified and divided just distal to the pulmonary branch, similar to the right side. Subcarinal lymph nodes (7 in AJCC and 107 in JES) can be removed at this point. Esophageal encircling with a traction band is not necessary because the third robotic arm can be used for retraction and lifting the esophagus during the entire procedure.

The most difficult part of the thoracic procedure is the left upper mediastinal dissection. This step requires sufficient experience to finish it completely without damaging the trachea or left RLN. We prefer to detach the esophagus completely from the trachea before lymph node dissection. This is why we perform left upper lymphadenectomy during the last stage of operation. A wide surgical view can be obtained after complete dissection of the entire esophagus. The trachea can be retracted in the anterior direction using Cadiere robotic forceps. Complete control of small vessel branches by monopolar robotic scissors along the left tracheal border before lymph node dissection is helpful for a bloodless surgical field. The left RLN is embedded inside of lymphatic tissue, therefore meticulous and fine dissection of tissue is necessary to find the left RLN. After identifying the RLN, the tracheobronchial lymph nodes can be removed first (10L and 5 in AJCC and 106tbL in JES). The most important aspect at this point is to preserve the left bronchial artery. Because the right bronchial artery has already been divided, cutting both arteries will induce significant ischemia in the airway and increase the possibility of tracheoenteric fistula postoperatively. Then, lymph nodes along the left RLN can be removed up to the inferior thyroidal artery. This step can remove whole lymph nodes in the left paratracheal area (2L and 4L in AJCC and 107recL in JES) and a portion of the left cervical paraesophageal lymph nodes (1L in AJCC and 101L in JES). Figure 3.5 presents a post-dissection view of the left paratracheal area.

As noted previously, RAMIE enables safe and complete lymphadenectomy in precarious anatomic regions. Its ability to do so is better than the thoracoscopic technique; and we feel that it is better than the open technique. The thoracic procedure is the most beneficial part of RAMIE in esophageal cancer surgery. The role of the assistant surgeon is limited in the thoracic procedure, and delivering suture material or retrieving lymph nodes is the major role of the assistant surgeon. Suctioning blood is sometimes necessary, but the amount of bleeding is minor in RAMIE.

Abdominal Procedure

The 4-arm technique can also be used for the abdominal procedure. The Cadiere forceps can be used for retraction of the liver and to hold the stomach during the abdominal procedure. After lifting the left lobe of the liver, the lesser omentum can be divided using the harmonic scalpel. A wide opening of the lesser curvature is necessary to gain a wide view around the celiac axis. The common hepatic artery lymph nodes (18 in AJCC map and 8a in JES), left gastric lymph nodes (17 in AJCC and 7 in JES), and celiac axis lymph nodes (20 in AJCC and 9 in JES) can be dissected at this point. The left gastric artery and coronary vein can be divided at the most proximal part of the celiac axis by robotic polymer clips. Lymph node dissection can be performed along the splenic artery (19 in AJCC and 9 in JES). At the level of the splenic hilum, short gastric vessels can be visualized and divided, and the left side of the cardia can be mobilized from the splenic hilum.

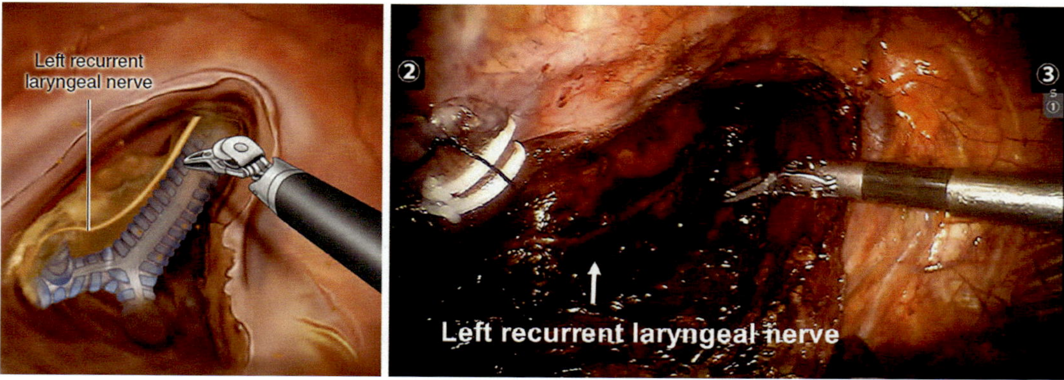

Fig. 3.5 Illustration of the paratracheal area after dissection of lymph nodes in the left upper mediastinum along the left recurrent laryngeal nerve and intraoperative image showing the left recurrent laryngeal nerve following lymph node dissection

After finishing the lesser curvature steps, the stomach can be lifted by the Cardiere forceps. The greater omentum is divided along the left gastroepiploic artery. To preserve collateral blood supply, sufficient omentum should remain with the stomach graft. On the right side, the gastrocolic ligament should be completely divided, and Kocher maneuver can be performed for maximum mobilization of the stomach. Pyloromyotomy is performed by sharp dissection at the pylorus. Grasping the pyloric muscle using the robotic dissecting grasper and severing the muscle with the scissors enable complete division of the pyloric muscle without damaging the gastric mucosa. Ramstedt-type pyloromyotomy is a routine procedure in our institute. The greater omentum is then divided along the right gastroepiploic artery to the level of the left gastroepiploic artery. Sufficient omentum should be preserved on the graft side at this point to preserve collateral blood flow. Attachments to the splenic hilum can be easily divided by gentle traction of the stomach. The hiatus should be opened only at the last stage of the abdominal procedure to prevent CO_2 pressure effects on the intrathoracic organs. The right diaphragmatic crus can be widened using the harmonic scalpel.

After finishing mobilization of stomach and the lymph node dissection, the gastric tube can be created intracorporeally. To maximize the advantages of the minimally invasive approach, we do not make additional laparotomy incisions or perform extracorporeal gastric tube formation. Close coordination with the assistant surgeon is important at this stage. The operator should hold the stomach with the robotic arms and should establish proper position for stapling. The assistant surgeon can divide the lesser curvature of the stomach using an endo-stapler. Stapling starts from 2 cm proximal to the pylorus and up to the level of the cardia. Lesser curvature lymph nodes (17 in AJCC and 3a/3b in JES) and cardiac lymph nodes (16 in AJCC and 1/2 in JES) can be removed during gastric tube formation. Usually five or six 60-mm-sized staplers are necessary for gastric tube formation. We usually make a 4 cm wide graft for the cervical anastomosis. The resected esophagogastic specimen is retrieved thorough the cervical wound and a Foley catheter is introduced into the abdomen. The gastric tube can be pulled up to the neck after suturing the tube to the Foley catheter. We routinely insert a feeding jejunostomy catheter in all patients. The jejunum is pulled out from the periumbilical port site, and a Stamm-type jejunostomy catheter can be inserted at the left port that is used for robotic arm 1.

Cervical Procedures

After pulling up the gastric tube, the esophagogastric anastomosis can be made by side-to-side anastomosis with linear staplers. The technique is a modification of the Orringer technique [16]. In the latter, the posterior walls are stapled and the anterior walls are sutured by interrupted or continuous suturing. Conversely, we close the anterior walls by stapling instead of suturing to maximize the size of anastomosis. Before stapling, the anterior walls are sutured by continuous suture with barbed sutures (V-Loc, Medtronic, MN) to approximate the esophageal and gastric mucosa. Then anterior walls are stretched laterally and stapled using a linear stapler (ECHELON FLEX GST-powered stapler with 60 mm size and 4.1 mm height, Ethicon, OH). This is a simple and fast technique that ensures wide esophagogastric anastomosis. We have performed this technique in 70 cervical anastomoses. The outcomes remain excellent with one occult anastomotic leakage (1.4%) and no anastomotic stricture over the past 2 years. The 2-year rate for our freedom from intervention for anastomotic stricture was 100% in our series.

Cervical lymph node dissection can be performed in indicated patients. Recently, we performed three-field lymph node dissections in advanced stage or upper and mid-thoracic esophageal cancer. Supraclavicular lymph nodes (level 3 and level 4 in the AJCC map, 101 and 104 in the JES map) can be removed during the cervical procedure.

Postoperative Management

Our institute started an enhanced recovery after surgery (ERAS) program 3 years ago. Because most patients were heavy smokers and chronic alcoholics, chronic obstructive pulmonary disease, chronic liver disease, and malnutrition were common in our series. We tried to optimize the ERAS program with modifications over this time period. Table 3.2 presents the ERAS program currently being used in our institute. Modifications to the program continue to be implemented with the goal of further improving postoperative outcomes.

We believe that early enteral nutrition is important for early recovery of patients. This issue has been emphasized in other studies [17–19], and early enteral feeding is related to reduced postoperative complications and early recovery of patients. In our practice, we begin jejunostomy feedings on postoperative day (POD) 1. Calorie intake can be escalated up to 100 kcal/hr by POD 5. Jejunostomy feedings can be maintained until 4 weeks postoperatively when oral calorie intake can be 80% of the feeding requirements.

We routinely use renal dose dopamine for 3 days postoperatively for the following reasons. Our fluid management protocol is to restrict postoperative fluid infusion to prevent pulmonary complications. Therefore, relative hypotension and transient renal insufficiency are expected, and decreased splanchnic blood flow may induce delayed healing of the esophagogastric anastomosis. To improve hemodynamic stability and maintain splanchnic blood flow, we therefore routinely use renal dose dopamine [20, 21].

Vocal cord evaluation is performed on POD 3 in all patients regardless of whether hoarseness is detected. Identifying the status of the vocal cord is important to prevent aspiration after starting oral feedings. Aspiration pneumonia is one of most serious complications after esophagectomy. Because very extensive lymph node dissection is carried out along both RLNs, transient vocal cord palsy is quite common. However, well-controlled management of vocal cord palsy can prevent aspiration pneumonia in most patients.

Early Postoperative Outcomes

From May 2008 to August 2017, a total of 186 patients underwent RAMIE at Seoul National University Hospital. There was one patient with 30-day mortality (0.5%) and three patients with 90-day mortality (1.6%). Overall in-hospital mortality occurred in five patients, and operation-related mortality rate was 2.7%. Thoracotomy conversion was necessary in two patients (1.1%) because of severe pleural adhesions even before docking the robot. However, in our series, we did not have any conversions after starting the robotic thoracic procedure. Our overall complication rate was 58%. The complications are listed in Table 3.3. The highest Clavien-Dindo grade of complications were grade 1 in 31 patients

Table 3.2 ERAS protocol at Seoul National University Hospital

ERAS items	Postoperative periods
ICU stay	POD 0 to POD 1
Pain management	IV PCA until POD 2
Chest tube removal	POD 1
Enteral feeding through jejunostomy	POD 1 to 4 weeks
Nasogastric tube removal	POD 3
Dopamine at renal dose (3 mcg/kg/min)	POD 0 to POD 3
Laryngoscopic evaluation of vocal cords	POD 3
Esophagography	POD 5
Initiation of oral feedings	POD 6
Hospital discharge	POD 8 to 12

PCA patient-controlled analgesia, *POD* postoperative day

Table 3.3 Postoperative complications after RAMIE

Complications	Number	%
Respiratory complication	16	8.6
Gastrointestinal complication	20	10.7
(Anastomotic leakage)	17	9.1
Neurologic complication	54	29.0
(Vocal cord palsy)	50	26.9
Cardiac complication	24	12.9
(Atrial fibrillation)	24	12.9
Chyle leakage	19	10.2

(16.7%), grade 2 in 47 patients (25.2%), grade 3 in 9 patients (4.8%), grade 4 in 5 patients (2.6%), and grade 5 in 5 patients (2.6%). The most common complication was vocal cord palsy at a rate of 26.9%. Because we did extensive lymph node dissection along the bilateral RLNs and evaluated vocal cord palsy in all patients, the incidence was relatively high. However, 24 of 50 patients (48.0%) with vocal cord palsy were asymptomatic by routine evaluation and most vocal cord palsies were transient and had improved at long-term follow-up. Respiratory complications occurred in 16 patients (8.6%) and anastomotic leakage occurred in 17 patients (9.1%). Although the respiratory complication rate did not change during the study period, the leakage rate decreased gradually. The leakage rate of the most recent 100 cases was 4.0%.

Long-Term Outcomes

Complete R0 resection was accomplished in 179 patients (96.2%). The mean number of dissected lymph nodes was 44.3 ± 21.2. A total of 32 patients died during the follow-up period and the overall 5-year survival rate in those who underwent RAMIE was 73.1%. Five-year survival rate of patients who underwent upfront surgery was 75.0% and for patients who underwent neoadjuvant chemoradiation followed by RAMIE was 59.0%. Survival rates according to pathologic stage in patients who underwent upfront surgery were 85.6% for stage 1, 66.0% for stage 2, and 62.2% for stage 3 (Fig. 3.6). We suspect that higher survival rates in patients who underwent upfront surgery were related to patient selection, because most of these patients had clinical stage 1 or 2 and a significant number of patients had stage migration after surgery. The patients who received neoadjuvant treatment had more advanced stage of disease, mostly clinical stage 3. Therefore, direct comparison between the upfront surgery and neoadjuvant treatment groups is not possible with our data. However, long-term survival of the patients who underwent RAMIE was excellent in both upfront surgery and neoadjuvant treatment groups.

Conclusions

RAMIE is based on more advanced technology when compared to thoracoscopic or laparoscopic surgery. It consists of more meticulous dissection of the upper mediastinal lymph nodes and safer

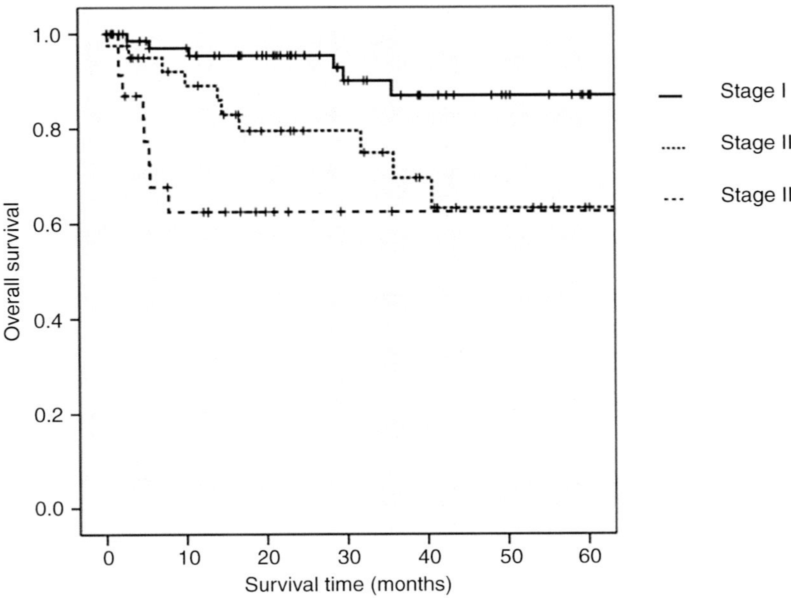

Fig. 3.6 Overall survival of patients who underwent RAMIE as upfront surgery stratified by pathologic stage

preparation of the gastric graft. Major complication rates are acceptable and postoperative mortality rates can be maintained at low levels. The most important advantage of RAMIE was the improved long-term survival when compared to historical reports. We believe that improved survival can be achieved by the combination effect of extensive lymphadenectomy and reduced postoperative mortality. Further studies on the RAMIE should be performed to clarify the oncologic role of RAMIE in the treatment of esophageal cancer.

References

1. Biere SS, van Berge Henegouwen MI, Maas KW, Bonavina L, Rosman C, Garcia JR, et al. Minimally invasive versus open oesophagectomy for patients with oesophageal cancer: a multicentre, open-label, randomised controlled trial. Lancet. 2012;379:1887–92.
2. Maas KW, Cuesta MA, van Berge Henegouwen MI, Roig J, Bonavina L, Rosman C, et al. Quality of life and late complications after minimally invasive compared to open esophagectomy: results of a randomized trial. World J Surg. 2015;39:1986–93.
3. Guo W, Ma X, Yang S, Zhu X, Qin W, Xiang J, et al. Combined thoracoscopic-laparoscopic esophagectomy versus open esophagectomy: a meta-analysis of outcomes. Surg Endosc. 2016;30:3873–81.
4. Wang H, Shen Y, Feng M, Zhang Y, Jiang W, Xu S, et al. Outcomes, quality of life, and survival after esophagectomy for squamous cell carcinoma: a propensity score-matched comparison of operative approaches. J Thorac Cardiovasc Surg. 2015;149:1006–14; discussion 14-5 e4
5. Yerokun BA, Sun Z, Yang CJ, Gulack BC, Speicher PJ, Adam MA, et al. Minimally invasive versus open esophagectomy for esophageal cancer: a population-based analysis. Ann Thorac Surg. 2016;102:416–23.
6. Straatman J, van der Wielen N, Cuesta MA, Daams F, Roig Garcia J, Bonavina L, et al. Minimally invasive versus open esophageal resection: three-year follow-up of the previously reported randomized controlled trial: the TIME trial. Ann Surg. 2017;266:232–6.
7. van Hillegersberg R, Boone J, Draaisma WA, Broeders IA, Giezeman MJ, Borel Rinkes IH. First experience with robot-assisted thoracoscopic esophagolymphadenectomy for esophageal cancer. Surg Endosc. 2006;20:1435–9.
8. van der Sluis PC, Ruurda JP, Verhage RJ, van der Horst S, Haverkamp L, Siersema PD, et al. Oncologic long-term results of robot-assisted minimally invasive thoraco-laparoscopic esophagectomy with two-field lymphadenectomy for esophageal cancer. Ann Surg Oncol. 2015;22(Suppl 3):S1350–6.
9. Park SY, Kim DJ, Do YW, Suh J, Lee S. The oncologic outcome of esophageal squamous cell carcinoma patients after robot-assisted thoracoscopic esophagectomy with total mediastinal lymphadenectomy. Ann Thorac Surg. 2017;103:1151–7.
10. Udagawa H, Ueno M, Shinohara H, Haruta S, Kaida S, Nakagawa M, et al. The importance of grouping of lymph node stations and rationale of three-field lymphoadenectomy for thoracic esophageal cancer. J Surg Oncol. 2012;106:742–7.
11. Tachimori Y, Nagai Y, Kanamori N, Hokamura N, Igaki H. Pattern of lymph node metastases of esophageal squamous cell carcinoma based on the anatomical lymphatic drainage system. Dis Esophagus. 2011;24:33–8.
12. Kim DJ, Park SY, Lee S, Kim HI, Hyung WJ. Feasibility of a robot-assisted thoracoscopic lymphadenectomy along the recurrent laryngeal nerves in radical esophagectomy for esophageal squamous carcinoma. Surg Endosc. 2014;28:1866–73.
13. Suda K, Ishida Y, Kawamura Y, Inaba K, Kanaya S, Teramukai S, et al. Robot-assisted thoracoscopic lymphadenectomy along the left recurrent laryngeal nerve for esophageal squamous cell carcinoma in the prone position: technical report and short-term outcomes. World J Surg. 2012;36:1608–16.
14. Rice TW, Ishwaran H, Ferguson MK, Blackstone EH, Goldstraw P. Cancer of the esophagus and esophagogastric junction: an eighth edition staging primer. J Thorac Oncol. 2017;12:36–42.
15. Japanese Classification of Esophageal Cancer, 11th Edition: part I. Esophagus 2017;14:1–36.
16. Orringer MB, Marshall B, Iannettoni MD. Eliminating the cervical esophagogastric anastomotic leak with a side-to-side stapled anastomosis. J Thorac Cardiovasc Surg. 2000;119:277–88.
17. Steenhagen E, van Vulpen JK, van Hillegersberg R, May AM, Siersema PD. Nutrition in peri-operative esophageal cancer management. Expert Rev Gastroenterol Hepatol. 2017;11:663–72.
18. Takesue T, Takeuchi H, Ogura M, Fukuda K, Nakamura R, Takahashi T, et al. A prospective randomized trial of enteral nutrition after thoracoscopic esophagectomy for esophageal cancer. Ann Surg Oncol. 2015;22(Suppl 3):S802–9.
19. Wang G, Chen H, Liu J, Ma Y, Jia H. A comparison of postoperative early enteral nutrition with delayed enteral nutrition in patients with esophageal cancer. Nutrients. 2015;7:4308–17.
20. Meier-Hellmann A, Bredle DL, Specht M, Spies C, Hannemann L, Reinhart K. The effects of low-dose dopamine on splanchnic blood flow and oxygen uptake in patients with septic shock. Intensive Care Med. 1997;23:31–7.
21. Gelman S, Mushlin PS. Catecholamine-induced changes in the splanchnic circulation affecting systemic hemodynamics. Anesthesiology. 2004;100:434–9.

Shaila Merchant, Owen Pyke, and Joseph Kim

Introduction

Gastrointestinal stromal tumors (GISTs) are the most common soft tissue tumors of the gastrointestinal tract. They originate from mesenchymal cells believed to be precursors of the interstitial cells of Cajal [1, 2]. While the estimated annual age-adjusted incidence of GISTs in the US was 0.78/100,000 in 2011 [3], the true incidence may be underreported [4]. Most of these GISTs occur within the stomach [5, 6] and although the exact locations within the stomach are variable, the majority of cases are detected in the antrum [7]. GISTs are predominantly initiated by gain-of-function mutations in *KIT* (c-KIT) [8], which is the target for the tyrosine kinase inhibitor imatinib that extends recurrence free survival and overall survival in the adjuvant setting [9, 10]. Resectable GISTs necessitate removal of the tumor with negative surgical margins [5], but there is no requirement for regional lymphadenectomy, given the low incidence of lymph node metastases [11].

Minimally Invasive Techniques for Resection of GIST

Open gastrectomy has been traditionally considered the gold standard operative approach for GISTs. However, the introduction of minimally invasive surgical techniques has shifted the trend towards utilizing laparoscopic and robotic surgical approaches with the benefits of decreased postoperative pain, shorter hospital length of stay, and quicker recuperation.

Multiple studies have evaluated the role of minimally invasive techniques for resection of gastric GIST. Laparoscopic surgery has been shown to be safe and effective for the surgical management of GISTs, including large tumors and tumors located in technically challenging locations (e.g., gastroesophageal junction, lesser curvature, and posterior wall of the stomach [12–16]. There are few studies that have examined robotic surgery for the resection of GIST. Small case series have reported the feasibility of robot-assisted techniques to remove gastric and duodenal GISTs [17–19]. The

Electronic Supplementary Material The online version of this chapter (https://doi.org/10.1007/978-3-030-18740-8_4) contains supplementary material, which is available to authorized users.

S. Merchant
Department of Surgery, Division of General Surgery and Surgical Oncology, Queen's University, Kingston, ON, Canada
e-mail: shaila.merchant@kingstonhsc.ca

O. Pyke
Department of Surgery, Stony Brook University Hospital, Stony Brook, NY, USA
e-mail: owen.pyke@stonybrookmedicine.edu

J. Kim (✉)
Department of Surgery, University of Kentucky, Lexington, KY, USA
e-mail: joseph.kim@uky.edu

enhanced maneuverability, improved visualization, and ergonomic ease afforded by the robotic platform compared to conventional laparoscopic surgery may allow the surgeon to perform resections in more challenging locations [18]. In this chapter, we outline the step-by-step surgical procedure in performing robotic segmental resection of a large GIST located near the junction of the cardia, fundus, and body.

Anatomy of the Stomach

The stomach has a rich vascular network of arteries and veins. The major arterial inflow originates from the branches of the celiac trunk, which gives off three branches including the left gastric artery, splenic artery and the common hepatic artery. The left gastric artery supplies primarily the lesser curvature of the stomach and the gastroesophageal junction. The splenic artery courses behind the superior border of the pancreas, and its branches include the short gastric vessels and the left gastroepiploic artery, which supplies the greater curvature of the stomach. Finally, the major branches of the common hepatic artery include the right gastric artery that supplies the lesser curvature and the pylorus and the gastroduodenal artery that joins the right gastroepiploic artery to supply the greater curvature of the stomach. Venous drainage follows that of the arterial network, emptying into the portal venous system via the splenic and superior mesenteric veins. The coronary vein (*aka* left gastric vein) runs adjacent to the left gastric artery and drains directly into the portal vein. The stomach has an extensive lymphatic drainage system; however, GISTs have very low risk of lymph node metastases, and regional lymphadenectomy is not required for these cancers [11].

Case Evaluation

The patient is a 40-year-old male with an 8-cm tumor originating from the submucosal layer of the anterior wall of the stomach near the borders of the cardia, fundus, and body of the stomach. The patient initially presented to the emergency department with hematemesis. Upper endoscopy was performed and identified a large bleeding tumor that appeared consistent with GIST. Endoscopic biopsies were performed and confirmed the diagnosis. Computed tomography (CT) imaging of the abdomen and pelvis demonstrated an 8-cm-wide based tumor in the proximal stomach with no evidence of distant metastatic disease (Fig. 4.1a, b). We considered the option of a neoadjuvant approach [20, 21]; however, given the bleeding and need for blood transfusions, we elected to proceed to the operating room.

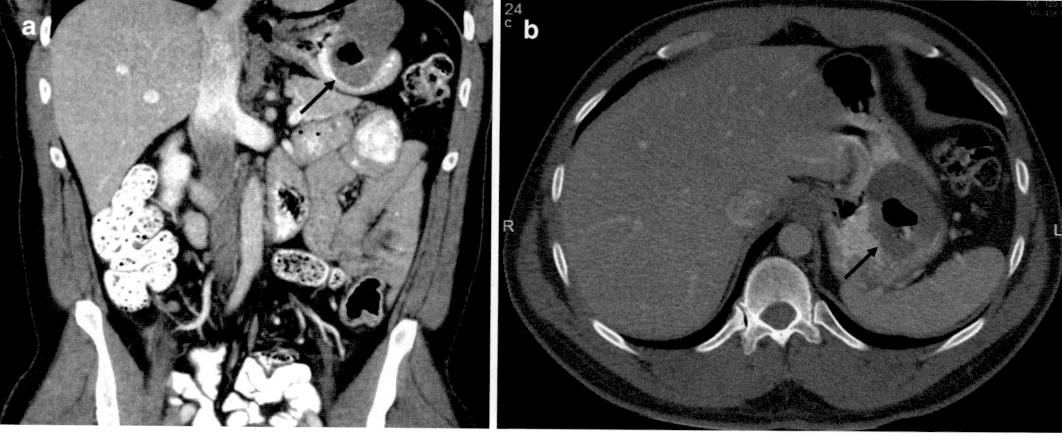

Fig. 4.1 (**a**) Coronal reconstruction of computed tomography scan demonstrating large proximal gastric cancer (black arrow). (**b**) Axial reconstruction of the same proximal gastric cancer (black arrow)

Pre-operative Considerations

After diagnosis of GIST has been confirmed, several steps are necessary prior to surgical intervention. This includes a staging workup consisting of endoscopic ultrasound (EUS) and CT scans of the chest, abdomen, and pelvis to evaluate the extent of disease and to rule out distant metastasis. Patients with unresectable or borderline resectable disease or GISTs in technically challenging locations (e.g., gastroesophageal junction) may benefit from neoadjuvant therapy with imatinib to downsize the tumor and increase the likelihood of complete surgical resection [20, 21]. Other tests may be required based on patient age and presence of comorbidities. No preoperative bowel prep is administered.

Surgical Technique

Patient Positioning and Setup

After transport to the operating room, the patient is placed in the supine position on the operating room table. We do not use the lithotomy position or split legs for gastrectomy. Prior to induction of general endotracheal anesthesia, sequential compression devices are placed on the bilateral lower extremities, and intravenous antibiotics are administered. After endotracheal intubation, a Foley catheter and orogastric tube are placed. We do not place central venous catheters, although radial artery catheters are often placed to facilitate accurate hemodynamic monitoring. Once these initial steps have been completed, both arms are tucked and the abdomen is prepped and covered with an Ioban drape.

Instruments

For this procedure, we used the following robotic instruments: fenestrated bipolar forceps, robotic hook with monopolar cautery, prograsp forceps, cadiere forceps, and needle driver. We used the following laparoscopic instruments: scissors, LAPRA-TY clip applier (Ethicon Endo Surgery), suction/irrigation, endo-GIA linear stapler, and thermal energy device.

Port Placement and Docking the Robot

For gastric resection, we favor placing five ports that are one hand-breadth apart in a semicircular line with the camera port at the umbilicus (Fig. 4.2). Initial entry at the umbilicus is established using a modified Hassan technique with placement of a 10/12-mm balloon port. Under direct visualization, an 8-mm robotic port for robotic arm 1 is placed in the left lateral abdomen in the mid-axillary line. We place a 10/12-mm assistant port in the right mid-abdomen in the mid-clavicular line. Robotic arms 2 and 3 are placed in mirror positions on the right and left sides of the abdomen. Once the trocars are placed, the Da Vinci robotic platform (Intuitive) is brought in over the left side of the patient's head (Si) or on the patient's left side (Xi). The Si platform was used for this procedure (Fig. 4.3).

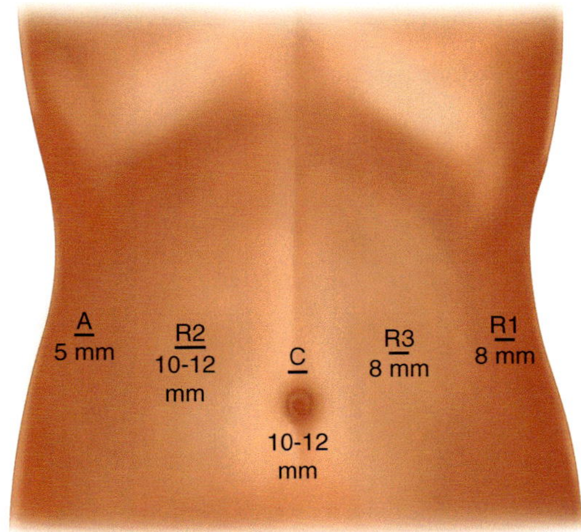

Fig. 4.2 Trocar placement for robotic wedge gastrectomy. Robotic arm #3 may be unnecessary under select conditions

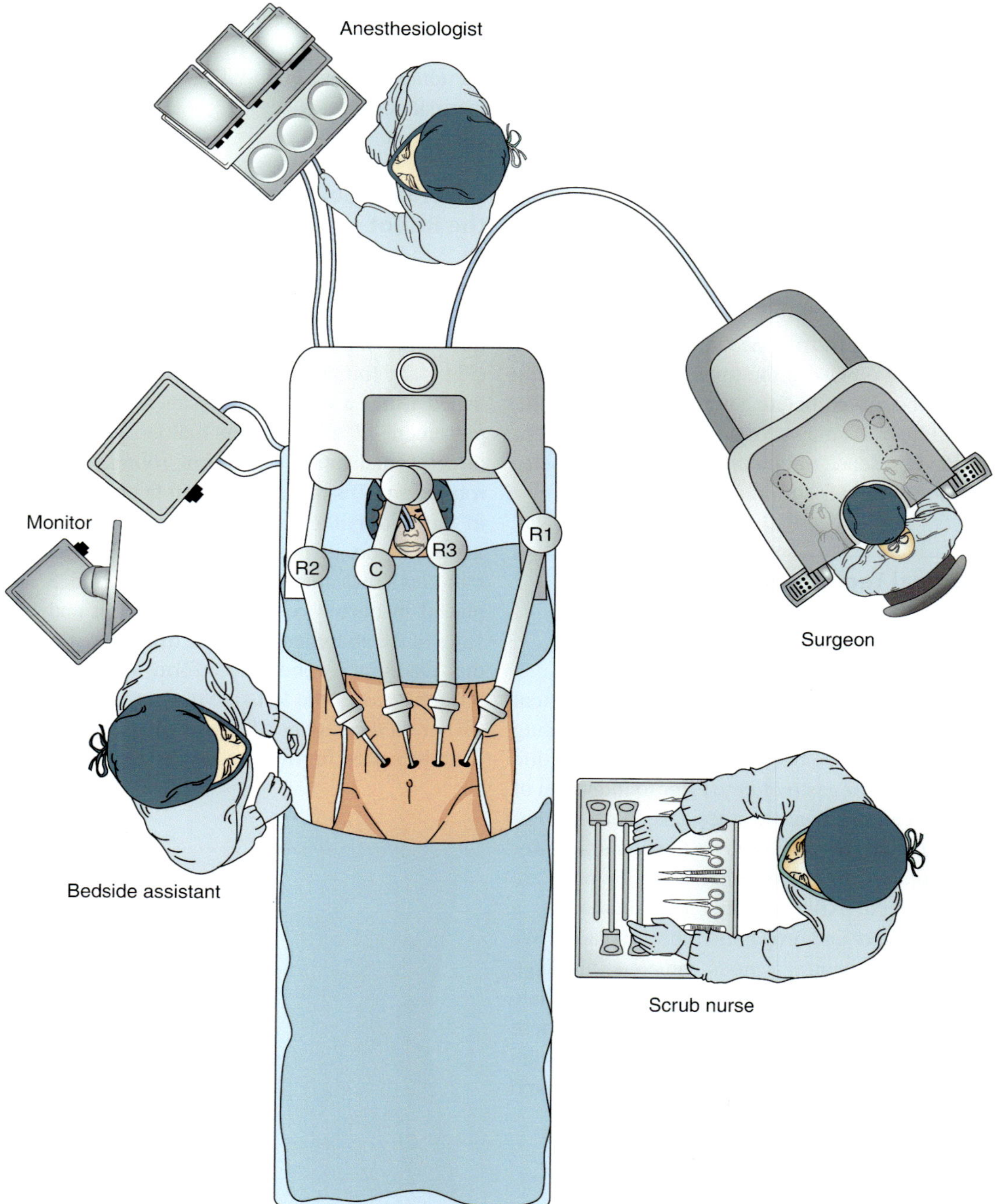

Fig. 4.3 Robotic setup for wedge gastrectomy using the Da Vinci Si platform

Surgical Steps (Video 4.1)

Upon entry into the abdominal cavity, an exploration was performed to assess for distant metastatic disease and none was identified. The approximately 8-cm tumor was visualized on the anterior aspect of the proximal stomach near the cardia (Fig. 4.4a, b). We considered surgical options including proximal gastrectomy and wedge resection. Given the size and location of the tumor, we were concerned about potentially narrowing the gastroesophageal junction with partial gastrectomy. However, proximal gastrectomy has considerable surgical risks including anastomotic leak and bile reflux. We elected to perform circumferential wedge resection of the tumor to minimize the amount of resected tissue, while obtaining negative surgical margins.

Although we did not utilize a dedicated liver retractor, other surgeons could employ one of several different options (e.g., Nathanson liver retractor). We used a prograsp in robotic arm 3 to retract the liver when needed. To minimize the amount of tissue necessary for resection of the GIST, the anterior aspect of the stomach was opened using monopolar cautery with the hook in robotic arm 1. Alternatively, the stomach could have been opened with the Ligasure (Covidien) through the assistant port. Opening the stomach is an oncologically acceptable step for GISTs, which are submucosal tumors, but it is not appropriate for gastric adenocarcinoma.

Fenestrated bipolar grasper in robotic arm 2 was used to retract the stomach, while an endoscopic GIA linear stapling device was placed through the assistant port. Serial firings of the stapler with 60-mm tan cartridges were used to circumferentially resect the tumor, ensuring grossly negative margins. We elected not to use the robotic stapler because of the lack of vascular cartridges and the need for a 15-mm trocar. Alternatively, cautery or a thermal sealing device can be employed to perform this resection. Once the tumor was completely resected, the tumor was placed in a specimen bag which was placed through the assistant port.

We closed the gastrotomy defect along a longitudinal plane rather than a transverse plan to avoid having the stomach fold over on itself. To avoid potentially narrowing the gastroesophageal junction with linear stapling devices, the closure was performed with robotic suturing in two layers with 3-0 PDS running suture. First, the two sides of the proposed incision line were loosely approximated with sutures that were secured with LAPRA-TY clips (Ethicon Endo Surgery). A running suture was then started with the needle driver in robotic arm 1 in a cranial to caudal direction. We placed a LAPRA-TY clip at both ends of the suture line instead of tying knots. A second 3-0 PDS running suture was placed as the second, outer layer. A final inspection for hemostasis was performed and the robot was undocked. The specimen bag is exteriorized by enlarging

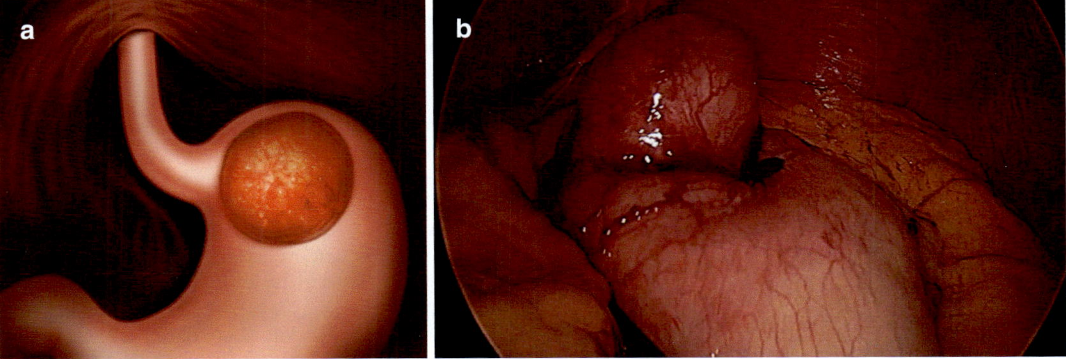

Fig. 4.4 (**a**) Illustration showing the location of the large, proximal gastric tumor on the anterior surface of the stomach. (**b**) Paired intraoperative image revealing only a small portion of the large gastric tumor

the assistant port. The fascial incisions of the 10/12-mm port sites were closed with the Carter-Thomason device using 0 Vicryl sutures and the skin was closed with subcuticular absorbable sutures. We did not leave an intraperitoneal drainage catheter.

Postoperative Care and Complications

Postoperative management after robotic wedge gastrectomy is the same as that after open surgery. Patients are generally managed on the regular surgical floors without need for intensive care units. It is our current routine to use nasogastric tubes (NGTs), which are removed on postoperative day #2. As we transition to enhanced recovery after surgery protocols, we will no longer use NGTs in the postoperative period. Furthermore, we do not perform upper gastrointestinal radiographic studies prior to removal of NGTs. After the NGT has been removed, a liquid diet is started and advanced as tolerated. Postoperative pain is controlled by non-narcotic analgesia which is supplemented as needed with patient-controlled analgesia and oral narcotic regimens. Patients are typically discharged home on postoperative day #4. Although patients may be at risk for the same postoperative complications observed with open gastric resection, we have never had anastomotic leak with wedge resection, and our rates of morbidity are quite low with zero mortality over the past decade.

Conclusions

Robotic wedge gastrectomy is feasible and safe for gastric GISTs in challenging locations. The greatest advantage with the robotic platform for our procedure was the ease in closing the resection defect with long running sutures. Straightforward robotic suturing can be performed safely by both experienced gastric surgeons and trainees alike.

References

1. Kindblom LG, Remotti HE, Aldenborg F, et al. Gastrointestinal pacemaker cell tumor (GIPACT): gastrointestinal stromal tumors show phenotypic characteristics of the interstitial cells of Cajal. Am J Pathol. 1998;152(5):1259–69.
2. Miettinen M, Sarlomo-Rikala M, Lasota J. Gastrointestinal stromal tumors: recent advances in understanding of their biology. Hum Pathol. 1999;30(10):1213–20.
3. Ma GL, Murphy JD, Martinez ME, et al. Epidemiology of gastrointestinal stromal tumors in the era of histology codes: results of a population-based study. Cancer Epidemiol Biomarkers Prev. 2015;24(1):298–302.
4. Choi AH, Hamner JB, Merchant SJ, et al. Underreporting of gastrointestinal stromal tumors: is the true incidence being captured? J Gastrointest Surg. 2015;19(9):1699–703.
5. DeMatteo RP, Lewis JJ, Leung D, et al. Two hundred gastrointestinal stromal tumors: recurrence patterns and prognostic factors for survival. Ann Surg. 2000;231(1):51–8.
6. Miettinen M, Lasota J. Gastrointestinal stromal tumors: pathology and prognosis at different sites. Semin Diagn Pathol. 2006;23(2):70–83.
7. Miettinen M, Sobin LH, Lasota J. Gastrointestinal stromal tumors of the stomach: a clinicopathologic, immunohistochemical, and molecular genetic study of 1765 cases with long-term follow-up. Am J Surg Pathol. 2005;29(1):52–68.
8. Hirota S, Isozaki K, Moriyama Y, et al. Gain-of-function mutations of c-kit in human gastrointestinal stromal tumors. Science. 1998;279(5350):577–80.
9. Dematteo RP, Ballman KV, Antonescu CR, et al. Adjuvant imatinib mesylate after resection of localised, primary gastrointestinal stromal tumour: a randomised, double-blind, placebo-controlled trial. Lancet. 2009;373(9669):1097–104.
10. Joensuu H, Eriksson M, Sundby Hall K, et al. One vs three years of adjuvant imatinib for operable gastrointestinal stromal tumor: a randomized trial. JAMA. 2012;307(12):1265–72.
11. Tokunaga M, Ohyama S, Hiki N, et al. Incidence and prognostic value of lymph node metastasis on c-Kit-positive gastrointestinal stromal tumors of the stomach. Hepato-Gastroenterology. 2011;58(109):1224–8.
12. De Vogelaere K, Hoorens A, Haentjens P, et al. Laparoscopic versus open resection of gastrointestinal stromal tumors of the stomach. Surg Endosc. 2013;27(5):1546–54.
13. MacArthur KM, Baumann BC, Nicholl MB. Laparoscopic versus open resection for gastrointestinal stromal tumors (GISTs). J Gastrointest Cancer. 2017;48(1):20–4.
14. De Vogelaere K, Van Loo I, Peters O, et al. Laparoscopic resection of gastric gastrointestinal

stromal tumors (GIST) is safe and effective, irrespective of tumor size. Surg Endosc. 2012;26(8):2339–45.

15. Lin J, Huang C, Zheng C, et al. Laparoscopic versus open gastric resection for larger than 5 cm primary gastric gastrointestinal stromal tumors (GIST): a size-matched comparison. Surg Endosc. 2014;28(9):2577–83.

16. Huang CM, Chen QF, Lin JX, et al. Can laparoscopic surgery be applied in gastric gastrointestinal stromal tumors located in unfavorable sites?: a study based on the NCCN guidelines. Medicine. 2017;96(14):e6535.

17. Vicente E, Quijano Y, Ielpo B, et al. Robot-assisted resection of gastrointestinal stromal tumors (GIST): a single center case series and literature review. Int J Med Rob Compu Assisted Surg. 2016;12(4):718–23.

18. Buchs NC, Bucher P, Pugin F, et al. Robot-assisted oncologic resection for large gastric gastrointestinal stromal tumor: a preliminary case series. J Laparoendosc Adv Surg Tech A. 2010;20(5):411–5.

19. Desiderio J, Trastulli S, Cirocchi R, et al. Robotic gastric resection of large gastrointestinal stromal tumors. Int J Surg. 2013;11(2):191–6.

20. Andtbacka RH, Ng CS, Scaife CL, et al. Surgical resection of gastrointestinal stromal tumors after treatment with imatinib. Ann Surg Oncol. 2007;14(1):14–24.

21. Eisenberg BL, Harris J, Blanke CD, et al. Phase II trial of neoadjuvant/adjuvant imatinib mesylate (IM) for advanced primary and metastatic/recurrent operable gastrointestinal stromal tumor (GIST): early results of RTOG 0132/ACRIN 6665. J Surg Oncol. 2009;99(1):42–7.

Minimally Invasive Gastric Wedge Resection

5

Sudeep Banerjee, Santiago Horgan, and Jason K. Sicklick

Introduction

Laparoscopic resection of gastric tumors has become increasingly adopted based upon numerous clinical series demonstrating equivalent oncologic outcomes as open resection [1–4]. The first report of laparoscopic gastric wedge resection was initially described in 1994 for the treatment of early gastric adenocarcinoma [5]. Minimally invasive gastric wedge resection has now evolved to become the standard approach for the surgical management of benign and malignant submucosal (i.e., non-adenomatous) gastric tumors [6–8].

The differential diagnosis of benign gastric tumors includes leiomyoma, schwannoma, pancreatic heterotopia, gastric cavernous hemangioma, lipomas, and plexiform fibromyxoma. Common malignant tumors include gastrointestinal stromal tumor (GIST), leiomyosarcoma, gastric carcinoid, and lymphoma. In contrast to gastric adenocarcinoma and certain gastric carcinoids, the safe treatment of the aforementioned tumors only requires obtaining clear gastric margins. Thus, formal lymphadenectomy and gastrointestinal anastomoses are usually avoided. This difference permits the use of a minimally invasive wedge resection approach where an approximately 1–2-cm cuff of normal gastric tissue is resected en bloc with both benign and malignant tumors. Thus, selecting patients for this type of operation relies upon accurate tissue diagnosis, thorough preoperative workup, and careful patient selection to yield best outcomes. Consequently, patients undergoing laparoscopic wedge resection as compared to larger, more formal resections may benefit from reduced hospital stays and postoperative recovery, as well as equivalent oncologic outcomes [9, 10]. For the present discussion, we will briefly address general preoperative principles, and primarily focus the discussion on the technical approach to laparoscopic gastric wedge resection for benign and non-adenomatous gastric tumors.

Electronic supplementary material The online version of this chapter (https://doi.org/10.1007/978-3-030-18740-8_5) contains supplementary material, which is available to authorized users.

S. Banerjee
Department of Surgery, University of California, Los Angeles, Los Angeles, CA, USA

Department of Surgery, University of California, San Diego, San Diego, CA, USA
e-mail: subanerjee@ucsd.edu

S. Horgan
Department of Surgery, Center for the Future of Surgery, University of California, San Diego, San Diego, CA, USA
e-mail: shorgan@ucsd.edu

J. K. Sicklick (✉)
Department of Surgery, University of California, San Diego, San Diego, CA, USA
e-mail: jsicklick@ucsd.edu

© Springer Nature Switzerland AG 2020
J. Kim, J. Garcia-Aguilar (eds.), *Minimally Invasive Surgical Techniques for Cancers of the Gastrointestinal Tract*, https://doi.org/10.1007/978-3-030-18740-8_5

Surgically Relevant Gastric Anatomy

The stomach is the beneficiary of many redundant arterial blood supplies from the celiac trunk. The lesser curvature of the stomach and the gastroesophageal junction (GEJ) are supplied by the left and right gastric arteries originating from the celiac axis and proper hepatic artery, respectively. The greater curvature of the stomach is supplied by the left and right gastroepiploic vessels originating from the splenic and gastroduodenal arteries, respectively. Additionally, the short gastric vessels originating from the splenic artery also supply the greater curvature and the posterior wall. Finally, the pylorus is supplied by the right gastric artery and gastroduodenal artery originating from the proper hepatic artery and common hepatic artery, respectively. The venous drainage mirrors the arterial anatomy and is delivered into the portal circulation via the splenic vein or the portal vein. This includes the coronary vein (also known as the right gastric vein), which drains directly into the portal vein. This rich blood supply and drainage makes the stomach less prone to ischemia following surgical resection of one or more gastric vessels. This absence of watershed zones makes it well suited for wedge resections.

The stomach is also innervated by parasympathetic nerves through the vagus nerve. The left vagal nerve forms the anterior gastric plexus along the antero-superior surface of the stomach, while the right vagal nerve forms the posterior gastric plexus along the postero-inferior gastric surface. Sympathetic innervation of the stomach is thru the celiac plexus originating from C5-9 nerve roots. The gastric vagal fibers provide for pyloric relaxation, whereas the sympathetic fibers control gastric acid secretion. The former innervation will be noteworthy when performing wedge resections of the lesser curve of the stomach, which can lead to impaired pyloric relaxation and gastric emptying.

Finally, the lymphatic drainage of the stomach is divided into 4 levels encompassing 16 stations. However, lymphadenectomy is not generally performed during most gastric wedge resection and is therefore not relevant to the current discussion.

Preoperative Patient Selection

Minimally invasive gastric wedge resection of tumors can be safely and effectively performed when the goals of oncologic resection are met. These include complete gross resection with microscopically negative margins, total extracapsular resection, and avoidance of tumor rupture or bleeding. In general, large or locally advanced tumors with adjacent organ involvement are generally treated with open resection as achievement of negative margins and avoidance of tumor fracture are often challenging with a minimally invasive approach. Moreover, adjacent organ preservation may be more feasible via a laparotomy incision. Ultimately, surgical decision-making must be a balance between applicability of these approaches and the individual surgeon's technical skill set, as well as maintaining oncologic principles and preserving adjacent organs when possible.

Appropriate patient selection is critical to minimally invasive wedge resection of gastric tumors. Although medical comorbidities among cancer patients are common, patients must be able to tolerate the cardiopulmonary strain associated with general anesthesia, as well as extended laparoscopy and pneumoperitoneum. Accurate tumor localization is also a major determinant of feasibility of wedge resection. Cross-sectional imaging techniques and upper endoscopy together can also provide valuable anatomic information that can guide the surgical approach. While the surgeon and patient may opt for a laparoscopic approach over an open approach, patients should be counseled about the possibility of conversion to laparotomy, as well as alternative approaches, including endoscopic mucosal resection. Herein, we focus on laparoscopic approaches to gastric wedge resection.

Tumor Diagnosis and Imaging

Tissue diagnosis is essential in the workup of gastric tumors in order to properly diagnose, stage, and determine a proper course of treatment. Gastric adenocarcinoma, some gastric carcinoids, and metastatic lesions would not be properly treated with a wedge resection. The remainder of the aforementioned submucosal gastric tumor types in the introduction may all be considered for wedge resection, and more specifically, minimally invasive surgery if technically feasible.

Cross-sectional imaging (e.g., computed tomography or magnetic resonance imaging) is often part of the initial identification of gastric tumors following symptomatic presentation or during workup of other medical conditions. Additionally, tumors may be identified during upper endoscopy, in which case additional imaging is usually obtained as part of the disease workup in order to assess for metastatic disease. Vice versa, patients with cross-sectional imaging demonstrating a gastric mass should undergo upper endoscopy as part of the initial tissue diagnosis. However, traditional upper endoscopy alone is often inadequate as it frequently fails to appreciate the submucosal tumor size and depth of gastric masses. Advanced imaging techniques including endoscopic ultrasound (EUS) provide the highest level of resolution of gastric wall penetration and neighboring structure involvement, and can be used as a determinant of eligibility for minimally invasive wedge resection [11]. Moreover, EUS-guided fine-needle aspiration and core-needle biopsy are often necessary to obtain adequate tissue for diagnosis, because superficial mucosal biopsies typically only identify normal mucosa and do not obtain tumor cells. Taken together, preoperative cross-sectional imaging and upper endoscopy with EUS are complementary parts of the preoperative workup of gastric tumors. These modalities are necessary for proper selection of patients for minimally invasive gastric wedge resection.

Operative Setup

In general, preoperative instructions include nothing by mouth for at least 8 hours prior to surgery, as well as discontinuation of antiplatelet or anticoagulant medications if deemed medically safe and appropriate. In the operating room, the patient is placed in the supine position with both arms either abducted or tucked. A split leg table is preferable as it allows for the operating surgeon to be positioned between the patient's legs. The patient should be securely strapped to the table to facilitate steep reverse Trendelenburg positioning. The surgical assistant is positioned on the patient's left side. Monitors are ideally positioned over the head of the bed in line with the operating surgeon and across from the first assistant (Fig. 5.1).

Upon induction of general endotracheal anesthesia, an orogastric tube may be placed to achieve gastric decompression. This should be removed prior to wedge resection in order to avoid accidental inclusion in the staple line. Alternatively, an upper endoscope can be later used to decompress the stomach. Urinary catheter may be placed and usually can be removed upon completion of the operation. This placement is dependent upon the anticipated operative time.

According to Surgical Care Improvement (SCIP) Guidelines, preoperative cefazolin should be administered within 1 hour of incision. Alternative agents in patients with β-lactam allergies include clindamycin, vancomycin plus aminoglycoside, aztreonam, or a fluoroquinolone. Following a time out or patient safety checklist review by the operating team, nursing staff, and anesthesia team, a supraumbilical 12 mm optical trocar is introduced in the left abdomen just offset from midline within the rectus muscle. At this time, a laparoscopic evaluation should be performed for preliminary tumor localization, assessment of additional disease (i.e., diaphragm, liver surfaces, peritoneal lining, omentum, and pelvis), and to determine optimal placement of additional trocars. Two 5-mm ports are placed in the left and right midclavicular positions approximately 5 cm inferior to the costal margins. These ports can be adjusted inferiorly if the tumor is located in the distal stomach. An additional 5-mm port is placed in the left midaxillary line approximately 2 cm inferior to the costal margin. If the tumor is partially or completely obscured by the left lateral section of the liver, a liver retraction system is necessary. A stab incision is made in the sub-xiphoid region just offset to the patient's left side. Using a hemostat, the peritoneal cavity is entered. A Nathanson liver retractor can then be placed thru this site (Fig. 5.2). Numbering the ports 1 thru 4 for the patient's right side, the

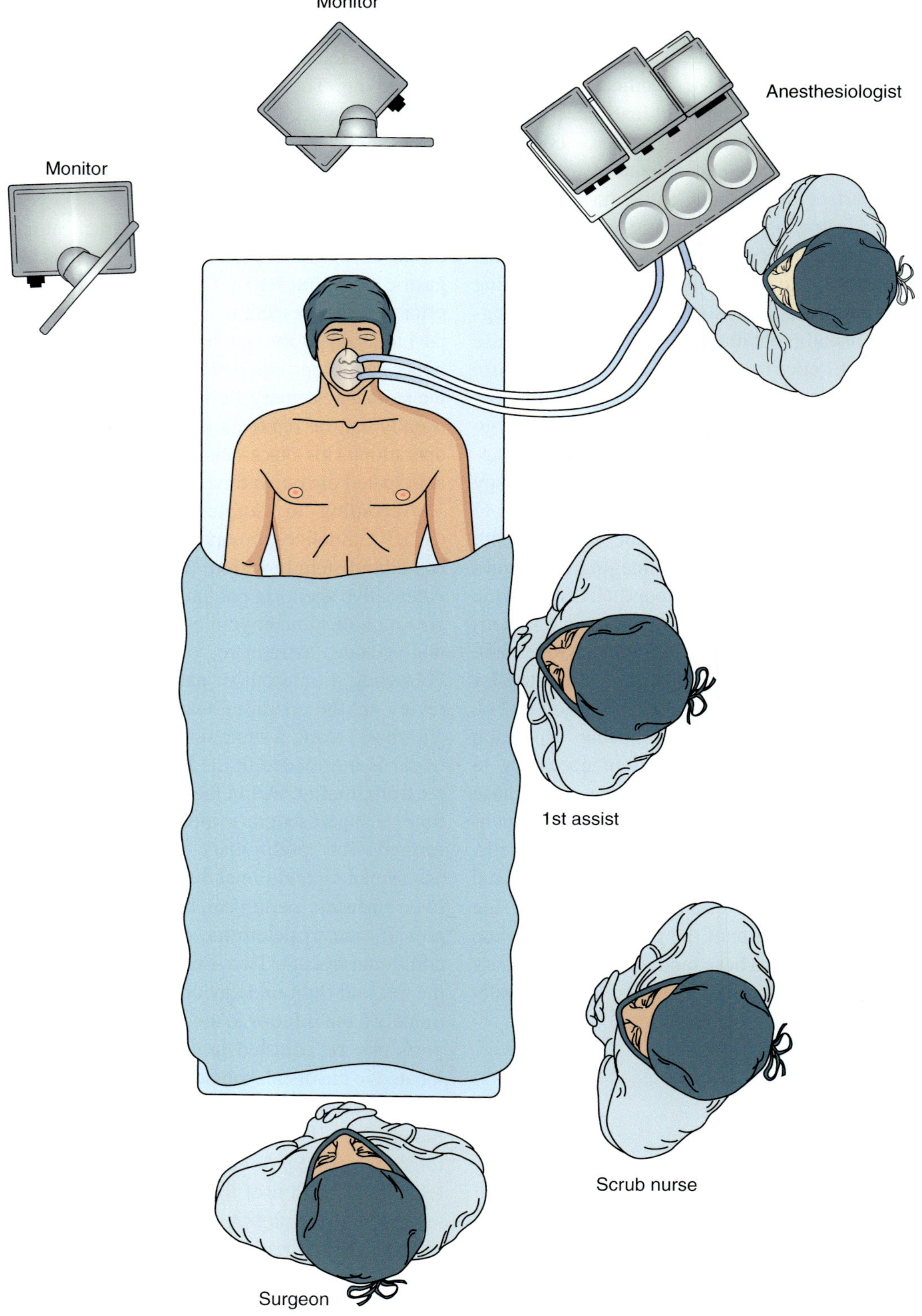

Fig. 5.1 Patient positioning and operating room setup

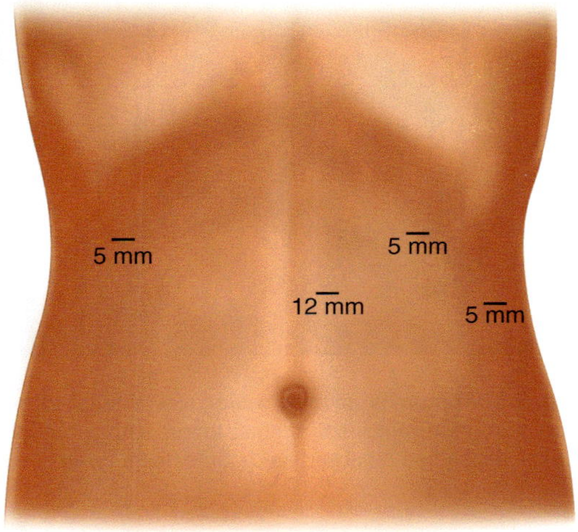

Fig. 5.2 Placement of laparoscopic trocars and Nathanson liver retractor

operating surgeon will generally use ports 1 (right midclavicular) and 3 (left midclavicular), while the assisting surgeon will generally use port 2 (periumbilical) for the camera and port 4 (left midaxillary) for lateral retraction. Additional trocars may be placed as deemed appropriate by the operating surgeon.

Intraoperative upper endoscopy is a useful adjunct to laparoscopic localization of gastric tumors, particularly when the mass is endophytic and difficult to appreciate from the extraluminal approach. Intraoperative endoscopy is also often utilized to confirm appropriate intragastric margins, adequate patency of the gastric lumen, and sufficient distance from the gastroesophageal junction (GEJ) or the pylorus for proximal or distal resections, respectively. Additionally, endoscopic insufflation at the end of the procedure can be useful to help re-confirm patency of the gastric lumen, as well as a lack of gastric volvulization (mesenteroaxial), which may occur following wedge resection of some pre-pyloric and antral tumors.

Operative Principles

The goals of complete resection for gastric tumors include microscopically negative margins (i.e., R0), total extracapsular resection, and avoidance

of tumor rupture or bleeding. The method for achieving these goals varies with tumor location, the mobility of the tumor, and whether the tumor has an endophytic or exophytic pattern of growth. In general, the most common and simple approach entails grasping normal gastric wall surrounding an exophytic tumor with an atraumatic instrument and elevating it toward the anterior abdominal wall. With an upper endoscope functioning as a bougie, anterior retraction is followed by dividing the normal adjacent stomach with a linear endoscopic gastrointestinal anastomosis (GIA) stapler just beyond the base of the tumor using the 12-mm port. Gastric masses that are not easily retracted and which are often endophytic can be mobilized by the placement of proximal and distal seromuscular sutures, which then can be retracted to elevate the tumor, thereby also facilitating GIA stapler placement. Alternatively, difficult to elevate masses (that are often endophytic) can be circumferentially excised with the use of ultrasonic coagulating shears followed by GIA stapler closure or laparoscopic suturing of the resultant gastrotomy in a transverse fashion. This approach may be useful for avoiding neighboring structures such as the GEJ or pylorus. Selection of GIA stapler cartridge is based on a subjective judgment on the thickness of the gastric wall. Normal appearing gastric wall is usually adequately sealed with a blue load (open height 3.5 mm; closed height 1.5 mm), while thickened gastric tissue can require a green load (open height 4.1 mm; closed height 2.0 mm). Intermediate thickness is handled with a gold load (open height 3.8 mm; closed height 1.8 mm). Additionally, bioabsorbable staple line reinforcement may be utilized to potentially reduce perioperative leaks and bleeding. Finally, a laparoscopic retrieval bag is used to safely remove the tumor from the peritoneal cavity using the 12-mm port.

Resection by Location

Surgical approach is often determined by the location of the tumor within the stomach. The following sections describe the techniques employed for each possible location.

Greater Curvature

Tumors located along the greater curvature of the stomach are accessed by first dividing the gastrocolic ligament. Thermal coagulating and cutting devices are often used to achieve hemostasis of gastroepiploic branches. Care should be taken to avoid unnecessary ligation of the right gastroepiploic artery. Continuing along the greater curve, division of the short gastric vessels allows for further mobilization of the lateral stomach enabling medial rotation of the greater curve. This is facilitated by gentle retraction on the gastrosplenic ligament by the surgical assistant, which improves visualization of these vessels. If necessary, this dissection can be taken up to the level of the superior pole of the spleen and left crus of the diaphragm. Ultimately, this dissection allows for anterior retraction of greater curvature tumors and facilitates resection as described above. These masses are usually resected with either a single fire of a GIA stapler or successive staple fires performed in a semi-perpendicular manner creating a "V"-shaped resected margin. If necessary, protrusion of the mass may be facilitated by using an endoscope to push the tumor towards the stapler.

Lesser Curvature

Tumors located on the lesser curvature of the stomach are slightly more difficult to access and require division of the gastrohepatic ligament for visualization. Early identification of the coronary vein and utilization of preoperative imaging for assessing the presence of a replaced/accessory left hepatic artery are important for avoiding iatrogenic injury. Division of the gastrohepatic ligament is generally performed with a hemostatic method to ligate branches of the left gastric artery, coronary vein, and vagal nerve fibers. Based on the location of the mass, division of the short gastric vessels along the greater curve of the stomach is sometimes necessary to achieve full anterior rotation of the lesser curve of the stomach. Mobilization of the lesser

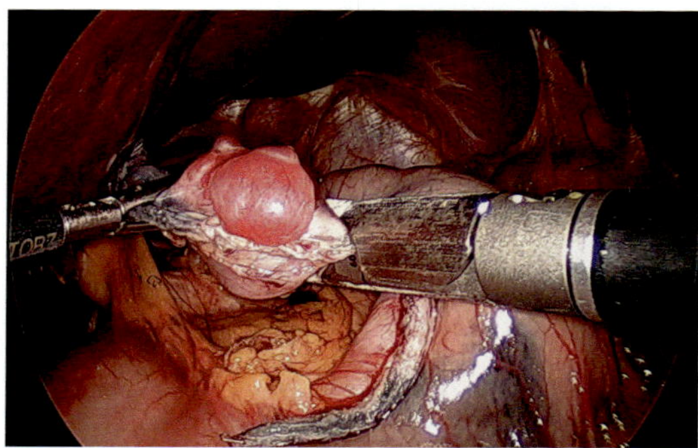

Fig. 5.3 Minimally invasive wedge resection of a lesser curvature gastrointestinal stromal tumor with an endoluminal stapler and bioabsorbable staple line reinforcement

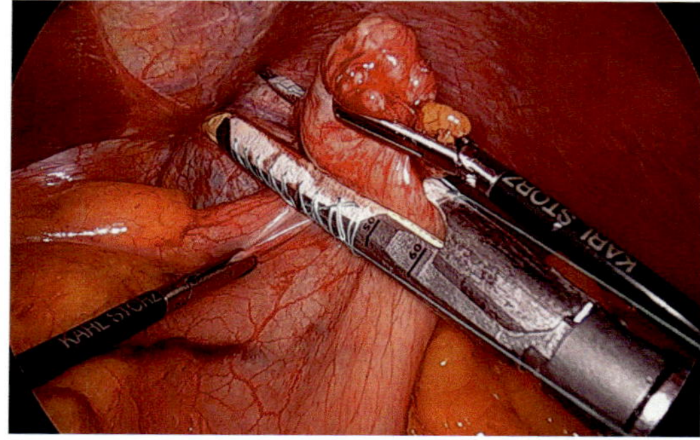

Fig. 5.4 Minimally invasive wedge resection of an anterior wall gastrointestinal stromal tumor

curvature permits rotation of the stomach to patient's left side and retraction of the tumor toward the anterior abdominal wall (Fig. 5.3, Video 5.1).

Anterior Wall

Anterior wall tumors are often readily visible upon creation of pneumoperitoneum. Occasionally, dissection of the greater omentum can help to appreciate the extent of inferiorly located masses. Tumors located on the anterior gastric wall are often mobile and it is not always necessary to divide the short gastric vessels to perform anterior retraction of these masses (Fig. 5.4, Video 5.1). In these cases, fewer laparoscopic ports may be needed.

Posterior Wall

Posterior wall tumors can be accessed by one of two approaches. The first method entails mobilization of the posterior gastric wall by organo-axial rotation of the stomach following mobilization of the lesser and greater curves of the stomach as discussed previously for the aforementioned tumors. This permits elevation of the posterior wall tumor toward the abdominal wall and resection as previously described. This approach is best suited for lesions that are located on the posterior surface of the stomach along either the lesser or greater curves. In these cases, care should be taken to avoid corkscrewing the stomach with staple firing as this can lead to narrowing or kinking of the gastric lumen.

An alternative approach is the creation of an anterior longitudinal gastrotomy through which tumors located on the posterior wall or posterior endophytic lesions can be accessed. It is often useful to place peripheral sutures along the margins of the tumor which are used to elevate the posterior wall mass through the anterior gastrostomy facilitating visualization of the tumor and placement of the GIA stapler. Closure of longitudinal gastrotomy should be performed horizontally to minimize luminal narrowing. This is usually performed with either a stapling device at the base of the gastrostomy or full-thickness suture closure of the defect.

Adjacent to Gastroesophageal Junction

Tumors located at the gastroesophageal junction must be approached cautiously to avoid proximal narrowing of the stomach and dysfunction of the lower esophageal sphincter (LES) complex. Tumors that are located at least 3 cm away from the GEJ can usually be safely resected using the techniques described above. Exophytic tumors located immediately adjacent to the GEJ are often amenable to treatment with wedge resection. The tumor must be easily elevated off the LES complex with a bridge of normal gastric tissue for linear GIA stapler placement. It is ideal to perform this with simultaneous upper endoscopy wherein an endoscope can function as a bougie and camera in order to avoid narrowing the GEJ (Video 5.1).

In contrast, endophytic lesions adjacent to the GEJ may be best treated through an intra-gastric laparo-endoscopic resection approach. In this method, one 12-mm trocar and one or two 5-mm trocars triangulating the location of the tumor are serially placed into the peritoneal cavity. An endoscope is placed into the stomach which is then insufflated. The stomach wall is penetrated with cuffed trocars, which are advanced full thickness thru the gastric wall and into the gastric lumen with concomitant endoscopic and laparoscopic visualization. The balloon cuffs are then insufflated and the trocars are retracted so that gastric wall is opposed to abdominal wall. This is somewhat analogous to the concept of the balloon (inside) and bumper (outside) apposition of a percutaneous endoscopic gastrostomy (PEG) tube. The tumor is then resected using the same principles of an intraperitoneal laparoscopic resection; however, a retroflexed endoscope can function as the camera in order to limit the number of trocars that must be introduced into the gastric lumen. The endophytic gastric mass is grasped intraluminally with normal gastric wall surrounding it. Intraluminal retraction is followed by dividing the normal adjacent stomach with a linear endoscopic gastrointestinal anastomosis (GIA) stapler just beyond the base of the tumor using the 12-mm port (Fig. 5.5). Typically, this is accomplished with serial gold stapler loads except at the last staple fire, which is either a white or gray load to minimize bleeding from the gastric mucosa. If bleeding occurs, clips can be placed on the staple line. The tumor may then be placed into a laparoscopic retrieval bag. For tumors less than 4 cm, the tail of the bag may be grasped with an endoscope and removed via the esophagus and mouth. For larger tumors, the 12-mm gastrostomy should be extended in order to allow for moving the tumor into the peritoneum and then out thru the abdominal wall

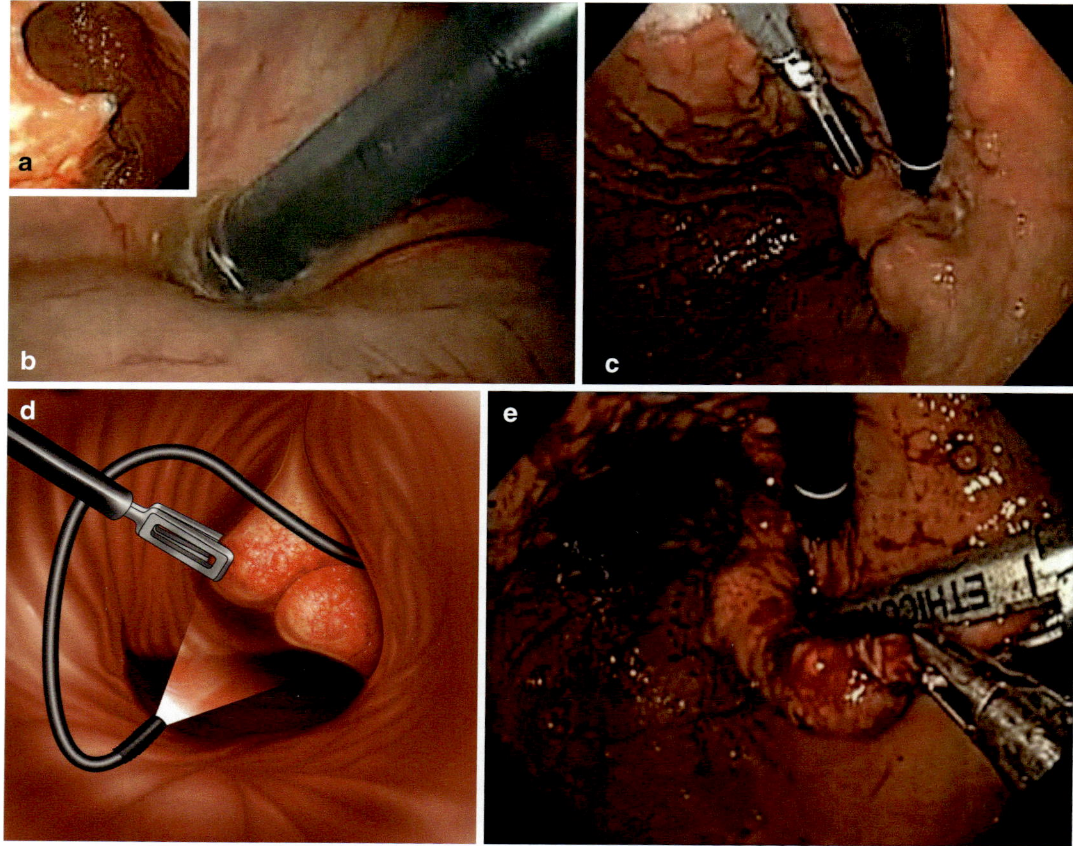

Fig. 5.5 Endoscopic-laparoscopic wedge resection of gastroesophageal junction gastrointestinal stromal tumor: (**a**) intragastric trocar placement, lumenal view; (**b**) intragastric trocar placement, intraperitoneal view; (**c**) retroflexed endoscopic view; (**d**) schematic depection of retroflexed endoscopic view; (**e**) intragastric stapler placement

defect. After the tumor is safely removed, the gastrostomies are closed with intracorporeal sutures or linear staple fires [12, 13]. A recent variant of this approach utilizes a single port to access the stomach. Entry to the stomach is accomplished through a 2.5-cm laparotomy followed by grasping and extracorporealizing the gastric body. A single port device is placed into the gastric body and the resection is performed. Upon completion, the gastrostomy is closed extracorporally [14]. While technically challenging with steep learn curves, these approaches are quite useful in cases where the tumor is not visible from the serosal surface.

An additional approach for benign tumors adjacent to the GEJ is enucleation off the LES complex. This can be accomplished by first entering the lumen of the stomach with a linear gastrotomy. The mass can then be carefully dissected, taking care to avoid fracture of the mass or full-thickness penetration of the stomach wall. After the mass is removed, the gastrotomy can be reapproximated with intracorporeal suturing. Injection of dilute epinephrine is often used to minimize mucosal oozing from the resection bed.

Antrum

Tumors of pre-pyloric region also pose a challenge due to the proximity of the pyloric muscle and tendency for luminal narrowing that can promote gastric outlet obstruction following resection. Analogous to the GEJ tumors, those located greater than 3 cm away from the pylorus can be safely resected using the approach specific to the surface of the stomach where the tumor occurs. Resection using GIA stapler should generally be performed in the perpendicular fashion to minimize luminal narrowing. Alternatively, it may be necessary to perform full thickness excision using ultrasonic shears to precisely avoid the pylorus. This may be performed with perpendicular closure of the resultant gastrotomy. Tumors that occur on the posterior pre-pyloric region can be approached through a longitudinal anterior gastrotomy that is generally made 5 cm proximally to the tumor to improve visualization of the pylorus. Particular caution should be exercised in the case of large tumors where closure of the resection defect may result in stenosis of the gastric outlet. In this case, laparoscopic or open distal gastrectomy should be considered with reconstruction (Bilroth I, Bilroth II or roux-en-Y gastrojejunostromy). In these situations, upper endoscopy is critical for assessing luminal patency and whether a more formal resection is necessary.

Postoperative Care

Postoperatively, patients may be started on sips of water or a clear liquid diet on the day of the operation. Ambulation is encouraged. The diet may be gradually advanced to full liquids with protein shakes and patients are discharged to home within 2–4 days. Further advancement to a soft diet occurs at home. At approximately 14 days postoperatively, a regular diet can be resumed. In contrast to anatomic gastric resections, permanent alterations to the patient's diet or dietary supplementation are usually unnecessary.

Complications

There are several potential complications associated with minimally invasive gastric wedge resection. Perioperative hemorrhage is generally due to staple line bleeding. Hematemesis should be promptly investigated with upper endoscopy taking care to avoid overinsufflation of the stomach to minimize tension on the fresh staple line. Staple line bleeding can usually be safely managed with endoscopic hemostatic methods (e.g., injection of epinephrine or placement of clips), as well as medical therapy with proton pump inhibitors. Alternatively, bleeding can rarely originate from unligated vessels encountered during the mobilization of the gastric body. If the patient is hemodynamically stable with laboratory evidence of anemia but no enteral blood, bleeding should be investigated with computed tomography with intravenous contrast to identify accumulation of intraabdominal blood or a hematoma. In select cases, this may be managed conservatively versus returning to the operating room for evacuation of the hematoma and ligation of any bleeding vessels. If the patient is hemodynamically unstable, they should be immediately resuscitated and return to the operation room for exploration and appropriate management.

Postoperative gastric leak is a feared, but fortunately rare complication of minimally invasive gastric surgery. Upper gastrointestinal series can be useful to confirming the presence of gastric leaks in ambiguous clinical scenarios. Prompt operative or percutaneous drainage of intraabdominal fluid collections along with initiation of broad spectrum antibiotics are important first steps. The decision about whether to attempt to close the gastric fistula is based on the presence of peritonitis, the size of leak, the rate drainage, the health of surrounding tissues, and the timing of the leak relative to the operation. Alternative approaches to operative closure include endoscopic over-the-scope clip (OTSC) devices [15] and more recently studies showing closure of gastric fistula with endoluminal vacuum (E-Vac) therapy [16].

Narrowing of the gastric lumen can cause a gastric outlet obstruction (GOO) due to mechanical narrowing of the stomach due to the amount of stomach resected. This is more likely in resections of the GEJ or pylorus and present early in the postoperative period. Performing upper endoscopy at the time of resection may be one approach to avoid this. GOO may also present in the subsequent weeks or months as scar tissue forms and stenosis of a partially narrowed gastric lumen occurs. Management should first include endoscopic balloon dilation followed by surgical revision if necessary.

Gastric wedge resection modifies the structure of the stomach anatomy. Although this change is generally benign, certain resections can place the stomach at high risk of mesentericoaxial gastric volvulus. This is most commonly seen in moderate to large wedge resections of the pre-pyloric region, which can cause the stomach to kink upon itself. This complication usually causes a functional gastric outlet obstruction. In cases where this may occur, the phenomenon can be replicated by overdistension of the stomach upon upper endoscopic insufflation. Immediate revision of the gastric resection to a formal distal gastrectomy with reconstruction should be performed if this kinking or gastric volvulus is identified. Thus, evaluation of the patency of the gastric lumen by endoscopy at the end of the operation is an important safeguard against development of this serious complication.

Lastly, interruption of the vagal innervation of the pylorus can result in pyloric tetany. This is usually due to transient disruption in vagal signaling caused by manipulation of the stomach during resection or due to resection of vagal fibers with a lesser curve resection. This is easily treated with endoscopic injection of botulinum toxin. Temporary paralysis of the pylorus enables restoration of normal pyloric regulation. Rarely, pyloric tetany can persist and may require a revision pyloromyotomy to restore normal gastric function.

Conclusions

Minimally invasive gastric wedge resection is a safe and effective approach for the management of benign and malignant non-adenomatous gastric tumors. Thorough preoperative diagnosis, workup, and patient selection are critical to the successful execution of this method. The oncologic principles including R0 resection and avoidance of tumor rupture or bleeding must be achievable through wedge resection in order to justify use of the approach. This must also be weighed with functional outcomes of partial gastrectomy. Surgical technique varies with tumor location in the stomach and the mobility of the tumor. Most regions of the stomach are easily resected after appropriate mobilization. Pre-pyloric and GEJ junction tumors present unique challenges that can be overcome by careful dissection and appropriate selection of surgical approaches.

Key Operative Steps

1. Place the patient in the supine position with both arms abducted on a split leg table in reverse Trendelenburg position.
2. Place a 12-mm located port in the periumbilical position and three additional 5-mm ports.
3. Perform a diagnostic laparoscopy to assess for metastatic disease.
4. Place a Nathanson liver retractor displacing the left lateral section of the liver in the cranial position.
5. Mobilize the greater curvature of the stomach by dissecting the short gastric vessels.
6. For lesser curvature tumors, open the gastro-hepatic ligament.
7. Identify the tumor and elevate it towards the anterior abdominal wall. Consider suture-assisted elevation if the tumor is endophytic or difficult to mobilize.
8. Place a GIA stapler at the base of the tumor overlaying an approximately 1-cm cuff of normal gastric tissue. The stapler should be positioned in a direction that maintains the patency of the gastric lumen. This can be ensured with simultaneous verification by upper endoscopy before firing the stapler.
9. Remove the tumor with a laparoscopic bag.
10. Use upper endoscopy to verify that the staple line is intact and without leakage or bleeding, to confirm adequate luminal patency, and to an absence of gastric mesenteroaxial volvulus.

References

1. Chi J-L, Xu M, Zhang M-R, Li Y, Zhou Z-G. Laparoscopic versus open resection for gastric gastrointestinal stromal tumors (GISTs): a

size–location-matched case–control study. World J Surg. 2017;41:2345–52. https://doi.org/10.1007/s00268-017-4005-8.

2. Koeda K, Nishizuka S, Wakabayashi G. Minimally invasive surgery for gastric cancer: the future standard of care. World J Surg. 2011;35:1469–77. https://doi.org/10.1007/s00268-011-1051-5.

3. Yang SY, et al. Surgical outcomes after open, laparoscopic, and robotic gastrectomy for gastric cancer. Ann Surg Oncol. 2017;24:1770–7. https://doi.org/10.1245/s10434-017-5851-1.

4. Ye L, et al. Meta-analysis of laparoscopic vs. open resection of gastric gastrointestinal stromal tumors. PLoS One. 2017;12:e0177193. https://doi.org/10.1371/journal.pone.0177193.

5. Ohgami M, et al. Laparoscopic wedge resection of the stomach for early gastric cancer using a lesion-lifting method. Dig Surg. 1994;11:64–7.

6. Mueller CL, et al. Application of an individualized operative strategy for wedge resection of gastric gastrointestinal stromal tumors: effectiveness for tumors in difficult locations. Surgery. 2016;160:1038–48. https://doi.org/10.1016/j.surg.2016.06.004.

7. Nguyen NT, et al. Laparoscopic enucleation or wedge resection of benign gastric pathology: analysis of 44 consecutive cases. Am Surg. 2011;77:1390–4.

8. Sicklick JK, Babicky M, DeMatteo RP. Resection of non-adenomatous gastric tumors. In: Jones DB, Schwaitzberg SD, editors. Operative endoscopic and minimally invasive surgery. Abingdon: CRC Press; 2019.

9. Lee S, et al. Oncologic safety of laparoscopic wedge resection with gastrotomy for gastric gastrointestinal stromal tumor: comparison with conventional laparoscopic wedge resection. J Gastric Cancer. 2015;15:231–7. https://doi.org/10.5230/jgc.2015.15.4.231.

10. Lee HH, et al. Laparoscopic wedge resection for gastric submucosal tumors: a size-location matched case-control study. J Am Coll Surg. 2011;212:195–9. https://doi.org/10.1016/j.jamcollsurg.2010.10.008.

11. Rösch T, et al. Accuracy of endoscopic ultrasonography in upper gastrointestinal submucosal lesions: a prospective multicenter study. Scand J Gastroenterol. 2002;37:856–62.

12. Conrad C, et al. Laparoscopic intragastric surgery for early gastric cancer and gastrointestinal stromal tumors. Ann Surg Oncol. 2014;21:2620. https://doi.org/10.1245/s10434-013-3432-5.

13. Barajas-Gamboa JS, et al. Laparo-endoscopic transgastric resection of gastric submucosal tumors. Surg Endosc. 2015;29:2149–57. https://doi.org/10.1007/s00464-014-3910-2.

14. Krenzien F, Pratschke J, Zorron R. Assessment of intragastric single-port surgery for gastric tumors. JAMA Surg. 2017;152:793–4. https://doi.org/10.1001/jamasurg.2017.1602.

15. Jacobsen GR, et al. Initial experience with an innovative endoscopic clipping system. Surg Technol Int. 2012;22:39–43.

16. Smallwood NR, Fleshman JW, Leeds SG, Burdick JS. The use of endoluminal vacuum (E-Vac) therapy in the management of upper gastrointestinal leaks and perforations. Surg Endosc. 2016;30:2473–80. https://doi.org/10.1007/s00464-015-4501-6.

Felix Berlth, Naoki Hiki, and Han-Kwang Yang

Introduction

While gastric cancer remains one of the most common causes of cancer-related deaths worldwide [1], countries with a high rate of early detection due to screening programs and general awareness, especially Japan and Korea, have developed advanced techniques to perform stomach- and function-preserving surgery. As such, pylorus-preserving gastrectomy (PPG) has been established as a good option for clinically early gastric cancer of the middle portion of the stomach [2, 3]. The principle of this operation is to combine luminal segmental resection of the stomach with preservation of pyloric function with an oncologically accurate extended D1+ lymph node dissection. Prospective studies have shown the long-term oncological safety of this approach compared to distal gastrectomy; and we await the results of a Korean prospective randomized trial regarding the functional outcome (KLASS-04).

The Japanese gastric cancer treatment guidelines list the PPG operation as an option for cT1N0 cancers of the middle portion of the stomach; however, the exact tumor location that is suitable for PPG is still under discussion, especially regarding the proximal extent of the tumor [4]. The distal extent of the tumor should be no closer than 4 cm from the pylorus to achieve a negative resection margin and to preserve sufficient antral tissue for pyloric function. Nevertheless, postoperative gastric stasis caused by pyloric spasm is one of the potential complications and challenges after PPG. Several technical alterations have been suggested to improve this particular outcome, which is a critical endpoint that is necessary to realize the clinical benefits of PPG. As laparoscopic surgery has been confirmed, in Japanese and Korean prospective randomized trials, to be an oncologically safe option for early gastric cancer, the PPG resection is widely performed by the minimally invasive approach followed either by intracorporeal or extracorporeal gastro-gastrostomy [5, 6]. This chapter describes the technical

Electronic supplementary material The online version of this chapter (https://doi.org/10.1007/978-3-030-18740-8_6) contains supplementary material, which is available to authorized users.

F. Berlth
Department of Surgery, Division of Gastrointestinal Surgery, Seoul National University Hospital, Seoul, Republic of Korea

Department of General, Visceral and Cancer Surgery, University Hospital of Cologne, Cologne, Germany

N. Hiki
Department of Upper Gastrointestinal Surgery, Kitasato University School of Medicine, Kanagawa, Japan
e-mail: nhiki@med.kitasato-u.ac.jp

H.-K. Yang (⊠)
Department of Surgery, Division of Gastrointestinal Surgery, Seoul National University Hospital, Seoul, Republic of Korea
e-mail: hkyang@snu.ac.kr

© Springer Nature Switzerland AG 2020
J. Kim, J. Garcia-Aguilar (eds.), *Minimally Invasive Surgical Techniques for Cancers of the Gastrointestinal Tract*, https://doi.org/10.1007/978-3-030-18740-8_6

steps of PPG for clinically early gastric cancer and suggests anastomotic techniques.

Approach, Placement of Trocars, and the Operative Field

For minimally invasive resection, the laparoscopic and robotic approaches represent possible options. Laparoscopic PPG is the most established and most standardized procedure; and much of the published evidence regarding minimally invasive PPG is based on the use of laparoscopic techniques. However, despite higher costs, the robotic approach may be safe and accurate for gastric cancer surgery as well, although a study comparing laparoscopic and robotic PPG did not reveal differences in outcomes [7].

In the laparoscopic setting, the patient is placed in supine, reverse Trendelenburg position with the legs elevated (Fig. 6.1). Typically, an 11-mm camera trocar is placed in the infra-umbilical position. Additional two 12-mm ports can be positioned right and left and cranial of the camera port followed by one 5-mm port each in the right and left upper lateral positions. If the operator stays on the right side of the patient and extracorporeal anastomosis is performed, two 5-mm trocars on the patient's left side are sufficient. The patient's position is similar for the robotic approach; but to achieve the longest distance between the external robotic arms, both 7-mm ports are placed more laterally (Fig. 6.2).

Operative Technique

Partial Omentectomy and Ligation of the Left Gastroepiploic Vessels

After diagnostic laparoscopy, the resection is started near the midline of the omentum. The stomach can be lifted to inflate air into the lesser sac to separate and provide distance between the stomach and the colon for safer division. After finding the correct plane in the lesser sac, omentectomy is proceeded towards the direction of the spleen. Typically, after visualization of the lower splenic pole, the left gastroepiploic vessels can be identified (Fig. 6.3a) and ligated with clips. Two clips on the patient side and one clip on the specimen side are recommended for safe ligation of all landmark vessels during gastrectomy. After ligation, the vessels can be followed to the stomach to prepare the greater curvature for cleaning.

The portion of the greater curvature that will be preserved is cleaned of tissues, vessels, and lymph nodes. This maneuver of cleaning the greater curvature is performed in a distal to proximal direction starting approximately at the location of the proposed transection plane of the stomach and heading proximal to the ligated left gastroepiploic vessels (Fig. 6.3b). To facilitate this step, the greater curvature of the stomach should be aligned with the direction of the energy device and proper traction and counter-traction should be maintained with the assistant's help. The greater curvature should be cleaned layer by layer (posterior and anterior layer) to remove lymphatic tissues close to or on the stomach surface while avoiding bleeding. These tissues remain in continuity with the omentum at the distal stomach. Upon completion of skeletonizing the proximal stomach, partial omentectomy is completed towards the right side of the patient until the infrapyloric area is approached. This first part of the operation is similar to standard laparoscopic distal gastrectomy for early gastric cancer.

Infrapyloric Dissection

The infrapyloric dissection is the most crucial and challenging part of the PPG operation. In order to maintain good pyloric function, both right gastroepiploic artery and vein should be clipped only after it has branched to the pylorus and antrum. On the other hand, the infrapyloric region must be cleared of lymphatic tissues for oncological accuracy and integrity. The partial omentectomy can be finished by heading towards the gallbladder and carefully separating the greater omentum from the underlying fused transverse mesocolon (Fig. 6.3c). In the last step of partial omentectomy, the second portion of the duodenum should be visualized (Fig. 6.3d). Now

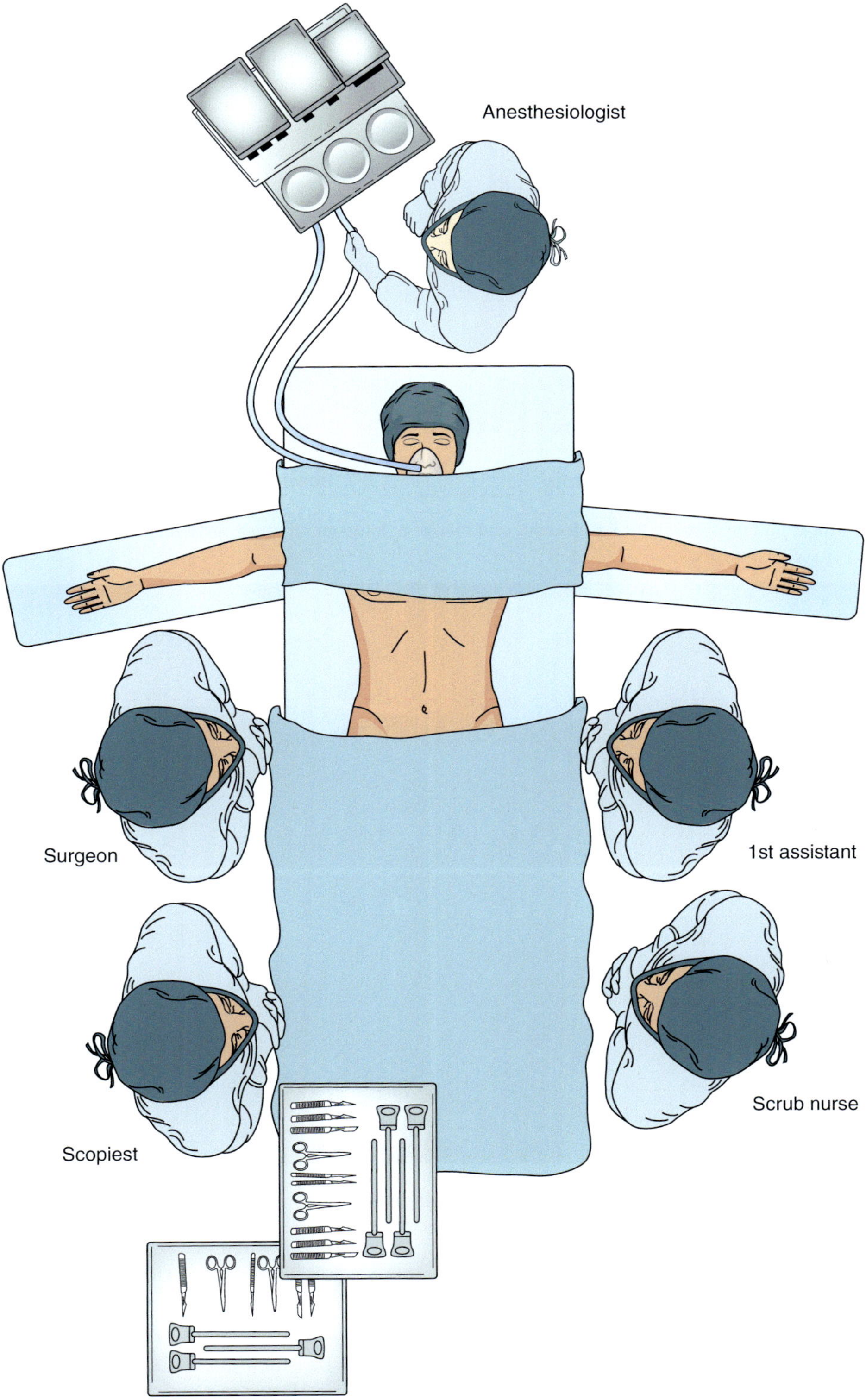

Fig. 6.1 Patient and surgeon positioning for minimally invasive pylorus-preserving gastrectomy

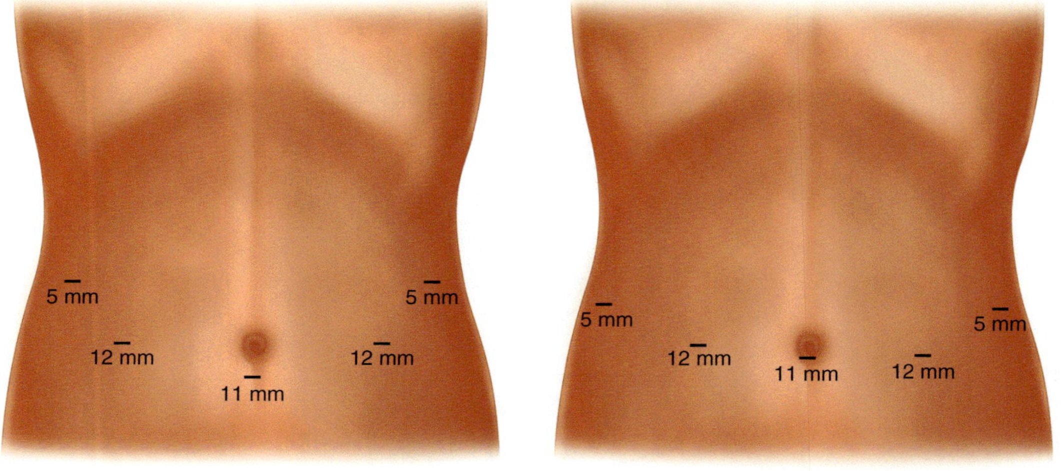

Fig. 6.2 Trocar/port positioning for laparoscopic and robotic pylorus-preserving gastrectomy

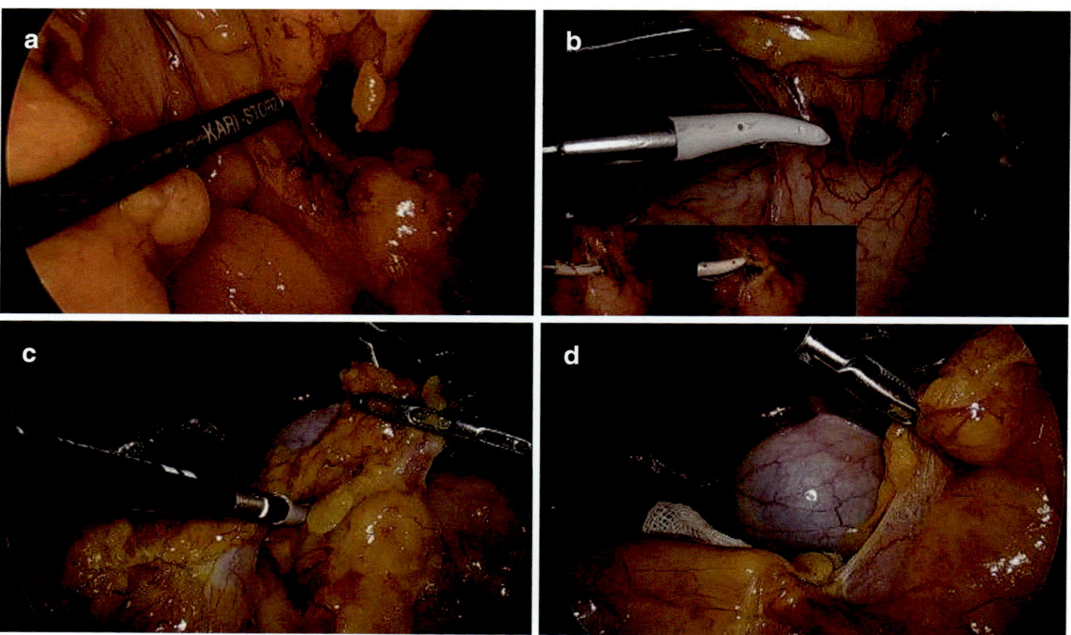

Fig. 6.3 Intraoperative image showing (**a**) isolation of the left gastroepiploic vessels, (**b**) cleaning the greater curvature, (**c**) completion of omentectomy, and (**d**) visualization of the duodenum

the fusion plane of infrapyloric tissue and meso-colon should be identified to initiate the infrapy-loric dissection. The assistant lifts up the antrum by gently grasping the posterior wall and care-fully retracting the mesocolon downward using gauze to maintain a proper operative field (Fig. 6.4a). The assistant's retraction of the stom-ach wall can facilitate effective counter-traction during the infrapyloric dissection by altering the direction of traction.

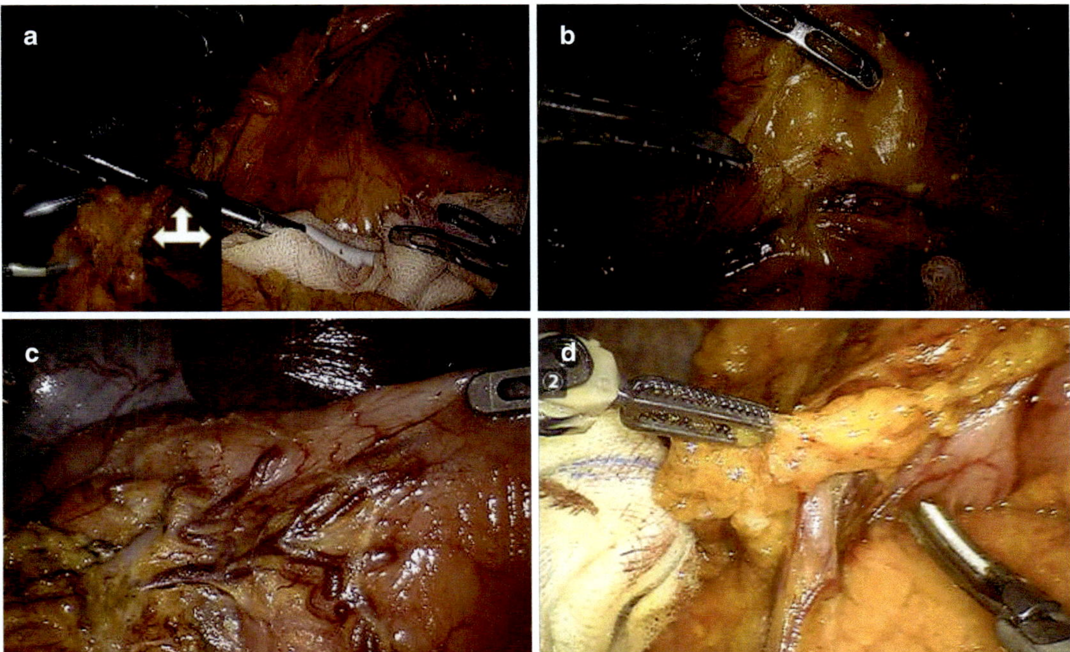

Fig. 6.4 Intraoperative image showing (**a**) the infrapyloric area prior to dissection, (**b**) the fusion plane between the mesocolon and right gastroepiploic vessels, (**c**) the anterior region of the infrapyloric area, and (**d**) dissecting along the right gastroepiploic vessels

The surgeon can approach the fusion plane by dissecting on the posterior aspect of the right gastroepiploic vessels in the direction of the gastroduodenal artery. Depending on its origin, the infrapyloric artery can be isolated and saved. There are several variations to this artery with the infrapyloric artery originating from the anterior superior pancreaticoduodenal artery (64.2%), the right gastroepiploic artery (23.1%), or the gastroduodenal artery (12.7%) [8]. Next, the fusion plane is dissected to separate the mesocolon from the tissues adherent to the stomach (Fig. 6.4b). At this point, the root of the right gastroepiploic vessels can be visualized. If the vessels appear during this step of dissection, it should be determined whether they supply blood to the pyloric region. To perform safe dissection of lymphatic tissues along the infrapyloric vessels, the assistant can retract the antrum towards the left upper quadrant which will place the infrapyloric vessels into a direction that is parallel to the direction of the energy device (Fig. 6.4b). Short bursts of coagulation with the energy device can preclude damage to the pyloric blood supply. As the dissection of the posterior side of the gastroepiploic vessels is completed, the peritoneal layer is opened on the anterior side of the vessels just proximal to the distal end (Fig. 6.4c). Small vessels supplying the pylorus are uncovered. If bleeding is encountered, we suggest compressing with gauze and avoiding thermal damage with an energy or bipolar device.

The distal resection line must be determined. The proximal pyloric branches of the greater curvature are cleaned of their lymphatic tissues. If the antrum cuff is too long, then stasis in this segment can occur due to impaired motility. As the posterior and the anterior sides are dissected, the infrapyloric lymphatic tissues are dissected and harvested along the gastroepiploic vessels in a distal to proximal direction (Fig. 6.4d). Now, the gastroepiploic vessels can be clipped after they have supplied the branches to the pylorus. We recommended saving both the arterial and venous branches to the pylorus to avoid postoperative edema which may lead to malfunction of the pylorus [9]. Before moving to the lesser curvature side, we recommend dividing the connection between lymph node station 5 and 8a under the stomach to facilitate later dissection of lymph node station 8a on the lesser curvature.

Distal Lesser Curvature

In order to elevate and stretch tissues and protect structures such as the common hepatic artery, we place three gauze sponges under the lesser omentum at the under surface of the stomach before approaching the anterior side of the lesser curvature. Lymph node station 5 along the right gastric artery is not harvested in PPG [10]. In this area, important perineural structures for the pyloric region are located, and oncologically, it is not mandatory to harvest nodes from this station for the indicated tumor location. However, if suspicious lymph nodes are visualized in the infrapyloric or suprapyloric regions, we advise dissecting the tissues for frozen section investigation or to abort the PPG procedure and convert to formal distal gastrectomy to achieve radical resection in this area. The right gastric artery arcade (Fig. 6.5a) should be clipped distal from its origin and approx-

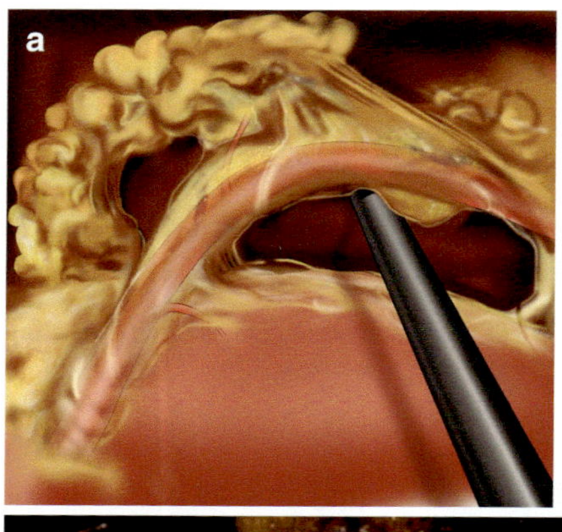

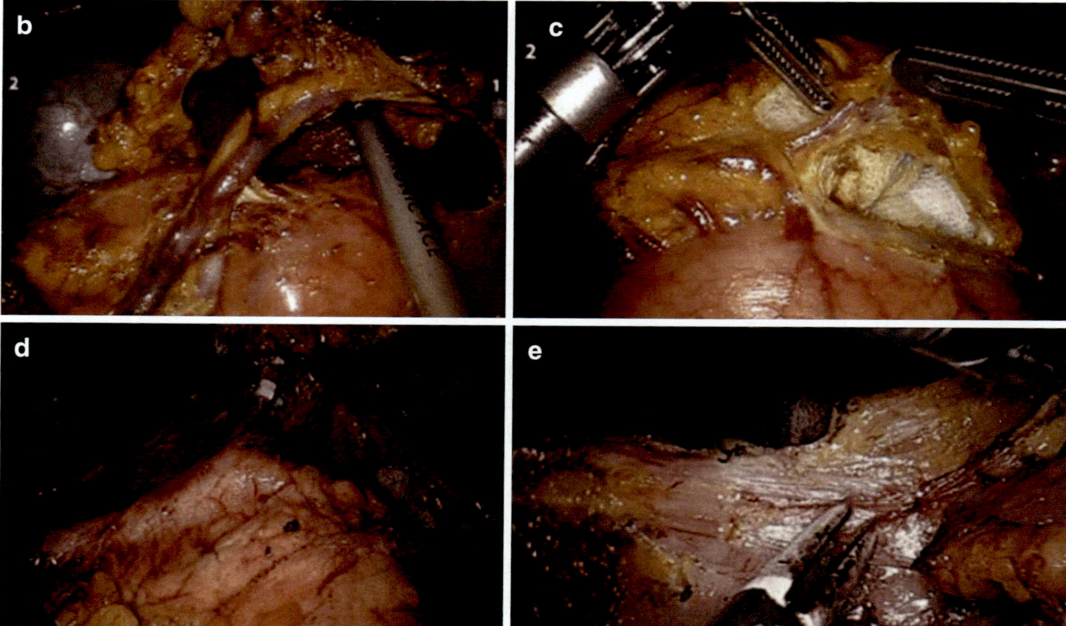

Fig. 6.5 (**a**) Illustration showing the right gastroepiploic vessels with preservation of the pyloric branches. (**b**) Paired intraoperative image with lifting of the right gastroepiploic vessels to highlight preservation of branches to the pylorus. Intraoperative images showing (**c**) the right gastric arcade, (**d**) clipped left gastric artery, and (**e**) cleaning the lesser curvature of the stomach

imately 3 cm from the pylorus. The assistant can place counter-traction on the lesser curvature by retracting the antrum in a caudal direction using gauze to maximize the force of retraction. Similar to dissection of the greater curvature, the lesser curvature can be skeletonized. The lesser omentum is divided in the direction of the gastroesophageal junction. During this step, preservation of the hepatic branches of nervi vagi can be achieved. Potential lymph nodes in this location or an aberrant left hepatic artery can complicate this step. With respect to oncological principles, the preservation of an aberrant left hepatic artery is an appropriate maneuver. The result of these steps now permits the suprapancreatic area to be visualized from above the lesser curvature of the stomach.

Supra-pancreatic Lymph Node Dissection

Lymph node station 8a dissection is performed along the common hepatic artery to the root of the left gastric artery. As mentioned above, it is better to separate tissues between lymph node station 5 and 8a on the posterior aspect of the distal stomach. If a coronary vein is visualized early, it should be clipped and divided. The assistant can grasp and lift the pedicle of the left gastric vessels in an orthogonal position to the supra-pancreatic border (Fig. 6.5b. The assistant's counter-traction on the pancreas using gauze sponge is optional. Attention should be paid to avoid excessive retraction on the pancreas which can lead to injury to the vessels [11]. The left gastric artery and vein are skeletonized and clipped at its roots (Fig. 6.5c). For D1+ dissection, harvesting lymph node station 11p is not mandatory; however, if dissection is desired it can be performed after the left gastric vessels are divided. The tissue behind the root of the left gastric artery should be harvested as part of lymph node station 9.

Lesser Curvature Dissection

After completion of the necessary steps for dissection along lymph node station 8a, the tissues of the supra-pancreatic area along the diaphragmatic crus are dissected towards the direction of the esophagogastric junction. The necessity of dissecting lymph node station 1 in middle stomach for early gastric cancer is controversial and deferring dissection of these nodal tissues could preserve vagal innervation to the pylorus. However, the guidelines for PPG suggest that these nodal tissues should be removed as part of the surgical specimen. The nodal tissues along the lesser curve (i.e., lymph node station 3) are dissected layer by layer similar to the dissection of the greater curvature up to the location of the proximal resection line (Fig. 6.5d). Gentle retraction by the assistant is crucial to stretch the tissues for clean dissection of lymphatic tissues while avoiding bleeding. The lesser curvature of the stomach can be quite thin and tearing or thermal penetration of the stomach should be avoided (Fig. 6.5e).

Gastro-gastrostomy

Extracorporeal Anastomosis

If an extracorporeal anastomosis is performed, a mini-laparotomy (5 cm) is sufficient in most cases. For the exact location of the incision, laparoscopic views can be helpful. For the most common location of early cancer in the middle portion of the stomach (i.e., lower body/corpus), a transverse incision represents a comfortable approach. For higher locations (i.e., mid-body), a vertical midline incision can be used.

After laparotomy, the mobilized stomach can be gently extracted. To easily determine the luminal extent of resection, preoperative endoscopic clipping is a good option. For extracorporeal anastomosis, the clips are palpable and can be located. Distal resection can be performed by clamping the proximal portion of the stomach and dividing the stomach layer by layer with electrocautery. The distal margin is sent for frozen section evaluation.

One maneuver to decrease postoperative pyloric spasm is manual dilatation of the pylorus, which can easily be achieved at this point in the procedure [12]. A ring forceps is inserted into the lumen and the pylorus is gently stretched for 10–15 seconds (Fig. 6.6a). For the proximal resection, an Allen clamp is applied across the

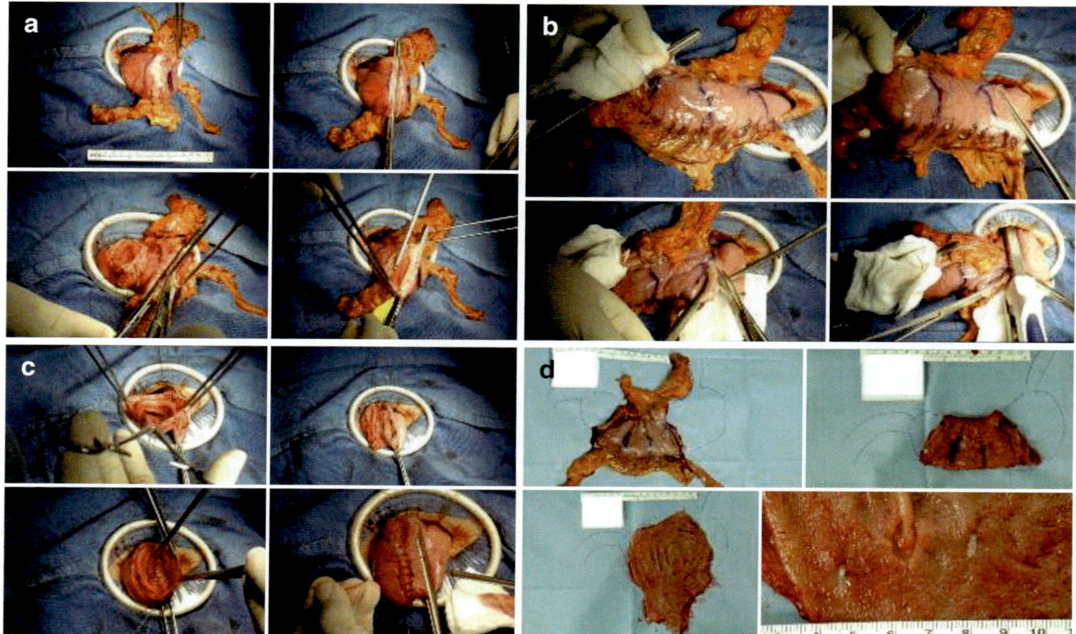

Fig. 6.6 Intraoperative images showing (**a**) distal resection of the stomach and dilatation of the pylorus, (**b**) proximal resection of the stomach, (**c**) creation of the gastro-gastrostomy, and (**d**) the pathologic specimen

proposed transection line from the greater to lesser curvature; and another clamp is placed in a similar fashion at the distal transection line. The proximal clip, the cancer, and the resection lines can all be marked with ink on the external surface of the stomach. Then, the middle portion of the stomach is resected using a linear stapler (Fig. 6.6b). After retrieving the resected stomach, we check the resection margin macroscopically. Then, a proximal margin can be sent for frozen section examination.

At last, the gastro-gastrostomy is performed with a single-layer continuous interlocking hand-sewn anastomosis using 3–0 polyfilament absorbable sutures (Fig. 6.6c). In case of tension or bleeding, the anastomosis can be reinforced with single sutures. Since the specimen without connective tissue represents a segmental resection, it is important to provide orientation for the pathologist to ensure precise documentation of appropriate resection margins before tissues are fixed (Fig. 6.6d).

Intracorporeal Anastomosis

If intracorporeal anastomosis is desired, the luminal extent of resection can be determined using different methods. Endoscopic clipping of the desired margins seems beneficial; and x-ray, ultrasound, or intraoperative gastroscopy can be used to localize the clips. A combination of clipping and intraoperative gastroscopy is a safe option for intracorporeal anastomosis [13]. This intracorporeal technique is performed using linear staplers. For reconstruction, the first option appears similar to the delta-shape intracorporeal anastomosis in Billroth I resection. Both parts of the remnant stomach are opened at the end of the stapler line along the greater curvature. A linear stapler is inserted first in the proximal stomach and followed by the distal stomach and both parts are gently brought together. The staple lines of both parts of the stomach (proximal and distal stomach) should be positioned parallel above the inserted stapler. Special care should be taken to ensure that the distal remnant stomach does not slip in the direction of the pylorus during this maneuver. After firing the linear stapler and connecting the proximal and distal stomach, the common channel/opening can be closed using another firing of the linear stapler, while carefully avoiding narrowing of the lumen.

The second option for intracorporeal anastomosis after PPG was developed by one of our authors (N.H.) as the "piercing method". This technique was developed since a linear stapler that is inserted in the distal remnant stomach cannot transversely reach the opposite side for the widest anastomoses when there are also large distances from the stapler line to the pylorus. For this technique, the distal part of the stomach is opened at both greater and lesser curvature sides and the stapler is gently pushed through both openings (Fig. 6.7). We recommend placing the stapler first in the distal stomach followed by placement in the proximal stomach. The staple lines of the resection are brought into parallel position above the inserted stapler. After firing the stapler and connecting both parts of the stomach, both common channels/openings and the parallel staple lines are closed/resected with another linear stapler (Fig. 6.8). For this purpose,

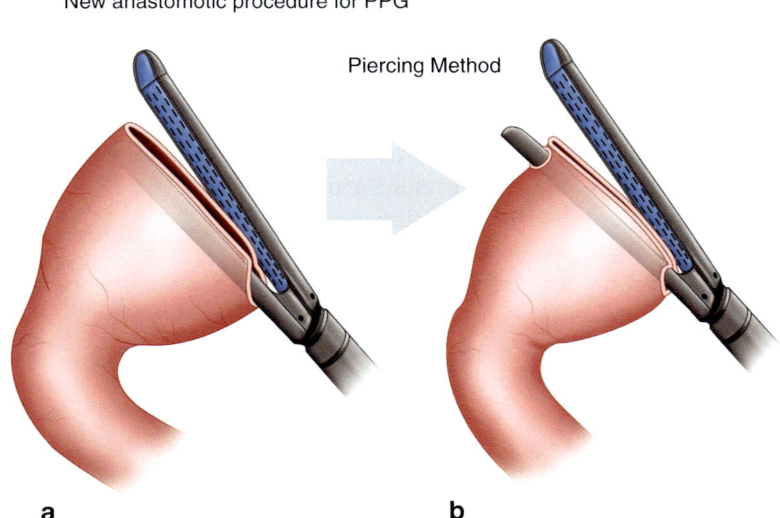

Fig. 6.7 Illustration demonstrating the piercing method. (**a**) For wide remnant antrum, the linear stapler may not fully reach from the greater to lesser curvatures. (**b**) If a small gastrotomy is made at the lesser curvature, the linear stapler can successfully reach from the greater curvature to the lesser curvature

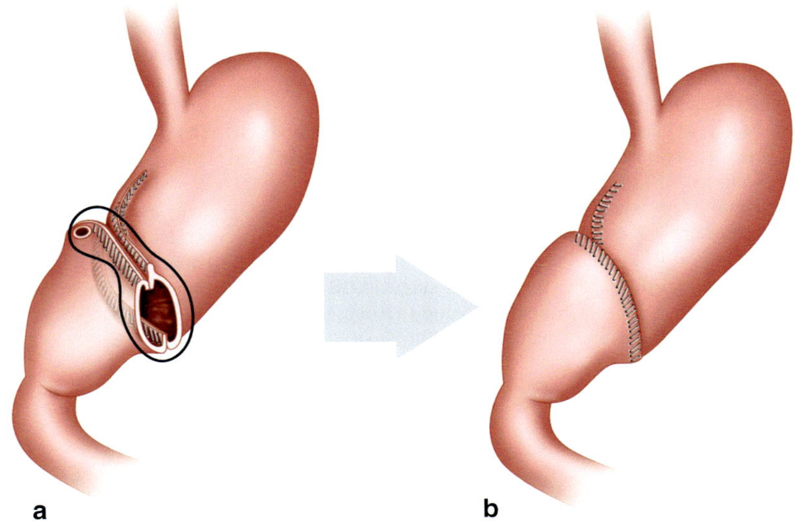

Fig. 6.8 Illustration showing end-to-end gastro-gastrostomy by the piercing method. (**a**) The posterior anastomosis is created by the piercing technique. (**b**) The two linear stapler lines and the common gastrotomy are closed/resected by 3 staple piercing method technique that results in a completed end-to-end gastro-gastrostomy

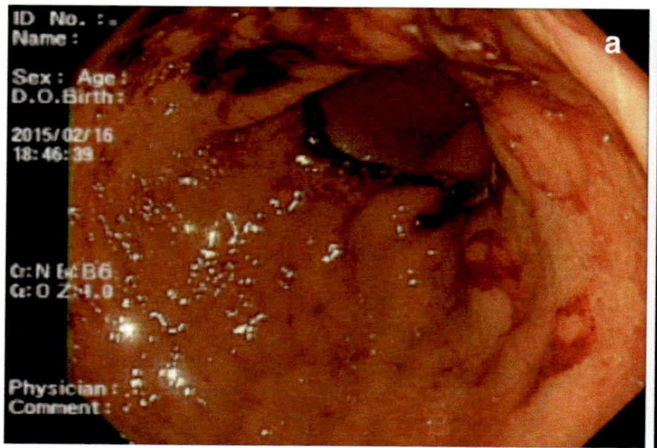

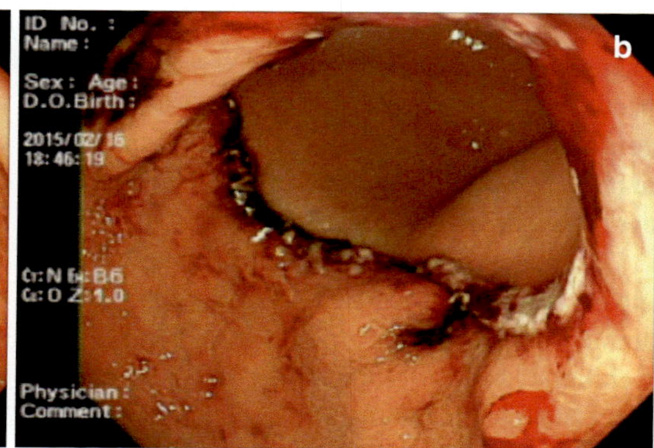

Fig. 6.9 Endoscopic images showing ideal end-to-end gastrogastrostomy by the piercing method. (**a**) There was no sign of bleeding with a widely patent anastomosis. (**b**) The piercing method created an end-to-end gastrogastrostomy using the full length of the transected antral edge

stay sutures should be placed on the edge of the greater and lesser curvature openings, as well as at the parallel staple lines to safely include these tissues/staples in the resected tissues. After applying at least two linear staple lines, the openings should be closed and the parallel staple lines should be replaced by a single one. Endoscopic views show a wide and sufficient anastomosis (Fig. 6.9).

References

1. Torre LA, Bray F, Siegel RL, et al. Global cancer statistics, 2012. CA Cancer J Clin. 2015;65:87–108.
2. Hiki N, Sano T, Fukunaga T, et al. Survival benefit of pylorus-preserving gastrectomy in early gastric cancer. J Am Coll Surg. 2009;209:297–301.
3. Suh YS, Han DS, Kong SH, et al. Laparoscopy-assisted pylorus-preserving gastrectomy is better than laparoscopy-assisted distal gastrectomy for middle-third early gastric cancer. Ann Surg. 2014;259:485–93.
4. Japanese Gastric Cancer Association. Japanese gastric cancer treatment guidelines 2014 (ver. 4). Gastric Cancer. 2017;20:1–19.
5. Katai H, Mizusawa J, Katayama H, et al. Short-term surgical outcomes from a phase III study of laparoscopy-assisted versus open distal gastrectomy with nodal dissection for clinical stage IA/IB gastric cancer: Japan Clinical Oncology Group Study JCOG0912. Gastric Cancer. 2017;20:699–708.
6. Kim W, Kim HH, Han SU, et al. Decreased morbidity of laparoscopic distal gastrectomy compared with open distal gastrectomy for stage I gastric cancer: short-term outcomes from a multicenter randomized controlled trial (KLASS-01). Ann Surg. 2016;263:28–35.
7. Han D-S, Suh Y-S, Ahn HS, et al. Comparison of surgical outcomes of robot-assisted and laparoscopy-assisted pylorus-preserving gastrectomy for gastric cancer: a propensity score matching analysis. Ann Surg Oncol. 2015;22:2323–8.
8. Haruta S, Shinohara H, Ueno M, et al. Anatomical considerations of the infrapyloric artery and its associated lymph nodes during laparoscopic gastric cancer surgery. Gastric Cancer. 2015;18:876–80.
9. Kiyokawa T, Hiki N, Nunobe S, et al. Preserving infrapyloric vein reduces postoperative gastric stasis after laparoscopic pylorus-preserving gastrectomy. Langenbeck's Arch Surg. 2017;402:49–56.
10. Kong SH, Kim JW, Lee HJ, et al. The safety of the dissection of lymph node stations 5 and 6 in pylorus-preserving gastrectomy. Ann Surg Oncol. 2009;16:3252–8.
11. Tsujiura M, Hiki N, Ohashi M, et al. "Pancreas-compressionless gastrectomy": a novel laparoscopic approach for suprapancreatic lymph node dissection. Ann Surg Oncol. 2017;24:3331–7.
12. Zhu C-C, Kim T-H, Berlth F, et al. Clinical outcomes of intraoperative manual dilatation of pylorus in pylorus-preserving gastrectomy: a retrospective analysis. Gastric Cancer. 2018;21:864. https://doi.org/10.1007/s10120-018-0814-1.
13. Kawakatsu S, Ohashi M, Hiki N, et al. Use of endoscopy to determine the resection margin during laparoscopic gastrectomy for cancer. Br J Surg. 2017;104:1829–36.

Hiroya Takeuchi and Yuko Kitagawa

Introduction

In East Asian countries such as Japan and Korea, early-stage gastric cancer [i.e., American Joint Committee on Cancer (AJCC), clinical T1 (cT1) T stage] is found in many asymptomatic patients due to recent advances in endoscopic diagnosis and surveillance programs; and the population at risk currently exceeds 50% in these major institutions [1]. Endoscopic submucosal dissection (ESD) has already been accepted as the most minimally invasive procedure for resection of early gastric cancer [1]. Laparoscopic gastrectomy represents an important intermediate option between ESD and distal or total gastrectomy by open laparotomy for patients with gastric cancer [2]. Currently, laparoscopic distal gastrectomy (LDG) is comparable with conventional open distal gastrectomy and can be performed in routine clinical practice [3, 4]. Many patients with

Electronic supplementary material The online version of this chapter (https://doi.org/10.1007/978-3-030-18740-8_7) contains supplementary material, which is available to authorized users.

H. Takeuchi (✉)
Department of Surgery, Hamamatsu University School of Medicine, Shizuoka, Japan
e-mail: takeuchi@hama-med.ac.jp

Y. Kitagawa
Department of Surgery, Keio University School of Medicine, Tokyo, Japan
e-mail: kitagawa@a3.keio.jp

early gastric cancer are currently treated with advanced laparoscopic gastrectomy procedures, such as LDG and laparoscopic total gastrectomy (LTG) with appropriate lymph node dissection in many countries [1–4]. LDG and LTG contribute to better aesthetics and earlier postoperative recovery [5]. However, patients' quality of life (QOL) is mainly affected by late-phase complications including dumping syndrome and body weight loss resulting from disturbances in oral intake due to the extent of gastric resection. Therefore, both minimal invasive techniques for early-phase recovery by laparoscopic surgery and late-phase function-preserving gastrectomy should be carefully considered in patients indicated for these procedures.

Function-preserving gastrectomy such as partial gastrectomy, segmental gastrectomy, and proximal gastrectomy with limited lymph node dissection is known to improve postoperative late-phase function. However, a certain incidence of skip metastasis in the second or third compartment of regional lymph nodes remains an obstacle to wider application of these procedures. To overcome these issues, the concept of sentinel lymph node (SLN) mapping may become a novel diagnostic tool for the identification of clinically undetectable lymph node metastasis in early gastric cancer.

SLNs are defined as the first draining lymph nodes from the primary tumor site [6, 7], and they are thought to be the first possible site of micrometastasis along the route of lymphatic drainage from the primary lesion. The pathological status of SLNs can theoretically predict the status of all regional lymph nodes. If SLNs are recognizable and negative for cancer metastasis, unnecessary radical lymph node dissection could be avoided. SLN navigation surgery is defined as a novel, minimally invasive surgery based on SLN mapping and the SLN-targeted diagnosis of nodal metastasis. SLN navigation surgery can prevent unnecessary lymph node dissection, thus preventing the associated complications and improving the patient's QOL.

SLN mapping and biopsy were first applied to melanoma and breast cancer patients and were subsequently extended to patients with other solid tumors [7–9]. The clinical application of SLN mapping for early gastric cancer has been controversial for years. However, single institutional results and a multicenter trial of SLN mapping and biopsy for early gastric cancer observed acceptable SLN detection rate and accuracy of determining the lymph node status [10, 11]. On the basis of these results, we are developing a novel, minimally invasive function-preserving gastrectomy technique combined with SLN mapping and biopsy.

Laparoscopic SLN Biopsy Procedures

A dual-tracer method that utilizes radioactive colloids and blue or green dye is currently considered the most reliable method for stable detection of SLNs in patients with early gastric cancer [10, 11]. An accumulation of radioactive colloids facilitates the identification of SLNs even in resected specimens by using a handheld gamma probe, and the blue dye is effective for intraoperative visualization of lymphatic flow, even during laparoscopic surgery. Technetium-99 m tin colloid, technetium-99 m sulfur colloid, and technetium-99 m antimony sulfur colloid are preferentially used as radioactive tracers. Isosulfan blue and indocyanine green (ICG) are the currently preferred choices as dye tracers.

In our institution, patients with cT1 tumors, primary lesions <4 cm in diameter, and cN0 gas-

tric cancer undergo SLN mapping and biopsy [10, 11]. In our procedures, 2 ml (150 MBq) of technetium-99 m tin colloid solution is injected the day before surgery into four quadrants of the submucosal layer of the primary tumor site using an endoscopic puncture needle. Endoscopic injections to the submucosal layer facilitate accurate tracer injection rather than laparoscopic injection from the seromuscular side of the gastric wall. Technetium-99 m tin colloid with relatively large particle size accumulates in the SLNs after local administration.

The blue or green dye is injected into four quadrants of the submucosal layer of the primary site using an endoscopic puncture needle at the beginning of surgery. Blue lymphatic vessels and blue-stained nodes can be identified by laparoscopy within 15 min after injection of the blue or green dye. Simultaneously, a handheld gamma probe is used to locate the radioactive SLN. Intraoperative gamma probing is feasible even in laparoscopic gastrectomy using a special gamma detector that can be introduced through trocar ports [10, 11].

For intraoperative SLN sampling, the "pickup method" is well established for the detection of melanoma and breast cancer. However, it is recommended that the clinical application of intraoperative SLN sampling for gastric cancer should include sentinel lymphatic basin dissection, which is a modified focused lymph node dissection involving hot and blue lymph nodes [10, 11]. The gastric lymphatic basins are divided in the following five directions along the main arteries: left gastric artery area, right gastric artery area, left gastroepiploic artery area, right gastroepiploic artery area, and posterior gastric artery area [12].

ICG is known to have excitation and fluorescence wavelengths in the near-infrared range [13]. Until now, some investigators have used infrared ray electronic endoscopy (IREE) to demonstrate the clinical utility of intraoperative ICG infrared imaging as a new tracer for laparoscopic SLN mapping [13, 14]. IREE might be a useful tool to improve visualization of ICG-stained lymphatic vessels and SLNs even in the fat tissues. More recently, ICG fluorescence imaging has been developed as another promising novel technique for SLN mapping [15, 16]. SLNs could be clearly visualized by laparoscopic ICG fluorescence imaging compared to the laparoscopic observation of ICG with normal light. Further studies would be needed to evaluate the clinical efficacy of ICG infrared or fluorescence imaging and to compare those with radio-guided methods in prospective studies. However these new technologies might revolutionize laparoscopic SLN mapping procedures in early gastric cancer.

Results of SLN Mapping in Gastric Cancer

To date, more than 100 single institutional studies have demonstrated acceptable outcomes of SLN mapping for early gastric cancer in terms of the SLN detection rate (90–100%) and accuracy (85–100%) in determining the lymph node status; these outcomes are comparable with those of SLN mapping for melanoma and breast cancer [11]. A large-scale meta-analysis, which included 38 relevant SLN mapping studies with 2128 gastric cancer patients, demonstrated that the SLN detection rate and accuracy of predicting lymph node metastasis based on SLN status were 94% and 92%, respectively [17]. They concluded that the SLN concept is technically feasible for gastric cancer, especially patients with early T stage (cT1) by combining tracers and submucosal injection methods during the SLN biopsy procedures.

Our group in Japan has conducted a multicenter prospective trial (UMIN ID: 000000476) of SLN mapping using a dual-tracer method with a radioactive colloid and blue dye [10]. In the trial, SLN mapping was performed between 2004 and 2008 for 397 patients with early gastric cancer at 12 comprehensive hospitals, including our institution. Eligibility criteria were that patients had cT1N0M0 or cT2N0M0 single tumor with diameter of primary lesion less than 4 cm and without prior treatments.

The SLN detection rate by using the dual-tracer method was 97.5% ($n = 387$ of 397), and lymph node metastasis was diagnosed in 57 (14.7%) of 387 patients. Of the 57 patients with lymph node metastasis, 53 (93.0%) had positive SLNs. The accuracy of determining the metastatic status based on SLN evaluation was 99.0% ($n = 383$ of 387). In 32 (60.4%) of 53 patients with positive SLNs, lymph node metastases were limited to only SLNs. Of 21 SLN-positive/non-SLN-positive patients, 15 (71.4%) had metastatic non-SLNs within SLN basins and 6 (28.6%) had metastatic non-SLNs located outside the SLN basins but within the extent of D2 lymph node dissection. Four patients had false-negative SLN biopsy results of whom three had pT2 and/or primary tumors more than 4 cm in size [10]. The results of that clinical trial are expected to provide us with perspectives on the future of minimally invasive SLN navigation surgery for early gastric cancer.

Clinical Application of SLN Navigation Surgery in Early Gastric Cancer

The distribution of sentinel lymphatic basins and the pathological status of SLNs would be useful in deciding on the extent of gastric resection and avoiding the universal application of distal or total gastrectomy with D2 dissection. Appropriate indications for laparoscopic surgery such as partial (wedge) resection, segmental gastrectomy, pylorus-preserving gastrectomy, and proximal gastrectomy (LPG) for cT1N0 gastric cancer could be individually determined on the basis of SLN status (Figs. 7.1 and 7.2a–c) [18–20]. Earlier recovery after surgery and preservation of QOL in the late phase can be achieved by limited laparoscopic gastrectomy with SLN navigation. Our study group in Japan has currently been conducting the multicenter prospective trial (UMIN ID: 000014401) which will evaluate function-preserving gastrectomy with SLN mapping in terms of long-term survival and patients' QOL. A Korean group is also conducting a multicenter prospective phase III trial to elucidate the oncologic safety including long-term survival of laparoscopic stomach-preserving surgery with

Fig. 7.1 Individualized function-preserving approaches for cT1N0M0 gastric cancer based on sentinel lymph node mapping. ESD, endoscopic submucosal dissection

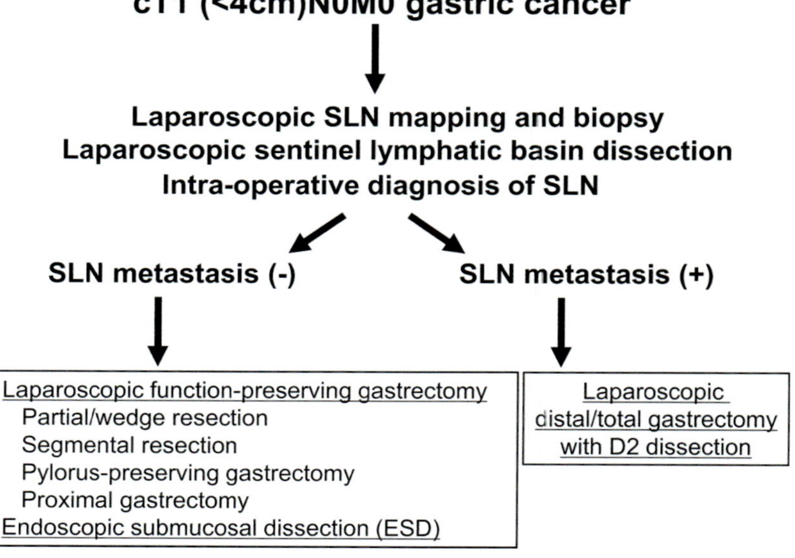

Fig. 7.2 Laparoscopic function-preserving gastrectomy with sentinel lymphatic basin dissection. (**a**) Partial (wedge) resection, (**b**) segmental (pylorus preserving) gastrectomy, (**c**) proximal gastrectomy, and (**d**) sentinel lymphatic basin dissection and ESD

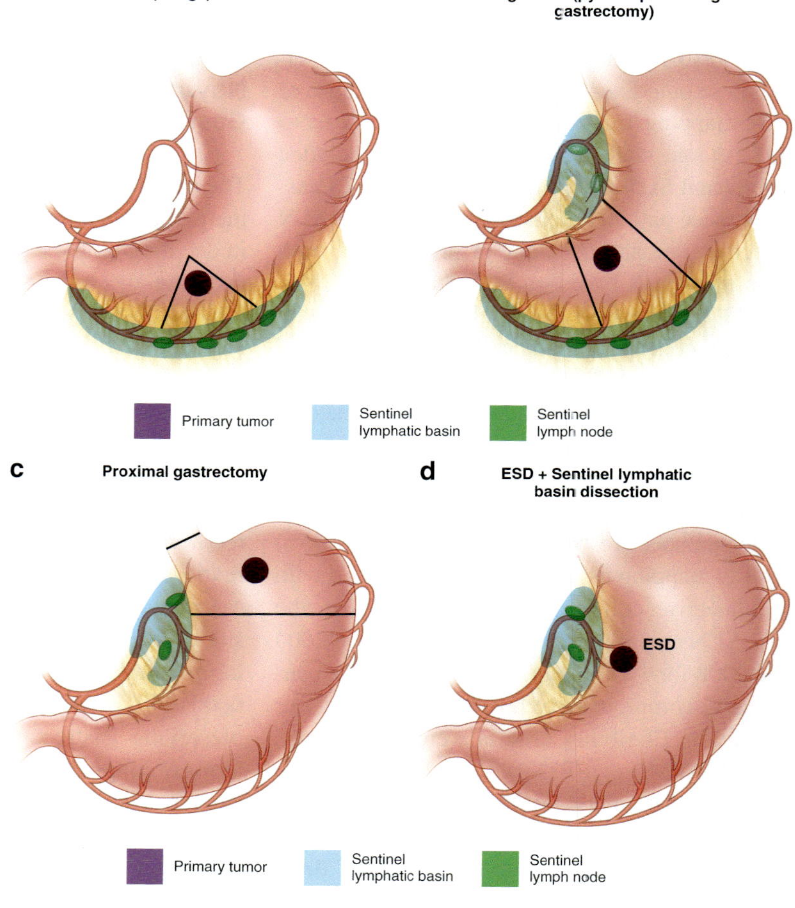

sentinel lymphatic basin dissection compared to a standard laparoscopic gastrectomy [21].

A combination of laparoscopic SLN biopsy and ESD for early gastric cancer is another attractive option as a novel, whole stomach-preserved, minimally invasive approach. If all SLNs are pathologically negative for cancer metastasis, then theoretically ESD instead of gastrectomy may be sufficient for the curative resection of cT1 gastric cancer beyond ESD criteria (Fig. 7.2d) [20, 22]. However, further studies are required to verify the safety and effectiveness of combined treatments involving laparoscopic SLN biopsy and ESD.

Currently, LDG or LPG are frequently applied to patients with early gastric cancer according to the results of pathological assessment of primary tumor resected by ESD. To date, it has not been clarified whether SLN mapping is even feasible after ESD. One of the most important issues is whether lymphatic flow from the primary tumor to the original SLNs might change after ESD. In our preliminary study, however, the sentinel lymphatic basin is not markedly affected by previous ESD [20, 22]. Thus, modified gastrectomy according to SLN distribution and metastatic status might be feasible even for the patients who underwent ESD prior to surgery.

Nonexposed Endoscopic Wall-Inversion Surgery Plus SLN Biopsy (Video 7.1)

In current function-preserving surgery such as laparoscopic local resection or segmental gastrectomy, the approach of gastrectomy is only from the outside of the stomach, in which the demarcation line of the tumor cannot be visualized at the line of resection. Therefore, the surgeon cannot limit resection of the stomach to prevent a positive surgical margin. The recent introduction of a new technique, referred to as nonexposed endoscopic wall-inversion surgery (NEWS), is a technique of partial gastric resection, which can minimize the extent of gastric

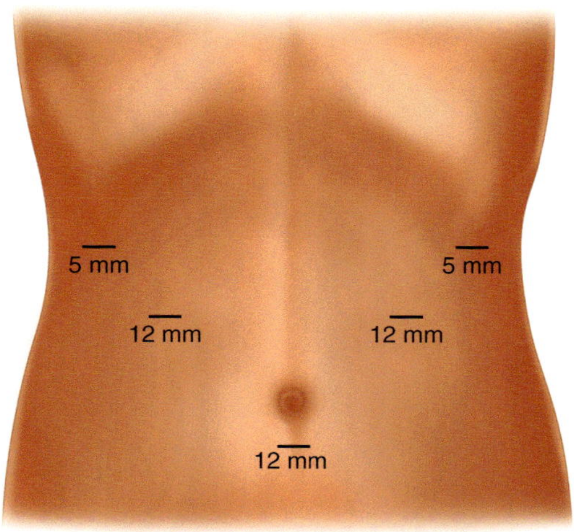

Fig. 7.3 Trocar/port placement for laparoscopic function-preserving gastrectomy with sentinel lymphatic basin dissection

resection using endoscopic and laparoscopic surgery without opening the gastric wall to treat gastric cancer. During this procedure, a gastrotomy penetrating the full stomach wall is not created, and cancer cells, which are on the mucosal surface, would be neither touched nor disseminated to the peritoneum. The NEWS is thought to be useful to prevent the peritoneal dissemination of cancer cells [23]. We have been accumulating cases of NEWS with laparoscopic SLN biopsy for early gastric cancer with the risk of lymph node metastasis in our clinical trial [23–25].

In brief, under general anesthesia, one camera port at the umbilicus and four trocars were inserted for laparoscopic surgery at four quadrants of the upper left, upper right, lower left, and lower right, respectively (Figs. 7.3 and 7.4) [23]. Subsequently, the primary lesion was clearly observed by conventional endoscopy, narrow band imaging with magnifying endoscopy, and chromoendoscopy to demarcate the tumor margin and to decide the resection area, and several circumferential mucosal markings of the primary tumor were placed approximately 5–10 mm outside the lesion using the tip of a 2.0-mm Dual knife (KD-650 L; Olympus Medical Systems,

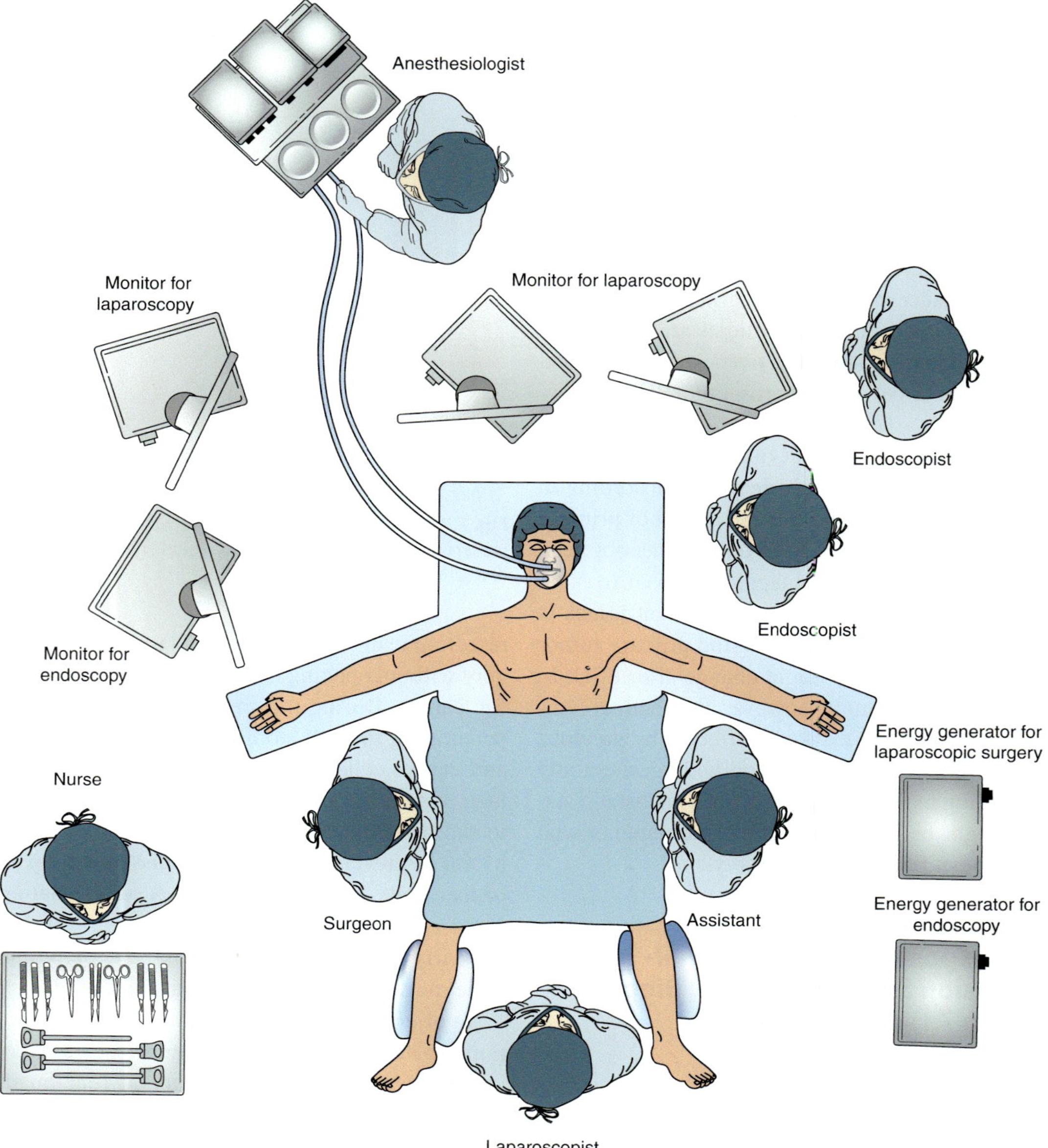

Fig. 7.4 Patient positioning and operating room setup

Co., Ltd., Tokyo, Japan). After placing mucosal markings, ICG was injected endoscopically into the submucosa around the lesion to examine SLNs (Figs. 7.5 and 7.6a–k) [23]. The SLN basin including hot or stained SLNs was dissected, and an intraoperative pathological diagnosis con-firmed that no metastasis had occurred. Subsequently, NEWS was performed for the primary lesion (Fig. 7.6f–k) [23].

In the placing of serosal markings using a spatula-type electrode (A6284; Olympus), mucosal markings were protruded toward the outer side

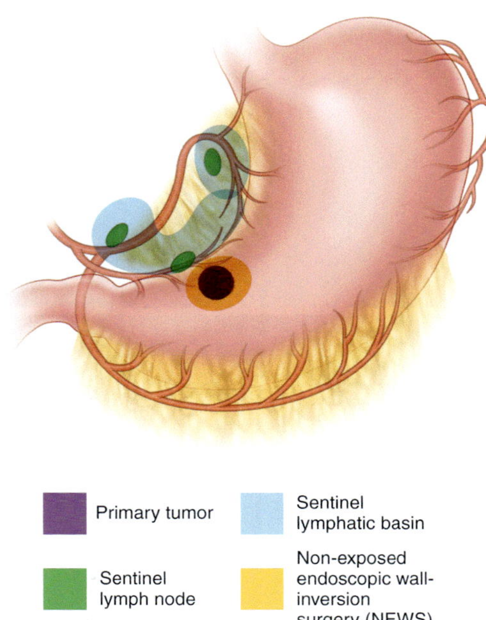

Fig. 7.5 Nonexposed endoscopic wall-inversion surgery (NEWS) with SLN mapping and sentinel lymphatic basin dissection. ESD, endoscopic submucosal dissection

using the Dual knife for the laparoscopist to recognize the location of these markings. A transparently visible shadow of the device from the opposite side was also used to make the serosal markings. Sodium hyaluronate solution (MucoUp; Seikagaku Corporation, Tokyo, Japan) with a small amount of ICG was additionally injected endoscopically into the submucosal layer around the circumference of the primary lesion, followed by a laparoscopic circumferential seromuscular incision 5 mm outside the serosal markings. In order to avoid perforating the mucosa from the outside, the seromuscular layer was cut carefully up to the level of the submucosa stained with green. After deeper cutting of the submucosa toward the outer side to create a flap, the seromuscular layers were linearly sutured, with the lesion inverted toward the inside of the stomach. On the way to the suturing, a laparoscopic surgical sponge (Securea; Hogy Medical Co., Ltd., Tokyo, Japan) that was cut elliptically according to the size of the lesion was inserted between the serosal layer of the inverted lesion and the suture layer, in order to provide a counter-traction to the mucosa and to prevent cutting the suture during the subsequent endoscopic procedure. Finally, the circumferential mucosal and submucosal incision was made endoscopically 5 mm outside of the mucosal markings around the inverted lesion using the Dual knife, while the inserted spacer was dug out. The detached primary lesion and the sponge were retrieved perorally, and the mucosal edges were closed with several endoscopic clips (HX-610-90 L; Olympus). After confirming no air leakage by pooling with normal saline on the serosal side of the suture, endoscopy and laparoscopic devices were withdrawn and scars were sutured (Fig. 7.6f–k).

The NEWS combined with laparoscopic SLN biopsy can minimize not only the area of lymphadenectomy but also the extent of gastric resection with full-thickness partial gastrectomy for patients with negative SLNs [24, 25]. Furthermore, NEWS does not require iatrogenic perforation of the stomach, which enables us to apply this technique to cancers without risk of cancer dissemination. The combination of NEWS with laparoscopic SLN biopsy is expected to become a promising, minimally invasive, function-preserving surgery to cure cases of cN0 early gastric cancer.

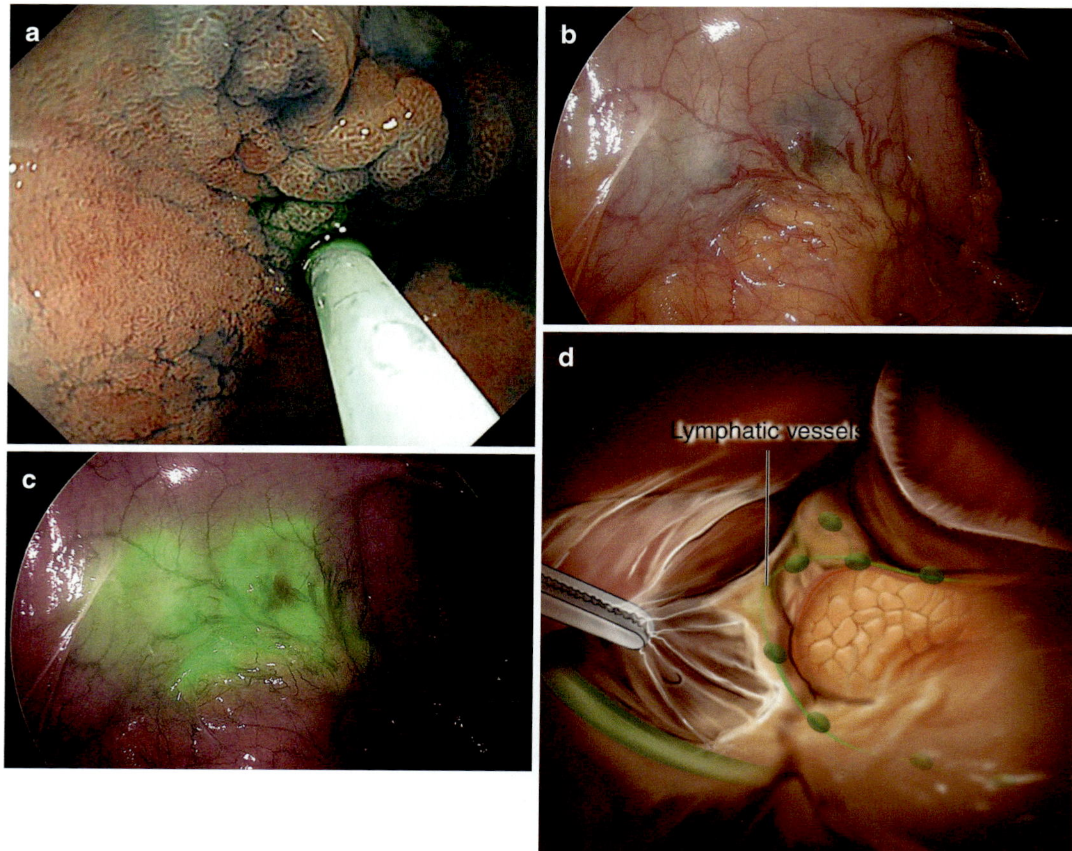

Fig. 7.6 Technique for nonexposed endoscopic wall-inversion surgery (NEWS) with SLN biopsy and sentinel lymphatic basin dissection. (**a**) Indocyanine green (ICG) was endoscopically injected into the gastric submucosal layer surrounding the primary tumor, (**b**) laparoscopic observation of ICG with normal light, (**c**) observation of ICG with infrared ray electronic endoscopy, (**d**) illustration showing ICG within lymphatic vessels and a sentinel lymph node, (**e**) paired intraoperative image showing that infrared ray electronic endoscopy can clearly visualize SNs and lymphatics, (**f**) serosal markings on the primary tumor, (**g**) laparoscopic seromuscular incision around the circumference of the lesion, (**h**, **i**) laparoscopic seromuscular suturing for closure of the circumferential incision and inversion of the primary lesion, (**j**) endoscopic circumferential mucosal incision, and (**k**) endoscopic retrieval of the primary tumor

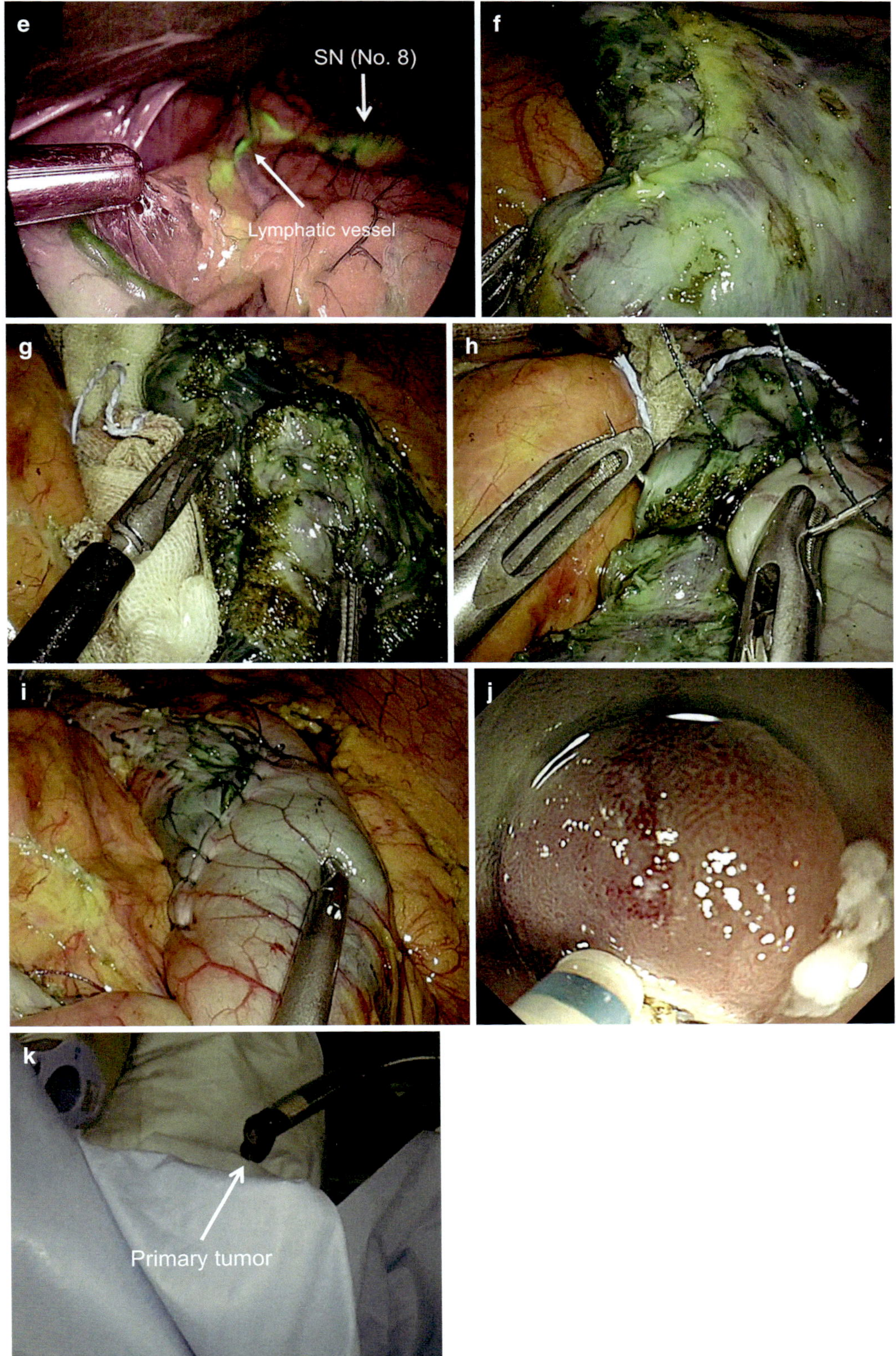

Fig. 7.6 (continued)

Conclusion

For early-stage gastric cancer, the establishment of individualized, minimally invasive treatments that may retain the patients' QOL should be the next surgical challenge. Although further studies are needed for careful validation, function-preserving gastrectomy such as full-thickness partial gastrectomy along with minimally invasive SLN navigation surgery could be a promising strategy for this goal.

References

1. Sano T, Hollowood K. Early gastric cancer. Diagnosis and less invasive treatments. Scand J Surg. 2006;95:249–55.
2. Kitano S, Iso Y, Moriyama M, Sugimachi K. Laparoscopy-assisted Billroth I gastrectomy. Surg Laparosc Endosc. 1994;4:146–8.
3. Adachi Y, Shiraishi N, Shiromizu A, et al. Laparoscopy-assisted Billroth I gastrectomy compared with conventional open gastrectomy. Arch Surg. 2000;135:806–10.
4. Shinohara T, Kanaya S, Taniguchi K, et al. Laparoscopic total gastrectomy with D2 lymph node dissection for gastric cancer. Arch Surg. 2009;144:1138–42.
5. Kim YW, Baik YH, Yun YH, et al. Improved quality of life outcomes after laparoscopy-assisted distal gastrectomy for early gastric cancer: results of a prospective randomized clinical trial. Ann Surg. 2008;248:721–7.
6. Kitagawa Y, Fujii H, Mukai M, et al. The role of the sentinel lymph node in gastrointestinal cancer. Surg Clin North Am. 2000;80:1799–809.
7. Morton DL, Wen DR, Wong JH, et al. Technical details of intraoperative lymphatic mapping for early stage melanoma. Arch Surg. 1992;127:392–9.
8. Giuliano AE, Kirgan DM, Guenther JM, et al. Lymphatic mapping and sentinel lymphadenectomy for breast cancer. Ann Surg. 1994;220:391–401.
9. Bilchik AJ, Saha S, Wiese D, et al. Molecular staging of early colon cancer on the basis of sentinel node analysis: a multicenter phase II trial. J Clin Oncol. 2001;19:1128–36.
10. Kitagawa Y, Takeuchi H, Takagi Y, et al. Sentinel node mapping for gastric cancer: a prospective multicenter trial in Japan. J Clin Oncol. 2013;31:3704–10.
11. Takeuchi H, Kitagawa Y. New sentinel node mapping technologies for early gastric cancer. Ann Surg Oncol. 2013;20:522–32.
12. Kinami S, Fujimura T, Ojima E, et al. PTD classification: proposal for a new classification of gastric cancer location based on physiological lymphatic flow. Int J Clin Oncol. 2008;13:320–9.
13. Tajima Y, Murakami M, Yamazaki K, et al. Sentinel node mapping guided by indocyanine green fluorescence imaging during laparoscopic surgery in gastric cancer. Ann Surg Oncol. 2010;17:1787–93.
14. Ishikawa K, Yasuda K, Shiromizu T, et al. Laparoscopic sentinel node navigation achieved by infrared ray electronic endoscopy system in patients with gastric cancer. Surg Endosc. 2007;21:1131–4.
15. Nimura H, Narimiya N, Mitsumori N, et al. Infrared ray electronic endoscopy combined with indocyanine green injection for detection of sentinel nodes of patients with gastric cancer. Br J Surg. 2004;91:575–9.
16. Miyashiro I, Miyoshi N, Hiratsuka M, et al. Detection of sentinel node in gastric cancer surgery by indocyanine green fluorescence imaging: comparison with infrared imaging. Ann Surg Oncol. 2008;15:1640–3.
17. Wang Z, Dong ZY, Chen JQ, et al. Diagnostic value of sentinel lymph node biopsy in gastric cancer: a meta-analysis. Ann Surg Oncol. 2012;19:1541–50.
18. Takeuchi H, Saikawa Y, Kitagawa Y. Laparoscopic sentinel node navigation surgery for early gastric cancer. Asian J Endosc Surg. 2009;2:13–7.
19. Takeuchi H, Oyama T, Kamiya S, et al. Laparoscopy-assisted proximal gastrectomy with sentinel node mapping for early gastric cancer. World J Surg. 2011;35:2463–71.
20. Takeuchi H, Kitagawa Y. Sentinel node navigation surgery in patients with early gastric cancer. Dig Surg. 2013;30:104–11.
21. Park JY, Kim YW, Ryu KW, et al. Assessment of laparoscopic stomach preserving surgery with sentinel basin dissection versus standard gastrectomy with lymphadenectomy in early gastric cancer-A multicenter randomized phase III clinical trial (SENORITA trial) protocol. BMC Cancer. 2016;16:340.
22. Mayanagi S, Takeuchi H, Kamiya S, et al. Suitability of sentinel node mapping as an index of metastasis in early gastric cancer following endoscopic resection. Ann Surg Oncol. 2014;21:2987–93.
23. Goto O, Takeuchi H, Kawakubo H, et al. First case of non-exposed endoscopic wall-inversion surgery with sentinel node basin dissection for early gastric cancer. Gastric Cancer. 2015;18:440–5.
24. Takeuchi H, Kitagawa Y. Sentinel lymph node biopsy in gastric cancer. Cancer J. 2015;21:21–4.
25. Takeuchi H, Goto O, Yahagi N, et al. Function-preserving gastrectomy based on the sentinel node concept in early gastric cancer. Gastric Cancer. 2017;20(Suppl 1):53–9.

Vanessa Palter, Laz Klein, and Natalie Coburn

Introduction

Gastric cancer is highly fatal with an overall 5-year survival of approximately 30–50% [1–3]. In North America, gastric cancer tends to be detected at a later stage than in Asia; with stage at presentation, variations in adherence to surgical guidelines and tumor biology likely lead to poor overall survival. In Japan and Korea, survival is much higher reflecting earlier detection through population-based screening and a more aggressive surgical approach. Stage-matched series show that through appropriate surgical technique, Western surgeons are able to achieve surgical outcomes equivalent to Asian series [4–7].

Surgical resection, either alone or in combination with chemotherapy and/or radiation, offers

Electronic Supplementary Material The online version of this chapter (https://doi.org/10.1007/978-3-030-18740-8_8) contains supplementary material, which is available to authorized users.

V. Palter (✉)
St. Michael's Hospital, Toronto, ON, Canada
e-mail: paltervane@smh.ca

L. Klein
Department of General Surgery,
University of Toronto, Toronto, ON, Canada
e-mail: l.klein@utoronto.ca

N. Coburn
Sunnybrook Health Science Centre,
Toronto, ON, Canada
e-mail: Natalie.Coburn@sunnybrook.ca

the only possibility of cure for gastric cancer. The extent of resection for gastric adenocarcinoma is determined by the location of the tumor in the stomach, the stage at presentation, and the need to obtain microscopically negative margins. The majority of tumors in the antrum and pylorus can be adequately resected with a distal or subtotal gastrectomy, whereas lesions proximal to this, diffuse histology, or patients with familial gastric cancer often require total gastrectomy [8, 9].

Minimally invasive approaches for gastrectomy offer several advantages over the open approach including less blood loss, decreased analgesia requirements, fewer wound complications, and shorter hospital stay, yet at the cost of longer operative time [10, 11]. In early gastric cancers (EGC), which are cancers limited to the mucosa or submucosa regardless of lymph node status, it is well established that laparoscopic distal gastrectomy offers several short-term advantages over the open technique with equivalent lymph node harvest, morbidity, and perioperative mortality [12, 13–15]. EGC has a predicted lymph node involvement of 5% for mucosal cancers and 20% for submucosal cancers, with series from Japan and Korea having a 5-year overall survival of EGC of over 95% [16–19]. Although the final 5-year results from the KLASS-01 trial, a randomized controlled trial (RCT) comparing laparoscopic to open distal gastrectomy for clinical stage 1 gastric cancer, are not yet published, the interim results are encouraging. In Asia, laparoscopic distal gastrectomy for EGC, which represents up to 57% of all gastric cancers, is routinely performed [9, 14, 20].

The role of laparoscopic gastrectomy for more advanced tumors has not yet been established. The KLASS-2 trial, an ongoing Korean multi-institutional RCT, seeks to provide large-scale prospective data to help answer this question for distal tumors [21]. Tumors included in the KLASS-2 trial include cT2-T4a lesions, with at most limited perigastric nodal metastases [21]. Data from retrospective studies investigating patients with more advanced gastric cancer, however, are encouraging. A recent case-matched study investigating total gastrectomy for gastric cancer in over 3000 patients demonstrated no difference in long-term survival rates between laparoscopic and open conventional gastrectomy [22]. In addition, several nonrandomized studies support both the oncologic and clinical safety of laparoscopic D2 lymphadenectomy for advanced gastric cancer [10, 12, 23–28].

As surgeon experience grows both in Asia and North America, there is interest in applying minimally invasive techniques to total gastrectomy for both early and advanced gastric cancer. Creating the anastomosis and performing D2 lymph node dissection are significantly more technically demanding for total gastrectomy than for distal gastrectomy [10]. With experience, however, the results seem promising. Several meta-analyses comparing laparoscopic to open gastrectomy for advanced gastric cancer showed no statistical difference in overall survival and disease-free survival between the laparoscopic and open groups [29, 30]. In addition, a single-institution retrospective study assessing 336 patients who received either open or laparoscopic gastrectomy with D2 lymph node dissection for advanced gastric cancer showed no difference in morbidity, survival, or pattern of recurrence [31]. In Asia, other published studies have shown comparable 5-year survival rates for laparoscopic gastrectomy to open gastrectomy [32, 33]. The results from the KLASS-03 trial, a large-scale RCT comparing open to laparoscopic total gastrectomy for early gastric cancer, will provide additional critical information to help with patient selection for this technically demanding operation [34].

As evidence and experience in minimally invasive techniques develop, minimally invasive gastrectomy appears to be an attractive option for appropriately selected cases. This chapter will discuss appropriate patient selection and learning curve of the procedure, the technique of laparoscopic gastrectomy with D2 lymphadenectomy, and considerations for postoperative management.

Learning Curve

Several earlier studies have assessed the learning curve of laparoscopic distal gastrectomy. Using a composite score looking at postoperative complications, operating room time, as well as adequacy of lymph node dissection, Jin et al. showed a learning curve of approximately 40 cases [35]. Moreover, Kunisaki et al. demonstrated that outcomes for laparoscopic distal gastrectomy approached that of open distal gastrectomy after 60 cases [36]. There is little data in the literature regarding the learning curve for laparoscopic total gastrectomy. In a study assessing 256 sequential laparoscopic total gastrectomies at a single institution, Jung et al. describe a learning curve of 100 cases, after which point operative time and blood loss stabilize [37]. Interestingly, in this study, when assessing lymph node harvest as the outcome, learning curves seem somewhat shorter, with a significant improvement in lymph node retrieval rate between the first 33 cases compared to the next 21 cases [37]. A second study assessing 203 sequential laparoscopic total gastrectomies for early gastric cancer among two surgeons showed a slightly shorter learning curve of approximately 45 cases [38].

These aforementioned studies are limited by the fact that they do not describe the surgeons' experience with open gastrectomy, nor their experience with other advanced minimally invasive operations. Additionally, they do not report oncologic outcomes. Since an examination of the learning curve for open gastrectomy suggests that oncologic outcomes are improved after 100 cases, short- and long-term outcomes should be examined for programs incorporating a new technique, such as laparoscopic gastrectomy for cancer [39]. Finally, to date, all learning curve data are from Asia where both open and laparoscopic surgeries for gastric cancer are performed more frequently than in North America. Some of these centers perform 700–1000 gastrectomies annually, by a team of surgeons with fellowship training in gastric cancer, while the median annual number of gastrectomies reported in the National Cancer Database (NCDB) is 9 [40]. In the Western context where tumors are more advanced, patients tend to have a higher body mass index and less favorable anatomy, and surgeons have less laparoscopic experience with gastrectomy for cancer, the learning curve is likely to be more significant.

There is data suggesting that robotic gastrectomy may have a shorter learning curve compared to laparoscopic gastrectomy. In a single-institution study, the learning curve for robotic surgery was between 12 and 14 cases for two experienced surgeons, each of whom had performed more than 250 laparoscopic gastrectomies [41]. This learning curve is shorter than that described by others with learning curves between 20 and 25 cases [42–44]. In all situations, however, these reported learning curves apply to surgeons who have significant experience with both open and laparoscopic gastrectomy.

Exposure to this procedure, not just as a surgeon but also as an assistant, has been shown to shorten the learning curve for the procedure. A Japanese study demonstrated that surgical trainees who had assisted in over 60 cases, either as the camera operator or as the first assistant, had learning curves shortened to 6 cases (while under the assistance of an experienced surgeon) [45]. In addition, in an educational system where trainees had significant exposure to laparoscopic gastrectomy, there was no difference in morbidity, blood loss, or lymph node harvest when comparing cases at the early and late phases of the learning curve [46]. Training opportunities either through assisting in the operating room or in simulated environments, therefore, have potential to shorten the learning curve for this technically demanding procedure.

Patient Selection

Appropriate patient selection is essential when deciding whether to perform laparoscopic or open gastrectomy for adenocarcinoma. Although the only patient-related contraindication for the procedure is inability to tolerate pneumoperitoneum, other patient factors should be considered including experience of the surgeon, location of the tumor, and degree of lymph node dissection. Indeed, especially when surgeons are in the early phase of their experience, selecting patients with few medical comorbidities, low body mass index, and small early tumors is critical.

Preoperative Planning and Diagnostic Laparoscopy

Prior to surgical intervention for gastric cancer, patients should have a complete work-up. At minimum, this includes upper endoscopy and biopsy of the tumor and CT scan of the chest and abdomen and pelvis to assess for T stage, the potential for nodal involvement, and for metastatic disease. Endoscopic ultrasound may be of benefit to differentiate between early and more advanced lesions. A meta-analysis, which included 5601 patients, demonstrated that endoscopic ultrasound had good sensitivity and specificity (0.86 and 0.91, respectively) to differentiate between T1 and T2 lesions with T3 and T4 tumors [47]. The accuracy of the endoscopic ultrasound, however, is highly operator dependent and likely related to the volume performed, which is very institution dependent, especially in the West where gastric cancer is infrequently assessed using endoscopic techniques.

Frequently, preoperative imaging is inaccurate in advanced gastric cancer and can miss radiologically occult metastatic disease [48]. Therefore, if a patient has no evidence of metastatic disease on imaging, has T3 or T4, or nodal involvement, then we recommend performing staging laparoscopy with peritoneal washings for cytology. This approach is supported by various national and society guidelines including Cancer Care Ontario (CCO), Society of American

Gastrointestinal and Endoscopic Surgeons (SAGES), and the Scottish Intercollegiate Guidelines Network (SIGN) [49, 50]. Positive cytology at diagnostic laparoscopy is a significant predictor of mortality and is defined as pM1 disease [51]. If peritoneal deposits or positive cytology are identified at diagnostic laparoscopy and the patient has no symptom, the REGATTA RCT demonstrated that chemotherapy provides equivalent survival with fewer complications compared to resection [52].

Technique of Diagnostic Laparoscopy

For diagnostic laparoscopy, the patient is positioned in the supine position with arms extended and padded appropriately. A minimum number of ports are placed (one camera port and either one or two working ports). The camera port (12 mm) is created using an open Hassan technique at the umbilicus. The working ports (5 mm) are in the right upper and left upper quadrant, respectively. Once pneumoperitoneum is established, then the abdominal cavity is systematically inspected for any signs of metastatic disease. The pelvis, liver, right and left paracolic gutters, greater and lesser omentum, as well as transverse mesocolon are all systematically assessed. If the tumor is located on the posterior wall of the stomach, then the gastrocolic omentum is opened and the retrogastric space assessed. If any lesions are identified that are concerning metastatic disease, they are biopsied and sent for pathological analysis. If ascites is identified, then it is sampled and sent for cytology.

Washings for cytology are then performed. Warmed normal saline (250 ml) is infused sequentially into the left upper quadrant, right upper quadrant, and pelvis. The patient is gently agitated after each infusion of warmed saline to allow contact over all organs and tissues. Saline (30 ml) is then sequentially collected from each area and sent separately for cytology. Once pathological analysis has confirmed no metastatic disease, then we plan for definitive surgery.

Patient Positioning and Operating Room Setup for Laparoscopic Gastrectomy

The patient is positioned supine on a split-leg table. The arms are extended from the body and secured on arm boards or tucked at the sides of the patient. All pressure points are padded. Safety straps ensure that the patient is secured to the table, and footboards are used to avoid the patient sliding when in reverse Trendelenburg position. Monitors for the laparoscopic camera are positioned near the patient's head.

Various positions for the surgeon and assistants have been described. These include (1) the surgeon operating from between the legs, the first assistant on the patient's right side, and the second assistant holding the camera on the patient's left side or (2) the camera operator standing between the patient's legs, the surgeon initially standing on the patient's left side with the first assistant on the right side, and then the surgeon switching to the patient's right side as the case progresses [53–55] (Fig. 8.1). We prefer the latter approach as it gives the greatest amount of flexibility.

Port Placement

Access to the abdomen is gained either via Veress needle technique under the left costal margin or via open Hassan technique at the superior aspect of the umbilicus [55]. Pneumoperitoneum is then established. Various port placement strategies have been described; however, general principles include having the camera port just superior to the umbilicus and working ports approximately 5 cm or a hands-breadth apart. Our practice is to place the camera just superior to the umbilicus through a Hassan port, place a 5/12-mm right upper quadrant port and a 5/12-mm left upper quadrant port, and then place two more 5-mm ports. One in the left upper quadrant and one in the right upper quadrant (Fig. 8.2). We place a liver retractor (Nathanson) through a small

Fig. 8.1 Patient positioning and operating room setup

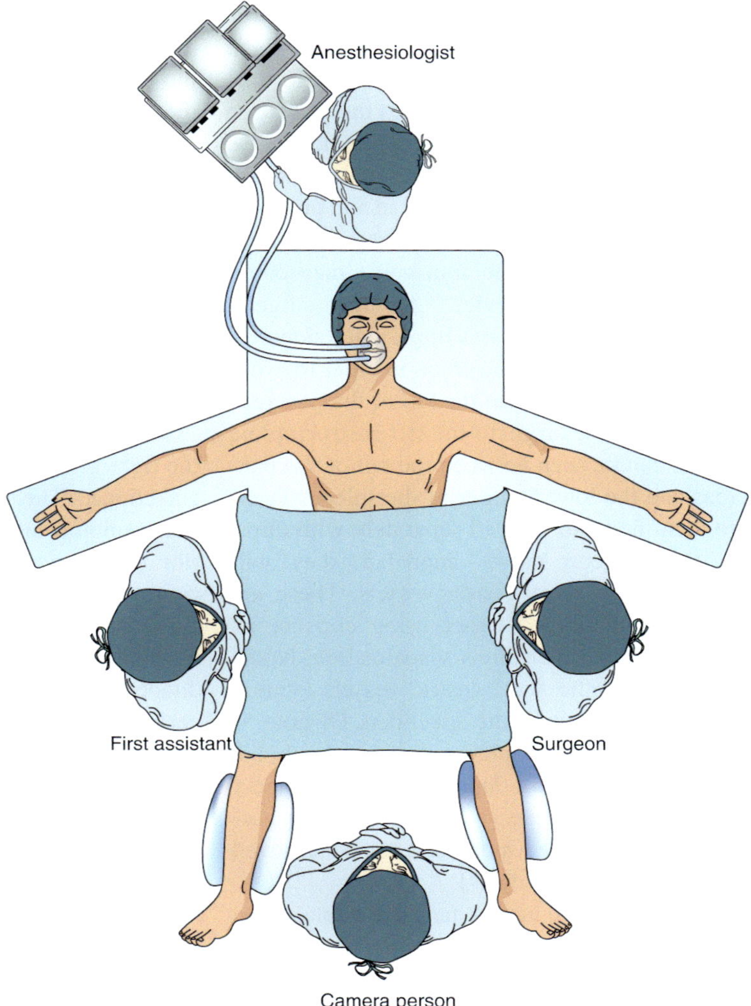

incision just under the xyphoid process and use this to retract the liver during the operation. Alternatively, the liver can be suspended with a sponge over a suture, bringing it up to the anterior abdominal wall [56].

Gastrocolic Omentum and Station 4sb and 4sa Lymph Nodes

After diagnostic laparoscopy to ensure no metastatic disease, definitive resection commences (Video 8.1). The patient is placed in reverse Trendelenburg position. The assistant retracts the transverse colon inferiorly, and the surgeon retracts the greater omentum cephalad using

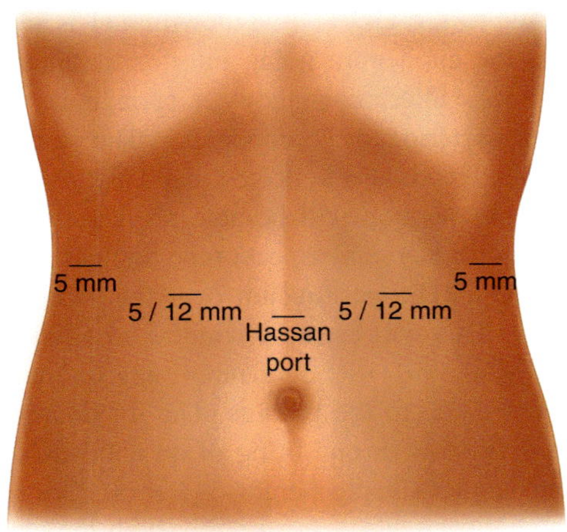

Fig. 8.2 Trocar/port placement for laparoscopic total gastrectomy

atraumatic bowel graspers. Using hook electrocautery, the surgeon incises the avascular plane between the colon and greater omentum, thus entering the lesser sac. Entry into the lesser sac is usually around the midpoint of the transverse mesocolon. The surgeon then retracts the stomach and greater omentum cephalad and proceeds toward the spleen taking down the attachments of the omentum to the transverse mesocolon using an energy device. As the surgeon approaches the spleen, it is important to identify the splenic flexure of the colon in order to avoid inadvertent injury. Once the tail of the pancreas is identified, the origin of the left gastroepiploic vessels can be seen between the tail of the pancreas and the lower border of the spleen. These are identified and divided separately with clips. As the surgeon moves cephalad, they will encounter the short gastric vessels. These are isolated and divided either using clips or an energy device under direct visualization. Nodal tissue around the short gastric vessels (station 4sa) is included with the specimen. Of note, if there is clinical suspicion for involved 4sb nodes, then the 2014 Japanese Gastric Cancer Association guidelines advocate for total gastrectomy even if the lesion itself can be removed with distal gastrectomy [9].

Dissection continues as far as possible to the left crus of the diaphragm. Without performing a splenectomy, it can be very technically challenging for station 10 nodes (splenic hilar nodes) to be included with the specimen due to the complex and variable anatomy of the splenic vessels. Should a complete station 10 lymphadenectomy be required for tumor factors, then local technical expertise should be taken into consideration when deciding whether or not to perform a spleen-preserving procedure. Our practice is to perform a splenectomy if we plan to include a complete station 10 lymphadenectomy in our dissection.

Greater Curve, Right Gastroepiploic Vessels, and Station 4d and 6 Lymph Nodes

The surgeon then reverses direction and continues the omentectomy toward the patient's right side. The stomach continues to be retracted cephalad and the transverse colon retracted caudally. The surgeon continues to take the omentum off the transverse colon mesentery working toward the gallbladder, thus including nodal tissue along the greater curvature of the stomach (station 4d).

Posterior attachments of the stomach to the anterior surface of the pancreas are divided as the surgeon moves toward the pylorus. This maneuver facilitates anterior retraction of the stomach and exposes the second part of the duodenum and head of the pancreas. This step is facilitated by gentle traction on the pancreas with a small sponge.

In order to retrieve infra-pyloric nodal tissue, the right gastroepiploic vein is cleared at its root and clipped. Then the same is done with the right gastroepiploic artery. If possible, the anterosuperior pancreaticoduodenal vein is identified to confirm the limit of dissection for station 6 nodal tissue. Nodal tissue is then meticulously removed from the head of pancreas working up toward the duodenum and infra-pyloric area. Dissection is performed keeping in mind the borders of the station 6 nodal area (the first branch of the right gastroepiploic artery, the lower border of the pancreas, and the anterosuperior pancreaticoduodenal vein).

Division of Duodenum

The gastroduodenal artery (GDA) is identified as it travels posterior to the duodenum. Staying anterior to the GDA, a window/tunnel is made under the duodenum going inferior to superior. From this inferior window, a sponge is then placed posterior to the duodenum. The stomach and duodenum are reflected caudally. At this point, the surgeon will be able to visualize the sponge on the cranial aspect of the first part of the duodenum. The peritoneum over the sponge is incised. This will create a window to allow for the division of the duodenum approximately 1–2 cm distal to the pylorus. The duodenum is then divided with one firing of an endovascular linear stapler (staple height 3–4 mm). Prior to duodenal transection, ensure that both the nasogastric tube and temperature probe (if inserted by anesthesia) have been removed. Our practice is to oversew the duodenal stump.

Right Gastric Vessels and Station 5 Lymph Nodes

After the duodenum is divided, the stomach is retracted caudally. The hepatoduodenal ligament is dissected, and the pars flaccida is opened. Carefully follow the GDA from where it was identified posterior to the first part of the duodenum and trace it to the hepatic artery proper. The left lateral aspect of the hepatic artery proper is exposed, and the root of the right gastric artery is identified as it comes off the hepatic artery proper. Clip and divide the right gastric artery at its origin.

Left Gastric Vessels and Station 7, 9, and 11 Nodes

Retract the stomach superiorly and cranially to patient's right side. Incise the peritoneum over the superior border of the pancreas with the assistant retracting the pancreas caudally with a sponge. Using a closed instrument, the assistant gently retracts the pedicle containing the left gastric vessels. The left gastric vein will be visualized at the intersection of the common hepatic artery and the splenic artery. We clear the left gastric vein and divide it at the point of drainage into the portal or splenic vein. Then we continue the dissection toward the patients' left side and carefully dissect nodal tissue from the proximal portion of the splenic artery and vein (11p) using an energy device. We clear soft tissue from around the left gastric artery (station 7) and isolate and clip it at its origin. Proceed toward the hiatus posteriorly on the stomach clearing station 9 nodes.

We clear the splenic vessels going toward the splenic hilum (including nodal station 11d). In over 50% of patients, there is a posterior gastric artery originating from the splenic artery. Be cognizant of this anatomy and identify and divide it formally if present or the surgeon risks running into troublesome bleeding.

Computed tomography (CT) scans should be reviewed preoperatively to determine if there is an accessory or replaced left hepatic artery. If possible, the surgeon should attempt to preserve these during the D2 dissection. This necessitates avoiding dividing the left gastric artery at its ori-gin; however, studies have shown that nodal harvest is equivalent if the accessory or replaced vessel is skeletonized and preserved [57].

Lesser Curve and Station 12 and 8a Nodes

Staying on the GDA and the divided right gastric artery, clear off the anterior surface of the hepatic artery proper, reflecting nodal tissue to the specimen and to the patient's left-hand side. Be mindful of the portal vein posteriorly. This step will enable inclusion of station 12a lymph nodes with the specimen. Continue reflecting nodal tissue toward the patient's left side and clear station 8a nodes (from the anterior aspect of the common hepatic artery) with the specimen.

Hiatal Dissection and Station 1 and 2 Lymph Nodes

At this point, the only remaining attachments of the stomach are at the hiatus. The pericardial lymph nodes (stations 1 and 2) are resected en bloc with the specimen. Station 2 lymph nodes should be preserved if performing subtotal gastrectomy. The anterior fat pad of the distal esophagus is cleared and the esophagus circumferentially dissected. The esophagus is then divided with one firing of an endovascular linear stapler. The specimen is either placed into an appropriately sized endocatch bag (usually 15 cm) or it can be removed from the abdomen after extending the supra-umbilical port site or by creating a Pfannenstiel incision. Margins are sent for frozen section analysis dependent upon tumor type and location.

Reconstruction

Laparoscopic reconstruction from total gastrectomy is made with a Roux-en-Y esophagojejunostomy. This is a technically challenging anastomosis and can be classified as intra- or extracorporeal and further classified as a side-to-side anastomosis with linear staplers or end-to-side anastomosis with circular staplers.

Intracorporeal End-to-Side Anastomosis

Our preference is the intracorporeal end-to-side anastomosis with the transorally inserted Anvil (OrVil, Medtronic). Following esophageal transection, the OrVil tube (consisting of a nasogastric tube attached to an anvil) is inserted transorally. Once the tube reaches the esophageal stump, an esophagotomy is made on the stump using electrocautery. The nasogastric tube is delivered through the esophagotomy and the anvil thus deployed in the distal esophagus. The nasogastric tube is cut from the anvil and removed from the abdominal cavity. The temperature probe and nasogastric tube should be removed from the esophagus prior to placement of the OrVil device.

A loop of jejunum from the ligament of Treitz that comes up easily to the esophageal stump is chosen. The jejunum is then divided with a linear stapler. The staple line is then removed with electrocautery and four stay sutures placed around the open roux limb. The 5/12-mm port in the left upper quadrant is upsized and the EEA stapler inserted through the abdominal wall. Using the stay sutures, the open end of the small bowel is manipulated over the stapler. After the end-to-side anastomosis is created intracorporeally with the jejunum in an antecolic position (Fig. 8.3), the circular stapler is withdrawn and the jejunal stump is closed laparoscopically with an endolinear stapler.

The jejuno-jejunostomy is then performed in the usual fashion, choosing a point approximately 40–60 cm distal from the esophagojejunostomy to prevent bile reflux. The anastomosis is made with one firing of a linear stapler, and then the common enterotomy is sewn closed. The resulting mesenteric defects are conventionally sutured closed to prevent internal hernias.

Postoperative Care

In general, we do not recommend nasogastric tube or intraperitoneal drainage tubes [58]. Patients may begin clear fluids on postoperative day one. As the patient progresses, their diet is advanced to a post-gastrectomy diet. Dietician referral and counseling regarding post-gastrectomy diet is helpful prior to discharge. We do not routinely perform gastrograffin swallow to evaluate for a leak if a patient is clinically well. Should there be clinical concern for a leak, however, prompt resuscitation and CT scan with oral contrast or an oral contrast study is required. After discharge, close follow-up to ensure adequate nutrition and supplementation for vitamin B12, iron, and calcium are indicated as required [59].

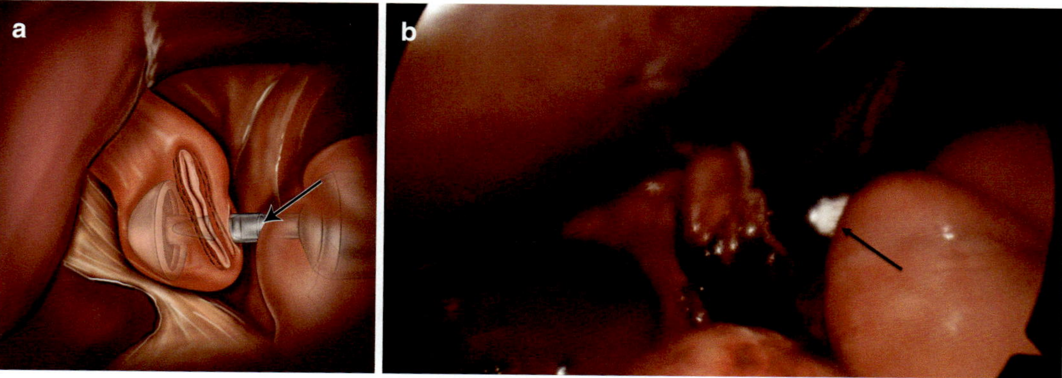

Fig. 8.3 (**a**) Illustration of the EEA stapler within the Roux limb. The trocar/pin of the EEA stapler is attached to the anvil within the distal esophagus. (**b**) Paired intra-operative image showing the white base of the anvil (black arrow) attached to the trocar/pin of the EEA stapler

References

1. Kim JP. Surgical results in gastric cancer. Semin Surg Oncol. 1999;17(2):132–8.
2. McCulloch P, Nita ME, Kazi H, et al. Extended versus limited lymph nodes dissection technique for adenocarcinoma of the stomach. Cochrane Database Syst Rev. 2003;(4):1–33.
3. Ferro A, Peleteiro B, Malvezzi M, et al. Worldwide trends in gastric cancer mortality (1980–2011), with predictions to 2015, and incidence by subtype. J Cancer. 2014;50(7):1330–44.
4. Cascinu S, Labianca R, Barone C, et al. Adjuvant treatment of high-risk, radically resected gastric cancer patients with 5-fluorouracil, leucovorin, cisplatin, and epidoxorubicin in a randomized controlled trial. J Natl Cancer Inst. 2007;99(8):601–7.
5. Noguchi M. Racial factors cannot explain superior Japanese outcomes in stomach cancer. Arch Surg. 1997;132(1):99.
6. Strong VE, Russo A, Yoon SS, et al. Comparison of young patients with gastric cancer in the United States and China. Ann Surg Oncol. 2017;24(13):3964–71.
7. Krijnen P, Dulk den M, Meershoek-Klein Kranenbarg E, et al. Improved survival after resectable non-cardia gastric cancer in The Netherlands: the importance of surgical training and quality control. Eur J Surg Oncol. 2009;35(7):715–20.
8. Lewis FR, Mellinger JD, Hayashi A, et al. Prophylactic total gastrectomy for familial gastric cancer. Surgery. 2001;130(4):612–7; discussion 617–9.
9. Japanese Gastric Cancer Association. Japanese gastric cancer treatment guidelines 2014 (ver. 4). Gastric Cancer. 2016;20(1):1–19.
10. Son T, Hyung WJ. Laparoscopic gastric cancer surgery: current evidence and future perspectives. World J Gastroenterol. 2016;22(2):727–35.
11. Viñuela EF, Gonen M, Brennan MF, et al. Laparoscopic versus open distal gastrectomy for gastric cancer: a meta-analysis of randomized controlled trials and high-quality nonrandomized studies. Ann Surg. 2012;255(3):446–56.
12. Huscher CGS, Mingoli A, Sgarzini G, et al. Laparoscopic versus open subtotal gastrectomy for distal gastric cancer: five-year results of a randomized prospective trial. Ann Surg. 2005;241(2):232–7.
13. Aoyama T, Yoshikawa T, Hayashi T, et al. Randomized comparison of surgical stress and the nutritional status between laparoscopy-assisted and open distal gastrectomy for gastric cancer. Ann Surg Oncol. 2014;21(6):1983–90.
14. Kim W, Kim HH, Han SU, et al. Decreased morbidity of laparoscopic distal gastrectomy compared with open distal gastrectomy for stage I gastric cancer: short-term outcomes from a multicenter randomized controlled trial (KLASS-01). Ann Surg. 2016;263(1):28–35.
15. Sakuramoto S, Yamashita K, Kikuchi S, et al. Laparoscopy versus open distal gastrectomy by expert surgeons for early gastric cancer in Japanese patients: short-term clinical outcomes of a randomized clinical trial. Surg Endosc. 2013;27(5):1695–705.
16. An JY, Baik YH, Choi MG, et al. Predictive factors for lymph node metastasis in early gastric cancer with submucosal invasion: analysis of a single institutional experience. Ann Surg. 2007;246(5):749–53.
17. Lai JF, Kim S, Kim K, et al. Prediction of recurrence of early gastric cancer after curative resection. Ann Surg Oncol. 2009;16(7):1896–902.
18. Strong VE, Song KY, Park CH, et al. Comparison of disease-specific survival in the United States and Korea after resection for early-stage node-negative gastric carcinoma. J Surg Oncol. 2013;107(6):634–40.
19. Kitano S, Shiraishi N, Uyama I, et al. A multicenter study on oncologic outcome of laparoscopic gastrectomy for early cancer in Japan. Ann Surg. 2007;245(1):68–72.
20. Shimizu S, Tada M, Kawai K. Early gastric cancer: its surveillance and natural course. Endoscopy. 1995;27(1):27–31.
21. Hur H, Lee HY, Lee HJ, et al. Efficacy of laparoscopic subtotal gastrectomy with D2 lymphadenectomy for locally advanced gastric cancer: the protocol of the KLASS-02 multicenter randomized controlled clinical trial. BMC Cancer. 2015;15(1):355.
22. Kim HH, Han SU, Kim MC, et al. Long-term results of laparoscopic gastrectomy for gastric cancer: a large-scale case-control and case-matched Korean multicenter study. J Clin Oncol. 2016;32(7):627–33.
23. Du XH, Li R, Chen L, et al. Laparoscopy-assisted D2 radical distal gastrectomy for advanced gastric cancer: initial experience. Chin Med J. 2009;122:1404–7.
24. Hur H, Jeon HM, Kim W. Laparoscopy-assisted distal gastrectomy with D2 lymphadenectomy for T2b advanced gastric cancers: three years's experience. J Surg Oncol. 2008;98(7):515–9.
25. Hwang Il S, Kim HO, Yoo CH, et al. Laparoscopic-assisted distal gastrectomy versus open distal gastrectomy for advanced gastric cancer. Surg Endosc. 2009;23(6):1252–8.
26. Cai J, Wei D, Gao CF, et al. A prospective randomized study comparing open versus laparoscopy-assisted D2 radical gastrectomy in advanced gastric cancer. Dig Surg. 2011;28(5–6):331–7.
27. Strong VE, Devaud N, Allen PJ, et al. Laparoscopic versus open subtotal gastrectomy for adenocarcinoma: a case–control study. Ann Surg Oncol. 2009;16(6):1507–13.
28. Wei HB, Wei B, Qi CL, et al. Laparoscopic versus open gastrectomy with D2 lymph node dissection for gastric cancer: a meta-analysis. Surg Laparosc Endosc Percutan Tech. 2011;21(6):383–90.
29. Choi YY, Bae JM, An JY, et al. Laparoscopic gastrectomy for advanced gastric cancer: are the long-term

results comparable with conventional open gastrectomy? A systematic review and meta-analysis. J Surg Oncol. 2013;108(8):550–6.

30. Zou ZH, Zhao LY, Mou TY, et al. Laparoscopic vs open D2 gastrectomy for locally advanced gastric cancer: a meta-analysis. World J Gastroenterol: WJG. 2014;20(44):16750–64.

31. Shinohara T, Satoh S, Kanaya S, et al. Laparoscopic versus open D2 gastrectomy for advanced gastric cancer: a retrospective cohort study. Surg Endosc. 2013;27(1):286–94.

32. Park DJ, Han S-U, Hyung WJ, et al. Long-term outcomes after laparoscopy-assisted gastrectomy for advanced gastric cancer: a large-scale multicenter retrospective study. Surg Endosc. 2012;26(6):1548–53.

33. Lee JH, Ahn SH, Park DJ, et al. Laparoscopic total gastrectomy with D2 lymphadenectomy for advanced gastric cancer. World J Surg. 2012;36(10):2394–9.

34. Cho GS. Laparoscopy-assisted total gastrectomy for clinical stage I gastric cancer (KLASS-03). ClinicalTrials.Gov. https://clinicaltrials.gov/ct2/show/NCT01584336. Accessed 30 Nov 2017.

35. Jin SH, Kim DY, Kim H, et al. Multidimensional learning curve in laparoscopy-assisted gastrectomy for early gastric cancer. Surg Endosc. 2007;21(1):28–33.

36. Kunisaki C, Makino H, Yamamoto N, et al. Learning curve for laparoscopy-assisted distal gastrectomy with regional lymph node dissection for early gastric cancer. Surg Laparosc Endosc Percutan Tech. 2008;18(3):236–41.

37. Do Hyun Jung SSY, Park YS, et al. The learning curve associated with laparoscopic total gastrectomy. Gastric Cancer. 2016;19(1):264–72.

38. Jeong O, Ryu SY, Choi WY, et al. Risk factors and learning curve associated with postoperative morbidity of laparoscopic total gastrectomy for gastric carcinoma. Ann Surg Oncol. 2014;21(9):2994–3001.

39. Kim CY, Nam BH, Cho GS, et al. Learning curve for gastric cancer surgery based on actual survival. Gastric Cancer. 2016;19(2):631–8.

40. Enzinger PC, Benedetti JK, Meyerhardt JA, et al. Impact of hospital volume on recurrence and survival after surgery for gastric cancer. Ann Surg. 2007;245(3):426–34.

41. Zhou J, Shi Y, Qian F, et al. Cumulative summation analysis of learning curve for robot-assisted gastrectomy in gastric cancer. J Surg Oncol. 2015;111(6):760–7.

42. Yang SY, Roh KH, Kim YN, et al. Surgical outcomes after open, laparoscopic, and robotic gastrectomy for gastric cancer. Ann Surg Oncol. 2017;24(7):1770–7.

43. Huang KH, Lan YT, Fang WL, et al. Initial experience of robotic gastrectomy and comparison with open and laparoscopic gastrectomy for gastric cancer. J Gastrointest Surg. 2012;16(7):1303–10.

44. Park SS, Kim MC, Park MS, et al. Rapid adaptation of robotic gastrectomy for gastric cancer by experienced laparoscopic surgeons. Surg Endosc. 2012;26(1):60–7.

45. Nunobe S, Hiki N, Tanimura S, et al. The clinical safety of performing laparoscopic gastrectomy for gastric cancer by trainees after sufficient experience in assisting. World J Surg. 2013;37(2):424–9.

46. Tokunaga M, Hiki N, Fukunaga T, et al. Learning curve of laparoscopy-assisted gastrectomy using a standardized surgical technique and an established educational system. Scand J Surg. 2011;100(2):86–91.

47. Mocellin S, Marchet A, Nitti D. EUS for the staging of gastric cancer: a meta-analysis. Gastrointest Endosc. 2011;73(6):1122–34.

48. Seevaratnam R, Cardoso R, McGregor C, et al. How useful is preoperative imaging for tumor, node, metastasis (TNM) staging of gastric cancer? A meta-analysis. Gastric Cancer. 2012;15(Suppl 1(S1)):S3–S18.

49. Hori Y, SAGES Guidelines Committee. Diagnostic laparoscopy guidelines: this guideline was prepared by the SAGES Guidelines Committee and reviewed and approved by the Board of Governors of the Society of American Gastrointestinal and Endoscopic Surgeons (SAGES), November 2007. Surg Endosc. 2008;22(5):1353–83.

50. Coburn N, Cosby R, Klein L, et al. A quality initiative of the program in evidence-based care (PEBC), Cancer Care Ontario (CCO); January 2017. https://www.cancercareontario.ca/sites/ccocancercare/files/guidelines/summary/pebc2-19s_0.pdf. Accessed 30 Nov 2017.

51. Ajani JA, Bentrem DJ, Besh S, et al. Gastric cancer, version 2.2013: featured updates to the NCCN Guidelines. J Natl Compr Cancer Netw. 2013;11(5):531–46.

52. Fujitani K, Yang HK, Mizusawa J, et al. Gastrectomy plus chemotherapy versus chemotherapy alone for advanced gastric cancer with a single non-curable factor (REGATTA): a phase 3, randomised controlled trial. Lancet Oncol. 2016;17(3):309–18.

53. Cassidy MR, Gholami S, Strong V. Minimally invasive surgery. Surg Oncol. 2017;26:193–212.

54. Kim J, Garcia-Aguilar J. In: Kim J, Garcia-Aguilar J, editors. Surgery for cancers of the gastrointestinal tract. New York: Springer; 2014.

55. Strong VE. In: Strong VE, editor. Gastric cancer. Cham: Springer; 2015.

56. Vargas-Palacios A, Hulme C, Veale T, et al. Systematic review of retraction devices for laparoscopic surgery. Surg Innov. 2016;23(1):90–101.

57. Kim HI, Han SU, Yang HK, et al. Multicenter prospective comparative study of robotic versus laparoscopic gastrectomy for gastric adenocarcinoma. Ann Surg. 2016;263(1):103–9.

58. Kim J, Lee J, Hyung WJ, et al. Gastric cancer surgery without drains: a prospective randomized trial. J Gastrointest Surg. 2004;8(6):727–32.

59. Nussbaum DP, Pappas TN, Perez A. Laparoscopic total gastrectomy in the western patient population: tips, techniques, and evidence-based practice. Surg Laparosc Endosc Percutan Tech. 2015;25(6):455–61.

Minimally Invasive Gastrectomy

9

Jenny Lam, Catherine Tsai, Santiago Horgan,
and Kaitlyn J. Kelly

Introduction

Utilization of minimally invasive approaches, including laparoscopic and robotic platforms, for resection of gastric cancer has been increasing rapidly in recent years. The benefit for patients of minimally invasive compared with open gastrectomy is improvement in short-term outcomes like narcotic requirements, time to return of bowel function, length of hospitalization, postoperative morbidity, and likelihood of receipt of adjuvant systemic therapy when indicated [1, 2].

There are a variety of techniques available for the different steps of the operation, such as gastric mobilization, lymphadenectomy, and reconstruction. Anastomoses can be performed by either intracorporeal or extracorporeal methods [3–5]. These include circular stapling, linear stapling, and hand-sewing, with or without construction of a jejunal pouch in cases of total gastrectomy. While no single technique has been shown to be superior, this chapter will provide a detailed description and video of the techniques adopted at a high-volume center for minimally invasive gastrectomy (MIG) in the USA. The majority of the procedure is performed laparoscopically, and the robot is utilized for the modified D2 lymphadenectomy.

Technical Aspects of Minimally Invasive Gastrectomy

Patient Positioning

MIG is performed with the patient positioned supine on a split-leg table with a bean bag or non-slip pad to prevent slippage with reverse Trendelenburg and Trendelenburg positioning. Patient arms can be tucked or left abducted on arm boards with appropriate padding of elbows and hands and other pressure points. The patient is secured to the table at the arms and calves with tape and at the thighs with safety straps. Once patient positioning is completed, it is important to place the patient in steep reverse Trendelenburg as a test to assure stability on the table (Fig. 9.1).

Port Placement

Port placement for MIG follows the same principles as for any laparoscopic or robotic procedure.

Electronic supplementary material The online version of this chapter (https://doi.org/10.1007/978-3-030-18740-8_9) contains supplementary material, which is available to authorized users.

J. Lam · C. Tsai · S. Horgan (⊠) · K. J. Kelly
Department of Surgery, Center for the Future of Surgery, University of California, San Diego, San Diego, CA, USA
e-mail: jel028@ucsd.edu; cat042@ucsd.edu; shorgan@ucsd.edu; k6kelly@ucsd.edu

© Springer Nature Switzerland AG 2020
J. Kim, J. Garcia-Aguilar (eds.), *Minimally Invasive Surgical Techniques for Cancers of the Gastrointestinal Tract*, https://doi.org/10.1007/978-3-030-18740-8_9

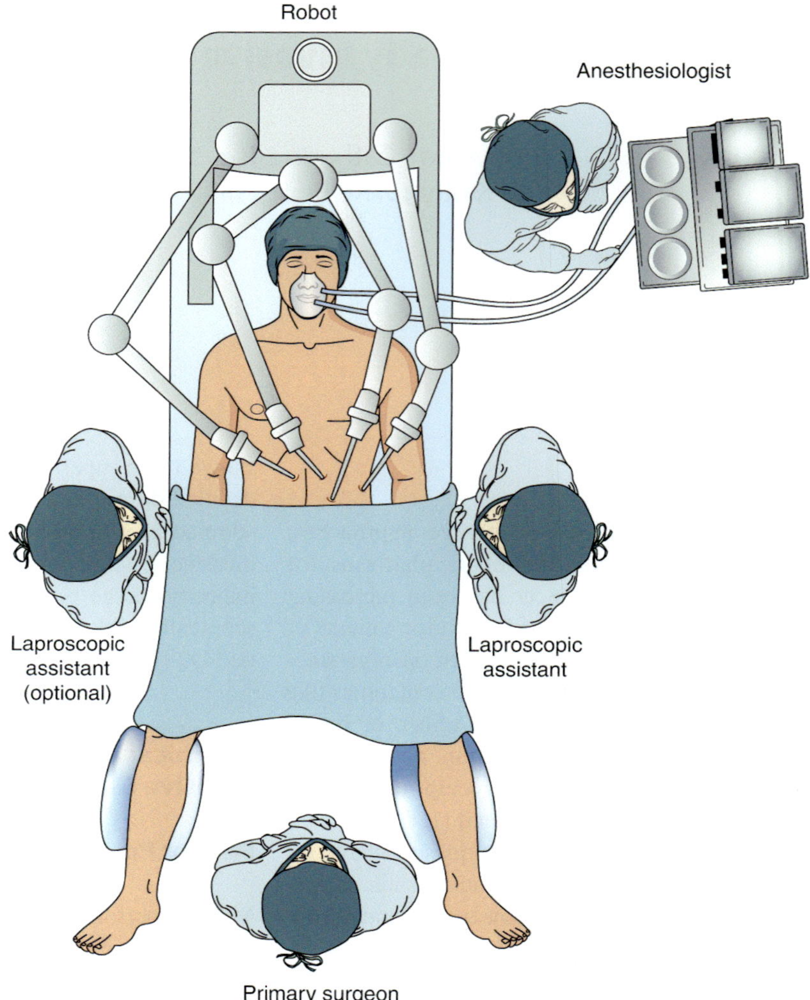

Fig. 9.1 Operating room setup for robotic gastrectomy

This includes placement of the camera port at a distance of 15–20 cm from the target anatomy and placement of ports 5–8 cm apart. Initial access is obtained with a 5-mm optical viewing trocar placed through the left rectus abdominus muscle approximately 1 inch cephalad and 1 inch left of the umbilicus. This port is later converted to a 12-mm port once the others are placed and is used for the camera. Two additional robotic ports are then placed on either side of and slightly cephalad to the camera port, both approximately 5–8 cm away from it. The one to the left of the camera port should be at about the level of the left mid-clavicular line or slightly lateral to it, and the one to the right of the camera port should

be at or slightly to the right of the midline of the abdomen. An additional 12-mm port is placed as far laterally as possible off the left costal margin. An optional additional 5- or 12-mm assistant port can be placed caudal to and between the left-sided robotic port and this left lateral port if necessary. A laparoscopic self-retaining retractor is placed in the epigastrium slightly to the left of the midline to retract the left lobe of the liver and expose the esophageal hiatus (Fig. 9.2).

The operating surgeon stands between the patient's legs and utilizes the two robotic ports. The first assistant stands on the patient's left side and uses the left lateral port. If available, an optional second assistant stands on the patient's

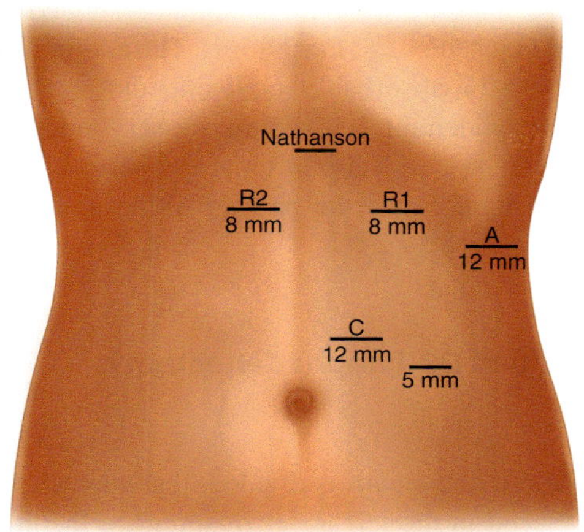

Fig. 9.2 Trocar/port placement for robotic gastrectomy

right side to hold the camera. This can alternatively be done by the first assistant.

Procedural Steps

Video 9.1

The abdomen is explored for adhesions and for evidence of peritoneal or other metastatic disease, although ideally patients would have had a previous staging laparoscopy with peritoneal washings to evaluate for metastatic disease. If the lesion is not appreciable on the extraluminal surface, an endoscope is passed to verify the location of the lesion. For gastroesophageal junction (GEJ) tumors, the distal esophagus and Z-line should be carefully examined to localize the proximal extent of the lesion. It is critical to ensure that an adequate esophageal resection margin (2–4 cm from the lesion) can be obtained from the transabdominal approach. Once this is confirmed, the patient is placed in reverse Trendelenburg position.

Mobilization of Greater Curvature and Partial Omentectomy

The procedure commences by identifying the gastroepiploic vessels coursing along the greater curvature of the stomach and incising the greater omentum approximately 1 inch from these vessels in a clear area to ensure that the level 4 perigastric lymph nodes remain with the specimen [6]. This can be done with hook cautery or an energy sealing device (ESD) such as the laparoscopic Harmonic Scalpel or Ligasure. Visualization of the posterior wall of the stomach confirms entry into the lesser sac. The posterior wall of the stomach is then grasped by the operating surgeon and retracted anteriorly and to the patient's right side. The assistant utilizes the left lateral port to provide counter-traction on the peri-splenic fatty tissues and splenic flexure. This dissection is carried out toward the spleen and short gastric vessels. The short gastric vessels are preserved when distal subtotal gastrectomy is being performed but are ligated with the ESD for total gastrectomy. This maneuver provides exposure up to the left crus of the diaphragm.

Hiatal Dissection for Total Gastrectomy

The peritoneum overlying the left crus is incised with cautery or ESD. Gentle blunt dissection is then performed between the crus and the posterolateral aspect of the esophagus. The edge of the left crus is dissected down to the level where crossing fibers from the right crus are seen. Attention is then turned to the lesser omentum. The pars flaccida is incised sharply or with hook cautery, and the lesser omentum is divided with ESD until the right diaphragmatic crus is visualized. The peritoneum overlying the right crus is then incised and opened up over the anterior aspect of the hiatus keeping the gastroesophageal fat pad with the specimen. Blunt dissection is then performed between the right crus and the esophagus to enter the mediastinum, and the aorta is identified.

Once this step is complete, a grasper is passed posteriorly behind the distal esophagus and a penrose drain is introduced via the left lateral 12-mm port. The penrose is secured around the distal esophagus with an Endoloop tie and is used for retraction. The distal esophagus is then mobilized for a short distance. The vagus nerves are divided both anteriorly and posteriorly with the ESD.

Mobilization of the Distal Stomach

Attention is turned back to the greater curvature. The posterior wall of the stomach is now grasped by the first assistant and is elevated. The posterior attachments between the stomach and pancreas are then divided sharply or with cautery in the direction of the pylorus. The gastrocolic ligament/greater omentum is incised in the direction of the origin of the right gastroepiploic vessels. Complete omentectomy is not routinely performed [7]. Once this area is reached, the vessels are identified and dissected circumferentially at the level of the superior border of the pancreas. The vessels are then ligated with clips or vascular stapler. It is for this portion of the operation where the additional optional assistant port placed caudally in the left mid abdomen may be helpful. The remaining fatty tissue between the proximal duodenum and colon mesentery is then divided until the wall of the duodenum is reached just distal to the pylorus.

Division of Proximal Duodenum

Attention is then turned toward the suprapyloric region. The previously made opening in the pars flaccida is carried over to the peritoneum overlying the porta hepatis with the ESD, and the right gastric artery is divided. The peritoneum and vascular tissue along the superior border of the duodenum are carefully divided. A laparoscopic gastric band passer can be useful at this point in the dissection to develop a window around the proximal duodenum for subsequent passage of a stapler. The lap band passer is placed under the proximal duodenum at the level where the inferior wall was cleared and is then flexed to bluntly develop the plain between the superior aspect of the duodenum and the underlying portal structures. An endovascular stapler with thick tissue (approx. 3.0 mm height) staple load is then intro-

duced, and the proximal duodenum is stapled and divided just distal to the pylorus. The authors prefer to use bioabsorbable staple line reinforcement on the duodenum. It is often necessary to temporarily change to a 5-mm laparoscope to use the 12-mm camera port for passage of the stapler for this step.

Modified D2-lymphadenectomy (D1 + β)

Once the duodenum is divided, the stomach can be placed in the left upper quadrant to facilitate exposure of the N2 lymph nodes [6]. The robot is docked at this time (directly over the patient's head for the Si system and from the patient's right side for the Xi system). In most cases, only two of the robot instrument arms are necessary. A fenestrated bipolar grasper is placed in the surgeon's left hand, and the hook cautery is placed in the right hand. The bedside assistant utilizes the left lateral 12-mm port for introducing the suction irrigator device or graspers to assist with retraction as needed.

The peritoneum overlying the proper hepatic artery is opened with the hook cautery starting in the region where the right gastric artery was divided previously. The fatty and nodal tissue from the left side of the porta hepatis is then carefully dissected away from the hepatic artery and portal vein (Fig. 9.3). Hook cautery is usually sufficient to control the small crossing vessels and lymphatics in this tissue. The peritoneum along the anterior border of the pancreas is then similarly incised with hook cautery, and the underlying hepatic artery lymph node and common hepatic artery are identified. The dissection is continued along the common hepatic artery toward the origin of the left gastric artery. The coronary, or left gastric, vein is encountered and is ligated with clips placed by the bedside assistant and is divided sharply. Once the left gastric artery is identified, the dissection is carried further to the patient's left side to clear the fatty and nodal tissue from the proximal aspect of the splenic artery. This tissue is swept up toward the specimen. It is helpful to

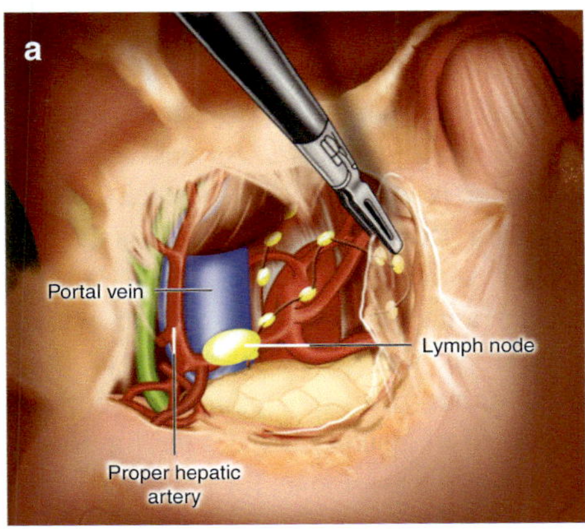

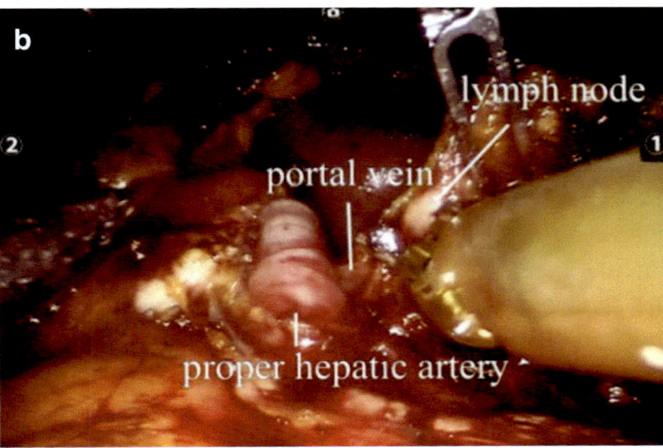

Fig. 9.3 (**a**) Illustration showing exposure of the proper hepatic artery and left lateral aspect of the portal vein. (**b**) Paired intraoperative image showing the starting point for modified D2-lymphadenectomy. The peritoneum overlying the porta hepatis was incised, and the fatty and nodal tissue from the left lateral aspect of the proper hepatic artery is swept over toward the specimen

ask the bedside assistant to elevate the stomach either directly or with the Penrose around the esophagus so that the left gastric artery is running straight up (i.e., anteriorly) and down (i.e., posteriorly). The artery is then circumferentially dissected and ligated with large clips or is stapled at its origin.

Division of Distal Esophagus or Proximal Stomach

If distal subtotal gastrectomy is being performed, the fatty and nodal tissue from the proximal stomach on the lesser curve side is dissected down off of the esophagus and stomach to the level where the stomach will be divided. This is done with hook cautery as there is usually minimal bleeding once the left gastric artery has been divided. This step is not necessary in total gastrectomy. At this point, the robot is undocked and the 8-mm robotic trocar on the patient's left side (corresponding to the surgeon's right hand working port) is upsized to a 12-mm trocar. The distal esophagus or proximal stomach is divided with a linear stapler depending on the extent of gastrectomy being performed. It is important to ensure that no orogastric or nasogastric tube or temperature probe is in place before stapling.

Reconstruction

In distal subtotal gastrectomy, an ante-colic Billroth II gastrojejunostomy is created if over one-half of the stomach is remaining and a Roux-en-Y gastrojejunostomy is preferred if less than one-half of the stomach remains. For total gastrectomy, a Roux-en-Y esophagojejunostomy is performed. The patient is placed in Trendelenburg position, and the transverse colon is elevated in a cephalad direction. The ligament of Treitz (LOT) is identified. A mobile piece of jejunum approximately 30–40 cm downstream from the LOT is selected based on mobility and tension-free reach to the gastric remnant or distal esophagus. For Billroth II reconstruction, the jejunum is sutured to the posterior wall of stomach at least 2 cm from the gastric staple line with two interrupted silk stay sutures. The bowel is oriented so that the afferent limb is on the patient's left side and the efferent limb is on the right. A marking suture is placed on the afferent aspect of the bowel to maintain orientation. Small enterotomies are then made in both the stomach and the jejunum at the efferent aspect of the anastomosis, and a linear stapler (60 mm preferred) is advanced into the lumens and fired. The remaining enterotomy from the staple passage is closed in a single layer with an absorbable barbed suture.

For Roux-en-Y esophagojejunostomy, a single quadrant technique is utilized to minimize the number of ports and repositioning required. Again, the bowel is brought into proximity to the divided distal esophagus as a continuous loop, so that the afferent limb is on the patient's left side and the efferent limb is on the right. A marking stitch is again placed on the afferent side between the esophagogastric or esophagojejunal anastomosis and the LOT. A trans-oral anvil (OrVil, Covidien) is then passed, usually by the anesthesiologist. Once the tip of the tubing is visible against the stapled off distal esophagus, a small hole is made in the esophagus with electrocautery to facilitate passage of the tubing through the wall of the esophagus. Care is taken to minimize contact between the contaminated tubing and the abdominal viscera. The tubing is grasped with a grasper and is pulled out of the abdomen via the 12-mm port. The tubing is then gently detached from the anvil by cutting the suture and is removed through the 12-mm port. A large enterotomy is then made at the anti-mesenteric border of the afferent limb of bowel, near the marking suture. The left lateral port site is then enlarged, and a circular stapler is passed directly through the abdominal wall and is advanced into the bowel through the enterotomy. It is advanced into the bowel, and a stapled, end-to-side esophagojejunostomy is created. The stapler is then removed keeping it closed as it is brought back out through the abdominal wall. A 15-mm port is then placed through that port site, and a penetrating towel clip is used to maintain pneumoperitoneum. Two reinforcing 2-0 silk sutures are then placed on either side of the esophagojejunal anastomosis.

Next, the Roux limb is run 50–70 cm distal to the esophagojejunal anastomosis, and a silk stay suture is placed between the afferent limb, proximal to the enterotomy, and the Roux limb at this site. These two loops of bowel should be directly adjacent to each other in the left upper quadrant. The tails of this stay suture are left long enough that they can be used for retraction. The first assistant grasps them and retracts the two bowel loops in the cephalad direction. Two small enterotomies are then made, and a linear 60-mm laparoscopic stapler is advanced into them. A side-to-side stapled anastomosis is created. The remaining enterotomy is closed in a single layer with a barbed absorbable suture. Lastly, the segment of bowel between the two anastomoses containing the enterotomy created for passage of the circular stapler is excised. For subtotal gastrectomy where a Roux-en-Y anastomosis is performed, this same technique is used, but the gastrojejunal anastomosis is performed with a linear stapler if the gastric remnant is large enough. In either case, an upper endoscopy is then performed to visually inspect the intraluminal aspect of the anastomosis for hemostasis and to assess for any leakage of insufflated air.

Specimen Retrieval

Both the segment of jejunum and the stomach are placed in a specimen bag and are removed from the abdomen via the left lateral port site that was enlarged for the circular stapler. The specimen extraction site is then thoroughly irrigated and the fascia usually closed with an open technique in two layers. If there is concern for margin positivity, the specimen can be removed earlier in the operation to allow for frozen section examination and the extraction site can be managed with a gel port or can be partially closed with interrupted sutures around a 12- or 15-mm trocar to allow for the reconstruction to be done after specimen removal.

Summary

Numerous variations in technique for laparoscopic and robotic gastrectomy for cancer have been described, with no single approach being clearly superior. In the approach described here, the majority of the procedure is performed laparoscopically with full mobility to visualize and work in the upper abdomen. The robot is utilized for the celiac lymphadenectomy where the wristed instrumentation and stable camera allow for a more precise dissection than what can be achieved with standard laparoscopy. The authors have found this technique to be safe and effective and to routinely result in adequate lymph node retrieval.

References

1. Kelly KJ, Selby L, Chou JF, et al. Laparoscopic versus open gastrectomy for gastric adenocarcinoma in the west: a case-control study. Ann Surg Oncol. 2015;22:3590–6.
2. Bao H, Xu N, Li Z, et al. Effect of laparoscopic gastrectomy on compliance with adjuvant chemotherapy in patients with gastric cancer. Medicine (Baltimore). 2017;96:e6839.
3. Shim JH, Yoo HM, Oh SI, et al. Various types of intracorporeal esophagojejunostomy after laparoscopic total gastrectomy for gastric cancer. Gastric Cancer. 2013;16:420–7.
4. Corcione F, Pirozzi F, Cuccurullo D, et al. Laparoscopic total gastrectomy in gastric cancer: our experience in 92 cases. Minim Invasive Ther Allied Technol: MITAT. 2013;22:271–8.
5. Liu XX, Jiang ZW, Chen P, et al. Full robot-assisted gastrectomy with intracorporeal robot-sewn anastomosis produces satisfying outcomes. World J Gastroenterol: WJG. 2013;19:6427–37.
6. Hartgrink HH, van de Velde CJ, Putter H, et al. Extended lymph node dissection for gastric cancer: who may benefit? Final results of the randomized Dutch gastric cancer group trial. J Clin Oncol. 2004;22:2069–77.
7. Jongerius EJ, Boerma D, Seldenrijk KA, et al. Role of omentectomy as part of radical surgery for gastric cancer. Br J Surg. 2016;103:1497–503.

Minimally Invasive Hyperthermic Intraperitoneal Perfusion for Gastric Cancer

10

Timothy E. Newhook and Brian Badgwell

Introduction

The peritoneum is the most common site of metastases in gastric cancer and also of recurrence after potentially curative gastrectomy [1]. While the long-term survival rates for localized gastric cancer treated with multimodality therapy are approximately 60%, patients with stage IV metastatic disease are unlikely to survive beyond a few years [2]. Current National Comprehensive Cancer Network treatment recommendations for gastric cancer metastatic to the peritoneum include systemic chemotherapy alone or best supportive care [3]. Of note, patients with positive peritoneal cytology obtained at staging laparoscopy are classified as having Stage IV incurable disease [4]. Staging laparoscopy identifies disease metastatic to the peritoneum, either carcinomatosis or positive cytology, in approximately 30% of gastric cancer patients that appear to have localized disease on imaging [5]. Therefore, a regional technique of treating gastric adenocarcinoma metastatic to the peritoneum is appealing and could expand treatment options beyond traditional systemic therapy. Hyperthermic intraperitoneal chemotherapy (HIPEC) has many theoretical advantages in the treatment of gastric cancer, but the true benefit remains a question to be answered in the context of a clinical trial. Minimally invasive HIPEC may offer advantages in decreasing complications and allowing for the repeated use of HIPEC. The purpose of this chapter is to review the technique of laparoscopic HIPEC and our experience based on recently completed and ongoing clinical trials.

Historical Perspective

Administration of cytotoxic chemotherapy directly to the peritoneum is an accepted approach to offer relatively high doses of chemotherapy while limiting systemic effects. Hyperthermia also offers several theoretical advantages such as increasing the depth of chemotherapy penetration, heat-associated synergistic effects with chemotherapy, and a direct antitumor effect. Heated peritoneal chemotherapy has demonstrated effectiveness in appendiceal tumors and mesothelioma and is considered a standard of care treatment option [6, 7]. There has been increasing interest in peritoneal therapy for carcinomatosis from colon, ovarian, and, recently, gastric origins. There have been 13 randomized trials of *adjuvant* intraperitoneal chemotherapy for gastric cancer, and a recent meta-analysis demonstrated improved OS. Collectively, these studies displayed 40% improvement in survival (hazard ratio = 0.60; 95% confidence ratio [CI], 0.43–0.83) for patients

T. E. Newhook · B. Badgwell (✉)
The University of Texas MD Anderson Cancer Center, Houston, TX, USA
e-mail: tnewhook@mdanderson.org;
bbadgwell@mdanderson.org

© Springer Nature Switzerland AG 2020
J. Kim, J. Garcia-Aguilar (eds.), *Minimally Invasive Surgical Techniques for Cancers of the Gastrointestinal Tract*, https://doi.org/10.1007/978-3-030-18740-8_10

treated with adjuvant HIPEC [8, 9]. Further investigations into HIPEC for gastric cancer are also supported by recent trials of HIPEC in combination with gastrectomy and cytoreduction, demonstrating improvements in survival [10]. However, the complications from gastrectomy and debulking are considerable, with a recent US clinical trial failing to accrue, stopping after enrollment of 17 patients (out of 136 planned), and reporting a 89% morbidity rate, 33% reoperative rate, and 11% mortality rate [11]. Therefore, methods to diminish complications are warranted and may be enhanced by a minimally invasive approach.

Background and Indications for Laparoscopic HIPEC in Gastric Cancer

The use of HIPEC for gastric cancer, particularly for patients with peritoneal carcinomatosis, has shown to positively influence survival for patients with poor prognoses [8, 9, 12]. However, there is considerable morbidity and mortality associated with this procedure. Data exists suggesting that laparoscopic HIPEC without cytoreduction and gastrectomy is a low-risk procedure. A recent systematic review of laparoscopic HIPEC, primarily for palliation of malignant ascites, suggested that this is a safe procedure, with no mortality and <10% morbidity in 183 patients [13]. There is also a relatively large experience from a single center in Japan with laparoscopic HIPEC followed by neoadjuvant bidirectional induction chemotherapy in gastric cancer [14]. In this strategy, laparoscopic HIPEC is performed following laparoscopic diagnosis, and patients continue to receive systemic therapy along with intraperitoneal administration of cytotoxic therapy, followed by cytoreductive surgery (CRS) and HIPEC for patients who have had a good response. Utilizing this strategy in 194 patients, 78% of patients proceeded to CRS and HIPEC with an almost 16-month median survival [15]. Laparoscopic HIPEC is a crucial component of this option for patients, as pathologic response to the neoadjuvant bidirectional therapy was an independent predictor of better prognosis.

Our group recently published the first completed trial of HIPEC in gastric cancer and also the first of laparoscopic HIPEC in the USA [16, 17]. Although the laparoscopic HIPEC procedure was associated with survival beyond that expected from previous reports for patients with peritoneal disease, any statement regarding survival benefit will require comparative analysis. Nonetheless, we were able to clearly demonstrate that the procedure was safe with a major morbidity rate of 3%, and no mortality in 38 procedures performed in 19 patients. Importantly, 26% of patients went on to undergo gastrectomy in this trial. Strategies affording these patients potential CRS, such as laparoscopic HIPEC, may lead to better survival with low morbidity.

Preoperative Work-Up

Patient preparation for laparoscopic HIPEC first requires similar preoperative workup undertaken for standard laparoscopic operations. Patient candidacy to tolerate general anesthesia and the systemic effects of pneumoperitoneum must be ascertained, including cardiopulmonary evaluation and electrocardiogram. A thorough surgical history, including previous operations that may preclude safe laparoscopic surgery due to adhesive disease, must be completed. Standard preoperative laboratory testing should be performed, including a complete blood count, metabolic panel, and coagulation indices.

Confirmation of the diagnosis of gastric adenocarcinoma, including a review of existing pathologic specimens should be performed to ascertain candidacy for laparoscopic HIPEC. Cross-sectional imaging of the abdomen and pelvis should be performed, most commonly via CT scan, as well as either CT scan of the chest or chest X-ray to identify nonperitoneal metastatic cancer. Once the diagnosis has been confirmed and degree of metastatic disease has been ascertained, if any, the operation may be offered to the patient.

Discussion regarding the risks and benefits of laparoscopic HIPEC should occur with patients, despite this typically being a low-risk procedure. Risks of general laparoscopy should be mentioned, along with the risks of anesthesia. Moreover, risks relating to the chemotherapeutic agent utilized for HIPEC should be discussed. Lastly, and perhaps most importantly, the risks of disease recurrence and the need for additional HIPEC procedures to control disease must be made clear to the patient and their caregivers.

Chemotherapy

A number of therapeutic strategies have been utilized in various studies of laparoscopic HIPEC. Currently, cytotoxic chemotherapeutic agents are used most often. Multiple investigators have reported single-agent or combination strategies of mitomycin C and cisplatin at varying dosages [17–20]. Also, 5-fluorouracil and oxaliplatin have also been used in the palliative setting for gastric cancer with laparoscopic HIPEC [21]. Yonemura and colleagues have reported extensively on laparoscopic HIPEC as part of a bidirectional chemotherapeutic strategy in the neoadjuvant setting for peritoneal metastases from gastric cancer utilizing a regimen of docetaxel and cisplatin, along with oral administration of S1 [22]. Reported studies can be reviewed in Table 10.1.

Table 10.1 Reported therapeutic regimen of laparoscopic HIPEC for gastric cancer

Study	Setting	Therapy
Badgwell [17]	Neoadjuvant	Mitomycin-C 30 mg, cisplatin 200 mg
Ba et al. [21]	Palliative	5-Fluorine 1.5 g, oxaliplatin 200 mg
Valle et al. [20]	Palliative	Mitomycin-C 12.5 mg/m^2
Facchiano et al. [19]	Palliative	Mitomycin-C 120 g/m^2, cisplatin 200 mg/m^2
Chang et al. [18]	Neoadjuvant	Mitomycin-C 8 mg/L perfusate, cisplatin 250 mg/m^2
Yonemura et al. [22]	Neoadjuvant	Docetaxel (30 mg/m^2), cisplatin (30 mg/m^2)

Port Placement and Operative Details

Following induction of general anesthesia and successful endotracheal intubation, the entire abdomen is prepped and draped. A Foley catheter is advised for accurate urine output. Pneumoperitoneum may be established in a fashion according to surgeon preference; however, our practice is direct entry via Hassan technique in the supraumbilical position. The abdomen is insufflated to 15 mm Hg, and diagnostic laparoscopy is performed to ascertain the extent of carcinomatosis or other metastatic disease. Patients may have undergone previous laparoscopy to diagnose their disease and thus may have prior port sites in the lateral abdominal wall. Bilateral, mid-abdominal 12-mm working ports are placed. Peritoneal washing is next performed for cytology, and biopsies are obtained from suspicious lesions.

Following the diagnostic phase of the operation, the bilateral working ports are exchanged for inflow and outflow catheters (Sorin, USA) and are placed under laparoscopic visualization as shown in Fig. 10.1. The patient's right port is utilized to position the outflow cannula into the patient's right upper quadrant over the liver

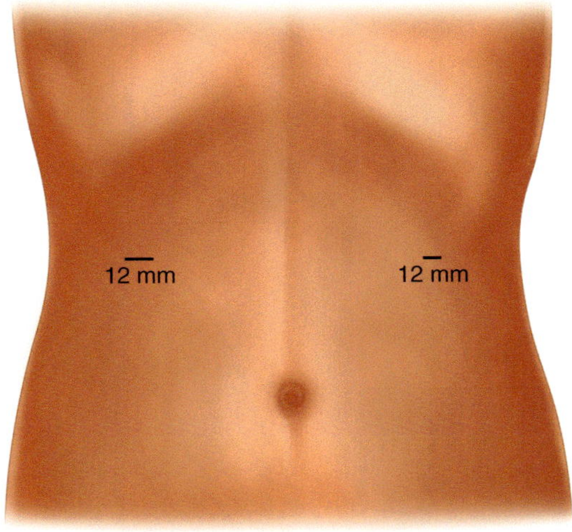

Fig. 10.1 Cannula placement for laparoscopic hyperthermic intraperitoneal perfusion with chemotherapy

(Fig. 10.2). An inflow cannula is placed into the patient's left upper quadrant, anterior to the stomach, via the patient's left-sided port.

To initiate HIPEC, crystalloid perfusate is then circulated using an extracorporeal circulation device (Medtronic COBE Century Heart Lung Machine, Minneapolis, MN, USA) at a flow rate of 700–1500 mL/min. Figure 10.3 demonstrates the operating room setup for HIPEC. Once the flow rate and outflow temperature are optimized (typically >39 °C), the appropriate chemotherapeutic agents are added to the peritoneal perfusion circuit. Target inflow temperatures are 41–42 °C, and target outflow temperatures are 39–40 °C. The abdomen is consistently manipulated over the course of 60 min to effectively distribute the perfusate (and chemotherapy) evenly throughout the abdomen.

After 60 min, abdominal washout is performed with 3 L of crystalloid solution. Pneumoperitoneum is then re-established, the peritoneal cavity is re-inspected, and any structures (typically, omentum)

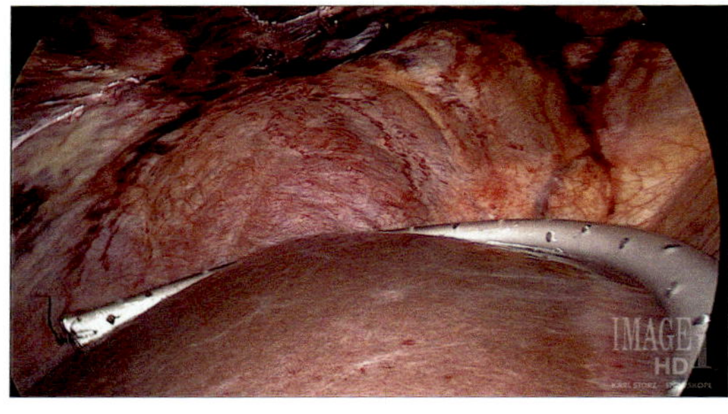

Fig. 10.2 Image demonstrating the location of the outflow cannula over the dome of the liver

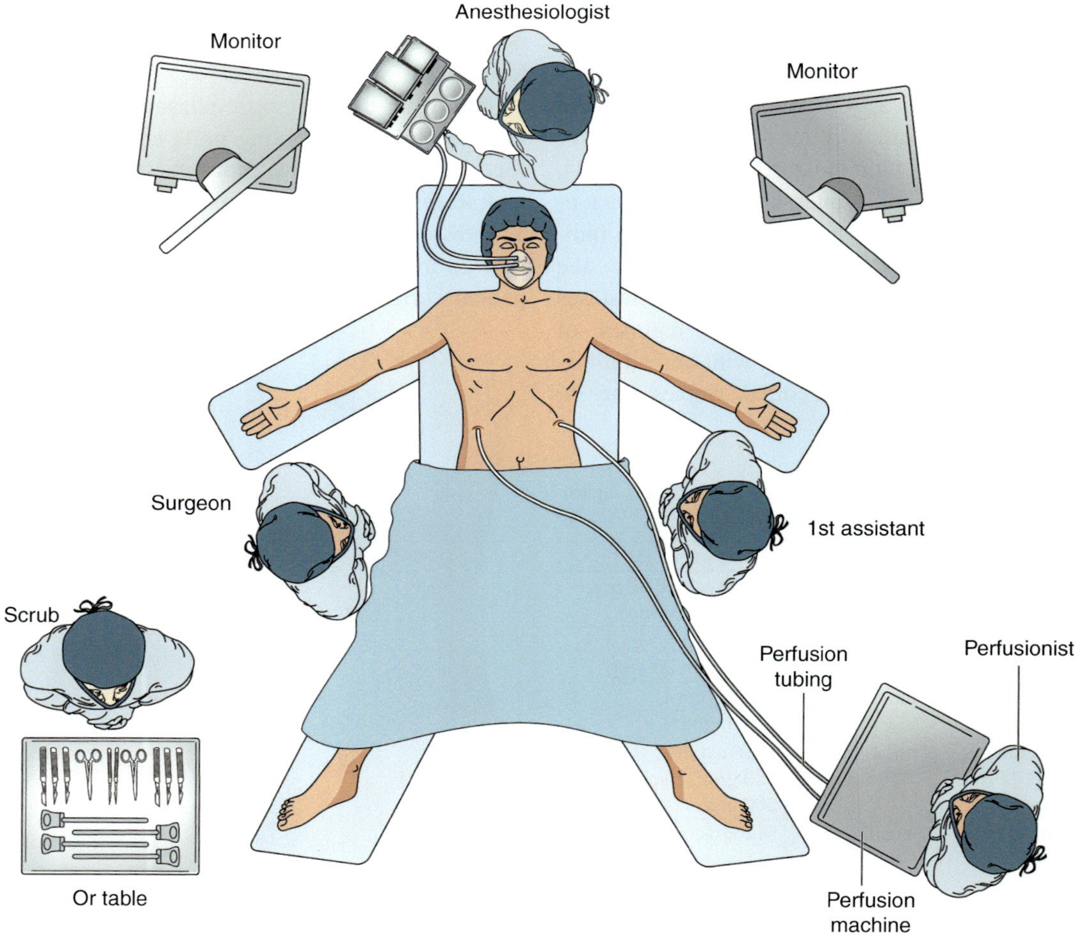

Fig. 10.3 Operating room setup for hyperthermic perfusion utilizing an extracorporeal circulation device

adherent to the cannulas are removed. Lastly, the cannulas are removed under direct visualization.

Perioperative Management and Complications

Patients typically receive a 1-L bolus of normal saline fluid preoperatively as prehydration in the holding area. To limit the systemic toxicity of cisplatin, a loading dose of 7.5 g/m^2 of sodium thiosulfate is given to the patient prior to addition of cisplatin to the perfusion circuit. Sodium thiosulfate 25.56 g/m^2 is administered as a continuous infusion over the next 12 h. As compared to traditional cytoreductive surgery and HIPEC for gastric cancer, patients require less resuscitative volume postoperatively, and thus, maintaining urine output greater than 30 cc/h is sufficient.

Patients should expect an approximate 2-day length of stay in the hospital following laparoscopic HIPEC for gastric cancer. A clear liquid diet beginning immediately postoperatively is advanced as tolerated quickly to regular over the subsequent 24 h. Careful attention must be paid to avoiding renal insufficiency via adequate resuscitation and maintenance of urine output.

The use of HIPEC may improve survival following resection for gastric cancer; however, an open approach following cytoreductive surgery has significant morbidity [8–11]. Benefits of laparoscopy, including lack of a large incision, lower postoperative pain, and faster recovery make laparoscopic HIPEC an attractive modality. Systematic review of the literature for laparoscopic HIPEC for any indication demonstrates an approximate 7% rate of complications, all of which were minor and not requiring reoperation [12]. Moreover, laparoscopic HIPEC is a low-risk operation for gastric cancer. In a randomized controlled phase II trial of laparoscopic HIPEC with mitomycin C and cisplatin following systemic therapy for patients with stage IV gastric cancer, the procedural complication rate was 11% with 0% 30-day mortality rate [17].

Results from our recently reported Phase II clinical trial show an overall complication rate of 11% for laparoscopic HIPEC covering 38 procedures in patients with peritoneal carcinomatosis or positive peritoneal cytology from gastric cancer [17]. Most complications were minor, including transient rise in creatinine and intraoperative arrhythmia.

Variation in Technique

Minimally invasive laparoscopic HIPEC is a relatively novel surgical procedure, and there are multiple variations of this technique among different centers, including varying strategies to deliver therapy locally to the peritoneum. Pressurized intraperitoneal aerosol chemotherapy (PIPAC) has been only very recently described as a novel technique to deliver chemotherapy to the peritoneum for patients with peritoneal metastases from gastric cancer [23]. In this technique, diagnostic laparoscopy is performed as previously described, followed by administration of pressurized aerosol of doxorubicin (1.5 mg/m^2) followed by cisplatin (7.5 mg/m^2). Utilizing this minimally invasive technique, a total of 24 patients underwent 60 PIPAC procedures with 50% of patients having an objective tumor response [23].

Further, laparoscopic HIPEC is a component of a recently reported protocol of neoadjuvant laparoscopic HIPEC followed by neoadjuvant intraperitoneal/systemic chemotherapy for patients with gastric cancer metastatic to the peritoneum [22]. Neoadjuvant laparoscopic HIPEC utilizing docetaxel and cisplatin (both 30 mg/m^2) is performed, followed by a series of 3-week cycles of docetaxel and cisplatin administration via a peritoneal port system (NIPS). Systemic therapy is administered in conjunction with NIPS in a bidirectional fashion. Patients then proceeded to undergo laparotomy and cytoreductive surgery. Utilizing this strategy, the Peritoneal Cancer Index score at the time of laparotomy was significantly lower than at the time of initial laparoscopic HIPEC; and 57.6% ($n = 30$) of patients subsequently underwent complete cytoreduction.

Summary

As the peritoneum is commonly involved in patients with metastatic gastric cancer, there is increasing support for direct delivery of chemotherapy to the peritoneum via HIPEC. Laparoscopic HIPEC allows patients to have their peritoneal disease treated directly yet avoid the typical high morbidity associated with HIPEC via laparotomy. Moreover, as laparoscopic HIPEC is a procedure that can be performed serially, eradication of low-volume peritoneal disease may lead to gastrectomy for some patients, as demonstrated in recent clinical trials. Laparoscopic HIPEC thus remains a safe and attractive option for patients with peritoneal carcinomatosis or positive peritoneal cytology from gastric cancer.

References

1. Ikoma N, Chen HC, Wang X, et al. Patterns of initial recurrence in gastric adenocarcinoma in the era of preoperative therapy. Ann Surg Oncol. 2017; 24:2679.
2. Badgwell B, Blum M, Estrella J, et al. Predictors of survival in patients with resectable gastric cancer treated with preoperative chemoradiation therapy and gastrectomy. J Am Coll Surg. 2015;221(1):83–90.
3. National Comprehensive Cancer Network Guidelines Version 1.2017. Gastric Cancer. Available at www.nccn.org. Accessed 1 May 2017.
4. Amin MB, et al., editors. American joint commission on cancer, staging manual, eighth edition. Stomach Cancer, p. 203–220.
5. Ikoma N, Blum M, Chiang YJ, et al. Yield of staging laparoscopy and lavage cytology for radiologically occult peritoneal carcinomatosis of gastric cancer. Ann Surg Oncol. 2016;23:4332.
6. Chua TC, Moran BJ, Sugarbaker PH, et al. Early- and long-term outcome data of patients with pseudomyxoma peritonei from appendiceal origin treated by a strategy of cytoreductive surgery and hyperthermic intraperitoneal chemotherapy. J Clin Oncol. 2012;30(20):2449–56.
7. Yan TD, Deraco M, Baratti D, et al. Cytoreductive surgery and hyperthermic intraperitoneal chemotherapy for malignant peritoneal mesothelioma: multi-institutional experience. J Clin Oncol. 2009;27(36):6237–42.
8. Yan TD, Black D, Sugarbaker PH, et al. A systematic review and meta-analysis of the randomized controlled trials on adjuvant intraperitoneal chemotherapy for resectable gastric cancer. Ann Surg Oncol. 2007;14(10):2702–13.
9. Sun J, Song Y, Wang Z, et al. Benefits of hyperthermic intraperitoneal chemotherapy for patients with serosal invasion in gastric cancer: a meta-analysis of the randomized controlled trials. BMC Cancer. 2012;12:526.
10. Yang XJ, Huang CQ, Suo T, et al. Cytoreductive surgery and hyperthermic intraperitoneal chemotherapy improves survival of patients with peritoneal carcinomatosis from gastric cancer: final results of a phase III randomized clinical trial. Ann Surg Oncol. 2011;18(6):1575–81.
11. Rudloff U, Langan RC, Mullinax JE, et al. Impact of maximal cytoreductive surgery plus regional heated intraperitoneal chemotherapy (HIPEC) on outcome of patients with peritoneal carcinomatosis of gastric origin: results of the GYMSSA trial. J Surg Oncol. 2014;110(3):275–84.
12. Gill RS, Al-Adra DP, Nagendran J, et al. Treatment of gastric cancer with peritoneal carcinomatosis by cytoreductive surgery and HIPEC: a systematic review of survival, mortality, and morbidity. J Surg Oncol. 2011;104(6):692–8.
13. Facchiano E, Risio D, Kianmanesh R, et al. Laparoscopic hyperthermic intraperitoneal chemotherapy: indications, aims, and results: a systematic review of the literature. Ann Surg Oncol. 2012;19(9):2946–50.
14. Yonemura Y, Canbay E, Li Y, et al. A comprehensive treatment for peritoneal metastases from gastric cancer with curative intent. Eur J Surg Oncol. 2016;42(8):1123–31.
15. Canbay E, Mizumoto A, Ichinose M, et al. Outcome data of patients with peritoneal carcinomatosis from gastric origin treated by a strategy of bidirectional chemotherapy prior to cytoreductive surgery and hyperthermic intraperitoneal chemotherapy in a single specialized center in Japan. Ann Surg Oncol. 2014;21(4):1147–52.
16. Badgwell B, Blum M, Das P, et al. Lessons learned from a phase II clinical trial of laparoscopic HIPEC for gastric cancer. Surg Endosc. 2018;32(1):512.
17. Badgwell B, Blum M, Das P, et al. Phase II trial of laparoscopic hyperthermic intraperitoneal chemoperfusion for peritoneal carcinomatosis or positive peritoneal cytology in patients with gastric adenocarcinoma. Ann Surg Oncol. 2017;24:3338.
18. Chang E, Alexander HR, Libutti SK, et al. Laparoscopic continuous hyperthermic peritoneal perfusion. J Am Coll Surg. 2001;193(2):225–9.
19. Facchiano E, Scaringi S, Kianmanesh R, et al. Laparoscopic hyperthermic intraperitoneal chemotherapy (HIPEC) for the treatment of malignant ascites secondary to unresectable peritoneal carcinomatosis from advanced gastric cancer. Eur J Surg Oncol. 2008;34(2):154–8.
20. Valle M, Van der Speeten K, Garofalo A. Laparoscopic hyperthermic intraperitoneal peroperative chemotherapy (HIPEC) in the management of refractory malignant ascites: a multi-institutional retrospective analysis in 52 patients. J Surg Oncol. 2009;100(4):331–4.

21. Ba MC, Cui SZ, Lin SQ, et al. Chemotherapy with laparoscope-assisted continuous circulatory hyperthermic intraperitoneal perfusion for malignant ascites. World J Gastroenterol. 2010;16(15):1901–7.
22. Yonemura Y, Ishibashi H, Hirano M, et al. Effects of neoadjuvant laparoscopic hyperthermic intraperitoneal chemotherapy and neoadjuvant intraperitoneal/ systemic chemotherapy on peritoneal metastases from gastric cancer. Ann Surg Oncol. 2017;24(2):478–85.
23. Nadiradze G, Giger-Pabst U, Zieren J, et al. Pressurized intraperitoneal aerosol chemotherapy (PIPAC) with low-dose cisplatin and doxorubicin in gastric peritoneal metastasis. J Gastrointest Surg. 2016;20(2):367–73.

Palanisamy Senthilnathan,
S. Srivatsan Gurumurthy, and C. Palanivelu

Introduction

Minimally invasive surgery, a widely adopted tool for most domains of gastrointestinal surgery, has been relatively slow to evolve in the field of pancreatic surgery. The reasons include proximity to the great vessels, retroperitoneal location, need for advanced intracorporeal suturing skills, and increased risk of complications associated with these procedures. With enormous development in surgical technology coupled with improved anatomical knowledge and refined skills, minimally invasive pancreatic surgery has grown out of its infancy and is an established speciality in hepatopancreatobiliary surgery today. As a result, the initial skepticism and reluctance associated with minimally invasive pancreatic resection have decreased, and many surgeons are now attempting to enter this difficult terrain [1–6]. Recent publications highlight potential advantages of minimally invasive pancreatic resection (MIPR) over open pancreatic resection (OPR) which include reduced pain, decreased blood loss and need for transfusion, earlier return of bowel function, decreased wound infection rates, and shorter intensive care unit and overall hospital stays [7–

Electronic supplementary material The online version of this chapter (https://doi.org/10.1007/978-3-030-18740-8_11) contains supplementary material, which is available to authorized users.

P. Senthilnathan (✉) · S. Srivatsan Gurumurthy
C. Palanivelu
Gem Hospital and Research Centre,
Coimbatore, India

10]. Although the number of MIPRs performed for benign and malignant diseases of the pancreas has increased in recent years, cost considerations and financial implications of these new approaches need to be well defined. Furthermore, clear guidelines and standardization of surgical technique are paramount for the safe and steady expansion of this novel surgical approach [11, 12].

Evolution of Minimally Invasive Pancreaticoduodenectomy

The first description of laparoscopic pancreatic head resection was reported in 1994 by Gagner and Pomp, where they used a hybrid approach using a right subcostal hand port for tumor assessment and for the anastomosis [13]. In their first attempt at laparoscopic pancreaticoduodenectomy (LPD) in a patient with chronic pancreatitis, they wrote with great skepticism questioning the benefit of a laparoscopic approach to surgery of this magnitude. They also voiced their concerns regarding the significant technical challenges demanded by the procedure. Given the respect for Gagner's technical skills with minimally invasive techniques in the surgical community, LPD was mostly abandoned. Palanivelu in India continued working on LPD, and he presented his early experience in 2001 and later published additional experience with LPD in 42 patients, demonstrating a complication rate of 31% with no surgical death or conversion to open procedure. This report showed that in select patients, the procedure may be performed safely with good oncologic outcomes and acceptable perioperative results [14]. Over the years, technical modifications in energy source, radicality of surgery, type of reconstruction, and specimen extraction were made. These refinements in technique resulted in better outcomes as reported with a 75-patient series in 2009 [15]. Oncologically, margin status and lymph nodal yield were comparable to the open approach which translated to equal survival rates. Palanivelu's group also reported in 2015 that the radicality of LPD is comparable to the open approach when performed by experienced minimal access surgeons [16]. They have also assessed long-term survival outcomes following LPD in 130 patients with pancreatic and periampullary cancers, showing excellent short-term results and acceptable long-term survival [17]. More recently, Palanivelu and colleagues published the first RCT comparing LPD and OPD for periampullary tumors demonstrating a significant reduction in hospital stay and trends toward decreased blood loss, fewer transfusions, and reduced wound infection rates in the LPD arm [18].

Laparoscopic Pancreaticoduodenectomy

Indications

Patient selection is extremely important for successful application of the laparoscopic approach. It is prudent to select early, small lesions for beginners; and later, with experience, larger tumors can be attempted. Associated conditions like obesity, previous upper abdominal surgery, and borderline resectable tumors should be avoided. The preferred indications early in the learning curve include ampullary tumors, distal common bile duct tumors, early carcinoma of the head of pancreas, and duodenal carcinoma.

Port Position

A total of seven trocars are used for this procedure (Fig. 11.1). The exchange of the camera between the midline and right lateral 10-mm port facilitates performance of critical steps like the

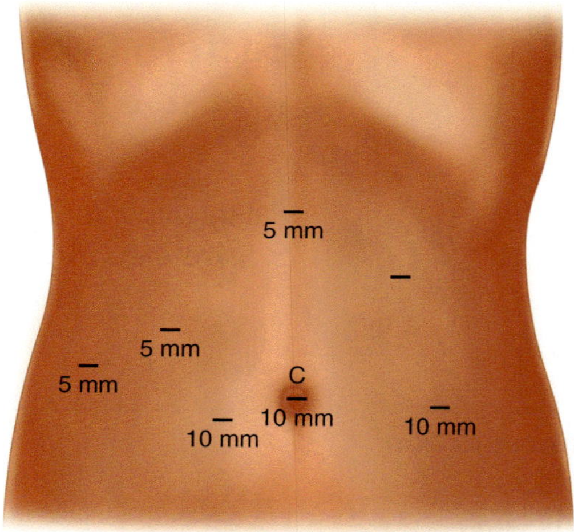

Fig. 11.1 Trocar/port positioning for laparoscopic pancreatectomy

extended Kocher maneuver, parenchymal transection, and uncinate dissection.

Team Setup, Patient Positioning, and Instrumentation

The patient is placed supine with split legs and in reverse Trendelenburg position. The monitor is placed at the head end of patient. The position of the surgeon varies depending on the area of dissection and reconstruction.

Position of the Surgeon

The position of the operating surgeon varies depending on the area of dissection or reconstruction. Mostly, the surgeon stands between the legs of the patient (Fig. 11.2). For certain steps like hepatic flexure mobilization and hepaticojejunostomy (HJ) anastomosis, the surgeon moves to the left side of the patient with the camera surgeon standing between the legs of the patient.

Phase 1: Resection

Video 11.1

For descriptive purposes, the procedure can be divided into two phases: resection and recon-

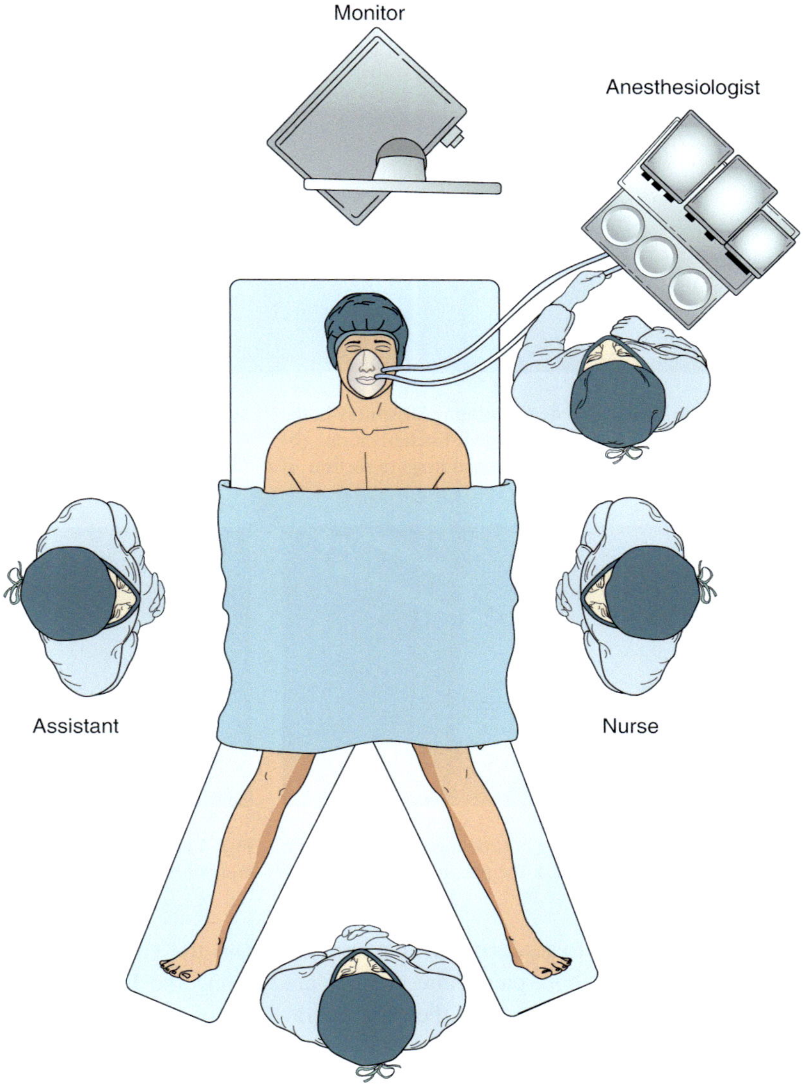

Fig. 11.2 Patient positioning and operating room setup for laparoscopic pancreatectomy

struction. After staging laparoscopy to rule out intra-abdominal distant metastasis, the procedure is started by taking down the hepatic flexure and exposing the entire duodenum (Fig. 11.3). The gastrocolic ligament is divided and the lesser sac is entered. The head of the pancreas is completely exposed by dividing the right gastroepiploic vessels and gastrocolic trunk. The resectability of the lesion is assessed by two important maneuvers. The first is extended Kocherization which allows the surgeon to assess the tumor in relation to the superior mesenteric artery (SMA) (Fig. 11.4). The second is tunneling behind the

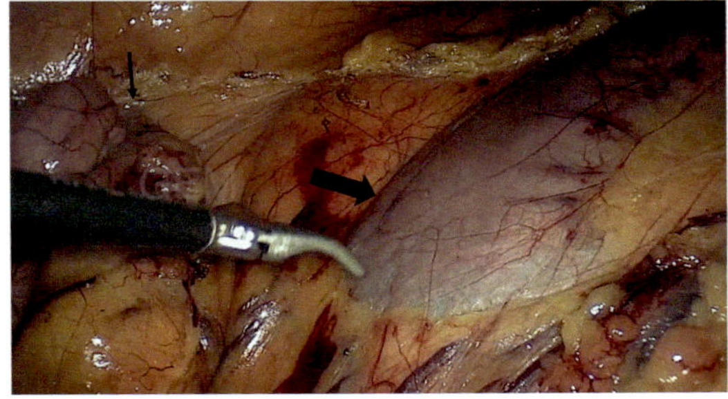

Fig. 11.3 Intraoperative image showing takedown of the hepatic flexure (thin black arrow) adjacent to the duodenum (thick black arrow)

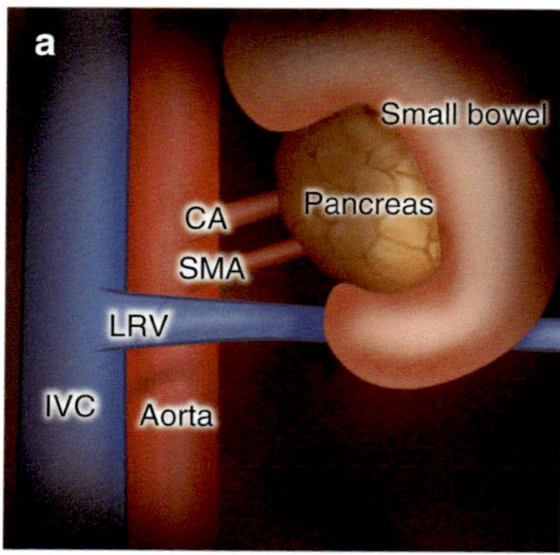

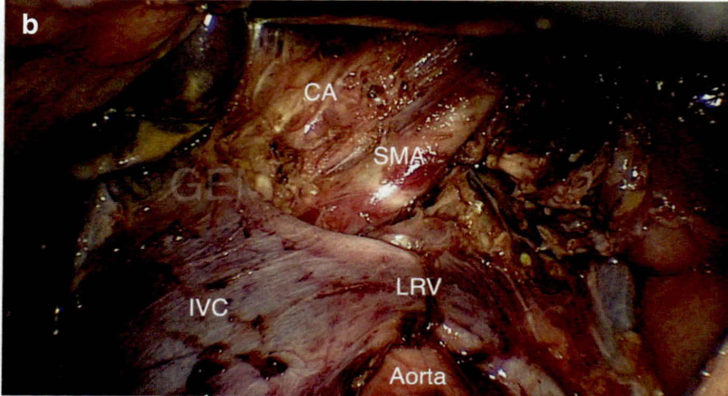

Fig. 11.4 (**a**) Illustration demonstrating structures in the retroperitoneum following extended Kocherization. (**b**) Paired intraoperative image demonstrating retraction of structures to the left, exposing the inferior vena cava (IVC), left renal vein (LRV), superior mesenteric artery (SMA), and celiac axis (CA)

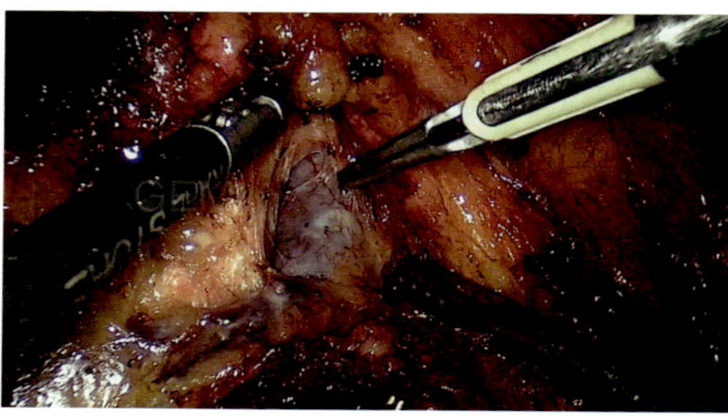

Fig. 11.5 Intraoperative image showing the creation of a tunnel posterior to the neck of the pancreas

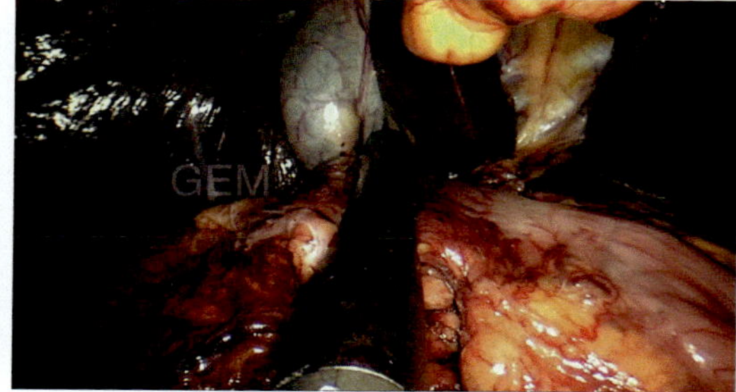

Fig. 11.6 Intraoperative image showing duodenal division with a laparoscopic linear stapler

neck of the pancreas to assess portal vein involvement (Fig. 11.5). If those pancreatic margins are both free of disease infiltration, then the operation proceeds.

If the decision is made to proceed, the antrum or first part of the duodenum is transected using an Endo GIA stapler, thus exposing the entire field of dissection (Fig. 11.6). The dissection of portal structures begins with decompression of the gallbladder since this step provides better visualization of the structures in the porta hepatis. Calot's triangle is dissected, and the cystic artery and duct are clipped and divided. The gallbladder is left attached to the liver until the reconstruction is completed, since it will provide good retraction of the liver.

The common bile duct (CBD) is then transected above the level of the cystic duct junction, and the entire fibro-fatty and lymphatic tissues along the hepatoduodenal ligament are cleared exposing the common hepatic artery and portal vein. Bile spillage from the opened CBD is avoided by applying an endoscopic bulldog clamp. The common hepatic artery is traced along the superior border of the pancreas in the gastrohepatic omentum, where the gastroduodenal artery is identified and ligated at its origin from the common hepatic artery (Fig. 11.7). Dissection continued toward the celiac axis along the superior border of the pancreas taking down lymphatic tissues with the specimen.

The mobilization of the duodenum continues toward the third and fourth parts, including the proximal 15 cm of jejunum. Attention is taken to ligate the first jejunal branch followed by transection of the jejunum with the Endo GIA stapler with

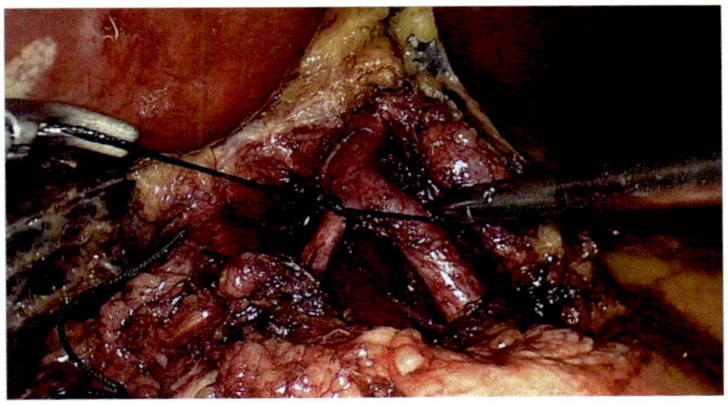

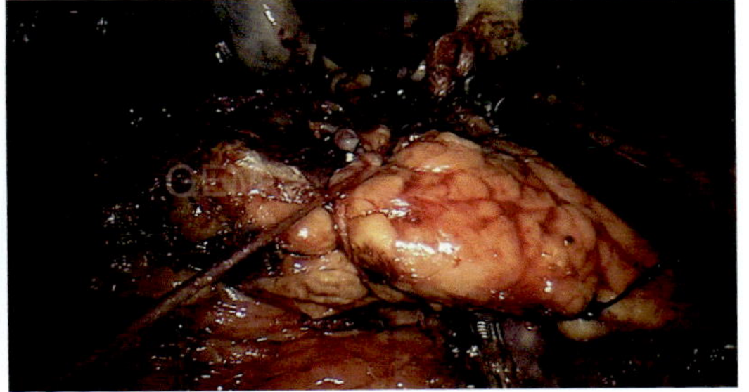

Fig. 11.7 Intraoperative image showing silk suture ligation of the gastroduodenal artery

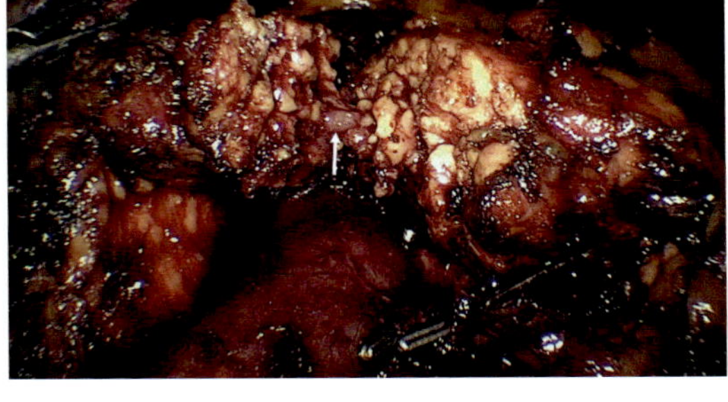

Fig. 11.9 Intraoperative image demonstrating the identification of the pancreatic duct (white arrow)

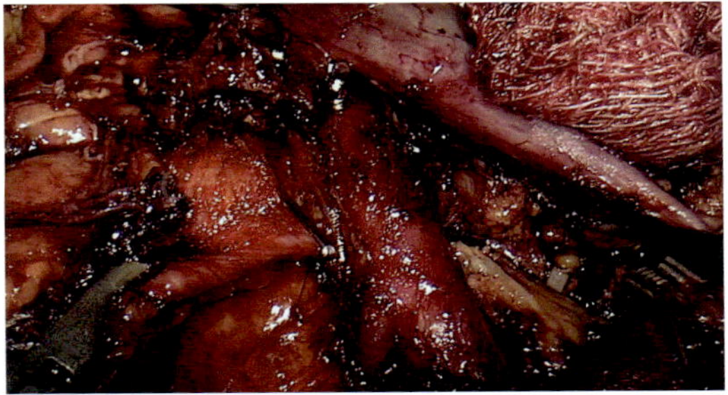

Fig. 11.8 Intraoperative image showing an umbilical tape that has been tied around the neck of the pancreas

Fig. 11.10 Intraoperative image demonstrating clips that have been placed on the inferior pancreaticoduodenal artery

a white cartridge. This facilitates delivery of the transected jejunum toward the specimen side. Alternatively, after dissecting the ligament of Treitz and completely mobilizing the duodenojejunal flexure, the jejunum may be transected in the supracolic compartment. This technical modification, which is now our preference, facilitates clear delineation of the first jejunal artery and vein.

Pancreatic transection at the neck begins after placing stay sutures on the superior and inferior borders on either side of the proposed transection line which helps for retraction and hemostasis (Fig. 11.8). The pancreas is transected using the harmonic shears, while the suspected area of the pancreatic duct is divided with scissors to avoid injury to the ductal mucosa (Fig. 11.9). The attachments of the uncinate process to the SMA are visualized including the inferior pancreaticoduodenal vessels which are clipped and divided ensuring complete removal of the gland along the right border of SMA (Fig. 11.10). This remains one of the most important and technically chal-

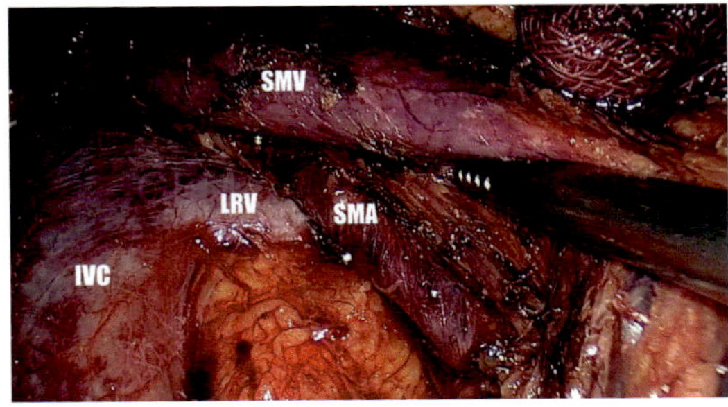

Fig. 11.11 Intraoperative image demonstrating completion of resection phase with exposure of the inferior vena cava (IVC), left renal vein (LRV), superior mesenteric artery (SMA), and superior mesenteric vein (SMV)

lenging steps of the operation (Fig. 11.11). Once completed, the specimen is placed into an endoscopic specimen bag and delivered through a Pfannenstiel incision at the end of the procedure.

Steps to achieve adequate exposure and proper handling of the pancreas

- Attach the falciform ligament to the anterior abdominal wall
- Adequate takedown of hepatic flexure and extended Kocherization
- Create wide tunnel posterior to the neck of the pancreas
- Divide gastrocolic trunk at its junction with the superior mesenteric vein
- SMA-first approach to assess resectability
- Early ligation of inferior pancreaticoduodenal artery decreases bleeding during pancreatic division
- Tie umbilical tape around the neck of the pancreas early to facilitate duct dilatation and easy identification of the duct during neck transection
- Use hemostatic and traction sutures to avoid direct handling and bleeding of pancreas
- Dissect pancreatic parenchyma with harmonic shears for bloodless dissection followed by slow side-to-side movements to tease apart pancreatic tissues
- Use scissors to divide midportion of pancreatic parenchyma when nearing the pancreatic duct
- Leave 3-mm cuff of pancreatic duct beyond divided parenchymal transection line to facilitate duct-to-mucosa anastomosis
- Use laparoscopic vessel retractor and switch camera to the right 12-mm port for uncinate dissection
- Use laparoscopic 3-mm instruments for handling pancreatic duct and suturing over small feeding tube
- Leave gallbladder attached to the liver until final steps to facilitate traction for HJ anastomosis

Phase 2: Reconstruction

Video 11.2

The jejunum is brought to the supracolic compartment in retrocolic fashion. The pancreatic stump is mobilized for a length of 2–3 cm to facilitate the pancreatic anastomosis. A duct-to-mucosa pancreaticojejunal (PJ) reconstruction is done by modified Blumgart technique. Up to

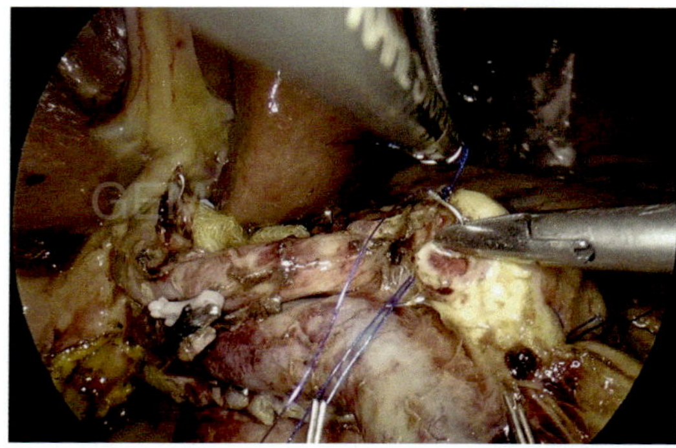

Fig. 11.12 Intraoperative image demonstrating sutures placed across the pancreatic duct in preparation for duct-to-mucosa suturing of the modified Blumgart technique

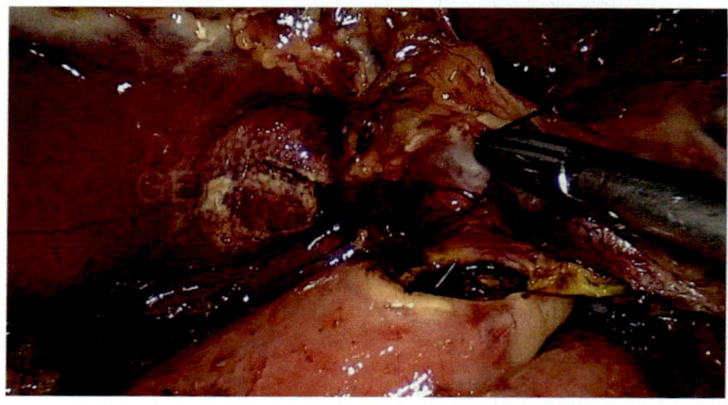

Fig. 11.13 Intraoperative image demonstrating suturing of the anterior layer of the hepaticojejunal anastomosis

three 3-0 Prolene trans-pancreatic sutures are taken from the anterior to posterior capsule of the pancreas, then taking a horizontal mattress bite on the jejunum, and reversing direction from posterior to anterior through the pancreas and finally tying the suture. About 4–6 duct-to-mucosa 4-0 PDS sutures are taken along the diameter of the pancreatic duct (Fig. 11.12). The mucosal anastomosis is reinforced using 3-0 polypropylene seromuscular to pancreatic capsule sutures anteriorly.

Approximately 7–8 cm distal to the PJ anastomosis, the HJ is performed by creating an enterotomy in the jejunum that is anastomosed with the cut end of the hepatic duct in single layer with 4-0 PDS interrupted sutures. If the duct is dilated, the anterior layer can be completed using a continuous suture (Fig. 11.13).

Distal to the HJ anastomosis, duodenojejunostomy is performed in antecolic fashion using 2-0

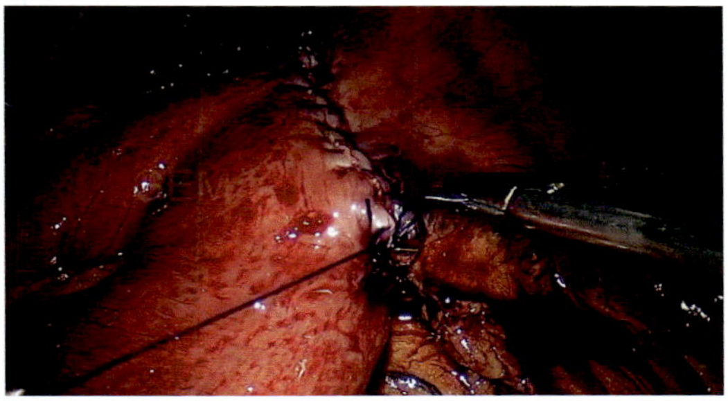

Fig. 11.14 Intraoperative image demonstrating near completion of the duodenojejunostomy

PDS for continuous, extramucosal sutures (Fig. 11.14). When the antrum is resected, a gastrojejunostomy is performed using an Endo GIA stapler on the dependent posterior aspect of the stomach. Nasojejunal and nasogastric tubes are used for feeding and decompression, respectively. A 24-Fr drain is routinely placed close to the PJ.

Conclusion

The question remains as to what the future holds for MIPR. Evolution in MIPR techniques has enabled performance of technically demanding steps like SMA-first approaches and major vessel resection and reconstruction during pancreatic resections. The addition of the robot to the pancreatic surgeon's armamentarium may facilitate adoptability and expansion of MIPR. Large-scale, multi-institutional randomized controlled trials are essential to demonstrate the safety, non-inferiority, and possible advantages of MIPR over the open approach. Focused training programs, dedicated fellowship courses, proficiency-based virtual training, and video analysis and proctorship are essential for large-scale penetrance of MIPR among the surgical fraternity.

References

1. Song KB, Kim SC, Hwang DW, et al. Matched case-control analysis comparing laparoscopic and open pylorus-preserving pancreaticoduodenectomy in patients with periampullary tumors. Ann Surg. 2015;262(1):146–55.
2. Stauffer JA, Coppola A, Villacreses D, et al. Laparoscopic versus open pancreaticoduodenectomy for pancreatic adenocarcinoma: long-term results at a single institution. Surg Endosc. 2017;31(5):2233–41.
3. Boggi U, Amorese G, Vistoli F, et al. Laparoscopic pancreaticoduodenectomy: a systematic literature review. Surg Endosc. 2014;15:15.
4. Liao CH, Wu YT, Liu YY, et al. Systemic review of the feasibility and advantage of minimally invasive Pancreaticoduodenectomy. World J Surg. 2016;40(5):1218–25.
5. Delitto D, Luckhurst CM, Black BS, et al. Oncologic and perioperative outcomes following selective application of laparoscopic pancreaticoduodenectomy for periampullary malignancies. J Gastrointest Surg. 2016;20(7):1343–9.
6. Kendrick ML, Cusati D. Total laparoscopic pancreaticoduodenectomy: feasibility and outcome in an early experience. Arch Surg. 2010;145(1):19–23.
7. Kooby DA, Chu CK. Laparoscopic management of pancreatic malignancies. Surg Clin North Am. 2010;90(2):427–46.
8. Zureikat AH, Breaux JA, Steel JL, et al. Can laparoscopic pancreaticoduodenectomy be safely implemented? J Gastrointest Surg. 2011;15(7):1151–7.
9. Asbun HJ, Stauffer JA. Laparoscopic vs open pancreaticoduodenectomy: overall outcomes and severity of complications using the accordion severity grading system. J Am Coll Surg. 2012;215(6):810–9.
10. Correa-Gallego C, Dinkelspiel HE, Sulimanoff I, et al. Minimally-invasive vs open pancreaticoduodenectomy: systematic review and meta-analysis. J Am Coll Surg. 2014;218(1):129–39.
11. Vollmer CM, Asbun HJ, Barkun J, et al. Proceedings of the first international state-of-the-art conference on minimally-invasive pancreatic resection (MIPR). HPB. 2017;8(17):015.
12. Palanivelu C, Takaori K, Abu Hilal M, et al. International summit on laparoscopic pancreatic resection (ISLPR) "Coimbatore summit statements". Surg Oncol. 2017. https://doi.org/10.1016/j.suronc.2017.12.001. pii: S0960-7404(17)30282-7. [Epub ahead of print].
13. Gagner M, Pomp A. Laparoscopic pylorus-preserving pancreatoduodenectomy. Surg Endosc. 1994;8(5):408–10.
14. Palanivelu C, Jani K, Senthilnathan P, et al. Laparoscopic pancreaticoduodenectomy: technique and outcomes. J Am Coll Surg. 2007;205(2):222–30.
15. Palanivelu C, Rajan PS, Rangarajan M, et al. Evolution in techniques of laparoscopic pancreaticoduodenectomy: a decade long experience from a tertiary center. J Hepato-Biliary-Pancreat Surg. 2009;16(6):731–40.
16. Senthilnathan P, Chinnusamy P, Ramanujam A, et al. Comparison of pathological radicality between open and laparoscopic pancreaticoduodenectomy in a tertiary Centre. Indian J Surg Oncol. 2015;6(1):20–5.

17. Senthilnathan P, Srivatsan Gurumurthy S, Gul SI, et al. Long-term results of laparoscopic pancreaticoduodenectomy for pancreatic and periampullary cancer-experience of 130 cases from a tertiary-care center in South India. J Laparoendosc Adv Surg Tech A. 2015;25(4):295–300.

18. Palanivelu C, Senthilnathan P, Sabnis SC, et al. Randomized clinical trial of laparoscopic versus open pancreatoduodenectomy for periampullary tumours. Br J Surg. 2017;104(11):1443–50. https://doi.org/10.1002/bjs.10662.

Patrick Varley, Amr Al-Abbas, and Melissa E. Hogg

Development of the Robotic Approach

Although several iterations of the pancreaticoduodenectomy (PD) existed dating back to the 1890s, the first recorded one-stage procedure for the complete excision of the head of the pancreas and duodenum by Whipple was reported in 1941 [1, 2]. In the minimally invasive era, the first laparoscopic PD (LPD) was reported in 1994 by Gagner [3], but widespread adoption of this minimally invasive procedure has not caught on and is only practiced at high-volume specialized centers [4–7]. Laparoscopy has several limitations for procedures requiring complex reconstruction, such as two-dimensional imaging, tremor with long instruments, difficulty to be ambidextrous for difficult suture angles, and lack of wrist articulation in laparoscopic instrumentation. Hand assistance with laparoscopic resection and partial open reconstruction has been used in some centers but has failed to gain popularity [6, 8, 9].

Electronic supplementary material The online version of this chapter (https://doi.org/10.1007/978-3-030-18740-8_12) contains supplementary material, which is available to authorized users.

P. Varley · A. Al-Abbas · M. E. Hogg (✉)
University of Pittsburgh Medical Center,
Pittsburgh, PA, USA
e-mail: varleypr@upmc.edu; alabbasa@upmc.edu;
mhogg@northshore.org

Using the robotic platform overcomes many of the shortcomings of laparoscopy with improved three-dimensional imaging, 540° movement of surgical instruments, improved dexterity, and precision in complex tasks like vascular dissection and intracorporeal suturing [10–12]. In 2010, Giulianotti and colleagues reported the first large series of robotic pancreatic resections where 134 patients underwent various pancreatic procedures of which 60 patients underwent robotic PD (RPD) [6].

At the University of Pittsburgh, we performed our first RPD in 2008 and published the first description of our technique in 2011 [11, 13]. Since that time, our approach to the operation has undergone continuous refinement and has shifted from utilizing a hybrid of laparoscopic mobilization and robotic resection to a completely robotic procedure. Zureikat et al. reported the first 250 consecutive robotic procedures which included 132 RPD with low mortality and morbidity rates [7]. These encouraging early results have allowed the robotic approach to pancreatic surgery to become our preferred approach. Subsequently, Boone et al. reported that based on 200 consecutive RPD, the learning curve was 80 cases [14]. After 20 cases, there was an improvement in estimated blood loss and conversion; and after 40 cases, there was an increase in lymph node yield. However, time was the most difficult outcome to improve and an inflection point was noted using cumulative sum control chart (CUSUM) analysis at 80 cases. As of

2017, over 60% of PDs at our institution are completed using the robotic approach; and we recently completed the 500th RPD in September 2017.

Lessons from this evolution and prospective scrutiny of outcomes have allowed us to identify the learning curve for RPD and ultimately lead to the development of a standardized curriculum for training surgeons at all training levels [15, 16]. As RPD has matured as a technique, it has also been possible to perform multi-institutional analysis of its outcomes as compared to OPD. In 2016, Zureikat et al. reported a comparison of 211 RPDs from 2 institutions and 817 OPD from 8 high-volume institutions [17]. While operative times for RPD were longer than OPD, there were no difference in 90-day mortality, clinically relevant postoperative pancreatic fistula (POPF), wound infection, length of stay, 90-day readmission, or oncologic-related factors such as margin status or suboptimal lymphadenectomy.

Indications

Indications for RPD are the same as for OPD with the exception of patients who cannot tolerate pneumoperitoneum. Though our initial experience also excluded patients requiring vascular reconstruction, we have concluded that limited vascular resection and reconstruction can be performed safely through the robotic approach. The indications include, but are not limited to, cholangiocarcinoma, duodenal cancer, ampullary cancer, pancreatic adenocarcinoma, pancreatic acinar cell carcinoma, pancreatic neuroendocrine tumor, intraductal papillary mucinous neoplasm (IPMN), mucinous cystic neoplasm (MCN), chronic pancreatitis, and other less common etiologies.

All patients must have a preoperative pancreatic protocol, triple-contrast computed tomographic (CT) scan to stage the tumor, identify the configuration of the arterial anatomy, and determine whether there is tumor freedom or abutment or encasement of the portal vein (PV), superior mesenteric vein (SMV), superior mesenteric artery (SMA), and hepatic arteries. This CT scan also identifies anomalous or aberrant hepatic arteries which can aid in operative planning. Endoscopic ultrasound (US) allows fine needle aspiration (FNA) for cytologic diagnosis, demonstration of nodal disease, and characterization of vascular involvement of the tumor. Endoscopic retrograde cholangiopancreatogram (ERCP) allows brushings for cytology, provides a cholangiogram to delineate ductal anatomy, and offers therapeutic decompression of the biliary tree using plastic stents, covered metal stents, and uncovered metal stents. Serum CA19-9 levels, once bilirubin has normalized, are obtained preoperatively for all patients as a prognostic marker for pancreatic cancer and cholangiocarcinoma.

Based on preoperative work-up, patients with pancreatic cancer are classified as resectable, borderline resectable, locally advanced, or metastatic [18–20]. Resectable patients are either taken to surgery or given neoadjuvant therapy. Borderline resectable patients are all given neoadjuvant chemotherapy ± radiotherapy. Locally advanced patients are given systemic therapies, and if they respond, these patients will be reevaluated for surgical consideration. Patients with venous encasement that need portal vein resection with interposition graft are not approached robotically.

Anatomic Highlights and Landmarks

Ligament of Treitz

The identification and division of the ligament of Treitz are performed robotically following the Kocher maneuver. This dissection is critical for freeing the retroperitoneal attachments to the duodenum and pancreas. It is of critical importance to dissect directly onto the duodenum and not into the mesentery encompassing the SMV and SMA. This dissection is complete when the proximal portion of the jejunum can be pulled into the right upper quadrant (RUQ).

Hepatic Artery Lymph Node

This lymph node is large even when it is not pathologically involved and it is easy to identify.

Once identified and removed, the common hepatic artery (CHA), the PV, and the gastroduodenal artery (GDA) can be easily identified. This lymph node is highly vascular and friable, and removing it whole with the "no touch" technique is recommended to avoid venous oozing.

Superior Pancreaticoduodenal Vein or Vein of Belcher

This vessel is usually located at the superior aspect of the pancreas and enters the PV posteriorly. It is easy to avulse and may create significant bleeding from the PV. It is best to locate this vessel after the pancreatic neck dissection but to defer ligation until the end of pancreatic resection. This allows for ease of ligation to avoid potential hemorrhage.

First Jejunal Branch of the SMV

This branch is usually quite large and may have several branches to the uncinate process (Fig. 12.1). Ligating these branches without injuring the primary trunk is tedious but critical to free the inferior border of the uncinate from the small bowel mesentery allowing for better visualization of the lateral wall of the SMA.

Preoperative Preparation

Recent paradigm shifts in the preoperative preparation of patients undergoing major abdominal surgery have led us to adopt an enhanced recovery after surgery (ERAS) protocol for patients undergoing RPD. While patients still receive a bowel preparation the day before surgery, they are permitted to continue drinking clear liquids up until 2 h prior to surgery. As part of this protocol, patients also receive intrathecal morphine and an oral dose of extended-release opioid (e.g., OxyContin) prior to induction of anesthesia to facilitate postoperative pain management. Using this pathway, narcotics are limited in favor of other non-narcotic supplements (i.e., acetaminophen, ketamine, lidocaine, gabapentin, etc.). Prophylaxis includes sequential compression devices, 5000 units of subcutaneous heparin, and intravenous antibiotics which are re-dosed throughout the case. Arterial line placement is routinely used for blood pressure monitoring, while central venous access is placed at the discretion of anesthesiology. A Foley catheter and gastric decompression tube are also placed. While a nasogastric tube may be used, our ERAS protocol does not employ routine postoperative gastric decompression, and a temporary orogastric tube is therefore acceptable.

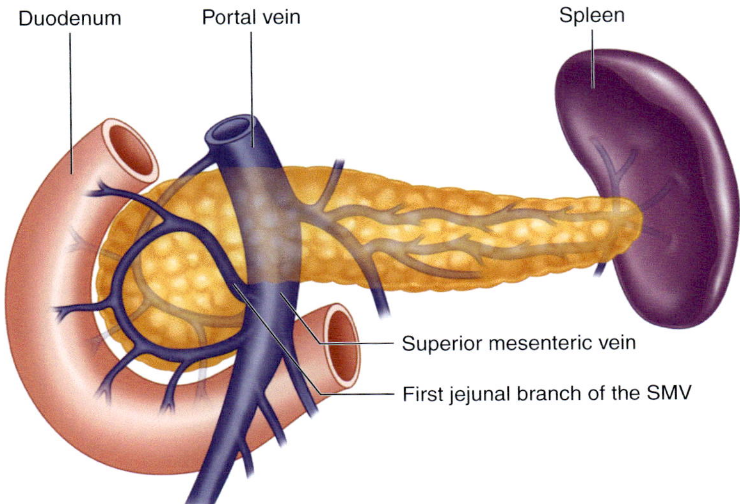

Fig. 12.1 Important venous anatomy of the pancreas, including the first jejunal vein

Positioning

A split-leg table is utilized with the patient's right arm tucked and the left arm extended at 60 ° (Fig. 12.2a). To minimize patient movement during the case, the table is padded with Pigazzi pads (Xodus Medical). If this is not available, crate sponges may be used as an alternative. Pressure

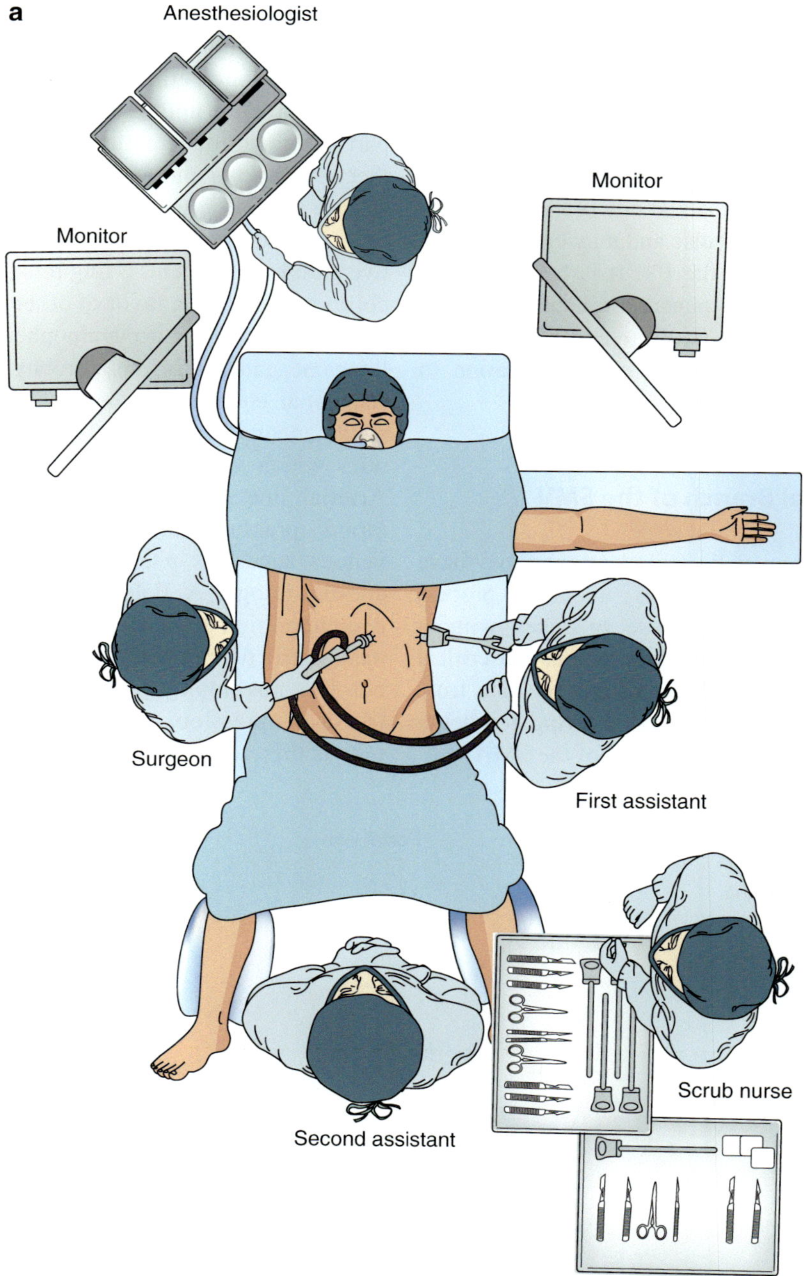

Fig. 12.2 Patient positioning and operating room setup for (**a**) laparoscopic mobilization and (**b**) robotic pancreatectomy

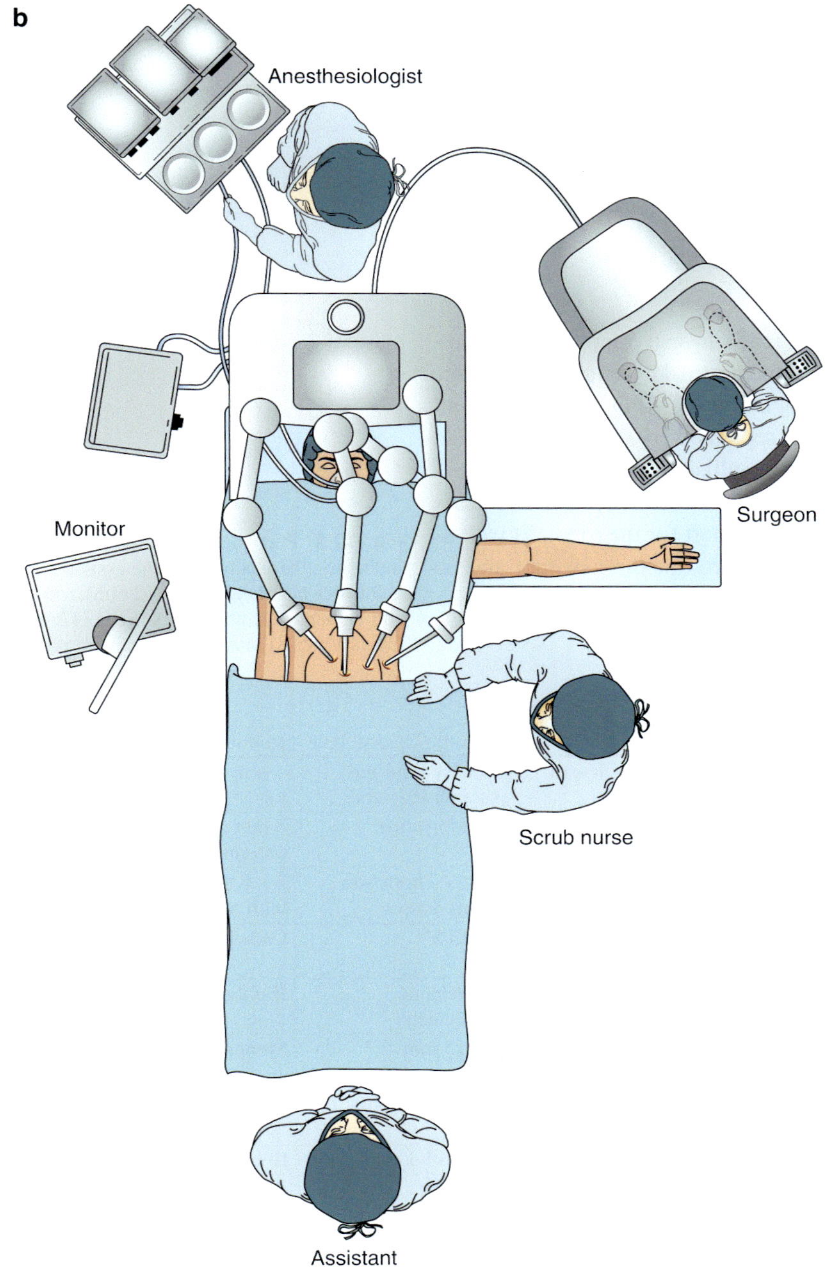

Fig. 12.2 (continued)

points are padded with additional crate sponges, and the patient is secured to the bed with a chest strap. Once the patient is secured, the legs are abducted, knees are padded to prevent hyperextension, and footboards are placed. To assist in maintaining euthermia throughout the case, the legs are covered with blankets and secured by tape; and the upper body is covered with a forced-air warming blanket positioned above the nipple line. Once the patient is appropriately positioned, the table is rotated to allow robot docking directly over the head (Si) or over the right shoulder (Xi) (Fig. 12.2b).

The preference of our group is the Si platform due to better visual optics within the high-definition 12-mm camera of the Si compared to the chip-on-tip technology of the 8-mm camera of the Xi which does not allow manual focus. Supplies for positioning and steps of RPD are listed in Table 12.1.

Port Placement

As with all minimally invasive approaches to surgery, port placement is a key component to the successful completion of RPD. In general, all ports should be separated by at least 5–6 cm to prevent instrument collisions. Standard port selection includes three 8-mm robotic working ports and a 12-mm camera port for the robot, as well as 5-mm and 12-mm ports for the assistant and an additional 5-mm port for the self-retaining liver retractor (Fig. 12.3). When using the Xi platform,

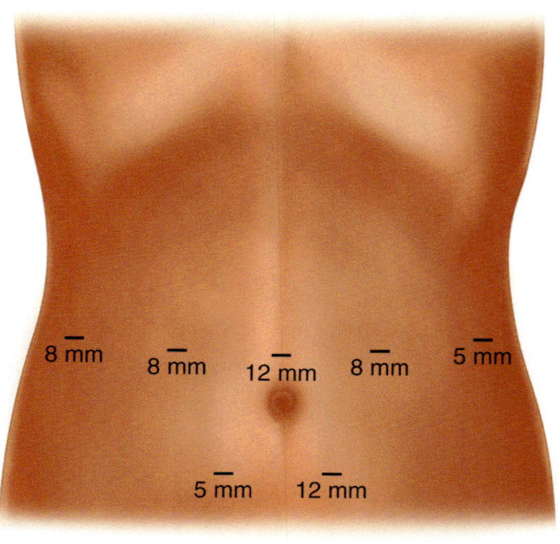

Fig. 12.3 Port placement for robotic pancreatectomy, indicating the positions of the assistant ports in the bilateral lower quadrants (5 and 12 mm), robotic ports (8 mm), and camera port at the umbilicus (12 mm). When using the da Vinci Xi platform, the camera port is an 8-mm port

Table 12.1 Equipment

Positioning	General laparoscopic	Specific laparoscopic	Robotic[a]	Open
Split-leg bed	5 mm 0 and 30° lenses[b]	Battery-powered suction-irrigator[c]	4-arm da Vinci drape kit	2 × 19-Fr Round Blake[d]
3″ silk tape	10 mm 0 and 30° lenses[b]	Bulldog clips[e]	8 mm disposable obturator	Bovie[f]
Blue foam rolls	5 and 10 mm Endoclip appliers[f]	Carter-Thomason suture passer[g]	3 × 8 mm ports (4 with Xi)	Pancreatic stents (4-, 5-, or 7-Fr)[h]
Egg crate	5 and 12 mm bladeless Versaports[f]	DHELP[f]	Cadiere forceps	Slush drape
Foot boards	2 × Alligator grasper	2 × 10 mm Endocatch[f]	Bipolar cord	SureClose
Left arm board	4 × Duckbill grasper (2 short, 2 long)	1 × 15 mm Endocatch[f]	Monopolar cord	Surgicel, Nu-Knit, Gelfoam[d]
Pigazzi Pink Pad[i]	Camera and light cord[b]	Gelpoint gelport[j]	Fenestrated bipolar	Thompson retractor[k]
Velcro chest strap	5 mm Blunt tip LigaSure[f]	Hem-o-lok appliers[e]	Hook cautery	Triad[f]
Forced-air warming blanket[l]	2 × insufflation tubing	Lapra-Ty (Applier-KA200/Clips-XC200)[d]	2 × Large needle driver	Ultrasound machine[m]
Warm blankets	Mediflex retractor[n]	Endo-GIA stapler[f]	2 × Prograsp forceps	6″ Umbilical tapes[f]
	Optical separator[j]	Angle-tipped gold staple loads (45 and 60 mm)[f]	Scissor cautery	6″ Yellow vessel loops
	General laparoscopic instruments	Purple staple loads (45 and 60 mm)[f]	Suture cut needle driver	General open instruments
			General robotic instruments	

Suppliers: [a]Intuitive, [b]Storz, [c]Stryker, [d]Ethicon, [e]Aesculap, [f]Covidien, [g]Cook Surgical, [h]Hobbs Medical, [i]Xodus Medical, [j]Applied Medical, [k]Thompson, [l]Arizant Healthcare, [m]Aloka, [n]Velmen

the 12-mm robotic camera port is exchanged for an 8-mm robotic port. Access is first gained in the left upper quadrant (LUQ) utilizing an optical trocar. After exploration, if no metastatic disease is found, additional ports are placed.

To provide the best visualization during the uncinate dissection, the 12-mm or 8-mm robotic camera port should be placed 2–3 cm above and approximately 2–3 fingerbreadths to the right of the patient's umbilicus in an "average"-sized patient. These may be adjusted for body habitus. When using a 12-mm camera port, a Carter Thomason suture-passing device (Cooper Surgical) is used to place a "figure of eight" suture around the 12-mm port prior to docking the robot. Two additional 8-mm robotic working ports are placed in the mid-clavicular line and anterior axillary line on the right. Assistant ports are positioned in the right lower quadrant (5-mm) and left lower quadrant (12-mm) on a line which bisects the distance between the camera port and its neighboring port on each side. The 12-mm LLQ assistant port will eventually serve as the specimen extraction site. Finally, a LUQ self-retaining liver retractor (Mediflex Surgical Products) is placed in the left anterior axillary line and the LUQ optical trocar is exchanged for an 8-mm robotic working port. It should be noted that port placement must be tailored to the patient, specifically in patients with shorter or longer torsos where the ports can be adjusted caudally or cranially, respectively.

Operative Steps

Video 12.1

Mobilization

When we first adopted the robotic-assisted technique, the mobilization steps were carried out laparoscopically. With refinement of our technique, however, the procedure is now completed entirely with a robotic approach. Following port placement, the robot is docked and instruments passed into the abdomen. Most of the operation is completed with the monopolar hook cautery in the right (R1) hand, fenestrated bipolar in the left (R2) hand, and the cadiere or prograsp in R3. We utilize a 30° robotic laparoscope, and when using the Si platform, it is oriented in the "down" position. The assistant uses an energy sealing device (LigaSure, Covidien) and suction-irrigator and a laparoscopic stapler when indicated.

To begin the dissection, the hook electrocautery or LigaSure is used to enter the lesser sac through the gastrocolic omentum sparing the gastroepiploic vessels. Congenital adhesions from the posterior body of the stomach to the pancreas are common and should be carefully lysed with a combination of blunt dissection and electrocautery. During this dissection, care is taken to remain in the appropriate plane, thereby avoiding injury to the gastroepiploic and middle colic veins. This dissection continues to the right side facilitating takedown of the hepatic flexure.

Once the hepatic flexure has been taken down, full Cattell-Braasch maneuver is performed by mobilizing the right colon along the white line of Toldt to the level of the appendix. Once this is completed, the right colon may be medialized allowing excellent exposure of the duodenum. Mobilization continues with Kocherization of the duodenum to the level of the left renal vein, which provides exposure of the inferior vena cava (IVC), SMA, and ligament of Treitz. During this dissection, anteromedial retraction of the duodenum is provided by R3, while the assistant can use the suction-irrigator to keep the dissection plane free of blood and the LigaSure to control larger vessels. When the Kocher maneuver is complete, resectability can be determined. With resectable tumors, the procedure proceeds with mobilization of the posterior duodenum, pancreatic head, and uncinate to the level of the root of the small bowel. A key maneuver is to release the ligament of Treitz from the patient's right side through an extended Kocher maneuver, thereby allowing delivery of the jejunum under the small bowel mesentery and into the RUQ.

After the proximal jejunum is delivered into the right supracolic compartment, a window is made in the jejunal mesentery approximately 10 cm from the uncinate and the jejunum is transected from the assistant's 12-mm port utilizing a laparoscopic linear stapler with a 60-mm hook-tipped gold load (Covidien). The assistant then uses the LigaSure to transect the jejunal mesentery on the specimen side to the level of the uncinate process. Care must be taken to stay very close to the intestine and immediately under it to avoid injury to the vascular supply within the small bowel mesentery. Any remaining retroperitoneal attachments to the duodenum and jejunum are the transected to allow "linearization" of the specimen.

With pancreaticoduodenal mobilization and distal intestinal transection complete, attention is then turned to the proximal extent of resection. The gastrohepatic ligament is entered through the pars flaccida using electrocautery or the LigaSure with care taken to avoid injury to a replaced left hepatic artery if present. The LigaSure is then used to ligate the right gastric artery (RGA) at the point of planned antral transection. Though pylorus-preserving PD can be performed as part of RPD, we generally favor the classic PD. A position immediately opposite to the ligation of the RGA is identified on the greater curvature, and the LigaSure is used to divide the gastrocolic omentum and ligate the gastroepiploic artery. This dissection is continued for a few centimeters proximally along the greater curvature to facilitate future anastomosis. After anesthesia has withdrawn the gastric tube, the stomach is transected using a purple load of the linear stapler (Covidien).

Portal Dissection

The first step of the portal dissection is identification and excision of the hepatic artery lymph node, which allows excellent exposure of structures within the porta hepatis. The node is excised using a combination of hook electrocautery and LigaSure. This node can cause bothersome bleeding refractory to coagulation, but which stops with gentle pressure and application of Surgicel (Ethicon). After excision, the node is sent for permanent pathology. R3 can then be used to grasp and retract the specimen staple line and retract it laterally, providing a window for dissection of

the CHA. The tissue overlying the CHA/GDA junction can be dissected with electrocautery, followed by gentle anterior traction with R2 and careful blunt dissection with the hook to develop the plane between the CHA and portal vein. With the anterior surface of the portal vein identified, its attachments to the superior border of the pancreas are divided to provide an adequate landing zone for future pancreatic transection.

Attention then returns to the arterial dissection, where the RGA is identified in the plane anterior to the CHA/GDA confluence and divided with a combination of titanium clips and LigaSure. We believe that lateral portal dissection with identification of the CBD prior to GDA transection is an important safety consideration as it allows identification of aberrant vascular anatomy prior to GDA transection. If there is any concern regarding adequate hepatic flow, we perform a Doppler ultrasound exam of the CHA before and after test clamping the GDA. The lateral aspect of the porta hepatis is approached by using R3 to retract the gallbladder cephalad, and the lateral and posterior nodal tissue along the CBD is dissected toward the specimen side. Once the lateral aspect of the CBD has been cleared, careful medial dissection from the PV follows. The GDA and CBD are then encircled with yellow vessel loops to facilitate provision of counter-tension and transected with angle-tipped gold loads of the linear stapler (Covidien). The GDA stump is marked with a titanium clip for later identification.

Uncinate Dissection

The uncinate dissection begins with identification of the inferior border of the pancreas at the SMV. The first goal of this dissection should be to identify the SMV both superiorly under the pancreatic neck and inferiorly as it enters the mesocolon. Dissection of the SMV from the pancreatic neck is then facilitated with both gentle anterior retraction using R2 and use of the assistant's suction-irrigator to provide counter-traction and to perform blunt dissection. During this dissection, several small pancreatic venous branches may be encountered which can bleed significantly. These may be controlled with bipolar cautery or LigaSure.

Once the retro-pancreatic tunnel has been completed, an umbilical tape may be passed underneath the pancreatic neck to provide a handle during pancreatic transection. R1 is exchanged for a monopolar scissor, and the assistant places the suction-irrigator within the retro-pancreatic tunnel to protect the portal venous confluence during transection. The scissors are then used with monopolar cautery to partially transect the pancreas on the anterior and inferior borders. Bipolar or LigaSure is used to control bleeding from the transverse pancreatic arteries when encountered. After transection has proceeded approximately halfway through the gland from caudal to cranial and halfway from anterior to posterior, the cold scissors are used to transect until the pancreatic duct is identified. Following division of the duct, transection may be completed with electrocautery.

The SMV dissection is completed through identification of the origin of the gastroepiploic vein, middle colic vein, trunk of Henle (if present), and the first jejunal branch. This is accomplished by completely dissecting both the medial and lateral borders of the SMV and then transecting the gastroepiploic vein at its origin using the LigaSure. If feasible, the middle colic vein is preserved. This allows the portal vein to be "rolled" medially off the uncinate, exposing the first jejunal branch. While this is generally preserved, the recurrent branches to the uncinate are coagulated with the fenestrated bipolar. With the uncinate free from the first jejunal branch, R3 can be used to roll the specimen "up and out" to expose the SMA.

The final dissection of the specimen begins with approach to the vascular groove of the SMV to the backside of the pancreas. The approach to this dissection can depend not only on gland texture but on potential for portal vein or SMV involvement. With a soft glad, we favor the "medial to lateral" approach where the layers are sequentially taken from anterior to posterior. In the case of a hard gland or suspected vein involvement requiring potential robotic vein resection, we prefer an "artery first" approach facilitated by a "hanging maneuver." To accomplish this, the SMV is dissected above and below the first jejunal branch which is then ligated. The SMV, which is still attached to the pancreas, is then suspended off the retroperitoneum with gentle traction of the pancreas, which allows medial to lateral dissection of the SMA from under the SMV (Fig. 12.4). During either of these approaches, close coordination is required between the robotic surgeon and assistant since it requires a combination of monopolar and bipolar electrocautery as well as the LigaSure to complete the maneuver safely. Unlike open PD, the inferior and superior pancreaticoduodenal arteries can be visualized during dissection with the help of the high-definition optics and magnification provided by the robotic platform. When encountered, these should be ligated with titanium clips in addition to the LigaSure. Once the uncinate dissection is complete, the specimen should be completely free, and it is placed into an extraction bag, removed from the abdomen, and sent to pathology for frozen section analysis of the common bile duct and pancreatic margins.

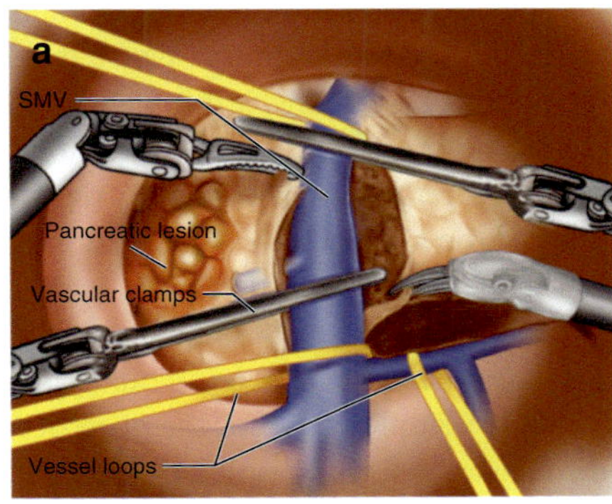

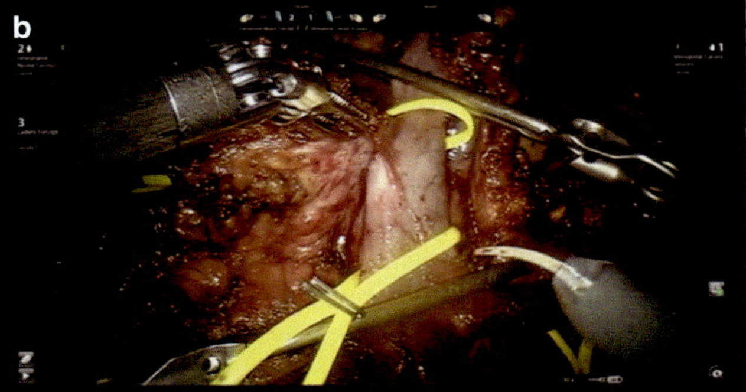

Fig. 12.4 (**a**) Illustration demonstrating pancreatic cancer with invasion of the side wall of the superior mesenteric vein (SMV). Vascular clamps have been placed transversely across the SMV above and below the level of the lesion. Vessel loops have been placed on the SMV above and below the lesion. (**b**) Paired intraoperative image showing robotic vein resection for locally advanced pancreatic cancer

Cholecystectomy

Robotic cholecystectomy can be performed in either an antegrade or retrograde manner. The cystic artery is ligated with 5-mm clips and the energy sealant device; and the cystic duct is ligated with 5- or 10-mm clips. In the case of a distal cholangiocarcinoma, the CBD may be reexcised above the cystic duct as part of the gallbladder specimen and sent as an additional margin. The gallbladder is placed into a 10-mm extraction bag and removed.

Pancreaticojejunostomy

To begin reconstruction, the proximal jejunum in the supracolic compartment is oriented with the mesentery facing the SMA/SMV. R1 and R2 are exchanged for needle drivers, and a duct-to-mucosa modified Blumgart pancreaticojejunostomy (PJ) is then created over a pancreatic duct stent (4, 5, or 7 Fr, Hobbs Medical). The anastomosis begins with three 8 in 2-0 silk sutures on a V-20 needle which forms the back row. These stitches are taken full thickness through the pancreas from anterior to posterior, then seromuscular through the jejunum near the mesenteric border, then posterior to anterior back through the pancreas. The middle stitch should straddle the pancreatic duct, and care must be taken that this stitch does not go through the duct itself. The stitches are tied with care being taken that the pancreatic duct is not occluded by tying the middle stitch too tightly, which can be confirmed by gently moving the stent in and out of the duct. The needles are left attached to these stitches as they will be used to complete the anterior outer layer. A small enterotomy in the jejunum is made opposite the pancreatic duct and the pancreatic duct stent temporarily removed. The duct-to-mucosa anastomosis is completed in anterior and posterior layers with interrupted 5-0 PDS (Ethicon) suture. The first suture is taken inside-outside on the pancreatic duct at the 7-o'clock position and then outside-inside on the jejunum ensuring that mucosa is included in the bite. Prior to tying, the second posterior suture is taken in the same fashion at the 5-o'clock position. Both stitches are then tied. The pancreatic duct stent

is replaced and the anterior row of the anastomosis is completed. This anterior duct-to-mucosa row is composed of two to five sutures depending on duct size which are taken outside-inside on the jejunum and inside-outside on the pancreas duct. The silk sutures from the posterior outer layer are then used to create an anterior outer layer by taking seromuscular bites of the jejunum anterior to the anastomosis.

Hepaticojejunostomy

An appropriate site for the hepaticojejunostomy (HJ) is identified approximately 10 cm downstream from the PJ at a point that will not create tension on the PJ. For normal or larger caliber ducts, we prefer a running anastomosis in anterior and posterior layers utilizing two 6 inches, 4-0 V-Loc sutures (Covidien). An enterotomy is made on the jejunum to match the size of the CBD, and the staple line is removed sharply from the CBD. Beginning at the lateral (9-o'clock) edge of the CBD, the posterior row is completed inside-outside on the duct and outside-inside on the jejunum, again ensuring that mucosa is included in each bite. The anterior layer is completed in the same lateral-to-medial direction but is taken outside-inside on the duct and inside-outside on the jejunum. When completed, the anterior and posterior layer sutures are tied to each other. For smaller ducts, the anastomosis can be completed over the stent with interrupted 5-0 PDS suture. A corner stitch is first taken outside-inside on the bile duct and inside-outside on the jejunum at the lateral 9-o'clock position. This stitch is left long but not tied. The tails of the corner stitch are then grasped in R3 and retracted anteriorly to set up the remainder of the anastomosis. The posterior stitches of the anastomosis continue from lateral to medial with bites taken inside-outside on the duct and outside-inside on the jejunum, tying each stitch as it is completed. After the posterior aspect of the anastomosis is completed, the stent is placed and the anterior row is completed from lateral-to-medial with stitches outside-inside on the duct and inside-outside on the jejunum.

Gastrojejunostomy

With the jejunum in the supracolic compartment, two 2-0 silk marking stitches are placed in the jejunum to provide a way of easily identifying the proper orientation for the gastrojejunostomy (GJ). The transverse colon is then retracted anteriorly and the jejunum reduced back to the left side of the abdomen. With the marking stitches identified, the loop of jejunum is grasped and brought up to the stomach anterior to the transverse colon. Though we have occasionally utilized a stapled anastomosis for the GJ, we prefer a four-layer hand-sewn end-to-side anastomosis. A 2-0 silk Lembert suture which imbricates the gastric staple line is placed medially and is then taken as a seromuscular bite through the jejunum. This corner stitch is tied and left long for retraction with R3. A posterior row of interrupted 3-0 silk Lembert sutures is then placed, and the gastric staple line removed for a distance of 6 cm. The inner, posterior layer is completed with a continuous 3-0 9-inches, V-Loc suture (Covidien) beginning at the medial aspect of the anastomosis and taken in full-thickness bites through the stomach and jejunum. This layer continues around the lateral corner of the anastomosis and then continued in a Connell fashion anteriorly. With the anterior portion approximately three-quarters complete, a second V-Loc suture is started medially and continued laterally until it meets the first suture. The sutures are tied together, and the anastomosis is completed with an anterior outer layer of 3-0 silk Lembert sutures.

After reconstruction, we thoroughly irrigate with normal saline and then create a falciform flap that is used to cover the GDA stump. The integrity of all three anastomoses is ensured, and we inspect for adequate hemostasis. A 19-Fr round blake drain is placed through the R3 port site and positioned anterior to the PJ and HJ and posterior to the GJ. The drain is secured to the skin with a 2-0 nylon suture, the robot is undocked, and all ports are removed under direct vision. The 12-mm port site is closed with the previously placed 0-Polysorb stitch, and the extraction site is closed with interrupted #1 Polysorb. The skin incisions are closed with 4-0 absorbable subcuticular stitches and skin glue.

Postoperative Care

Though patients undergoing RPD were initially sent to the intensive care unit (ICU) postoperatively, our patients now go to a regular surgical floor postoperatively which has both reduced length of stay (LOS) and costs [21]. Postoperative care for RPD patients also incorporates ERAS principles. We do not routinely utilize postoperative gastric decompression, but patients are kept NPO on POD #0. On POD #1, they are permitted clear liquids in the absence of significant nausea and/or vomiting. Pain is initially managed with scheduled intravenous acetaminophen and intermittent intravenous opioids and transitioned to oral medications once tolerating clear liquids. We generally avoid the use of ketorolac in these patients as it has been our observation that this may be associated with increased risk for POPF (data in submission). Patients are encouraged to ambulate early on POD #1, and the Foley catheter is removed, a clear liquid diet is begun, and fluids are minimized. Fluids are ceased on POD #2, and diet is advanced if the patient is tolerating clear liquids. Though we have previously utilized a modified Verona protocol for drain management, drain amylase levels are measured on POD #1 and #3 with the drain removed if the POD #3 level is less than 5000 [22, 23]. Most patients are discharged by POD #5 if they have no complications, and they are seen in clinic at 2 and 4 weeks postoperatively.

Acute Complications

Morbidity after pancreaticoduodenectomy is documented to be about 40% [24–26], and recent multi-institutional analyses have confirmed the equivalence of RPD and OPD with respect to these outcomes [17, 27]. We use the International Study Group of Pancreatic Surgery grading system for classification of POPF, delayed gastric emptying (DGE), and postoperative pancreatic hemorrhage (PPH) [28–30]. Within our learning-curve optimized cohort, we have reported a clinically significant morbidity rate (Clavien-Dindo Grade $\geq$ 3) of 23.3%, 90-day mortality of 3.3%, and clinically significant POPF (Grade B/C) rate of 6.9%. We do not routinely place gastric tubes or jejunal feeding tubes. In older patients with poor functional status or patients with malnutrition, we will occasionally place an 18-Fr gastro-jejunal dual port tube. Treatment of DGE varies case by case, but we have found metoclopramide and erythromycin to be largely ineffective. For mild cases, we will sometimes allow oral feeds and manage vomiting with TPN support. For severe cases, nasogastrojejunal tubes or percutaneous gastrojejunal tubes are placed endoscopically to allow for gastric decompression and distal feeds.

We treat suspected PPH very aggressively. The typical time window is 3 weeks post-op; however, this complication can occur any time after POD #5 [31]. PPH typically presents as a decrease in hemoglobin/hematocrit, blood in the drain, or gastrointestinal bleeding. If clinical suspicion is high, patients are managed by interventional radiology (IR) for celiac and SMA angiography. The GDA stump is marked with a 10-mm clip, and the RGA stump is marked with a 5-mm clip intraoperatively. We do not leave a stump on these vessels so the clips aid with identification. We manage bleeding with covered stents. If no extravasation is identified, but our suspicion remains high for a sentinel bleed, we will prophylactically use a stent or leave the femoral access catheter in place and watch the patient for evidence of re-bleed. If the clinical suspicion is low, we will obtain a CT angiogram to look for pseudoaneurysm or extravasation of contrast. If IR and/or CT scan are both negative and they continue with gastrointestinal bleed, our gastroenterologists perform endoscopic evaluation of the GJ anastomosis and afferent limb to the HJ and PJ.

Education and Learning Curve

PD has a long learning curve. Tseng et al. looked at the outcomes of high-volume pancreatic surgeons from early in their career and found that outcomes did not improve significantly until they had performed more than 60 PDs [32]. Schmidt et al. showed that perioperative morbidity was higher in surgeons who had done less than 50 PDs [33]. Gagner and Pomp reported the first

laparoscopic PD, but laparoscopy was never adopted owing to the high technical demands. Introduction of RPD brings higher dexterity compared to laparoscopy but added technical difficulties due to the loss of haptic feedback. This has necessitated additional surgical training.

The low volume of RPDs during training and its long learning curve necessitate a deliberate proficiency-based approach to training surgeons. The University of Pittsburgh has developed a five-step curriculum for teaching advanced robotic hepato-pancreatico-biliary (HPB) procedures. It includes (1) proficiency-based virtual reality simulation curriculum, (2) inanimate biotissue curriculum, (3) HPB video library, (4) intraoperative evaluation, and (5) skills maintenance with ongoing assessments (Fig. 12.5). This program has graduated trainees with interest in HPB surgery, many of whom have developed robotic programs at their new institutions.

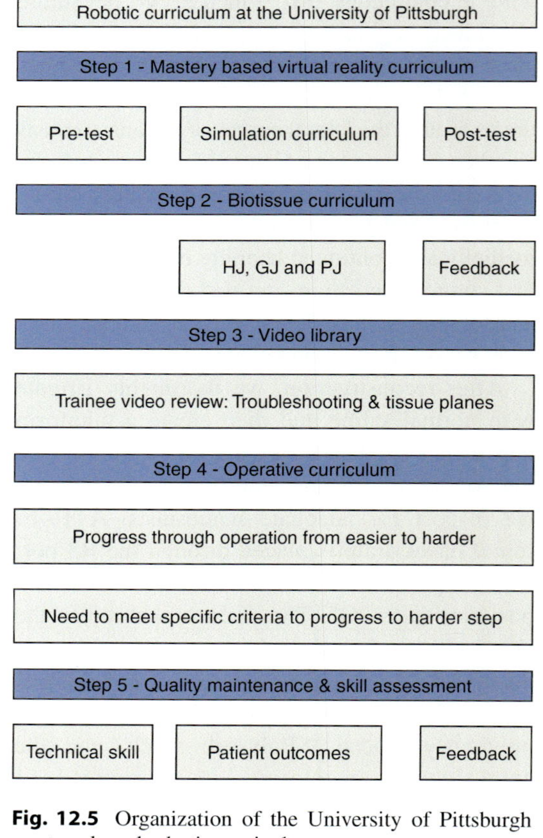

Fig. 12.5 Organization of the University of Pittsburgh mastery-based robotic curriculum

Conclusion

The robotic approach to pancreatic resections has been shown to be safe and feasible and has outcomes on par with the open approach. The training programs and the enhanced dexterity and stability of the platform make it superior to the laparoscopic approach for widespread dissemination of techniques. The RPD is our preferred approach for pancreatic head resection whenever indicated and feasible. Though learning RPD has an identified learning curve, an innovative, proficiency-based curriculum developed at our institution helps shorten the learning curve and could serve to facilitate further spread of RPD.

References

1. Whipple AO, Parsons WB, Mullins CR. Treatment of carcinoma of the ampulla of Vater. Ann Surg. 1935;102:763–79.
2. Whipple AO. Observations on radical surgery for lesions of the pancreas. Surg Gynecol Obstet. 1946;82:623–31.
3. Gagner M, Pomp A. Laparoscopic pylorus-preserving pancreatoduodenectomy. Surg Endosc. 1994;8:408–10.
4. Palanivelu C, Rajan PS, Rangarajan M, et al. Evolution in techniques of laparoscopic pancreaticoduodenectomy: a decade long experience from a tertiary center. J Hepato-Biliary-Pancreat Surg. 2009;16:731–40.
5. Kendrick ML, Cusati D. Total laparoscopic pancreaticoduodenectomy. Arch Surg. 2010;145:19–23.
6. Giulianotti PC, Sbrana F, Bianco FM, et al. Robot-assisted laparoscopic pancreatic surgery: single-surgeon experience. Surg Endosc. 2010;24:1646–57.
7. Zureikat AH, Moser AJ, Boone BA, et al. 250 robotic pancreatic resections. Ann Surg. 2013;258:554–9.
8. Gagner M, Pomp A. Laparoscopic pancreatic resection: is it worthwhile? J Gastrointest Surg. 1997;1:20–5; discussion 25-6.
9. Gagner M, Gentileschi P. Hand-assisted laparoscopic pancreatic resection. Semin Laparosc Surg. 2001;8:114–25.
10. Hanly EJ, Talamini MA. Robotic abdominal surgery. Am J Surg. 2004;188:19–26.
11. Zeh HJ, Bartlett DL, Moser AJ. Robotic-assisted major pancreatic resection. Adv Surg. 2011;45:323–40.
12. Gagner M, Palermo M. Laparoscopic Whipple procedure: review of the literature. J Hepato-Biliary-Pancreat Surg. 2009;16:726–30.
13. Nguyen KT, Zureikat AH, Chalikonda S, et al. Technical aspects of robotic-assisted pancreaticoduodenectomy (RPD). J Gastrointest Surg. 2011;15:870–5.
14. Boone BA, Zenati M, Hogg ME, et al. Assessment of quality outcomes for robotic pancreaticoduodenectomy. JAMA Surg. 2015;150:416.
15. Hogg ME, Tam V, Zenati M, et al. Mastery-based virtual reality robotic simulation curriculum: the first step toward operative robotic proficiency. J Surg Educ. 2017;74:477–85.
16. Tam V, Zenati M, Novak S, et al. Robotic pancreatoduodenectomy biotissue curriculum has validity and improves technical performance for surgical oncology fellows. J Surg Educ. 2017;74(6):1057–65.
17. Zureikat AH, Postlewait LM, Liu Y, et al. A multi-institutional comparison of perioperative outcomes of robotic and open pancreaticoduodenectomy. Ann Surg. 2016;264:640–9.
18. Varadhachary GR, Tamm EP, Abbruzzese JL, et al. Borderline resectable pancreatic cancer: definitions, management, and role of preoperative therapy. Ann Surg Oncol. 2006;13:1035–46.
19. Evans DB, Farnell MB, Lillemoe KD, et al. Surgical treatment of resectable and borderline resectable pancreas cancer: expert consensus statement. Ann Surg Oncol. 2009;16:1736–44.
20. Callery MP, Chang KJ, Fishman EK, et al. Pretreatment assessment of resectable and borderline resectable pancreatic cancer: expert consensus statement. Ann Surg Oncol. 2009;16:1727–33.
21. Cunningham KE, Zenati MS, Petrie JR, et al. A policy of omitting an intensive care unit stay after robotic pancreaticoduodenectomy is safe and cost-effective. J Surg Res. 2016;204:8–14.
22. Molinari E, Bassi C, Salvia R, et al. Amylase value in drains after pancreatic resection as predictive factor of postoperative pancreatic fistula: results of a prospective study in 137 patients. Ann Surg. 2007;246:281–7.
23. Ecker BL, McMillan MT, Allegrini V, et al. Risk factors and mitigation strategies for pancreatic fistula after distal pancreatectomy. Ann Surg. 2019;269(1):143–9.
24. Cameron JL, Riall TS, Coleman J, et al. One thousand consecutive pancreaticoduodenectomies. Ann Surg. 2006;244:10–5.
25. Hatzaras I, Schmidt C, Klemanski D, et al. Pancreatic resection in the octogenarian: a safe option for pancreatic malignancy. J Am Coll Surg. 2011;212:373–7.
26. Makary M, Winter J, Cameron J, et al. Pancreaticoduodenectomy in the very elderly. J Gastrointest Surg. 2006;10:347–56.
27. McMillan MT, Zureikat AH, Hogg ME, et al. A propensity score–matched analysis of robotic vs open pancreatoduodenectomy on incidence of pancreatic fistula. JAMA Surg. 2017;152:327–35.
28. Wente MN, Bassi C, Dervenis C, et al. Delayed gastric emptying (DGE) after pancreatic surgery: a suggested definition by the International Study Group of Pancreatic Surgery (ISGPS). Surgery. 2007;142:761–8.
29. Wente MN, Veit JA, Bassi C, et al. Postpancreatectomy hemorrhage (PPH)–an International Study Group of Pancreatic Surgery (ISGPS) definition. Surgery. 2007;142:20–5.

30. Bassi C, Dervenis C, Butturini G, et al. Postoperative pancreatic fistula: an international study group (ISGPF) definition. Surgery. 2005;138:8–13.
31. Lee JH, Hwang DW, Lee SY, et al. Clinical features and management of pseudoaneurysmal bleeding after pancreatoduodenectomy. Am Surg. 2012;78:309–17.
32. Eppsteiner RW, Csikesz NG, McPhee JT, et al. Surgeon volume impacts hospital mortality for pancreatic resection. Ann Surg. 2009;249:635–40.
33. Schmidt CM. Effect of hospital volume, surgeon experience, and surgeon volume on patient outcomes after Pancreaticoduodenectomy. Arch Surg. 2010;145:634.

Edward Cho, Spyridon Pagkratis, Houssam Osman, and D. Rohan Jeyarajah

Historical Perspective

Pancreatic head adenocarcinoma is a common solid malignancy with aggressive course and high mortality. Despite significant progress in chemotherapeutic regimens and other adjunctive treatments, its median survival remains less than 2 years with overall 5-year survival rate less than 10% [1]. Pancreaticoduodenectomy (PD) is considered to be the only potential cure, but unfortunately, only a minority of patients are candidates for resection at the time of diagnosis. In 1935, Dr. Allen Oldfather Whipple reported the first successful PD in a two-stage procedure in three patients [2], and 6 years later, he described the first single-stage PD [3]. Since then, more than 80 years have passed, but the technique has not

Electronic supplementary material The online version of this chapter (https://doi.org/10.1007/978-3-030-18740-8_13) contains supplementary material, which is available to authorized users.

E. Cho
Hepatobiliary Surgery, Methodist Richardson Medical Center, Richardson, TX, USA
e-mail: edwardc@tscsurgical.com

S. Pagkratis · H. Osman
HPB Surgery, Methodist Richardson Medical Center, Richardson, TX, USA
e-mail: HOsman@tscsurgical.com

D. R. Jeyarajah (✉)
Hepatopancreaticobiliary Surgery, Methodist Richardson Medical Center, Richardson, TX, USA

dramatically changed and PD is still considered one of the most complex and technically challenging abdominal operations with high perioperative morbidity and mortality.

In an effort to improve postoperative outcomes, less invasive approaches were adopted. Improvements in technology and technique over the last two decades have allowed us to perform laparoscopic and robotic pancreatic surgeries. These approaches have become popular for distal pancreatectomy, such that minimally invasive procedures are now considered to be the standard of care [4]. The first laparoscopic PD was reported by Ganger and Pomp in 1994 [5]. It was a 10 hour operation for chronic pancreatitis with prolonged postoperative hospital stay. Since then, the literature supports that laparoscopic PD is safe and feasible [6, 7]. Despite being performed in specialized centers, laparoscopic PD has not been widely adopted for numerous reasons including difficult anatomic location of the pancreas with close proximity to important vascular structures, limited working space of the retroperitoneum, complexity of the procedure requiring three anastomoses, and limitations of laparoscopy such as two-dimensional view, lack of depth perception, limited range of instrument motion, and long learning curve [8].

The introduction of the daVinci robotic system (Intuitive Surgical, CA) has helped to overcome some of these limitations. It offers improved ergonomics for the surgeon to decrease fatigue, offers fine motor control while eliminating tremor, provides 540° of articulating wrist movement and enhanced 3-D vision, and allows for more precise dissection and suturing on delicate tissues [9]. Using these advantages, Giulianotti in 2003 reported the first robotic-assisted PD (RAPD) [10]. Over the next 15 years, multiple pancreatic centers have incorporated the robot in their practice and have reported very promising results [4, 7–9, 11]. The paradigm has shifted from RAPD to hand-assisted robotic PD to purely robotic PD. Current literature supports when compared to open PD, the robotic approach provides comparable oncologic results in margin positivity and harvested lymph nodes, perioperative fistula rate, morbidity, and mortality and likely reduces blood loss, length of stay, pain, wound complications, and delayed gastric emptying [7–9, 11]. On the other hand, robotic PD is associated with longer operative times, especially for those at the beginning of the learning curve, and higher direct costs [8, 9, 11]. These results are better reproduced by highly trained and skilled surgeons in high-volume centers. It is our belief and experience that robotic PD is safe with equivalent technical and oncologic results in appropriately selected patients. In this chapter, we will present a reproducible step-by-step technique for robotic PD that follows the natural flow of open PD.

Indications

With experience, most patients who would qualify for open PD (OPD) would also qualify for robotic approach. It is our preference to reserve RAPD for patients that are felt to have clearly resectable tumors. Patient selection is critical, and the novice robotic surgeon should not engage in resecting a large periampullary tumor in a difficult abdomen early in the learning curve. Some groups have routinely performed robotic vein resection, but this is not our preference at this time. The robotic technique can be applied for pancreatic adenocarcinoma, neuroendocrine tumor (NET), intraductal papillary mucinous neoplasm (IPMN), common bile duct cholangiocarcinoma, duodenal lesion, pancreatitis, and others. At this time, our contraindications for this approach are patients with hostile abdomen from numerous previous operations and tumors that require vascular resection. As with OPD, patients with contraindications such as presence of metastatic disease, short life expectancy due to comorbidities, uncontrolled coagulopathy, and contraindications to general anesthesia should not be considered for robotic PD. Inability to tolerate pneumoperitoneum automatically excludes patients from this minimally invasive approach.

Preoperative Workup

For patients requiring PD, detailed history and physical exam are performed, including the onset of symptoms, presence of upper abdominal and/or back pain, jaundice, and symptoms of pancreatic insufficiency. Past medical history including onset of diabetes, cardiac disease, and respiratory comorbidities is pertinent, as well as family history, including first-degree cancer history and history of pancreatitis. Smoking and alcohol history is obtained and cessation counseling is held. Focused physical examination of the heart, lungs, and abdomen and exams for lymphadenopathy and peripheral vascular diseases are conducted.

Preoperative laboratory values including complete blood count, comprehensive metabolic panel, coagulation panel, cancer marker CA19-9, and HbA1C are obtained. Computed tomography (CT) of the chest is obtained to rule out metastatic disease to the lungs. CT of the abdomen and pelvis with triple phase contrast is also obtained to evaluate for metastatic disease and to assess for anatomic resectability. Routine endoscopic ultrasound (EUS)-guided biopsy of periampullary lesions is controversial. With the increased use of neoadjuvant chemotherapy, there has been a need to obtain tissue diagnosis prior to chemotherapy. It is imperative that the surgeon not insist on tissue diagnosis; the presence of a solid mass or distal CBD stricture in the appropriate clinical scenario should warrant PD. If there is any doubt of the diagnosis, liberal use of EUS is encouraged. If the patient has a duodenal mass requiring PD, esophagogastroduodenoscopy and colonoscopy are obtained.

Anesthesia, Patient Positioning, and Port Placement

Use of an Enhanced Recovery After Surgery (ERAS) pathway is encouraged in patients undergoing PD [12]. This will include high carbohydrate liquid intake until 2 h prior to surgery, use of aggressive pre-emptive pain regimen with acetaminophen and gabapentin, and use of alvimopan.

The patient is laid supine on a well-padded operating table. After induction of anesthesia, appropriate lines are placed. Arterial line is routinely used. For patients without many comorbidities, at least two large bore intravenous lines are sufficient for surgery. However, central lines are often placed in patients that require more invasive monitoring. After securing lines and pulse oximetry monitoring, both arms are tucked to the patient's side, using egg crate rolls to pad the elbows and hands. It is preferable to use a nonslip foam and restraint belts on the bed to prevent sliding when the patient is in reverse Trendelenburg position.

Positioning is Different for the Xi or Si Robotic Platforms

For the Si configuration, the patient is placed in split-leg position with the assistant surgeon between the legs. The patient's legs are secured well with straps and foot boards. Positioning is checked by both anesthesia and the surgeon to ensure that the patient does not move when placed into reverse Trendelenburg position.

For the Xi configuration, a foot board is secured at the bottom of the table, with the patient's feet in slight "V" configuration for ergonomic comfort, using appropriate foam rolls to pad the bottom and heel of the feet. Pillows are

used to pad the legs at the knees. The assistant stands at the patient's left side. Again, positioning is checked with the patient in reverse Trendelenburg position to ensure that the patient does not move.

The patient is prepped from mid-chest to the groin. Appropriate warming devices such as the Bair hugger and blankets are placed in the head/shoulder area and on the lower extremities. After appropriate draping and an operative timeout, we place a 5-mm port using an optical trocar and a 0 degree 5-mm camera at the midline in the supraumbilical area. Pneumoperitoneum is achieved with CO_2 insufflation to 15 mm Hg. Under direct visualization, two additional trocars on the patient's left are placed: an 8-mm port in the left midclavicular line one handbreadth away from the midline port and a second 8-mm robotic port in the left, anterior to the mid-axillary line that is one handbreadth away from the first 8-mm port (Fig. 13.1). Then an additional 12-mm camera port on the patient's right midclavicular line in the subcostal region that is one handbreadth away from the midline port (Fig. 13.1) is placed. The camera is placed to the patient's right of midline because it gives

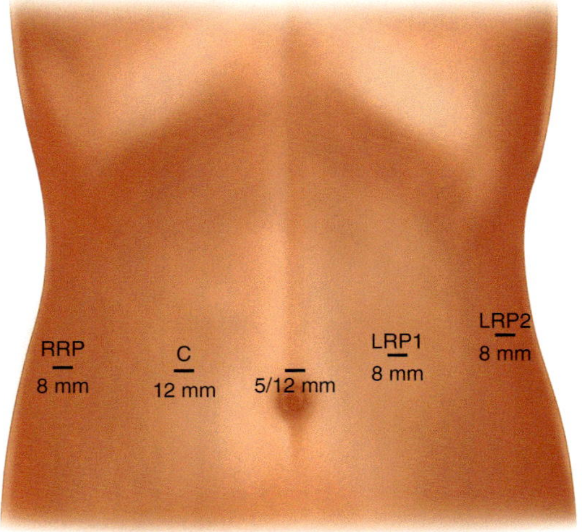

Fig. 13.1 Trocar placement for the Si system. RRP right robotic port, LRP left robotic ports 1 and 2. Arm 2 connects to RRP. Arm 1 to LRP 1, and Arm 3 to LRP 2

the best visualization of the superior mesenteric vein (SMV) and portal vein (PV) structure, which is the critical anatomic structure to identify and dissect around during PD. All ports are at least one handbreadth away from each other so that the robotic arms will not conflict with each other. Finally an 8-mm robotic port is placed on the patient's right, anterior to the mid-axillary line that is one handbreadth away from the last 12-mm midclavicular port. Subsequently, the original midline 5-mm port is upsized to a 12-mm air seal port (SurgiQuest Airseal, Medline) which can be used by the bedside assistant as an extra laparoscopic port (Fig. 13.1). Notably, the Airseal port must be placed last, because once Airseal mode is initiated, it becomes difficult to place additional trocars. Furthermore, for the Xi system, the trocars are placed in a more linear fashion, while the trocars for the Si system are placed in a more curvilinear fashion (Fig. 13.1). After an initial brief laparoscopic portion of the case, the patient is placed in slight reverse Trendelenburg position. The robot (Si system) is docked just above the patient's head. Figure 13.2 shows our typical port placements and robot docking position.

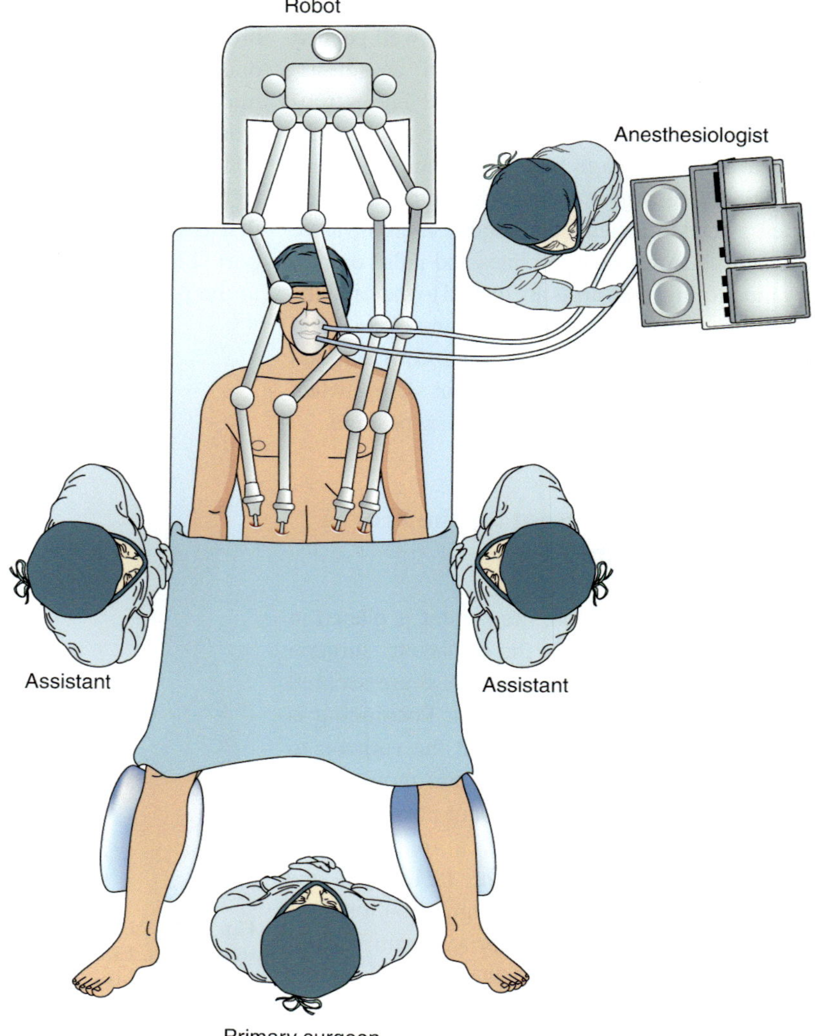

Fig. 13.2 Patient positioning for robotic pancreaticoduodenectomy with the Da Vinci Si system. The Si platform is docked from above the patient's head. The Xi platform can come from above the head or from the patient's left or right side. The authors prefer to position the Xi from the patient's left side

Operative Technique

Step 1: Laparoscopy and Robot Docking

The procedure starts laparoscopically by inspecting the abdomen for peritoneal disease. If there is no evidence of metastasis, the case continues. The greater curvature of the stomach is mobilized, entering the lesser sac through the gastrocolic ligament. The operating surgeon uses an atraumatic grasper (such as a DeBakey grasper) and a harmonic scalpel, and posterior gastric adhesions to the pancreas are taken down during this step. The transverse colon with its mesentery is retracted cephalad and the ligament of Treitz is identified. The small bowel is run distally and the anti-mesenteric side of the small bowel, approximately 40–60 cm distal to the ligament of Treitz, is sutured to the posterior wall of the stomach using 2-0 Ethibond and a Ti-KNOT device near the greater curvature, proximal to the future location of the gastrojejunostomy (Video 13.1 ref. 0:01″ to 0:30″). This step is performed before the robot is docked. Notably, the suture between the stomach and jejunum is placed toward the left of the patient with the small bowel traveling from left to right. This is important to prepare for the gastrojejunostomy at the end of the PD.

Robotic Resection

The robot is docked over the patient's head (Si) or over the patient's head or from the patient's left or right sides (Xi).

Instrument selection for initial dissection with Si system: arm 1, vessel sealer; arm 2, fenestrated bipolar; and arm 3, prograsp.

Instrument selection for initial dissection with Xi system: arm 1, fenestrated bipolar; arm 2, camera; arm 3, vessel sealer; and arm 4, prograsp.

Step 2: Identify SMV and Create the Tunnel

The next step is to identify and follow the right gastroepiploic vein to the superior mesenteric vein (SMV) at the inferior edge of the pancreas. The right gastroepiploic vein joins with the middle colic vein to form the gastrocolic trunk of Henle which leads the surgeon to the SMV and should be viewed as the key step to identifying the SMV. There is tendency to be far to the patient's right at this point of dissection.

The gastroepiploic vein may have to be sacrificed at this point with a single hemolock clip at its origin followed by ligating the vein with the vessel sealer. A tunnel is started under the neck of the pancreas using the vessel sealer, staying just anterior to the SMV (Fig. 13.3).

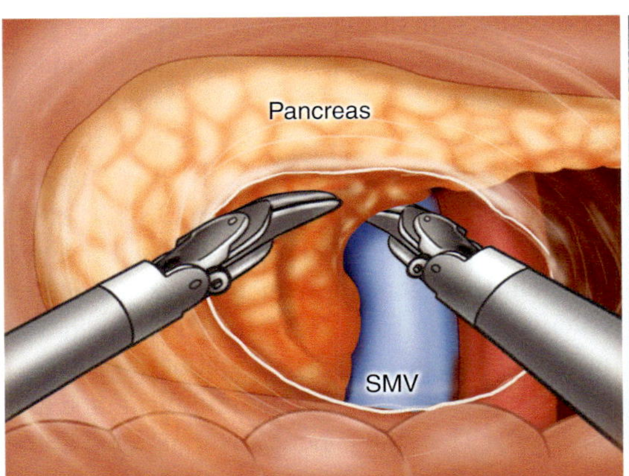

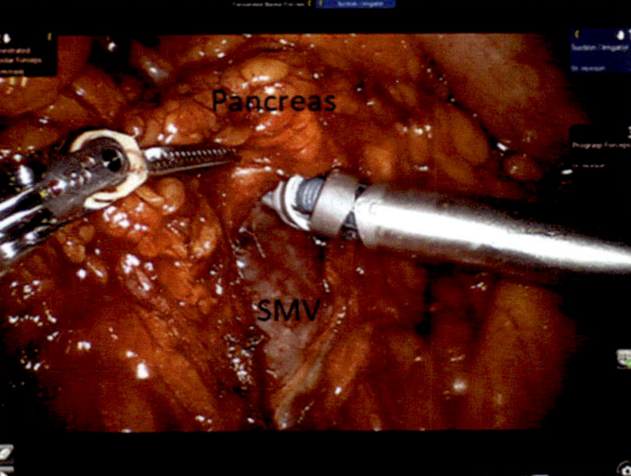

Fig. 13.3 Creation of the tunnel posterior to the neck of the pancreas

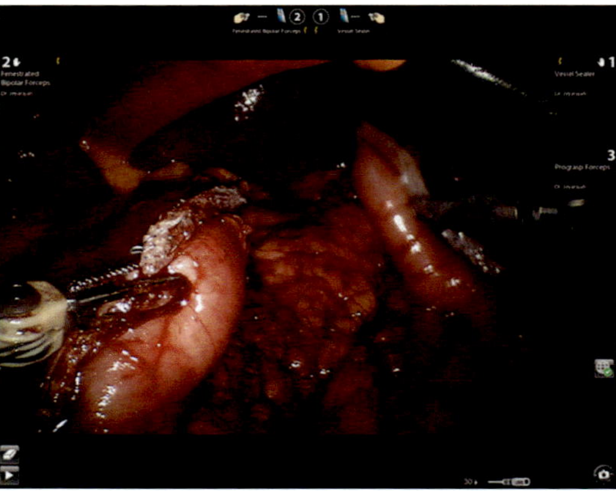

Fig. 13.4 Division of the stomach with the pancreas lying underneath

The assistant should use an atraumatic instrument to retract the transverse colon mesentery inferiorly and to provide counter-traction. The tunnel over the SMV is created for as long a distance as possible (Video 13.1 ref. 0:31″ to 0:50″). The assistant can also use the bedside suction to assist with development of this tunnel.

Step 3: Division of the Stomach

At this time, as long as the surgeon is certain that the SMV is free, it is reasonable to divide the stomach (Fig. 13.4). This is completed much earlier in RAPD than OPD, where our practice is to fully commit to PD only after all critical structures are dissected and isolated. The lesser and greater curvature vessels of the stomach are dissected and ligated using the vessel sealer device and the antrum is transected using a Flex 60-mm gold load stapler entered through the 12-mm Airseal port by the bedside assistant (Video 13.1 ref. 0:51″ to 1:10″). Care must be taken to ensure that the nasogastric tube is not included in the staple line. The proximal stomach is reflected toward the patient's left upper quadrant and the transected antrum toward the patient's right side.

Step 4: Hepatic Artery Dissection and Identification of the Gastroduodenal Artery

The lesser omentum is opened and the superior pancreatic node lying just anterior to the common hepatic artery (CHA) (station 8a) is identified. The superior pancreatic node is dissected and sent to pathology for permanent section only (Video 13.1 ref. 1:24″ to 1:57″). It is important to be aware that the CHA lies directly between this node and the superior aspect of the pancreas. If the portal vein is found directly underneath this node, this indicates replaced anatomy. The surgeon must be prepared for a replaced (and not accessory) right hepatic artery.

Then the CHA is traced to the patient's right side until the gastroduodenal artery is identified. It is important to practice good vascular technique and identify the correct "shiny white" plane of the artery to avoid bleeding. The gastroduodenal artery is carefully isolated (Fig. 13.5) and doubly clipped on the patient side and singly clipped on the specimen side with hemolock clips. The artery is transected with robotic scissors, whereas dissection of the vessels is performed using the vessel sealer. Other surgeons may find that the scissors can be useful for dissection.

Step 5: Creation of the Tunnel and Division of the Pancreas

The portal vein at the superior edge of the pancreas is identified. It is normally directly underneath the hepatic artery and to the patient's left of the gastroduodenal artery. The tunnel is completed starting inferiorly from the SMV toward the portal vein superiorly (Video 13.1 ref. 1:59″ to 2:20″) . An umbilical tape is passed through this tunnel so that the pancreas can be pulled anteriorly away from the vein. This is achieved using robotic arm 3 (Si) or robotic arm 4 (Xi) with the prograsp to hold the umbilical tape taut anteriorly. Then the pancreas is transected at the neck using the robotic scissors with electrocau-

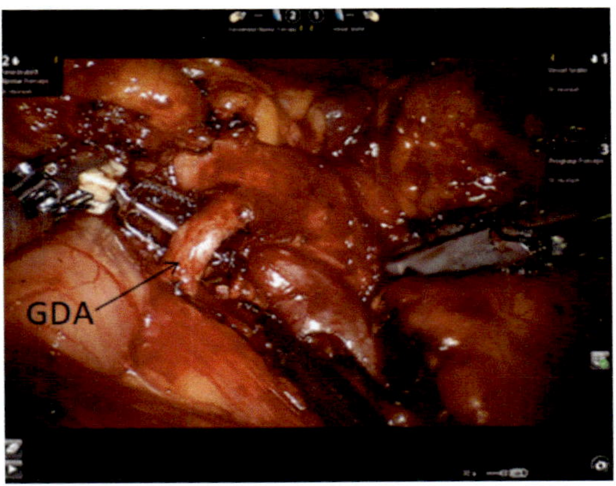

Fig. 13.5 Isolation of the gastroduodenal artery

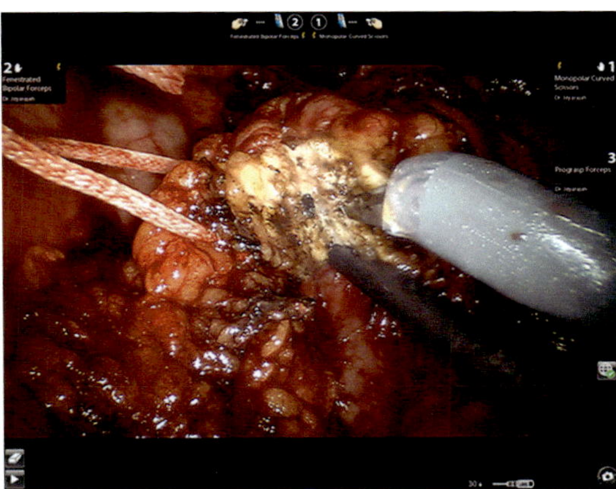

Fig. 13.6 Division of the pancreas, which is held anteriorly with an umbilical tape

tery (Fig. 13.6) (Video 13.1 ref. 2:23″ to 2:36″). The pancreatic duct is identified during the transection. Hemostasis is achieved with monopolar electrocautery attached to the scissors or bipolar energy attached to the fenestrated bipolar instrument. This technique can control bleeding effectively. Notably, some surgeons use the harmonic scalpel to transect the pancreas. While this may reduce bleeding, the pancreatic duct can be obstructed using this technique. In the instance that the pancreas is firm and the pancreatic duct is large, we may elect to use the harmonic scalpel.

Step 6: Kocher Maneuver and Division of the Jejunum

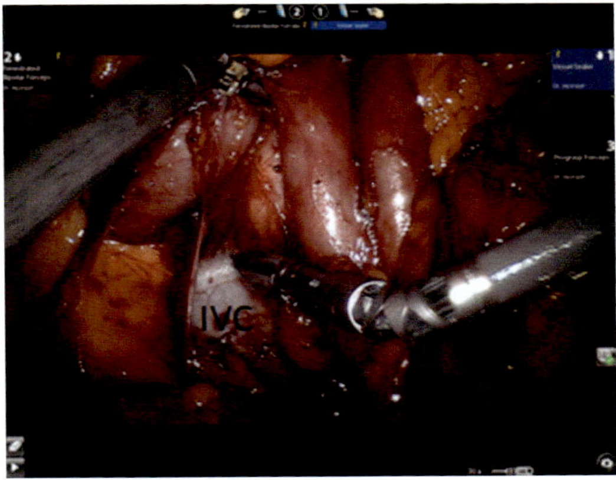

Fig. 13.7 Kocher maneuver exposing the inferior vena cava

A wide Kocher maneuver is started in retrograde fashion on the right side of the abdomen. This can be very difficult, so it is imperative to mobilize the hepatic flexure completely. In this manner, the duodenum is exposed and can be dissected away from the vena cava (Fig. 13.7). The duodenum is passed to robotic arm 3 (Si) or robotic arm 4 (Xi) using the prograsp to retract the duodenum up and toward the patient's head. The dissection is continued until the ligament of Treitz is reached from the right side of the patient and the proximal jejunum is prolapsed toward the patient's right side. The proximal jejunum is tran-

sected using a Flex 60-mm blue load stapler (Video 13.1 ref. 2:38″ to 3:20″). The proximal jejunal mesentery is divided using the vessel sealer and the fourth part of the duodenum is "unwound" such that the duodenum is now straightened and is in the right upper quadrant.

Step 7: Uncinate Process Dissection

At this point, only the uncinate pancreatic process and bile duct are left to be dissected. The uncinate is dissected off the SMA using the

Harmonic scalpel inserted through the assistant port (Video 13.1 ref. 3:22″ to 3:51″). The authors often utilize the SMA first approach, dissecting the mesopancreas off the SMA and then teasing the uncinate process away from the SMV.

Retraction of the uncinate process toward the patient's right side is best achieved with the fenestrated bipolar in robotic arm 2 (Si) or robotic arm 1 (Xi). The robotic suction can be placed to retract the SMV toward the patient's left side. This allows an excellent angle for the bedside assistant to use the harmonic scalpel to take the uncinate process off the SMA. Care must be taken to control the most superior venous branch off the SMV that is always at the most cranial portion of the specimen. This is usually controlled with hemoclips.

Step 8: Bile Duct Dissection

Next the common hepatic duct is dissected. This is located at the most superior aspect of the specimen, and the lateral common bile duct node will need to be taken to the patient's right of the common hepatic duct. Then, the common hepatic duct is isolated and transected using the robotic scissors. A margin is sent to pathology for frozen section examination at the time of transection of the duct. The entire specimen is placed in a large endocatch bag and placed in the left upper quadrant for later retrieval. It is our preference to leave the specimen in the endobag for the remainder of the operation which usually lasts about 1 hour.

Step 9: Pancreaticojejunostomy

The reconstruction now begins. The transected jejunum is already in the RUQ quadrant. The jejunum is oriented appropriately in a C-loop fashion in the RUQ. An end-pancreas to side-jejunal anastomosis is performed with the Blumgart technique [13]. Three 2-0 silk sutures on MH needles are placed through the pancreas near the transected neck, then to the anti-mesenteric side of the jejunum, and back through the pancreas again in a U stitch configuration. These three silk sutures with

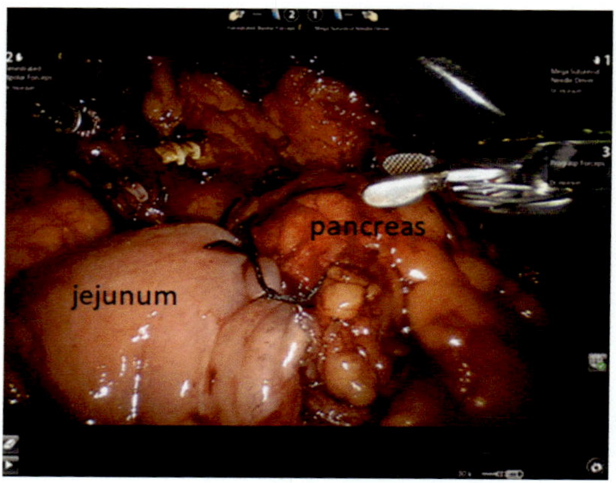

Fig. 13.8 Completed pancreaticojejunostomy with the Blumgart technique

needles are left in, and the cephalad most suture is retracted toward the patient's LUQ using the prograsp in robotic arm 3 (Si) or robotic arm 4 (Xi). The pancreatic duct-to-jejunal mucosa inner layer is completed using four 5-0 Monocryl sutures placed at the 3-, 6-, 9-, and 12-o'clock configurations (Video 13.1 ref. 3:55″ to 5:37″). It is useful to use a dyed suture in order to visualize it. We frequently insert a 5-Fr pediatric feeding tube cut at 10 cm into the pancreatic duct and passed through the enterotomy into the jejunum before the last monocryl suture is placed and tied. Then the Blumgart anastomosis is completed by using the three 2-0 silk sutures and taking a bite of the anti-mesenteric side of the jejunum again and tying the silk sutures, thus completing the outer anterior and posterior invaginating layers of jejunum over the transected pancreatic edge (Fig. 13.8).

Step 10: Hepaticojejunostomy

The hepaticojejunostomy is performed next. If the gallbladder remains in place, we use a 2-0 V-Loc suture to tie the fundus of the gallbladder to the anterior abdominal wall, using this method of liver retraction to help visualize the common hepatic duct. An enterotomy in the anti-mesenteric side of the jejunum distal to the pancreatic anastomosis is made, and an end-to-side

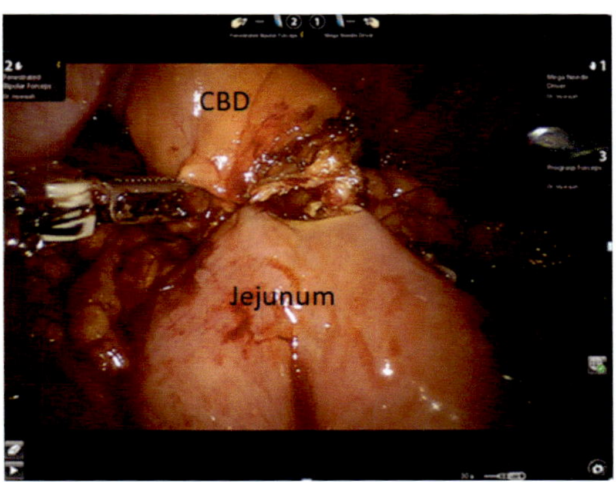

Fig. 13.9 Creation of the hepaticojejunostomy with running 4-0 monocryl suture

hepaticojejunostomy using running 4-0 monocryl suture is created (Fig. 13.9). Some surgeons will use two V-Loc 4-0 sutures for this anastomosis, but the barbs on the V-Loc can be traumatic so it has been our practice to use a 4-0 monocryl suture instead (Video 13.1 ref. 5:39″ to 6:18″) . Afterward, a cholecystectomy is performed. The gallbladder is dissected from the triangle of Calot using the robotic scissors, and the specimen is placed in another endocatch bag and placed in the patient's left upper quadrant for later retrieval.

Step 11: Gastrojejunostomy

The area where the distal jejunum was attached to the stomach is identified. A gastrotomy and enterotomy are made distally on the stomach and jejunum after the small bowel and stomach are lined up. A flex 60-mm blue load stapler is inserted by the bedside assistant, with each lip of the stapler entering into the two holes that were made, and the stapler is fired to create a gastrojejunostomy. The ensuing hole between the stomach and small bowel is closed with a running 2-0 V-Loc suture.

Step 12: Specimen Retrieval

The endocatch bags are retrieved through the 12-mm midline port and hemostasis is achieved. A drain is placed through the R1 port near the

pancreaticojejunostomy and hepaticojejunostomy anastomosis. The robot is undocked and moved away. Using laparoscopic camera visualization, the 12-mm camera port is closed with 0-Vicryl suture using an endoneedle device. The abdomen is then deflated, and all ports are removed. The midline 12-mm port site is enlarged to retrieve the specimens. Often, the final incision at this site is no more than 3 cm in length. The fascia at this site is closed with 0 PDS suture and skin is closed with 4-0 monocryl sutures and Dermabond is placed on the skin.

Postoperative Care Algorithm

The majority of the postoperative course after robotic PD is routine and consistent with the ERAS pathway; and most patients are admitted directly to the surgical ward. Patients with perioperative arrhythmia, hypotension, and increased blood loss requiring intraoperative transfusion or patients with significant comorbidities requiring close monitoring may warrant ICU admission. In our practice, patients do well when admitted directly to the floor. Patients are admitted from the OR with an abdominal drain, a nasogastric (NG) tube on low intermittent wall suction, and Foley catheter. Immediate postoperative blood work is obtained. Fluids at slightly higher than maintenance rate are given, and the urine output is trended along with vital signs to evaluate for resuscitation. Pain is controlled in multimodality fashion, with intravenous acetaminophen given for 24 h (Ofirmev, Mallinckrodt Pharmaceuticals), intravenous nonsteroidal anti-inflammatory agents given for 48 h (Caldolor, Cumberland Pharmaceuticals) and patient-controlled analgesia with a narcotic agent such as hydromorphone. Transverse abdominis plane (TAP) block is also administered by anesthesia during the preoperative period using a mix of Exparel (Pacira Pharmaceuticals), 0.25% marcaine, and saline in a 1:1:1 ratio. The patient is maintained nothing per os with limited oral intake, although alvimopan is given postoperatively and continued for 12 days. Pneumatic compression devices are used for deep vein thrombosis (DVT) prophylaxis, but chemical prophylaxis is held in the immediate postoperative period. Per ERAS pathway, patients are encouraged to walk with assistance 4–6 h postoperatively.

On postoperative day (POD) 1, the NGT is discontinued and the patient is placed on sips of liquids, gum, and hard candy. Unless contraindicated, the Foley catheter is removed and intravenous fluids are lowered. Chemical DVT prophylaxis, usually lovenox, is started. Activity is increased, often with help from physical and/or occupational therapy. Drain fluid is sent amylase analysis, and levels three times above normal or greater are considered positive for pancreatic leak [14].

On POD3, diet is slowly advanced to clears and full liquid diet. The patient is weaned from the PCA and started on oral pain medications. If the patient has symptoms of delayed gastric emptying, metoclopramide is given. A second drain fluid is sent for amylase analysis. If the amylase is lower than three times above normal levels, we often remove the drain at this time.

On POD5, the patient is tolerating regular diet. Postoperative pain should be controlled with oral pain medication. If the drain has not been removed, a third fluid sample is sent for amylase check. If the amylase level is lower than three times above normal values, the drain is removed. The patient will be normally discharged between POD4-6 unless complications arise. If drain amylase levels remain high, the patient will be discharged with the drain.

Conclusions

It is well documented that robotic PD is a safe technique in appropriately selected patients with good oncologic and perioperative results. Despite the fact that the daVinci surgical platform offers significant advantages compared to traditional laparoscopy, robotic PD still remains a very complex and challenging procedure with a long learning curve. This is the main reason that robotic PD has not been universally adopted. It is expected that with improved robotic technology, increased competition, and decreasing cost, the utilization of robotic techniques in pancreatic surgery will increase and surgeons will become more proficient and skilled [9]. Following the example of urology and gynecology, many general surgery residency programs provide robotic exposure and have adopted specialized training programs to teach their residents this new technology [9]. On the other hand, the benefit of this rapid adoption of robotic technology must be examined against the backdrop of an expensive health care system.

References

1. Jemal A, et al. Cancer statistics, 2006. CA Cancer J Clin. 2006;56(2):106–30.
2. Whipple AO, Parsons WB, Mullins CR. Treatment of carcinoma of the ampulla of Vater. Ann Surg. 1935;102(4):763–79.
3. Whipple AO. Observations on radical surgery for lesions of the pancreas. Surg Gynecol Obstet. 1946;82:623–31.
4. Mesleh MG, Stauffer JA, Asbun HJ. Minimally invasive surgical techniques for pancreatic cancer: ready for prime time? J Hepatobiliary Pancreat Sci. 2013;20(6):578–82.
5. Gagner M, Pomp A. Laparoscopic pylorus-preserving pancreatoduodenectomy. Surg Endosc. 1994;8(5):408–10.
6. Wang M, et al. Minimally invasive pancreaticoduodenectomy: a comprehensive review. Int J Surg. 2016;35:139–46.
7. Dai R, Turley RS, Blazer DG. Contemporary review of minimally invasive pancreaticoduodenectomy. World J Gastrointes Surg. 2016;8(12):784–91.
8. Peng, L et al. Systematic review and meta-analysis of robotic versus open pancreaticoduodenectomy. Surg Endosc. 2017;31(8):3085–97.
9. Baker EH, et al. Robotic pancreaticoduodenectomy for pancreatic adenocarcinoma: role in 2014 and beyond. J Gastrointes Oncol. 2015;6(4):396–405.
10. Giulianotti PC, et al. Robotics in general surgery: personal experience in a large community hospital. Arch Surg. 2003;138(7):777–84.
11. Kornaropoulos M, et al. Total robotic pancreaticoduodenectomy: a systematic review of the literature. Surg Endosc. 2017;31:4382.
12. Lassen K, et al. Guidelines for perioperative care for pancreaticoduodenectomy: enhanced recovery after surgery (ERAS(R)) society recommendations. Clin Nutr. 2012;31(6):817–30.
13. Blumgart LH. A new technique for pancreatojejunostomy. J Am Coll Surg. 1996;182(6):557.
14. Bassi C, et al. Postoperative pancreatic fistula: an international study group (ISGPF) definition. Surgery. 2005;138(1):8–13.

Implementation of the Robotic Technique in Pancreaticoduodenectomy

Georgios V. Georgakis, Hannah Thompson, and Joseph Kim

Introduction

A systematic approach to performing robotic pancreaticoduodenectomy has been developed over the past decade. Nevertheless, its application has been limited to a handful of centers around the world due to (1) requirements for advanced training of surgeons in complex surgery and use of robotic technology, (2) financial and time commitment from surgeons and their institutions to utilize the robotic platform, and (3) lack of adequate clinical volumes to ensure depth and breadth of training and development of expertise. In any event, it is clear that we are witnessing an increasing integration of computer assistance in the operating room with the emergence of surgeons who embrace these advanced technologies and have the technical skills to perform complex operative procedures at a computerized console. Although it is widely accepted that there is a lengthy learning curve for mastering new techniques and technologies, the questions of "what is required?" and "for how long?" remain unclear, especially when a program may already have both advanced hepatobiliary and robotic experiences. In this chapter, we share our experience and provide answers to these questions in the setting of having pre-existing hepatobiliary experience and advanced robotic skills.

The Stony Brook University Experience

The desire for a robotic pancreaticoduodenectomy program must be a component of a larger plan to develop a robotic gastrointestinal or hepatobiliary surgery program. The technical skills to perform robotic cholecystectomy, gastrectomy, small and large bowel resection, etc., are necessary and complementary to the performance of robotic pancreaticoduodenectomy and to the maintenance of skills to continue to safely perform all of these procedures. There must be commitment from three resources to establish a robotic program for complex gastrointestinal surgery: (1) surgeons, (2) operating room, and (3) institution.

Surgeon Commitment

Multiple levels of training are required for surgeons to develop initial comfort with and

Electronic supplementary material The online version of this chapter (https://doi.org/10.1007/978-3-030-18740-8_14) contains supplementary material, which is available to authorized users.

G. V. Georgakis · H. Thompson
Department of Surgery, Stony Brook University Hospital, Stony Brook, NY, USA
e-mail: Georgios.georgakis@stonybrookmedicine.edu; Hannah.Thompson@stonybrookmedicine.edu

J. Kim (✉)
Department of Surgery, University of Kentucky, Lexington, KY, USA
e-mail: joseph.kim@uky.edu

© Springer Nature Switzerland AG 2020
J. Kim, J. Garcia-Aguilar (eds.), *Minimally Invasive Surgical Techniques for Cancers of the Gastrointestinal Tract*, https://doi.org/10.1007/978-3-030-18740-8_14

subsequent mastery of the robotic platform. The initial training may involve the development of console and bedside skills, and subsequent training may require animal labs and observation of robotic procedures. The novice robotic surgeon should begin with less complex procedures and work toward performing the technically demanding operations later in the robotics learning curve. Additionally, the surgeon should anticipate that all robotic procedures will likely have longer length of surgery times than the corresponding laparoscopic or open procedures during this initial development of the robotic program.

For the most complex procedures, two specialty trained surgeons are required. The necessity of two surgeons is based on the need for surgeons to have both the clinical expertise and surgical skill for both operation and robotic platform (console and bedside). In our experience, neither the console nor the bedside is an appropriate setting for residents or fellows who have not completed formal robotic training curriculum.

Operating Room Personnel

The second level of commitment involves the operating room and its personnel. In addition to the commitment from surgeons, operating room staff require the appropriate training to utilize the robotic platform. The training is essential to maintain positive metrics for operating room safety and efficiency (e.g., room preparation, patient positioning, robotic docking time, instrument exchange, and overall flow of the operation). The necessity of proper training becomes especially evident when longer robotic procedures crossover into late work shifts with coverage by operating room personnel who may not have robotic experience.

Institutional Commitment

There must be strong commitment from the institution. The investment in new technologies is long term, and the implementation and use of new technology cannot be measured by single procedure productivity metrics, since robotic pancreaticoduodenectomy necessitates two attending surgeons, longer operative times, additional training, etc. With promising advances in surgical technology, the institution will also need to provide financial support to test and purchase new devices and instrumentation.

Our Current Environment

At Stony Brook University, we have recently embarked on performing robotic pancreaticoduodenectomy. In our division, we have an experienced surgical oncologist with experience using the robotic platform for gastrointestinal and foregut procedures over the past decade. A formal robotic training curriculum was not available during his early career, but he participated in several off-site training programs and received informal mentorship from senior robotic surgeons. The division recently recruited a surgical oncologist who had specialized training in complex robotic gastrointestinal surgery and who completed a formal robotic surgical oncology curriculum. Together, the two surgeons were the critical mass with combined experience in pancreatic surgery and robotic surgery to plan and perform the first robotic pancreaticoduodenectomy. In brief, our preoperative planning included discussion of the technique, review of previously recorded robotic procedures, and coordination with the operating room staff.

Operating Room Setup

General Preparations

On the day of surgery, plans are reviewed with operating room staff (anesthesia and nursing) regarding positioning, room setup, instruments, staff roles, etc. At our institution, we use the da Vinci Surgical System with Si platform. The patient is positioned in the supine position with the legs placed in split position, the right arm tucked, and the left arm placed on an arm board. The split legs enable the assistant to better access the assistant ports, especially in tall or morbidly obese patients. In smaller patients, standard supine position is also acceptable. The carts and tables are arranged as depicted in Fig. 14.1.

Trocar/Port Placement

We position our ports as depicted in Fig. 14.2. The peritoneum is accessed via a 5-mm left upper quadrant Optiview trocar (Ethicon), which is typically placed in the mid-axillary line. This port will be exchanged for robotic arm number 1, and the exact distance from the subcostal margin may vary depending on the patient's habitus. After excluding metastatic disease, the remaining ports are placed. For tall or obese patients, the ports are generally placed more cephalad because CO_2 insufflation of the abdominal cavity will increase the space/distance between the port insertion sites and target lesion. In contrast, port placement may require more inferior/caudal locations in smaller patients. We use a 12-mm blunt balloon trocar (Applied Medical) for our camera port, which is

typically placed two fingerbreadths cephalad and two fingerbreadths to the right of the umbilicus; an 8-mm robotic trocar in the right upper quadrant in

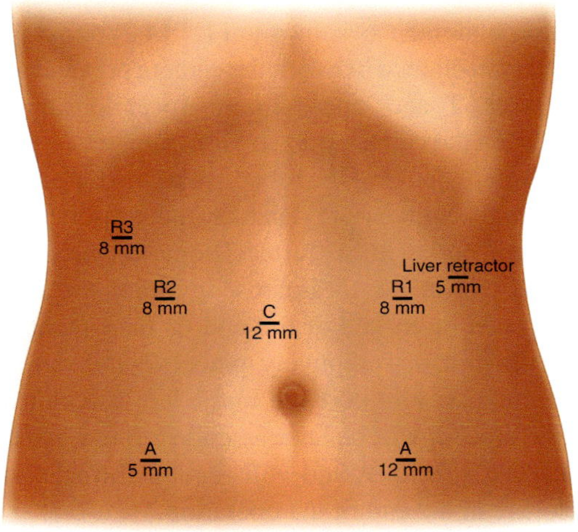

Fig. 14.2 Trocar/port placement for robotic pancreaticoduodenectomy

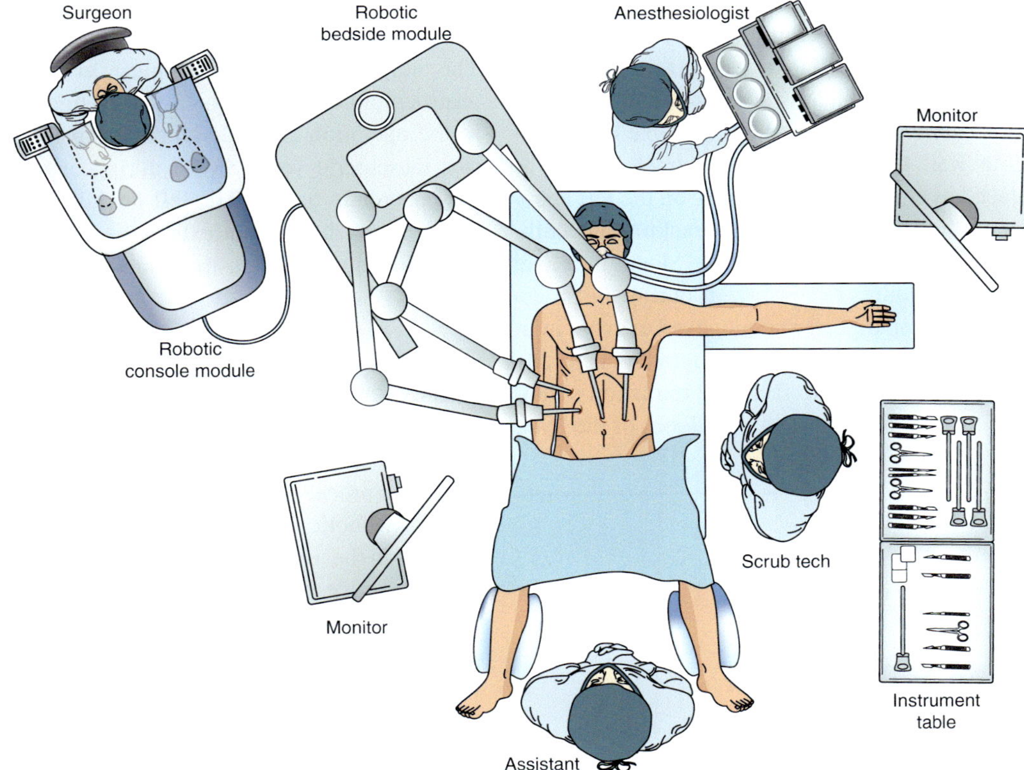

Fig. 14.1 Patient positioning and operative setup for robotic pancreaticoduodenectomy

the mid-clavicular line for arm number 2; and another 8-mm robotic trocar in the anterior axillary line for arm number 3, and we exchange the initial 5-mm trocar with a robotic 8-mm trocar for arm number 1. The assistant ports are placed in the lower abdomen as shown in Fig. 14.2: one 5-mm trocar positioned between the camera port and arm number 2 and one 12-mm trocar positioned between the camera port and arm number 1.

Before docking the robot, we routinely place a figure-of-eight 0-Vicryl suture in the fascia at the camera port with a Carter Thomason needle to avoid converting to laparoscopy after the robot has been undocked at the end of the operation. We do not pre-emptively place a suture at the 12-mm assistant port site in the left lower quadrant, since it will be later extended to remove the surgical specimen and will require formal open closure at the end of the operation.

Placement of Liver Retractor

We routinely use the liver retractor for robotic pancreaticoduodenectomy. We prefer to use the Snowden-Pencer® laparoscopic articulating triangular retractor that is stabilized at the bed rail by a Thompson Laparoscopic Flexible Holder for Elite Rail Clamp. The liver retractor must be placed as cephalad and laterally on the left abdomen as possible to avoid interaction and collisions with the robotic arms. Since the liver retractor requires readjustments during the procedure, we keep the left arm untucked to avoid injuries. We prefer to place the liver retractor centrally at the porta hepatis to facilitate retraction simultaneously of both left and right lobes of the liver.

Robotic Steps

Video 14.1

Entrance into Lesser Sac

Once the robot is docked over the patient's right shoulder (Fig. 14.1), we place the monopolar hook in robotic arm number 1, a fenestrated bipo-

lar grasper in robotic arm number 2, and a Cadiere or Prograsp forceps in robotic arm number 3. A suction-irrigator and energy sealing device (LigaSure™) are placed through the assistant ports. Dissection begins centrally at the gastrocolic ligament, at the level of the proposed antrectomy, by lifting the stomach anteriorly and cephalad with forceps in robotic arm number 3. We divide the avascular gastrocolic ligament using the robotic hook or LigaSure. Upon entrance into the lesser sac and identification of the posterior wall of the stomach, the forceps in robotic arm number 3 grasps the posterior stomach, and the attachments to the anterior surface of the pancreas are divided with the robotic hook or LigaSure. We separate the gastrocolic ligament from the transverse mesocolon at a location that enables easy identification of anatomic landmarks (lesser sac, posterior wall of the stomach, and anterior surface of the pancreas), which can be challenging in obese patients. Once we identify the avascular plane on the anterior surface of the pancreas, we follow it to the right all the way toward the hepatic flexure, staying anterior to the duodenum in preparation for Kocher maneuver. The surgeon must avoid injury to the right gastroepiploic vessels, which will be ligated later in the operation after identification of the superior mesenteric vein (SMV) during creation of the pancreatic tunnel. The left lateral dissection of the stomach does not extend beyond the proposed location of the gastrojejunostomy.

Cattell-Braasch Maneuver and Extended Kocherization

Our attention is turned to the right abdomen, where we proceed with take down of the hepatic flexure. Robotic arm number 3 and forceps or graspers in the assistant ports are used to continuously provide traction and counter-traction. Generally, robotic arm number 3 and assistant instruments are used to retract tissues in cephalad and caudal directions, respectively, thus avoiding collisions. Near-complete Cattell-Braasch maneuver (i.e., near-complete right medial visceral rotation) is required to facilitate extended Kocherization toward the ligament of Treitz

(LOT) entirely from the right side of the abdomen. The extent of this maneuver requires medialization of the cecum and terminal ileum to the axis of the inferior vena cava (IVC).

The extended Kocher maneuver is facilitated by gently grasping the duodenum with forceps in robotic arm number 3 and retracting it toward the patient's left side, while the forceps in robotic arm number 2 gently retracts the retroperitoneal tissues overlying Gerota's fascia in a lateral direction. With this exposure, the robotic hook in arm number 1 is used to divide the tissues as close to the duodenum as possible along its right lateral aspect. Dissection to separate the duodenum from the IVC proceeds cephalad toward the right lateral aspect of the porta hepatis. The porta hepatis must be separated from the retroperitoneum and the IVC to identify the lateral structures of the porta hepatis. In case of replaced right hepatic artery, this will be the most lateral structure in the porta hepatis.

During dissection of the porta hepatis, we expose the entire length of the common bile duct (CBD) on the lateral side. Additionally, lymph nodes on the posterolateral side of the porta hepatis (stations 12b1, 12b2, and 12c) are harvested, which facilitates exposure of the lateral aspect of the CBD. It is important to perform lymph node excision at this point of the procedure because the exposure to the right side of the porta hepatis will be obscured later in the procedure when the stomach is transected and retracted to the patient's right side. Isolation and identification of all portal structures, i.e., CBD, common hepatic artery, and portal vein, will be completed later in the procedure. We defer isolation and transection of the CBD until later in the operation when the porta hepatis is approached from the left side.

After completing dissection at the porta hepatis, our attention is turned in a caudal direction to complete the extended Kocher maneuver. A full, complete Kocherization is advised to facilitate complete mobilization of the third and fourth portions of the duodenum. Care must be taken to ensure that the dissection plane remains close to the duodenum to avoid vascular injury to the IVC or mesenteric vessels. Anatomically, the third portion of the duodenum follows a transverse course in the retroperitoneum from right to left and the fourth portion follows a slightly cephalad path, until the LOT, when it turns caudally and becomes the jejunum. During this step, we mobilize the third and fourth portions of the duodenum from its anterior, inferior, and posterior retroperitoneal attachments. On the anterior side, we free the duodenum from the root of the mesentery and the SMA/SMV. On the inferior side, we free the duodenum from the transverse mesocolon. On the posterior side, we free the duodenum from the aorta and the retroperitoneum. We perform these maneuvers to mobilize the duodenum using the robotic hook or LigaSure. Exposure for this step is facilitated by retracting the transverse mesocolon inferiorly which requires extended Cattell-Braasch maneuver. Since the SMA/SMV course in the root of mesentery in a craniocaudal fashion anterior to the third portion of the duodenum, the assistant must gently retract the root of the mesentery to the left to provide exposure (Fig. 14.3). Working in this space is one of the most challenging steps of this robotic operation.

Once the final fibers of the LOT are divided, the first portion of the proximal jejunum will be visible and can be drawn under the SMA/SMV into the right side of the abdomen. The monopolar hook in arm number 1 is exchanged with a grasper, and additional small bowel is gently pulled into the right side of the abdomen, where it is divided with a laparoscopic linear stapling device. The mesentery of the proximal jejunum is divided close to the serosa surface of the bowel with the LigaSure until the uncinate process is reached. The distal jejunum will remain in the right side of the abdomen until it is used later for reconstruction.

Transection of the Stomach

Our attention is then turned to the stomach. The grasper in robotic arm number 3 is then used to retract the lesser omentum anteriorly. The pars flaccida of the gastrohepatic ligament is opened, and the lesser omentum is divided along the lesser curvature of the stomach with the LigaSure or robotic hook to the proposed line of transection in the distal antrum. The greater omentum is similarly divided with the LigaSure to the proposed line of transection on the greater curvature of the stomach. We use a laparoscopic linear sta-

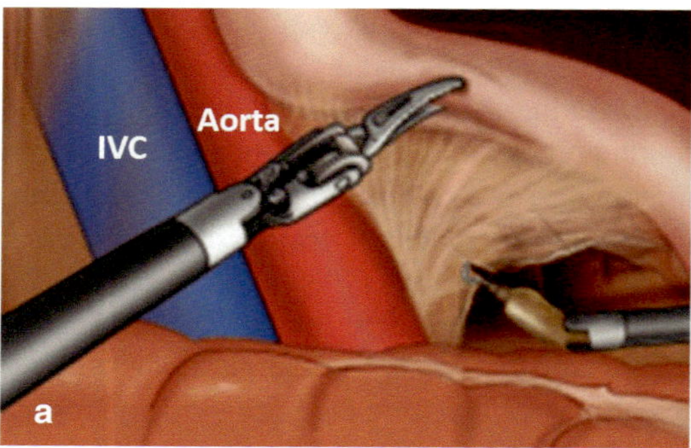

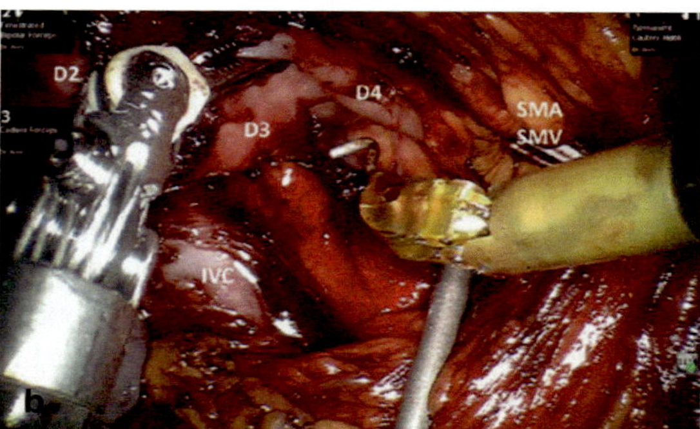

Fig. 14.3 (**a**) Illustration showing mobilization of the third and fourth portions of the duodenum. (**b**) Paired intraoperative image showing anterior retraction of the duodenum, inferior retraction of the transverse mesocolon, and left lateral retraction of the mesenteric root to expose the posterior aspect of the third and fourth portions of the duodenum

pler through the 12-mm assistant port to transect the stomach. The proximal stomach is then gently placed in the left upper quadrant, and the distal stomach is retracted to the right side with the grasper in robotic arm number 3, which exposes the anterior surface of the pancreas and the hepatic artery lymph node (station 8A).

Hepatic Artery Lymph Node and Gastroduodenal Artery

To fully identify the structures in the porta hepatis, the hepatic artery lymph node must be excised. The fibrinous tissues of the lymph node are gently grasped with forceps with arm number 2 and the lymph node is carefully separated from the anterior surface of the common hepatic artery (CHA) by dividing loose areolar tissues and vascular pedicles with the robotic hook and LigaSure device, respectively.

Dissection proceeds toward the gastroduodenal artery (GDA), which can be traced from the CHA and runs caudally on the anterior surface of the pancreas. The robotic hook is usually adequate to isolate the GDA, used as a right angle dissector, but the Maryland instrument can also be used, especially for dissection in the posterior aspect of the artery. Care should be taken to control the posterior branches of the GDA to the pancreas. Once the GDA is isolated to an adequate length, it is divided with the laparoscopic stapling

device with a vascular load. Other smaller vessels, including the right gastric artery, are divided with the LigaSure device.

Dissection with bipolar forceps in arm number 2 and hook in arm number 1 proceeds to fully delineate the structures in the porta hepatis. Now, we fully isolate the CBD from the left side and carefully separate the CBD from the CHA and portal vein. When all three structures are identified and isolated, the CBD is divided with the laparoscopic stapling device.

Finally, we turn our attention to the portal vein and create a landing zone on the anterior surface of the portal vein at the superior border of the pancreatic neck, by dividing the fibrinous tissues with the robotic hook. The superior border of the pancreas can be vascular, and attention must be paid to maintaining hemostasis.

Creating the Pancreatic Tunnel and Pancreatic Transection

We identify the SMV at the inferior border of the pancreatic neck. Identification of the right gastroepiploic vessels or middle colic vein may aid in locating the SMV. Once we identify the SMV, we ligate the right gastroepiploic vessels while preserving the middle colic vessels.

For creation of the pancreatic tunnel, we prefer to use closed graspers in robotic arm number 2 to carefully lift the pancreatic neck in an anterior direction to help create the tunnel space. While robotic arm number 2 provides anterior retraction, the robotic hook is used to gently separate the SMV from the fibers of the posterior pancreatic neck. Simultaneously, the assistant gently retracts the retropancreatic tissues to either side of the tunnel (Fig. 14.4). Both robotic arms are advanced together into the progressively enlarging tunnel until the landing zone on the superior border of the pancreas is reached. The pancreas is then divided using electrocautery while protecting the SMV from thermal injury. We prefer to place the LigaSure device across the anterior border of the SMV to protect the vessel.

This step concludes with the separation of the pancreas from the lateral aspect of the SMV and the separation of the uncinate process from the retroperitoneal tissues. Arm number 3 holds the head of the pancreas laterally and we prefer to use either the robotic hook or robotic scissors for the dissection. The assistant plays a key role by gently retracting the SMV medially and by using the suction-irrigator to keep the field dry for better hemostasis. There are multiple bridging vessels between the pancreas and the SMV that are controlled with either bipolar electrocautery or with the LigaSure. We advise having 4-0 and 5-0 Prolene sutures quickly available for repair of bleeding from the SMV. The first jejunal branch of the SMV is typically visible on the inferolateral side, and all attempts should be made for its preservation.

We perform the final dissection of the uncinate process with the Ligasure device, along the lateral course of the SMA. In this step, arm number 3 is important for holding the uncinate process cephalad and lateral, which straightens the retroperitoneal tissues and facilitates division of tissues along the SMA. With aberrant anatomy (e.g., replaced right hepatic artery from the SMA), care must be taken to preserve the vessels. Once the specimen is completely detached, it can be placed in a specimen bag.

If the gallbladder is still present, then it is removed at this step. All the specimens (lymph nodes, duodenum, pancreas, and gallbladder) can be placed in separate specimen bags through the 12-mm assistant port. Once the dissection is completed, the specimens can be removed from the abdominal cavity through a transverse extension of the left lower assistant (12-mm) port. Once specimen extraction is completed, the incision is covered with a Gelport to re-establish pneumoperitoneum and continue with the reconstruction. There is no need to undock the robot for this step, but it is important to remove the instruments for safety.

Reconstruction

For the reconstruction, we perform the pancreatojejunostomy, hepaticojejunostomy, and gastrojejunostomy in a sequential manner. The complexity of the procedure requires that during the dissection and transection of the pancreas, the operating surgeon and bedside assistant are highly experienced attendings. For reconstruction, there is no need for a second attending, and a skilled bedside assistant (resident or fellow) is adequate for the remainder of the operation, since there is no dissection and little retraction for the three anastomoses.

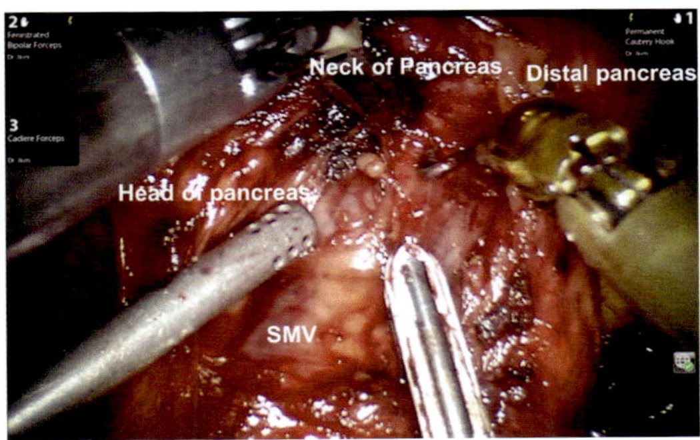

Fig. 14.4 Intraoperative image showing creation of the tunnel posterior to the neck of the pancreas. Robotic arm number 2 is used to gently provide anterior lift on the pancreas, while the robotic hook separates the fibers of the posterior pancreatic neck from the anterior surface of the superior mesenteric vein

Pancreaticojejunostomy

For the pancreaticojejunostomy, we utilize a modified duct-to-mucosa modified Blumgart technique, similar to the open Whipple procedure. We begin with three horizontal mattress 2-0 silk sutures with full-thickness bites of the pancreas and seromuscular bites of the small intestine. Before placing the central suture, we insert a 5 Fr pediatric feeding tube to stent the pancreatic duct to avoid inadvertent ligation of the pancreatic duct. We tie the sutures, but do not cut off the needles, because they will be used to incorporate an anterior seromuscular layer of jejunum. For these steps, we prefer robotic needle holders for arm numbers 1 and 2 and either a Cadiere or Prograsp forceps in arm number 3. For the duct-to-mucosa anastomosis, we create an enterotomy using robotic shears in the antimesenteric surface of the small intestine directly facing the open pancreatic duct. For the anastomosis, we use two posterior row 5-0 PDS interrupted sutures with the suture placed through the pancreatic duct first. Each suture is tied before another suture is placed. For the anterior row, we first place the pancreatic stent and then place three or more 5-0 sutures. At the completion of the anastomosis, we will have placed five to six 5-0 PDS sutures in an around the clock fashion. Finally, we use the previously placed 2-0 silk sutures to create the anterior layer of the pancreaticojejunostomy.

Hepaticojejunostomy

For sizeable common bile ducts (>1 cm), we use two running 4-0 V-Lock sutures (Ethicon). We first start with the anterior suture, placing it initially on the right posterolateral corner with outside-in bites. After three to four throws, when the suture is on the right anterolateral corner, we place the suture on gentle tension with arm number 3. Then we start the posterior row, exactly next to where the first suture was started, in a lateral-to-medial direction with inside-outside bites. Once this second suture reaches the left/medial corner, we take the first suture and sew it toward the second suture from a lateral-to-medial direction on the anterior wall. We do not tie the V-Lock suture at the meeting point.

Gastrojejunostomy

We use a stapled technique for the gastrojejunostomy. The robotic arm numbers 1 and 2 are equipped with graspers, and they are used to hold the transverse colon anteriorly. The assistant then identifies the proximal jejunum at the prior location of the LOT, gently retracting it in a left lateral direction to reduce redundant bowel out of the right upper quadrant. We then bring up the jejunum to the stomach in a tension-free manner and prepare for an antecolic retrogastric anastomosis. An enterotomy and gastrotomy are created, and the common channel is created with a laparoscopic linear stapler. The common enterotomy is then closed with a running 3-0 V-lock suture in a two-layer fashion.

At this point, we remove the arm number 3 robotic port, and a 19 Fr Blake drain is placed through this incision, anterior to the hepaticojejunostomy and laying superior to the pancreaticojejunostomy. A vascularized pedicle of the falciform ligament can be created and laid on the GDA stump.

The only incisions that require closure are the 12-mm camera port and the left lower quadrant extraction port. If the camera port is closed prior to docking of the robot, the only incision that remains to be closed after undocking the robot would be the extraction port. The skin is closed with routine techniques.

Conclusions

There remains much debate regarding the utility of implementing the robotic technique in hepatobiliary surgery. There are definitely challenges that must be overcome, including the ones that we described in the introduction. The performance of this operation requires a highly skilled surgeon with mastery of the open technique and the robotic platform and an equally skilled assistant. Currently, this procedure is mostly performed in high-volume, tertiary academic centers. However, it is clear that this technique can be performed by surgeons with considerable experience with open pancreaticoduodenectomy and mastery of the robotic technique. Our early experience with development of a complex gastrointestinal surgery robotic program suggests that robotic pancreaticoduodenectomy can be performed safely and efficiently. We have completed six totally robotic Whipples with no conversions, no mortality, and improved short-term outcomes with our two-surgeon experienced team.

Suggested Reading

1. Boone BA, Zenati M, Hogg ME, et al. Assessment of quality outcomes for robotic pancreaticoduodenectomy: identification of the learning curve. JAMA Surg. 2015;150:416–22.
2. Giulianotti PC, Mangano A, Bustos RE, et al. Operative technique in robotic pancreaticoduodenectomy (RPD) at University of Illinois at Chicago (UIC): 17 steps standardized technique: lessons learned since the first worldwide RPD performed in the year 2001. Surg Endosc. 2018;32:4329.
3. Hogg ME, Besselink MG, Clavien PA, et al. Training in minimally invasive pancreatic resections: a paradigm shift away from "see one, do one, teach one". HPB (Oxford). 2017;19:234–45.
4. Watkins AA, Kent TS, Gooding WE, et al. Multicenter outcomes of robotic reconstruction during the early learning curve for minimally-invasive pancreaticoduodenectomy. HPB (Oxford). 2018;20:155–65.
5. Zureikat AH, Postlewait LM, Liu Y, et al. A multi-institutional comparison of perioperative outcomes of robotic and open pancreaticoduodenectomy. Ann Surg. 2016;264:640–9.
6. Fujii T, Sugimoto H, Yamada S, et al. Modified Blumgart anastomosis for pancreaticojejunostomy: technical improvement in matched historical control study. J Gastrointes Surg. 2014;18:1108–15.

Ciro Andolfi and Konstantin Umanskiy

Indications

The laparoscopic technique has been adapted to essentially all operative approaches for small bowel resection. Specific indications include isolated small bowel Crohn's disease, ischemia or gangrenous segment of bowel, diverticula, benign strictures, vascular malformations, and neoplasms [1]. Approximately 75% of small intestinal tumors are malignant, with carcinoid tumors being the most common histological type, followed by adenocarcinoma, gastrointestinal stromal tumors (GIST), and lymphomas; altogether, these account for nearly 98% of all small bowel tumors [2].

Preoperative Work-Up and Perioperative Preparation

The preoperative work-up is guided by the underlying etiology and presenting symptoms. Imaging can help establish the diagnosis and

provide a "road map" for planned surgical intervention. An upper gastrointestinal series with small bowel follow-through (UGI-SBFT), computed tomography (CT), or magnetic resonance (MR) enterography can be quite useful as initial studies. An esophagogastroduodenoscopy (EGD) or colonoscopy with intubation of the terminal ileum can be beneficial to further characterize the lesion in question and obtain biopsies. Small bowel segments beyond the proximal jejunum and terminal ileum that are not easily accessible by conventional colonoscopy or EGD can be evaluated with double-balloon enteroscopy. Further imaging studies depend on the initial findings and may include ultrasound, positron emission tomography (PET), octreotide scan, or capsule endoscopy [2].

Mechanical bowel preparation and oral antibiotics may be administered preoperatively but are not essential unless colon resection is planned. A chlorhexidine shower is recommended the night before and the morning of the operation. Deep venous thrombosis prophylaxis with both sequential compression devices and subcutaneous heparin is advisable. Preoperative antibiotics are administered within an hour of initial incision using a first-generation cephalosporin and metronidazole; gentamicin and clindamycin are prescribed in patients with beta-lactam allergies [2, 3].

Electronic supplementary material The online version of this chapter (https://doi.org/10.1007/978-3-030-18740-8_15) contains supplementary material, which is available to authorized users.

C. Andolfi · K. Umanskiy (✉)
Department of Surgery, The University of Chicago
Pritzker School of Medicine, Chicago, IL, USA
e-mail: candolfi@surgery.bsd.uchicago.edu;
kumanskiy@surgery.bsd.uchicago.edu

Patient Positioning and Room Setup

The procedure is performed under general anesthesia. A nasogastric or orogastric tube and urinary catheter are placed following induction of anesthesia. The patient may be placed in either supine, split leg, or low lithotomy position with the arms padded and out or tucked by the patient's sides to allow more ergonomic positions for the surgeons, especially if two operators need to stand side-by-side. The surgeon usually stands across the table from the lesion, e.g., on the patient's right side for lesions in the patient's left abdominal cavity or for lesions involving the proximal bowel, and the surgeon stands on the patient's left side for lesions in the patient's right abdominal cavity or for lesions involving the terminal ileum. The camera operator stands on the same side as the surgeon. The assistant surgeon stands on the opposite side of the surgeon (Fig. 15.1). At least two monitors are required – one on each side of the patient. They should be easily movable toward the head and foot of the patient, as to be in line with the operating surgeon's direction of work. An ultrasound machine with laparoscopic probe may be needed in certain circumstances, such as intestinal ischemia or with neoplasm requiring hepatic assessment. Intraoperative endoscopy is occasionally needed to localize the lesion in question.

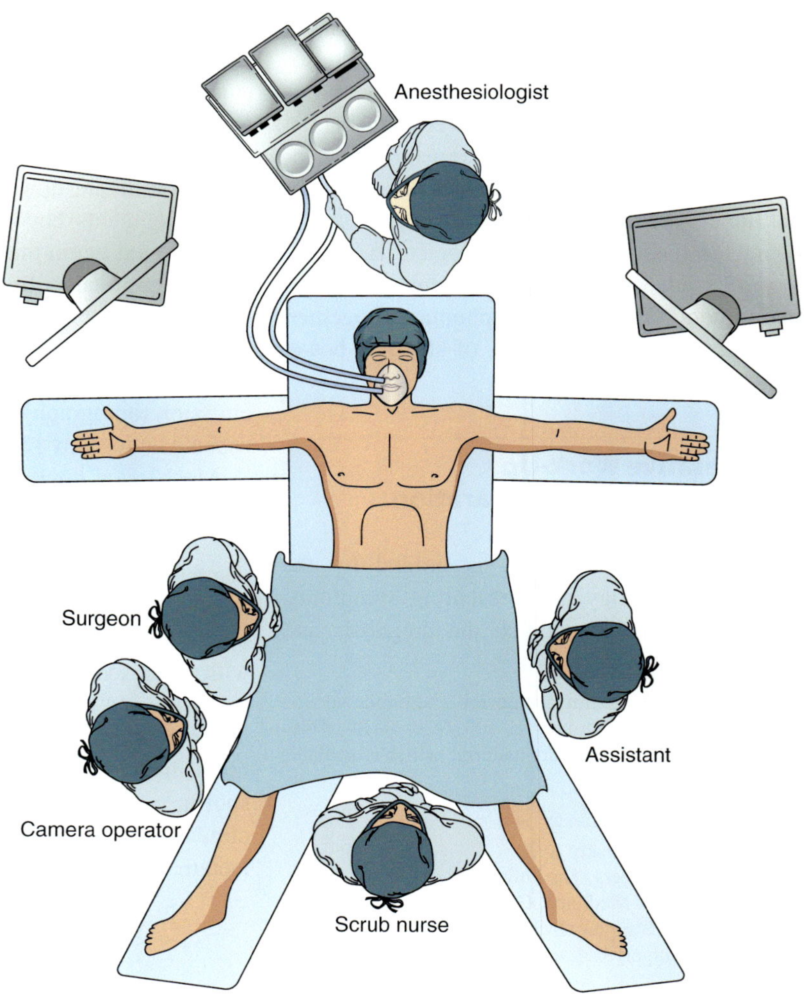

Fig. 15.1 Patient positioning and operating room setup for minimally invasive small bowel resection

Port Placement and Instrumentation

The first port is placed above or below the umbilicus to insufflate the abdomen and to introduce a laparoscope. The open Hasson technique is the preferred method to gain entry into the abdomen. Alternatively, the Veress needle and a trocar with Optiview technology can be used. An initial survey of the abdominal cavity is performed to evaluate the intestine and, if lesion is readily identified, additional port placement is planned accordingly. An angled (30 ° or 45 °) laparoscope provides the optimal view of the small bowel and its mesentery and is preferred over a 0 ° scope. The working ports should be positioned at the corners of an equilateral triangle across from the site of pathology with 8–9 cm length on each side (Fig. 15.2). In most circumstances, three ports are sufficient to accomplish the procedure. A fourth port in the supra-pubic area may be helpful for retraction or exposure. The size of trocars can be 5 mm or 10–12 mm depending on the instruments used during the case. Table 15.1 illustrates specific instruments recommended for laparoscopic small bowel resection, including atraumatic graspers, and laparoscopic linear staplers. Mesenteric vascular control may be accomplished by vascular endoscopic staplers, clips, or

Table 15.1 Instruments recommended for laparoscopic small bowel resection

No.	Instrument type
3–5	Trocars (10–12 mm and 5 mm)
2	Needle holders (optional)
2	Laparoscopic graspers
1	Laparoscopic dissector
1	Laparoscopic scissors
1	Laparoscopic vessel sealing device
1	Laparoscopic intestinal stapler
1	Laparoscopic vascular clips

bipolar energy devices. The choice of the device largely depends on individual surgeon's preference and experience. Laparoscopic scissors with monopolar cautery are helpful in performing enterolysis and fine dissection [3].

Techniques of Small Bowel Resection

Because of the potential for multifocal lesions or unsuspected disease in other parts of the abdomen, small bowel resection should be preceded by a thorough exploration and visualization of abdominal organs, particularly the liver, and the entire small bowel. If preoperative studies clearly localize the lesion, and there are extensive adhesions that preclude "running" the entire small bowel, then this recommendation may not apply [4, 5].

Laparoscopic-Assisted Small Bowel Resection

Video 15.1

The small bowel is typically evaluated laparoscopically, with the use of atraumatic graspers, from proximal to distal by placing the patient in slight reverse Trendelenburg position, with the left side elevated. This maneuver displaces the small bowel into the lower abdomen. The colon can be lifted cephalad, thereby exposing the ligament of Treitz. Beginning at the Treitz, the bowel is run by "hand over hand" technique. Once the proximal jejunum is evaluated, the patient's position

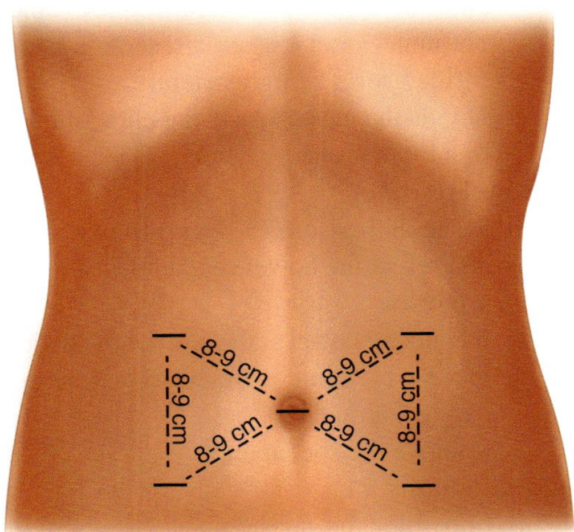

Fig. 15.2 Trocar/port placement for minimally invasive small bowel resection

is progressively changed to Trendelenburg position, with right side elevated to evaluate the distal half of the small intestine. Alternatively, a distal to proximal evaluation of the small bowel can be performed. Once the segment to be resected is identified, it can be marked and suspended by traction sutures on both sides of the lesion. It is helpful to use a 2-0 Prolene suture with a straight needle. The needle is passed through the tissue to be suspended, and the two ends of the suture are held together outside the abdominal wall with a small clamp. It is advantageous to divide the mesenteric vessels before exteriorization of the specimen through the abdominal incision using either an endoscopic linear stapler or a bipolar vessel sealer. This may be especially helpful in a patient with a thick abdominal wall. Once the specimen is fully mobilized, an incision measuring 3–5 cm is made in order to accommodate the section of the small intestine that will be resected. Depending on the size of the specimen, the location of the segment of the small bowel, and mobility of the mesentery, either a Pfannenstiel or a periumbilical midline incision is preferred. The wound is protected using a plastic wound protector, and the loop of the intestine with the lesion is drawn out through the incision. The exteriorization of the bowel before resection allows the palpation of the small bowel so that more subtle disease is not missed and avoids the contamination of the abdominal cavity. The resection and anastomosis are then performed in a standard extracorporeal fashion, by either hand-sewn or stapled method. The mesenteric defect can be left open or closed with a running absorbable suture either through the incision or intracorporeally after reestablishment of pneumoperitoneum. The abdomen is then copiously irrigated with warm sterile saline solution through the incision. After irrigation of the peritoneal cavity, the abdominal wall is closed. The peritoneal cavity can be finally inspected laparoscopically to assure hemostasis [6].

Technical tips for laparoscopic-assisted small bowel resection:

1. Evaluation of proximal small bowel
   (a) Surgeon and camera holder stand on the patient's right side.
   (b) Allow gravity to assist with retraction. Place patient in reverse Trendelenburg position. Small intestine will fall down to pelvis, away from the transverse colon.
   (c) Lift transverse colon to identify the ligament of Treitz.
   (d) Run the small intestine between a pair of atraumatic bowel clamps or endoscopic Babcock clamps.
2. Evaluation of distal small bowel
   (a) Small bowel is grasped by the assistant at the midpoint of its course.
   (b) Both surgeon and camera holder switch to the patient's left side to complete evaluation of the small bowel to the level of the ileocecal valve.
   (c) Identify the segment with the disease. Lyse adhesions to surrounding loops of bowel if necessary.
3. Prepare for bowel resection
   (a) Mark and suspend the section of bowel by placing traction sutures.
   (b) Use cautery to score the peritoneum overlying the mesentery on the side facing the surgeon along the line of intended resection. This outlines the V-shaped segment of small bowel and mesentery that is planned for resection. Make the V large enough for the intended purpose: for example, wide mesenteric excision is appropriate when operating for cancer but unnecessary when a resection is performed for a benign stricture.
   (c) Divide the mesentery using clips, staplers, or a bipolar energy device (Fig. 15.3).
4. Bowel resection
   (a) Make an incision (3–5 cm) to exteriorize and resect the bowel segment. Use wound protector.
   (b) Divide the bowel at the sites of the divided mesentery using a standard extracorporeal technique.
   (c) Remove the specimen.
5. Anastomosis
   (a) Construct the anastomosis extracorporeally using a standard technique (hand-sewn or stapled method).
   (b) Close the mesenteric defect (optional) extracorporeally or intracorporeally.

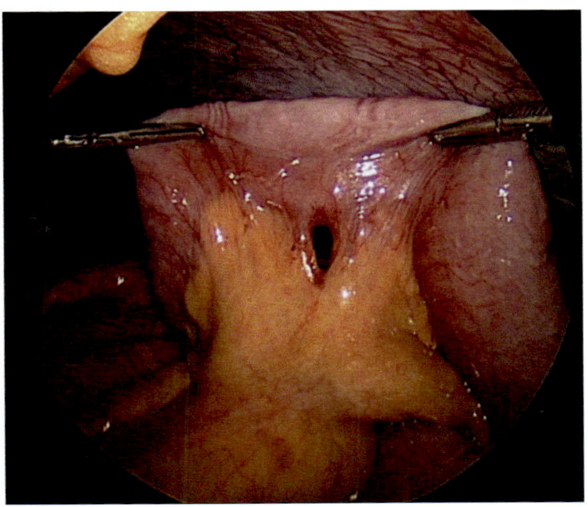

Fig. 15.3 Dissection to produce mesenteric defect in preparation for bowel resection

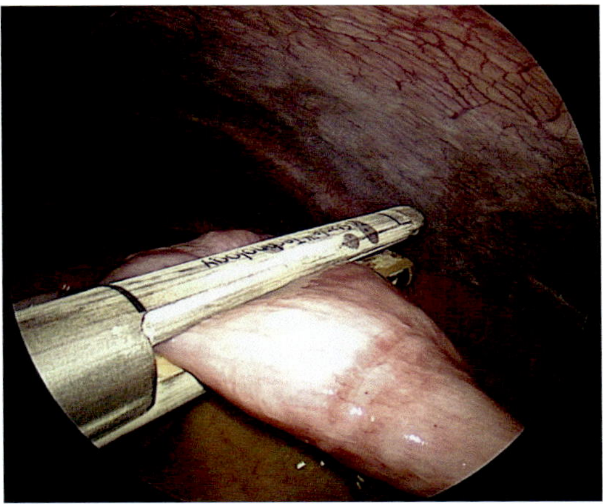

Fig. 15.4 Bowel resection using a laparoscopic linear stapler

(c) Return the anastomosed bowel to the peritoneal cavity.

(d) Close the small incision in layers, reestablish the pneumoperitoneum, confirm hemostasis, and inspect the bowel anastomosis.

Totally Laparoscopic Small Bowel Resection

The laparoscopic technique is similar to the laparoscopic-assisted technique described above except that resection and entero-enteric anastomosis is performed entirely intracorporeally [7].

1. Laparoscopic preparation for small bowel resection is outlined in steps 1 through 3 of the laparoscopic-assisted section.

2. Bowel resection

   (a) Divide the bowel at the sites of the mesenteric division using an endoscopic stapler (Fig. 15.4).

   (b) Make an incision (usually around 4 cm) to allow removal of the resected bowel segment.

3. Intracorporeal anastomosis

   (a) Align the divided bowel ends with stay sutures placed through the anti-mesenteric border of the bowel. The anastomosis can be constructed either in antiperistaltic

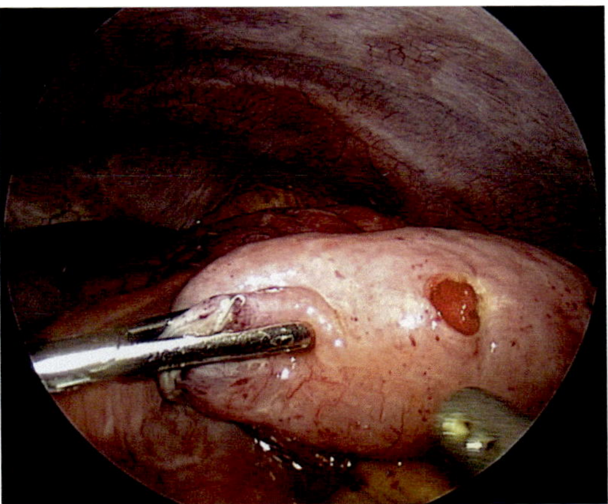

Fig. 15.5 Creation of enterotomy on the antimesenteric border of the small intestine

(side-to-side, functional end-to-end) or iso-peristaltic (side-to-side) fashion.

   (b) Create an enterotomy in both limbs of the bowel close to the antimesenteric borders (Fig. 15.5) with monopolar scissors or hook cautery, and then pass the limbs of the endoscopic gastrointestinal stapler into each enterotomy, approximating the segments. Close the stapler and verify the correct alignment (Fig. 15.6).

   (c) Fire and remove the stapler.

   (d) Use the traction sutures to inspect the anastomotic staple line for bleeding. The incidence of bleeding can be minimized by ensuring that the antimesenteric sides of each limb are used to construct the anastomosis. Control any bleeding sites. Bleeding areas at the staple line can be controlled with sutures or clips.

4. Closure of the enterotomies with stapled technique

   (a) Place three traction sutures (one at each end and one in the middle) to approximate the enterotomy defect and elevate the edges.

   (b) Place an endostapler (3.5 mm) or an Endo GIA with Tri-Staple technology (tan or purple) through a 12-mm port, just beneath the cut edges, and close it transversely. Be certain to ensure that both edges are completely enclosed within the stapler, but avoid including excessive amount of bowel.

   (c) Fire the stapler, and use scissors to remove excess tissue from the staple line.

5. Alternatively, a closure of the common enterotomy with intra-corporeal running V-Loc suture can be performed (Fig. 15.7) [8].

Complications

Anastomotic Leak

One of the most serious complications of any bowel anastomosis is anastomotic leak. Compared to the large intestine, the small bowel has a much lower leak rate. In fact, as long as the segments of bowel for anastomosis are well vascularized and the anastomosis is free of tension, small bowel leaks are exceedingly rare. Leaks in small bowel anastomosis most frequently result from technical error, excess tension on the anastomosis, or poor blood supply. A gross technical error can contribute to anastomotic leak, such as incomplete closure of the enterotomy with the linear stapler or if the enterotomy is hand-sewn and the sutures are not placed accurately.

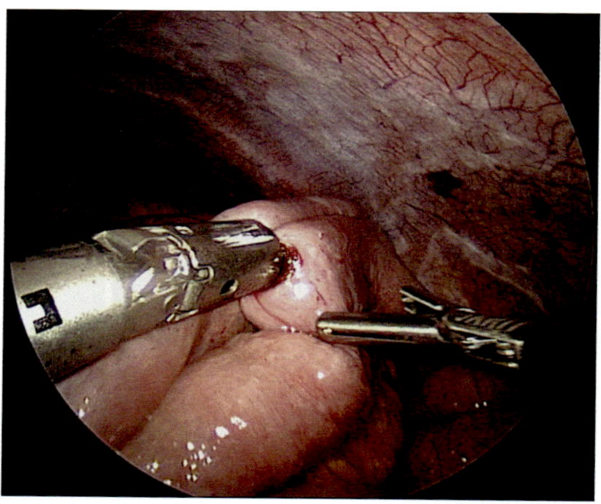

Fig. 15.6 The stapler is inserted into the two limbs of small for side-to-side functional end-to-end anastomosis

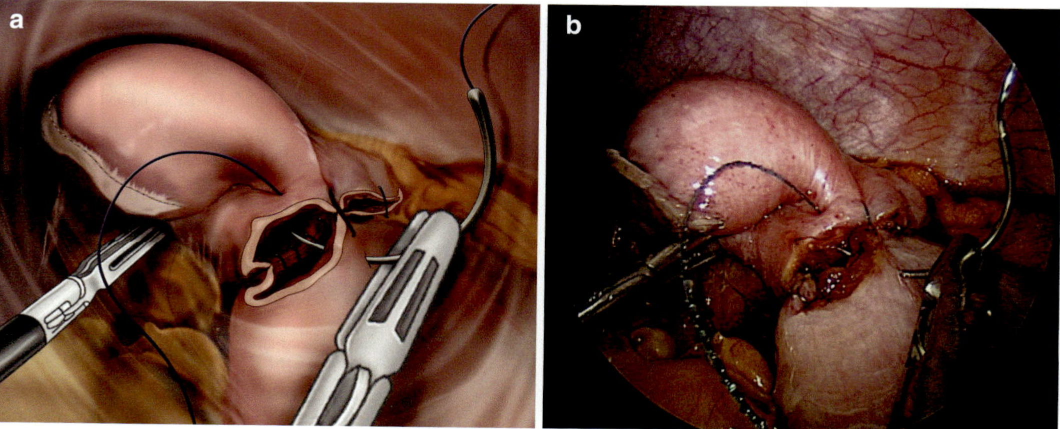

Fig. 15.7 (**a**) Illustration showing closure of the common enterotomy with laparoscopic suturing. (**b**) Paired intraoperative image showing laparoscopic suturing of the common enterotomy with V-Loc barbed sutures

If an anastomotic leak does occur, it may present with peritonitis, necessitating re-exploration, or the leak may decompress through the skin as an enterocutaneous fistula. An enterocutaneous fistula typically presents a few days after resection with what initially appears to be a wound infection. Once wound discharge becomes enteric, the diagnosis of enterocutaneous fistula can be established with certainty. Some enterocutaneous fistula will close spontaneously, although it may take several weeks of bowel rest and parenteral nutrition for complete resolution.

Anastomotic Stricture

The three factors thought to cause anastomotic stricture are technical error, ischemia, or tension on the anastomosis. The technical errors that most frequently result in anastomotic stricture include creation of an inadequate size opening (i.e., using short staple load), incorporating excess bowel wall in a stapled enterotomy closure, and bleeding with hematoma at the anastomotic site. Tension on the anastomosis may result in leakage or complete disruption. Occasionally, subclinical anastomotic leaks may result in anastomotic scarring and narrowing of the lumen.

Recognition of intraoperative technical errors is critical. If an error is recognized, it is highly recommended to redo the anastomosis. When anastomotic strictures are recognized during the postoperative period, the severity of the obstructive symptoms dictates whether reoperation and revision of the anastomosis is indicated. In some circumstances, anastomotic strictures can be dilated endoscopically.

Small Bowel Obstruction

Abdominal adhesions are one of the most common causes of postoperative small bowel obstruction. Even though adhesions can occur after any intra-abdominal operation, they tend to be less common following laparoscopic surgery. It is unknown why some patients form diffuse adhesions, while others remain adhesion-free even after multiple laparotomies. While there is no certain way to avoid this problem, limiting the amount of dissection and intraoperative hemorrhage may limit the extent of postoperative adhesions. Early postoperative small bowel obstruction after laparotomy should initially be managed with bowel rest, nasogastric tube decompression, and intravenous fluid support. Although cases of small bowel obstruction following laparoscopic surgery are rare, conservative management is not advised, as many of the cases are caused by a single adhesive band resulting in angulation or kinking of the bowel [9, 10]. Reoperative laparoscopic surgery is advised for early postoperative small bowel obstruction after laparoscopic surgery.

Prolonged Postoperative Ileus

Some degree of postoperative ileus is expected after small bowel surgery, but the minimally invasive approach often shortens its duration. The signs and symptoms of postoperative ileus may include a lack of intestinal peristalsis, abdominal bloating and distention, nausea, and vomiting. Prolonged postoperative ileus should raise the suspicion of a postoperative intra-abdominal infection, particularly an anastomotic leak. The condition must be differentiated from mechanical obstruction with physical examination and radiographic imaging (abdominal X-ray or computed tomography). Treatment for ileus is nonoperative and consists of intravenous fluids and bowel rest until bowel function resumes [11].

Short Bowel Syndrome

Short gut syndrome may develop as a result of excessive resection of the small bowel, leading to a malabsorptive state. The minimum length of bowel necessary to prevent short bowel syndrome is approximately 2 m, but this varies significantly among individuals. Children can adapt better than adults in tolerating massive bowel resection, since over time intestinal adaptation can occur allowing relatively normal intestinal function. A shorter length of small bowel can be tolerated if the ileocecal valve and pylorus remain intact. Tailored enteral diets have been created to maximize digestion, and total parenteral nutrition (TPN) can be used to supplement oral intake.

Conclusion

Small bowel resections are very common in the adult and pediatric general surgery practice. The reasons for performing a small bowel resection are numerous and include bowel obstruction, vascular damage, hemorrhage, neoplasms, inflammatory diseases, fistulas, and congenital anomalies. In spite of the numerous indications, the approach is generally similar for each situation. We usually prefer a totally laparoscopic approach. However, the main disadvantages of a complete laparoscopic small bowel resection are (1) the unavoidable contamination of the abdominal cavity when the bowel is transected, (2) the slightly longer operative times, and (3) the limited tactile feedback and intraluminal surveillance of the staple line for hemostasis.

References

1. Adams S, Wilson T, Brown AR. Laparoscopic management of acute small bowel obstruction. Aust N Z J Surg. 1993;63:39–41.
2. Bowles TL, Amos KD, Hwang RF, et al. Small bowel malignancies and carcinoid tumors. In: Feig BW, editor. The MD Anderson surgical oncology handbook. 5th ed. Philadelphia: Lippincott Williams & Wilkins; 2012.
3. Duh QY. Laparoscopic procedures for small bowel disease. Baillieres Clin Gastroenterol. 1993;7:833–50.
4. Lange V, Meyer G, Schardey HM, et al. Different techniques of laparoscopic end-to-end small-bowel anastomoses. Surg Endosc. 1995;9:82–7.
5. Schlinkert RT, Sarr MG, Donohue JH, et al. General surgical laparoscopic procedures for the "non-laparologist". Mayo Clin Proc. 1995;70:1142–7.
6. Scoggin SD, Frazee RC, Snyder SK, et al. Laparoscopic-assisted bowel surgery. Dis Colon Rectum. 1993;36:747–50.
7. Soper NJ, Brunt LM, Fleshman J Jr, et al. Laparoscopic small bowel resection and anastomosis. Surg Laparosc Endosc. 1993;3:6–12.
8. Waninger J, Salm R, Imdahl A, et al. Comparison of laparoscopic handsewn suture techniques for experimental small-bowel anastomoses. Surg Laparosc Endosc. 1996;6:282–9.
9. Chopra R, McVay C, Phillips E, et al. Laparoscopic lysis of adhesions. Am Surg. 2003;69:966–8.
10. Ibrahim IM, Wolodiger F, Sussman B, et al. Laparoscopic management of acute small bowel obstruction. Surg Endosc. 1996;10:1012–5.
11. Soybel DI, Landman WB. Ileus and bowel obstruction. In: Mulholland MW, Lillemoe KD, Doherty GM, Maier RV, Simeone DM, Upchurch GR, editors. Greenfield's surgery scientific principles and practice. 5th ed. Philadelphia: Lippincott Williams & Wilkins; 2011.

Kelsi Hirai, Miranda Lin, Georgios V. Georgakis, and Joseph Kim

Introduction

There are many indications for small bowel resection including obstruction, disorders such as Meckel's diverticulum or Crohn's disease, malignancy, and trauma. In this chapter, we will describe small bowel resection for malignancy. Primary small bowel malignancies, including adenocarcinoma, carcinoid, lymphoma, and stromal tumors, and small bowel metastases from distant sites are indications for small bowel resection [1, 2]. Malignancy can result in obstruction or bleeding, which was observed in our patient. In this chapter, we present a step-by-step approach to robotic small bowel resection.

Electronic supplementary material The online version of this chapter (https://doi.org/10.1007/978-3-030-18740-8_16) contains supplementary material, which is available to authorized users.

K. Hirai · G. V. Georgakis
Department of Surgery, Stony Brook University Hospital, Stony Brook, NY, USA
e-mail: kelsi.hirai@stonybrookmedicine.edu;
Georgios.georgakis@stonybrookmedicine.edu

M. Lin · J. Kim (✉)
Department of Surgery, University of Kentucky, Lexington, KY, USA
e-mail: joseph.kim@uky.edu

Preparation

Detailed patient history and physical examination are important measures for preoperative planning. Laboratory studies including complete blood count, coagulation status, and electrolytes help to determine perioperative risk factors. Prior to surgery, fluid and electrolyte balance should be established and blood volume should be optimized. Prophylaxis for deep venous thrombosis is initiated with subcutaneous heparin or enoxaparin and mechanical sequential compression devices. Perioperative antibiotics are administered to reduce the risk of surgical site infection [3].

Under select circumstances, early surgical planning may not be available. Emergent small bowel resection is mandatory for uncontrolled bleeding, while endoscopic and interventional radiologic procedures are typically ineffective. Under urgent conditions, it is important to obtain type and screen and cross-matching of blood, to administer perioperative antibiotics, and to expedite bringing the patient to the operating room while concurrently providing resuscitative care. Once in the operating room, a nasogastric tube is placed (if not already placed) for gastric and intestinal decompression, and a Foley catheter is recommended to monitor urinary output during the procedure. We do not advocate performing minimally invasive procedures when the patient is unstable and requires immediate exploration. We will consider robotic small bowel resection when the patient is hemodynamically stable. For this procedure, the patient will be placed supine with the legs split. It is our routine to have both arms tucked for all robotic procedures for patient safety when docking the robot.

Port Placement

We first place a 5-mm port in Palmer's point in the left lateral upper quadrant. This port will be replaced by a robotic 8-mm port. A second 5-mm port may be placed to verify the location of the lesion. Typically, we prefer placing five ports along a semicircular line with the base of the semi-circle near the right lower quadrant facing toward the left upper quadrant. Under direct visualization, ports are placed approximately 10–20 cm away from the area of interest with the periumbilical camera port in the middle of the semicircular line. Three robotic 8-mm ports are placed one handbreadth apart to avoid collisions of the robotic arms during surgery (Fig. 16.1). We use one 10-/12-mm assistant port, which is also placed in the semicircular line. Distances between the ports are measured after insufflation for improved accuracy. After placement of the ports, the robot is docked over the left shoulder with the Da Vinci Si [4].

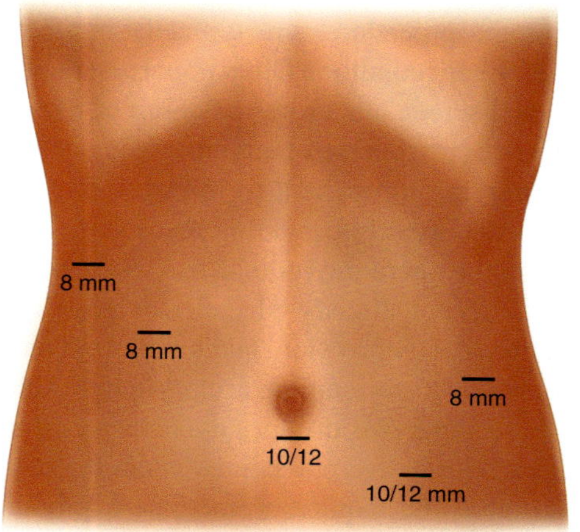

Fig. 16.1 Modified trocar/port placement for robotic small bowel resection

Instruments and Materials

We use a 5-mm 30 °-angled laparoscope for initial exam of the abdomen and a 10-mm 30 ° robotic camera. We use the following robotic instruments: fenestrated bipolar forceps, cadiere forceps, monopolar hook, the vessel sealer, and the mega needle driver. We also utilize the endoscopic gastrointestinal anastomosis (GIA) stapler and an endoscopic specimen bag. We employ two different techniques for intracorporeal suturing including 3-0 V-Loc 90 suture on a taper point needle and the Lapra-Ty Absorbable Suture Clip with 3-0 Vicryl sutures on a taper point needle. The Carter-Thomason device is used to close the fascia at the 10-mm ports with 0 Vicryl suture.

Small Bowel Resection

Video 16.1

First, the location of the cancer is verified by laparoscopy prior to docking the robot. After the robot is docked (Fig. 16.2), we utilize the fenestrated bipolar grasper in arm 2 and the cadiere forceps in arm 1 to lift up the intestine proximal and distal to the tumor. The robotic hook is placed into arm 1 to create a mesenteric defect proximal and distal to the location of the tumor at the proposed sites of small bowel transection [5]. We prefer to use the endo-GIA stapler to divide the small intestine, rather than creating a 15-mm port to utilize the robotic stapling device. We utilize 60-mm tan cartridges to divide the small intestine. The small bowel mesentery is then divided using the vessel sealer. For adenocarcinoma, we obtain generous margins (5 cm) and harvest lymphatic tissue in the mesentery at the base of the cancer. The surgical tissues are placed in a specimen bag and brought out through the 10-mm assistant port site.

Anastomosis

We perform a side-to-side, functional end-to-end anastomosis. First, the stapled ends of the proximal and distal bowel are aligned. Using the

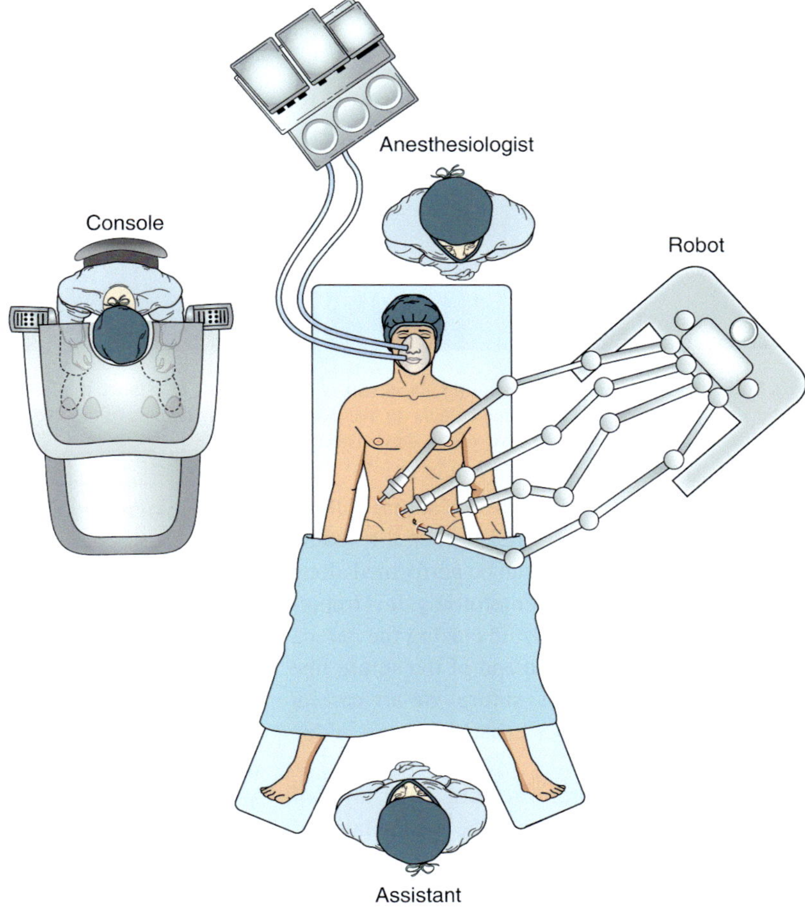

Fig. 16.2 Patient positioning and operating room setup for robotic small bowel resection

robotic hook, small bowel enterotomy is created approximately 1 cm from the stapled end on the superomedial aspect of the proximal and distal small bowel. The two jaws of the endo-GIA stapler are placed in each enterotomy, ensuring that the mesenteric borders of the proximal and distal small bowel are aligned (Fig. 16.3). The jaws are fully inserted to maximize the diameter of the anastomosis. Once the two ends of small bowel are parallel and the anti-mesenteric border is aligned, the stapler is fired to create a common channel. After stapling, the suture line is inspected for bleeding. Any bleeding is controlled with the fenestrated bipolar grasper or with sutures as necessary.

Closure of Common Enterotomy

We prefer to close the common channel with suturing rather than stapling. We employ two different techniques to close the common channel, either with robotic suturing using running suture with Lapra-Ty Absorbable Suture Clips or with V-loc sutures. When using the Lapra-Ty, we place one of these clips at the end of the suture and then perform standard serosa-to-mucosa and mucosa-to-serosa suturing in running fashion. Another Lapra-Ty Absorbable Suture Clip is placed on the completed end of the suture line. This precludes the need for robotic tying of knots. With the V-Loc suture, the needle must be threaded

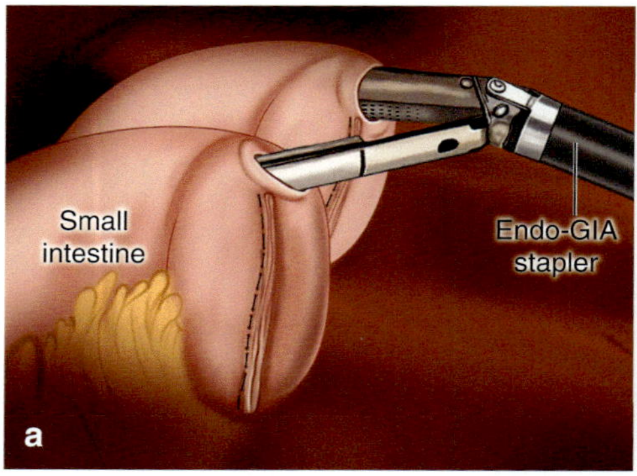

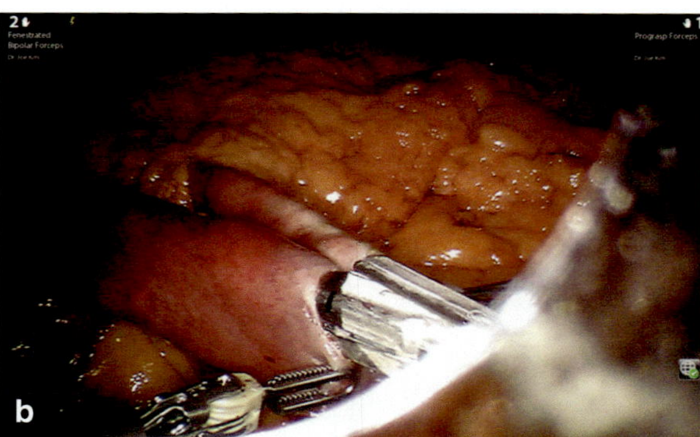

Fig. 16.3 (**a**) Illustration demonstrating placement of the linear stapler into the enterotomy defects in the small intestine. (**b**) Paired intraoperative photo demonstrating robotic assistance to place the linear stapler into the enterotomy defects of the two limbs of the small intestine

through the loop at the end of the suture following the first set of corner bites to lock the suture. Standard robotic suturing can be performed along the length of the common enterotomy. It is important to cinch the sutures while closing the defect. We do not tie a knot at the end of the suture line and instead simply cut the suture. We are careful to avoid leaving exposed barbs of the V-loc suture.

We typically perform a second, outer layer of the common channel closure. The second layer of the bowel wall anastomosis is completed in a similar fashion with running suture using either the Lapra-Ty or V-Loc techniques. However, we employ seromuscular bites for the outer layer. The small bowel mesenteric defect is approximated with running 3-0 Vicryl suture.

Fascial and Skin Closure

Once the anastomosis is complete, the laparoscope is used to view the abdominal cavity and ensure hemostasis. The fascia at the 10-/12-mm port site is re-approximated using the Carter-Thomason device. We do not close the fascia at the robotic port sites. The pneumoperitoneum is deflated, and ports are removed. Skin is then closed at all port sites with 4-0 Monocryl subcuticular interrupted sutures.

Postoperative Care

At the end of the operation and prior to leaving the operating room, the nasogastric tube is removed. Routine intravenous fluids are administered and a clear liquid diet is started on postoperative day 1. The diet is advanced to a regular diet as bowel function returns. Pain management with minimal narcotics and deep venous thrombosis prophylaxis are continued. Early ambulation is encouraged, and patients are routinely discharged in 2–3 days following robotic small bowel resection.

Conclusion

Robotic small bowel resection can be performed safely and effectively for small bowel malignancies. The robotic platform enables the common enterotomy to be closed securely and with ease. In our experience, the utilization of small incisions has resulted in less pain, quicker return of bowel function, and shorter hospital stays. Randomized studies to directly assess the benefits of the robotic platform for small bowel malignancies may be difficult to organize and complete due to the lower incidence of these cancers. Additional nonrandomized retrospective and prospective data will be important to provide outcome data.

References

1. Padussis JC. Open small bowel resection. Procedures Consult. 2016 Nov 24.
2. Townsend CM Jr, Evers BM, Beauchamp RD, et al. Sabiston textbook of surgery – the biological basis of modern surgical practice. 20th ed. Philadelphia: Elsevier; 2017. Print.
3. Kim J, Garcia-Aguilar J. Surgery for cancers of the gastrointestinal tract – a step-by-step Surgical approach. New York: Springer; 2015. Print.
4. Intuitive Surgical. Da Vinci Si surgical system user manual. Sunnyvale, CA, USA: Intuitive Surgical; 2014.
5. Zollinger RM Jr, Ellison EC. Zollinger's atlas of surgical operations. 9th ed. New York: McGraw-Hill; 2011. Print.

Part II

Colorectal

Jose L. Guerrero-Ramirez
and Maria Luisa Reyes-Diaz

Indications

A malignancy that appears in any location from the cecal appendix to the transverse colon is the main indication for resection of the right colon. Benign polyps are also an indication for right hemicolectomy, since the ascending colon has a relatively thin wall and endoscopists are more reluctant to perform resections, which is why surgery is recommended more frequently. Other indications are inflammatory bowel disease, diverticular disease, bleeding vascular ectasia, ischemic colitis, and large appendiceal neoplasms located in the appendicular base or with unfavorable pathological anatomy.

Operative Technique

Anatomical Considerations

The ascending colon, with an approximate size of 15 cm, is located at the right side of the abdominal cavity from the right iliac fossa to the liver; its

Electronic supplementary material The online version of this chapter (https://doi.org/10.1007/978-3-030-18740-8_17) contains supplementary material, which is available to authorized users.

J. L. Guerrero-Ramirez · M. L. Reyes-Diaz (✉)
General Surgery, Hospital Universitary Virgen del Rocío, Sevilla, Spain

posterior wall is fixed to the retroperitoneum, while the lateral and anterior walls are intraperitoneal structures. The nephrocolic ligament supports the hepatic flexure and is attached to the right kidney, duodenum, and hepatic hilum. The transverse colon measures about 45 cm in length, is suspended between the hepatic and splenic flexures, which constitute its fixation points, and is totally invested with visceral peritoneum.

The main arterial supply of the terminal ileum, cecum, and appendix comes from the ileocolic artery, a direct branch of the superior mesenteric artery. The right colic artery irrigates the ascending colon and has wide variability among patients, being absent in up to 20% of patients. The next important arterial branch to consider is the right branch of the middle colic artery. The arc of Riolan establishes communications between the middle colic artery and the left colic artery.

The main venous and lymphatic drainage runs parallel to the arterial vessel. The ileocolic lymphatic vessels drain into the para-aortic lymphatic system. Other important lymph nodes are the paracolic (located next to the marginal artery), the epicolic (on the wall of the colon), and the intermediate (located between the venous and arterial branches).

© Springer Nature Switzerland AG 2020
J. Kim, J. Garcia-Aguilar (eds.), *Minimally Invasive Surgical Techniques for Cancers of the Gastrointestinal Tract*, https://doi.org/10.1007/978-3-030-18740-8_17

Preoperative Planning

Right hemicolectomy is associated with considerable morbidity, making a proper preoperative evaluation mandatory. All patients should undergo a complete colonoscopy (identification, labeling, and biopsy), a thoracoabdominal scan (extension study), and an MRI or PET when distant metastases are suspected.

All patients should have medical clearance prior to surgery. The intestinal preparation prior to colectomy continues to be a controversial issue, and currently, it is often performed according to the preference of the surgeon, pending further evidence. Intravenous or even oral and intravenous antibiotic prophylaxis is always indicated.

Patient Positioning

The patient is placed in the supine position with a slight reverse Trendelenburg tilt and left lateral decubitus, with both arms folded toward the trunk (or at least the left arm must be folded). The pressure points are adequately protected, and a device is applied to hold the patient. Gastric decompression is recommended (only at the time of surgery), as well as bladder decompression (only for 24 h), unless it is needed to control the risk of intestinal injury or to improve the field of vision. The use of stirrups depends on the surgeon. The laparoscopic screen should be positioned on the right side at a suitable height to ensure proper ergonomics for the surgeon and the assistant, who will be located on the left side (Fig. 17.1). Placement of trocars should be arranged taking into account the dissection of the hepatic angle.

Trocar Positioning

Pneumoperitoneum is created with a Veress needle for initial insufflation to 12 mmHg. An umbilical trocar is placed in the periumbilical region. The peritoneal cavity is first examined for evidence of, in the case of malignant disease, peritoneal or hepatic metastasis. Under direct vision, in the left lower quadrant and left suprapubic region,

additional 5- and 12-mm trocars are inserted. A 5-mm assistant port is placed in the left upper quadrant (Fig. 17.1).

Surgical Technique

Several approaches have been proposed for right hemicolectomy, such as the lateral-medial approach, the medial-lateral approach, and the retroperitoneal approach [1–3]. The medial approach is the most commonly used, since, in addition to allowing a good exeresis of the mesocolon, the early proximal ligation of the vessels can prevent neoplastic cells from passing into the bloodstream; it also allows entry into a suitable retroperitoneal plane [4]. If there are adhesions present, they should be separated carefully, and the abdomen is scanned to assess metastasis and potential resectability. For a good surgical field, we must move the transverse colon toward the upper part of the abdomen and the small bowel to the left. The initial step is the identification of the ileocolic branch. To do this, medial exposure of the mesentery and the ileocolic region is performed, tracing the cecum to the iliac fossa, in the direction of the patient's right leg. If the traction is adequate, the vessels are clearly marked (Fig. 17.2). We must open the peritoneum using an electric scalpel, with an incision parallel to the vessels to be able to dissect them. Pulling the vessels upward and the retroperitoneum downward using tweezers will facilitate dissection of the correct retroperitoneal plane [5]. Before the ligation of the vessels, the duodenum should be identified (Fig. 17.3). The division can be performed with an endostapler or endoclips or sealed with energy devices (Fig. 17.4). This depends on the preference of the surgeon but always considering the thickness and state of atherosclerosis of the vessels.

After ligation, a careful dissection will be carried out in the duodenum and in the caudal portion of the pancreas for exposure of the middle colic vessels. The dissection around the trunk of Henle (union of the right gastroepiploic vein with the right branch of the middle colic vein or the main middle colic vein) can lead to the exposure

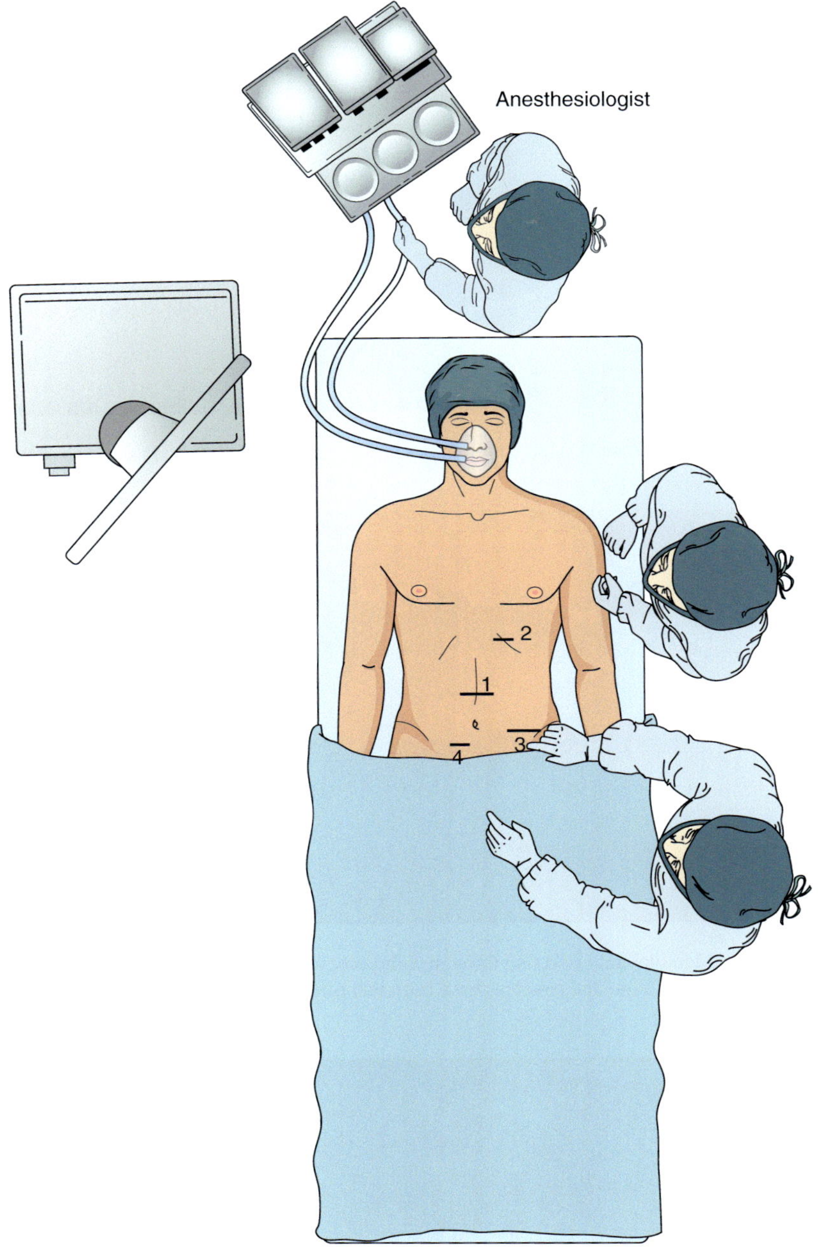

Fig. 17.1 Trocar positioning and operating room setup for the abdominal portion of laparoscopic right hemicolectomy

of an accessory right colic vein. The accessory right colic vein and the right branches of the middle colic vessels must be sealed or ligated (Fig. 17.5). Up to this point, the primary tumor has been minimally manipulated by the medial-to-lateral approach. Finally, the right flexure and the right colon, including the tumor-bearing segment, are separated laterally, which completes the mobilization of the entire right colon [6, 7]. During the dissection of the right parietocolic ligament (Fig. 17.6), it is not necessary to change the position of the patient; instead, the hepatic flexure portion of the procedure should always be performed with the patient in the Trendelenburg position. For dissection of this area, the assistant using the clamp in the trocar on the mid-clavicular

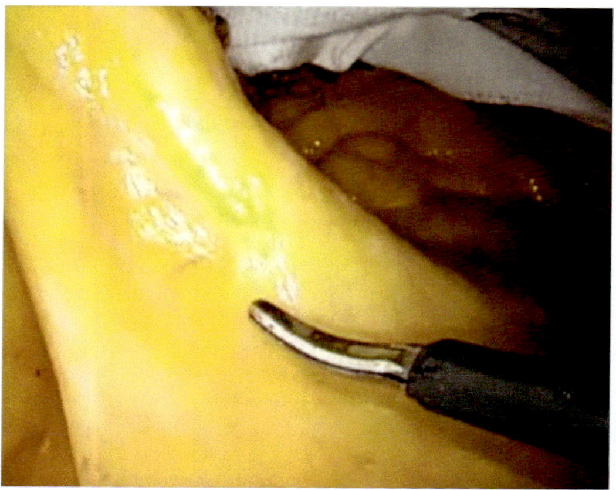

Fig. 17.2 Ileocolic vessels dissection

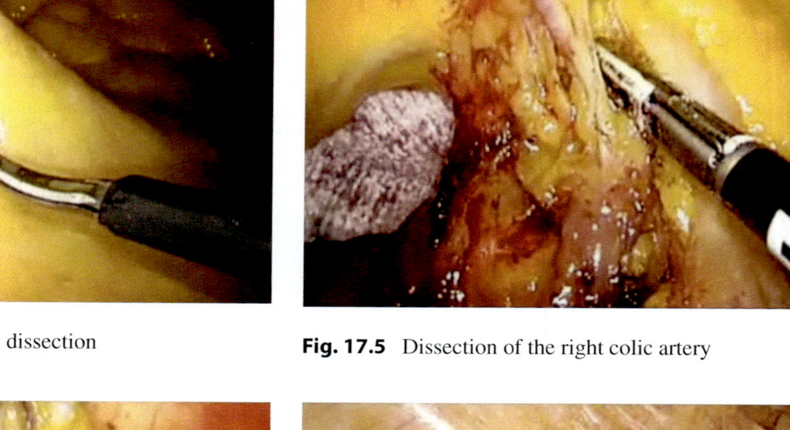

Fig. 17.5 Dissection of the right colic artery

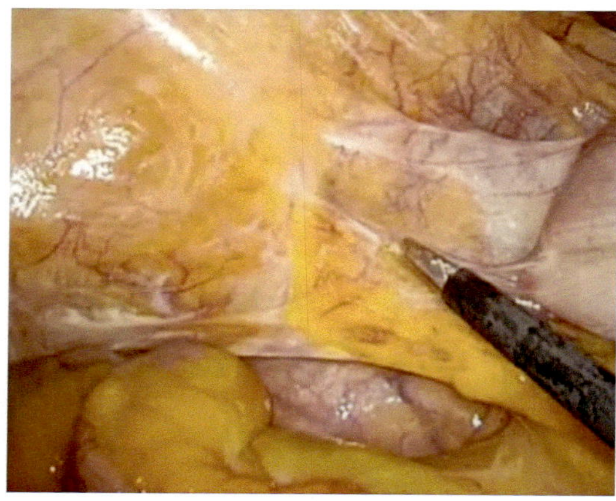

Fig. 17.3 Mediolateral dissection through embryological planes. The duodenum and pancreas have been identified

Fig. 17.6 Right colon lateral attachments

line presents it to the surgeon for dissection from the middle transverse colon to join the dissection of the parietocolic ligament. It is essential that the terminal ileum and right colon be well mobilized. In the laparoscopic approach, the creation of extra- or intracorporeal anastomosis is usually decided according to the laparoscopic experience of the surgeon or the form chosen for the extraction of the specimen (Video 17.1).

Extracorporeal Anastomosis

Once the entire right colon is mobilized, we must hold it with a clamp so that the mesentery does not twist and in order to facilitate extraction of

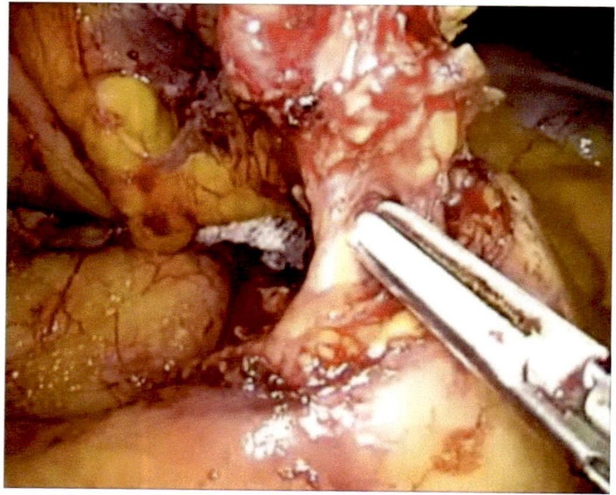

Fig. 17.4 Division of ileocolic vessels

the specimen by an enlargement of the port site in the umbilicus or a right subcostal incision. The wound should be covered with a wound guard. There are multiple anastomosis techniques, and the choice usually depends on the preference of the surgeon or a standardized approach in the institution. In many texts, lateral-lateral anastomoses, either manual or mechanical, are recommended. The anastomosis is returned to the peritoneal cavity with extreme care. The closure of the mesocolon is not mandatory, nor is a new laparoscopic view of the cavity, provided that we are sure that the mesocolon is not twisted.

with 3.5-mm staples (Fig. 17.9). The resulting enterotomy is closed with a running intracorporeal suture (3–0 Vicryl) or a fourth application of the GIA stapler (Fig. 17.10). The closure of the mesocolon is not mandatory. After deflation of the abdomen through the ports, a small Pfannenstiel incision is made in the suprapubic region, and after placement of a wound protector, the specimen is extracted.

The abdominal wound is closed, the peritoneal cavity is reinsufflated, and all trocars are removed under direct visualization. The fascia of any trocar larger than 5 mm is closed. All wounds are closed, and the operation is completed.

Intracorporeal Anastomosis

The transverse colon is transected with a laparoscopic linear stapler; we find a 60-mm load with 3.5-mm staples appropriate. The terminal ileum is divided 5–10 cm from the ileocecal junction with a second firing of the stapler (Figs. 17.7 and 17.8). The specimen is moved to the pelvis or left abdomen. The orientation of the terminal ileal and transverse colon stumps is confirmed, and the antimesenteric surfaces are approximated with a seromuscular suture. An enterotomy is created in each limb, and the limbs are anastomosed in a side-to-side fashion with a third firing of a 60-mm load of a laparoscopic linear stapler

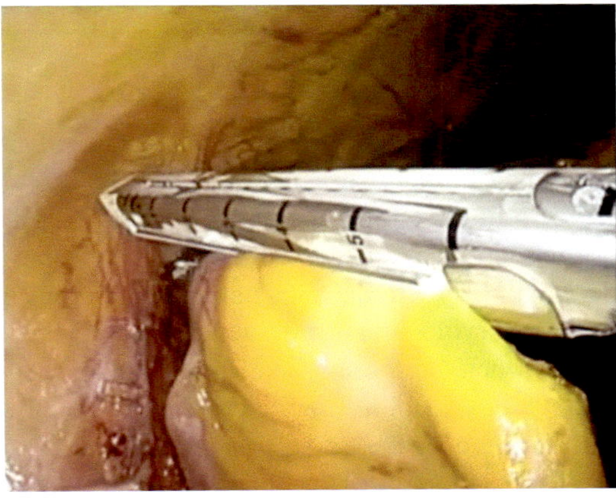

Fig. 17.8 Division of the small bowel with an endostapler

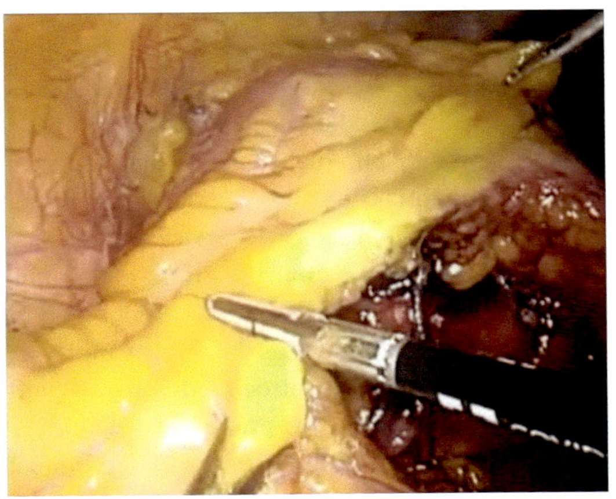

Fig. 17.7 Division of small bowel mesentery

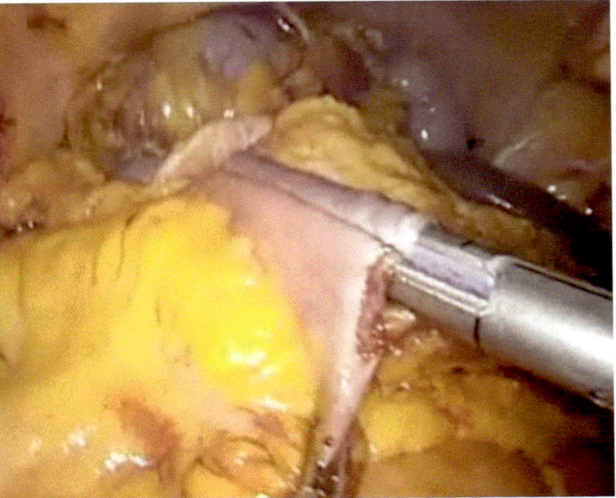

Fig. 17.9 Side-to-side anastomosis

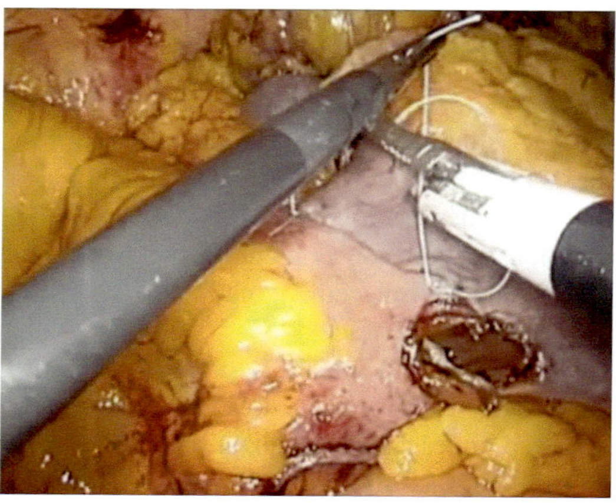

Fig. 17.10 Closure of the anastomosis

Oncological Objectives

The concept of total excision of the mesocolon, developed in open surgery by Hohenberger, [8] arose from the good oncological results secondary to the total excision of the mesorectum proposed by Heald. Mainly, it upholds the importance of the embryological planes, which should be followed when performing the dissection to adequately remove all the mesocolon and its ganglia, with ligature of the vessels at their origin. The quality of the surgical specimen has been shown to be related to a lower recurrence of disease and increased survival.

The three main concepts for an adequate technique are as follows:

1. Obtain an adequate plane of mesofascial or retrofascial dissection to fully mobilize the mesocolon, en bloc and without defects
2. Central ligation of the vessels, close to their roots to maximize the inclusion of vertical lymph nodes (central expansion of the disease)
3. Adequate and sufficient visceral resection to maximize the elimination of pericolic lymph nodes (longitudinal expansion of the disease).

With regard to the lymph nodes, at present, a minimum of 12 nodes are considered necessary in a specimen of oncological colon surgery for adequate staging.

Complications and Their Resolution

Correct knowledge about the potential complications associated with any surgical procedure is essential for early diagnosis and treatment. However, our priority should be to avoid such complications; therefore, it is vital to have an adequate knowledge of the abdominal anatomy, the tissue planes, and the steps of the procedure and to systematize all the actions that are carried out before, during, and after the procedure.

Injuries Associated with the Laparoscopic Approach

The most frequent complications are nerve lesions due to hyperextension and tissue injuries due to compression, especially in the upper extremities and in areas under pressure. Correct patient positioning to minimize the risk of complications is in the supine position, with the arms folded toward the trunk, protection of the wrists and fingers, the lower extremities maintained at an angle of 180 ° with respect to the trunk (avoiding hyperextension), and protection of the ankles. The patient must be positioned prior to the placement of the surgical drapes.

Injuries associated with the use of trocars and other surgical instruments are varied and can be avoided by exercising caution.

Creation of Pneumoperitoneum The abdominal cavity can be accessed using different techniques: a Veress needle, Hasson open technique, or optical trocar. The main lesions that we must avoid during this step are damage to vascular structures (mainly the aortic artery, vena cava, and iliac vessels) and injury to intra-abdominal organs. The use of the Hasson open technique or the optical trocar minimizes the risk of injury. A Veress needle can be introduced into the left hypochondrium, where the probability of damaging large vessels is lower, or at the umbilical level, where the abdominal wall is thin and the pressure that must be applied is lower, allowing adequate traction of the fascia and avoidance of the internal organs. Regardless of the method used, routine adherence to the following steps reduces the risk of injuring vital structures: visualization, stabilization of the abdominal wall, adequate incision, controlled penetration, and proper direction.

Injury During Placement of Trocars Lesions are more frequent in the small intestine than in the colon. Vascular lesions, although of low incidence, can have devastating consequences. To avoid these injuries, flat patient positioning, avoiding the great vessels during trocar insertion, and placement of trocars under direct vision are recommended.

Injuries Produced by Surgical Instruments and Thermal Injuries Dispersion of energy to neighboring tissues is more frequent with monopolar than bipolar instruments. Injuries can occur as a result of direct application, involuntary activation of the electrosurgical equipment, direct coupling to another metal instrument (so it is important to keep the instrument in the field of vision at all times and avoid metal trocars), or failure in the insulation of the instrument. Mechanical injuries can occur as a result of crushing when trying to extract a clamp that supports an intra-abdominal structure, penetration of the handle or a vessel, inadvertent tearing, or tearing during traction. To avoid these injuries, it is essential to be methodical and always check that the jaw of the clamp is free before removing it, insert the instrument in ventral direction and under direct vision, and not advance an instrument without visualization if resistance is found. As much as possible, have all the forceps within the field of vision and use atraumatic forceps.

Lesions Associated with Right Hemicolectomy

The main abdominal structures that can be damaged during a right colectomy, and that therefore must be well controlled, are the duodenum, the middle colic and ileocolic vessels, and the right ureter. As already mentioned, a systematic approach, adequate knowledge of the anatomy,

good exposure, and achievement of the correct plane of dissection from the beginning are essential to avoiding problems.

Exposure In any type of surgery, achieving adequate exposure is a basic requirement to avoid complications. The area on which the surgeon works should be the highest area of the patient to avoid interposition of handles or other structures. With the patient in the Trendelenburg and partial left lateral decubitus positions, it is important to have adequate fixation of the patient to the surgical table, which allows subsequent mobilization according to the technical needs. In this way, the transverse colon along with the greater omentum is directed cephalad, and the terminal ileum turns to the pelvis.

Identification of the Correct Dissection Plane One of the difficulties encountered with a medial-to-lateral approach is differentiation of the correct medial tissue plane, which can lead to entry into the retroperitoneum and, consequently, unnecessary bleeding and/or injury. To avoid entering the wrong plane, the right colon and its mesentery must be strongly tractioned in the ventral direction, while the retroperitoneum moves downward. The correct plane is usually a more superficial layer of the perceived plane. The difficulty of accessing this plane results from the embryological displacement of the colon from the midline to the lateral line, merging with the retroperitoneum. With the main vessels (ileocolic and superior mesenteric artery) medial to the fusion plane, unwanted entry into the retroperitoneum is possible. A lateral-to-medial approach is therefore easier from the anatomical-plane perspective.

Identification and Management of the Duodenum Identification of the duodenum is a key step in laparoscopic right colectomy. The relationship between the ileocolic vessels and the duodenum is the same in all patients, and the ileocolic artery constitutes the first branch of the inferior mesenteric artery under the duodenum. To ligate the ileocolic vessels, we must obtain adequate traction of the mesocolon at the ileocecal level until the vessels are identified. Subsequently, we must make a large window in the mesocolon and carefully dissect the field. At this point and prior to the ligation of the vessels, we must identify and keep the duodenum localized, to avoid injury. A common error is creating the mesocolon window too distal to the duodenum, which forces extension of the dissection superiorly until the duodenum is identified. Duodenal injury can occur unexpectedly if this structure is not controlled, or thermal injury can occur if the distal end of the instrument is kept very close while dissecting the ileocolic and/or middle colic pedicle. For this reason, it is essential to always direct visualization of the instrument and to minimize, as much as possible, direct manipulation of the duodenum. If injury occurs, it must be detected and treated immediately. If it is small, it can be repaired by laparoscopic suture. A more extensive injury requires conversion to open surgery for better control and appropriate treatment.

Another structure susceptible to being injured at this level is the gastrocolic trunk of Henle (arising from the confluence of the right gastroepiploic vein and the right branch of the middle colic vein). Injury of this structure can lead to severe bleeding, which is difficult to control, since it drains into the superior mesenteric vein. To prevent injury, dissection should be performed with great care near the pancreas and not move away from the mesocolon in the direction of the duodenum. If bleeding occurs, a broad exposure must be obtained, and by using a bipolar device, we usually manage to control the bleeding.

Ligation of Vascular Pedicles The main risk associated with ligation of vascular pedicles is subsequent bleeding due to an incorrect ligation [9]. Proper ligation can be achieved with multiple techniques: bipolar thermal energy, ultrasonic energy, endostaplers, or Endoloop. The limitations of each technique must be taken into account to prevent subsequent bleeding.

The right ureter and the gonadal vessels are usually removed from the plane of dissection, and their identification is not routinely necessary.

Injury to the right ureter may occur while incising at the base of the mesentery of the terminal ileum. The medial-to-lateral approach and adequate ventral and cephalic traction of the terminal ileum in this step can help avoid this complication.

Final Considerations

The use of the laparoscopic technique for right colectomy is widely accepted, both for benign and malignant pathologies. Multiple studies have demonstrated the noninferiority of the laparoscopic approach in terms of oncological results [10, 11]. In addition, this approach has benefits such as shorter postoperative hospital stay, the best aesthetic result, shorter duration of paralytic ileus, earliest onset of oral tolerance, the least postoperative pain (reducing the need for analgesics), and quicker return to work. However, we must take into account the learning curve associated with the laparoscopic approach, which can sometimes increase the duration and cost of surgery. Obese patients are a subgroup with a higher prevalence of postsurgical complications due to multiple comorbidities. In comparison with the open approach, laparoscopic colectomy is associated with lower morbidity (surgical site infection, intra-abdominal infection, wound dehiscence, pneumonia, urinary tract infection or sepsis, and renal failure) and lower postoperative mortality.

Conclusion

Laparoscopic surgery of the right colon is safe from the oncological point of view and is associated with multiple advantages in the short term compared to open surgery. However, complications are inevitable, regardless of the skill level of the surgeon, and it is necessary to take measures to avoid them, both those associated with the laparoscopic technique and those associated with colorectal surgery. Conversion may be necessary in certain situations, and although it is controversial, an early proactive conversion in patients with a high conversion risk will probably minimize the risk of complications, whereas reactive conversion at the end of the procedure in response to an unexpected injury will probably lead to worse results.

References

1. Siani LM, Garulli G. Laparoscopic complete mesocolic excision with central vascular ligation in right colon cancer: a comprehensive review. World J Gastrointes Surg. 2016;8(2):106–14.
2. Xu P, Ren L, Zhu D, Lin Q, Zhong Y, Tang W, et al. Open right hemicolectomy: lateral to medial or medial to lateral approach? PLoS One. 2015;10(12):e0145175.
3. Solon JG, Cahalane A, Burke JP, Gibbons D, McCann JW, et al. A radiological and pathological assessment of ileocolic pedicle length as a predictor of lymph node retrieval following right hemicolectomy for caecal cancer. Tech Coloproctol. 2016;20:545.
4. Jacobs M, Verdeja JC, Goldstein HS. Minimally invasive colon resection (laparoscopic colectomy). Surg Laparosc Endosc. 1991;1:144–50.
5. Milsom JW, Böhm B. Laparoscopic colorectal surgery. New York: Springer; 1996.
6. Darzi A, Hunt N, Stacey R. Retroperitoneoscopy and retroperitoneal colonic mobilization: a new approach in laparoscopic colonic surgery. Br J Surg. 1995;82:1038–9.
7. Okuda J, Tanigawa N. Colon carcinomas may be adequately treated using laparoscopic method. Sem Colon Rectal Surg. 1998;9:241–6.
8. Hohenberger W, Weber K, Matzel K. Standardized surgery for colonic cancer: complete mesocolic excision and central ligation – technical notes and outcome. Color Dis. 2009;11:354–65.
9. Lee SW, Shinohara H, Matsuki M, et al. Preoperative simulation of vascular anatomy by three-dimensional computed tomography imaging in laparo- scopic gastric cancer surgery. J Am Coll Surg. 2003;197:927–36.
10. Botoman VA, Pietro M, Thirlby RC. Localization of colonic lesions with endoscopic tattoo. Dis Colon Rectum. 1994;37:775–6.
11. Okuda J, Matsuki M, Yoshikawa S. Minimally invasive tailor-made surgery for advanced colorectal cancer with navigation by integrated 3D-CT imaging. Med View. 2002;86:6–13.

Robert K. Cleary and Warqaa M. Akram

Introduction

Adoption of the robotic platform as a minimally invasive option for right colectomy has not been as rapid as for robotic rectal resection, possibly because laparoscopic technical challenges are more evident in the narrow confines of the pelvis. Even outside of the pelvis, where laparoscopic colectomy has been conducted since 1991, adoption of the laparoscopic approach appears to have plateaued at 50–60%, suggesting the need for a minimally invasive option that surgeons are more willing to embrace than traditional open colectomy [1–5].

Interest in learning robotics for right colectomy appears to be increasing recently because of data suggesting short-term outcomes advantages for intracorporeal anastomosis when compared to extracorporeal anastomosis [6, 7]. Indeed, intracorporeal right colectomy is now part of the annual standardized National Association of Program Directors for Colon and Rectal Surgery Fellowship robotics course curriculum. For many surgeons, robotic instruments allow the skill set for complete colonic detachment from the retroperitoneum and an intracorporeal anastomosis that is considerably more challenging when attempted with the laparoscopic approach. In fact, most who perform laparoscopic right colectomy construct an extracorporeal anastomosis [8, 9]. The extracorporeal anastomosis for most laparoscopic and robotic surgeons is conducted by standard open techniques through a midline extraction incision, where incisional hernia rates are considerably higher than when extraction sites are off the midline [10–12]. Complete colonic mobilization followed by an intracorporeal anastomosis allows the specimen extraction site to be anywhere off the midline, most commonly the Pfannenstiel position.

Electronic supplementary material The online version of this chapter (https://doi.org/10.1007/978-3-030-18740-8_18) contains supplementary material, which is available to authorized users.

R. K. Cleary (✉)
Department of Surgery, St Joseph Mercy Hospital
Ann Arbor, Ann Arbor, MI, USA
e-mail: Robert.Cleary@stjoeshealth.org

W. M. Akram
Brody School of Medicine at East Carolina
University, Greenville, NC, USA
e-mail: akramw18@ecu.edu

Overview of Technique

As part of the enhanced recovery pathway, nutritional modulation is started 5 days prior to surgery and carbohydrate loading up to 2 hours prior to surgery. Multimodal pain management programs vary in composition with respect to oral acetaminophen, oral gabapentin, and transversus abdominis plane blocks in the preoperative suite. In the operating room, the patient is placed in the supine position. After induction of general anesthesia, upper extremities are placed at the side and pressure points are padded. A standard strap is placed across the waist, and a foam strap is placed across the chest. Urinary catheters are used selectively based on patient comorbidities and intraoperative fluids are goal-directed. The skin is prepped, and the patient is draped in a standard fashion. The following operative steps are those favored by the author and taught at the national colon and rectal surgery fellowship course. There are several reasonable and acceptable variations taught by other faculty not described in this chapter.

Da Vinci Si System

Pneumoperitoneum and Port Placement

There are several options to establish pneumoperitoneum including the use of a Veress® needle or Optiview® trocar either at the proposed camera trocar site or in the left upper quadrant to avoid midline vessel or small bowel injury. There are also several port placement options. After establishing pneumoperitoneum, we prefer to place the 8.5-mm or 12-mm camera trocar 2 cm to the left of the umbilicus and either at the level of the umbilicus or below depending on the craniocaudal level of the umbilicus. The camera trocar should be at or slightly below a point halfway between the subcostal midline and the symphysis pubis.

Under direct vision with the robotic camera, 8-mm robotic trocars are then placed in the suprapubic region and subcostal region just to the left of the midline. A 13-mm robotic trocar is then placed in the left upper quadrant on a "V" orientation between the camera and subcostal trocars as depicted in Fig. 18.1. External arm collisions for this operation are typically between the left upper quadrant (D1) and subcostal (D3) trocars and rarely between the camera and suprapubic (D2) trocar, so placing the camera and left upper quadrant (D1) trocars a few centimeters more caudal increases the distance from the subcostal D3 trocar, thereby avoiding collisions. When an

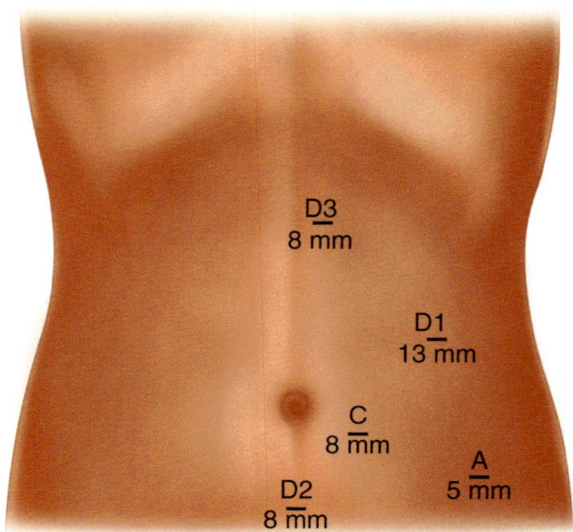

Fig. 18.1 Trocar/port placement for robotic right colectomy for Da Vinci Si platform

assistant port is used, a 5-mm trocar is typically placed in the left lower quadrant. An experienced assistant will recognize external collisions between D1 and D3 when they occur. Simply moving D3 about 2–3 cm away from D1 at the bedside often resolves the collision issue.

Docking the Robot

After port placement, the patient is placed in either slight Trendelenburg or slight reverse Trendelenburg and rotated right side up depending on surgeon preference. Complete laparoscopic abdominal exploration is more difficult after docking and is therefore performed prior to docking the robot. The small bowel is placed in the left side of the abdomen with the ileal mesentery splayed into the natural position, thereby exposing the ileocolic vessels. The robot is docked over the right side (Fig. 18.2). The robotic arms are attached to the respective trocars and the instruments passed under direct robotic camera vision. Instrument choice is based on surgeon preference. One option for the right-handed surgeon is to place the scissors, Vessel Sealer®, and the robotic stapler through the 13-mm trocar (D1) in the left upper quadrant. The fenestrated bipolar or cadiere instrument for fine retraction is placed in the 8-mm suprapubic trocar (D2), and

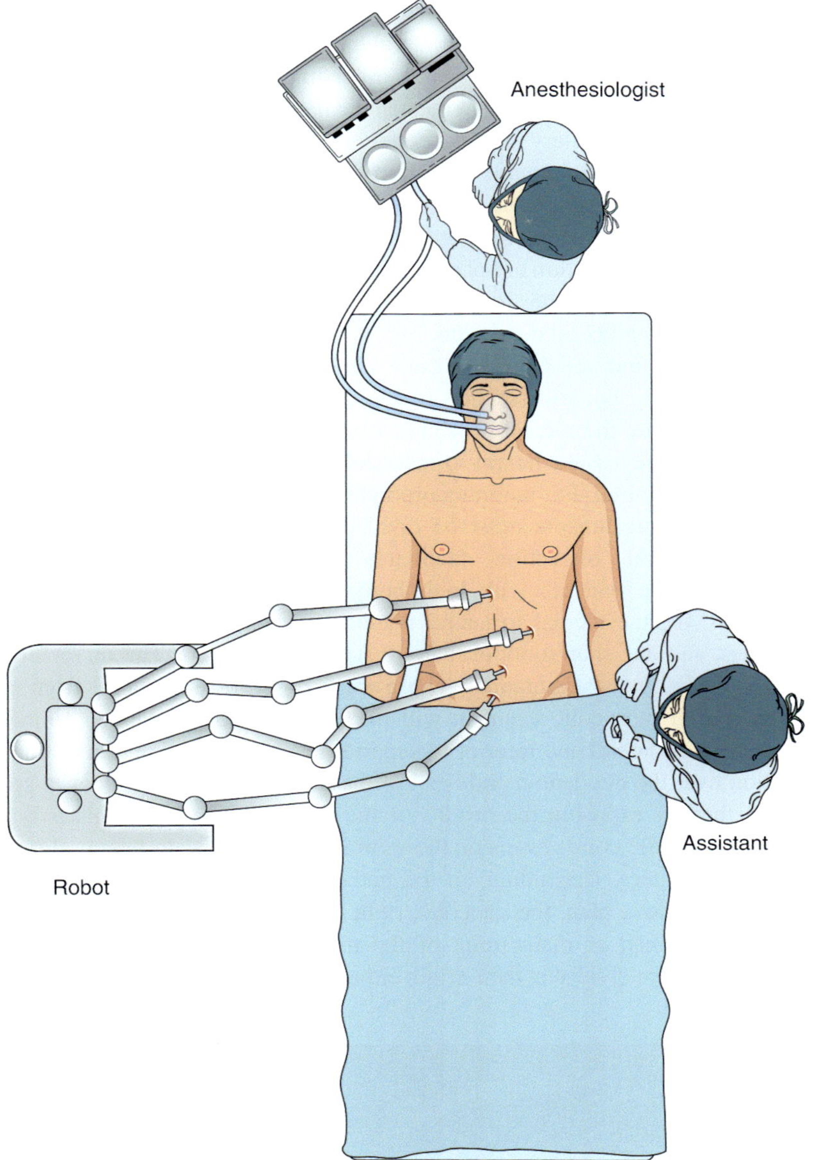

Fig. 18.2 Patient positioning and operating room setup for robotic right colectomy with Da Vinci Si/Xi platform

the third arm for fixed retraction (e.g., small grasper) is placed in the subcostal (D3) trocar.

Medial to Lateral Dissection and Division of Vascular Pedicles

Video 18.1

The order of operative steps depends on which are easiest to perform in a particular patient. It is best to proceed from what is anatomically clear rather than pursue a plane that is not obvious.

The operation starts with identification of the ileocolic vessels. The short grasper in subcostal D3 is used to lift the ileocolic vessels about 1/3 of the distance between the ileocecal wall and vessel origin. This maneuver provides exposure of the origin of the ileocolic vessels. A window is made in the mesentery beneath the ileocolic vessels about 2–3 cm distal to the origin with hot scissors, and the mesentery is dissected from the retroperitoneum in a medial to lateral fashion toward the terminal ileum, cecum, ascending colon, and over the duodenum to the hepatic flexure. Lifting the mesentery with closed fenestrated bipolar forceps in suprapubic D2 often demonstrates the plane between the mesentery and retroperitoneum. This medial to lateral dissection is done using a combination of hot and cold scissors for fine dissection and the closed tip of the Vessel Sealer® for broad blunt dissection.

The duodenum and Gerota's fascia are landmarks that help guide dissection in the correct plane. The more the medial-to-lateral dissection that is done, the less the lateral-to-medial dissection that is required. For the intracorporeal anastomosis, all attachments must be divided, and medial-to-lateral dissection facilitates these steps. In some patients with high body mass index (BMI), the medial to lateral plane is not obvious, and one should not hesitate to start lateral to medial in those situations. Those who perform central mesocolic excision will maximize the medial to lateral and inferior to superior dissection over the duodenum and head of the pancreas, thereby exposing the origins of the right colic and middle colic vessels on the ventral side of the mesentery. Depending on the pathology and the operative plan, the ileocolic, right colic, and right branch or main trunk of the middle colic vessels are divided at their origin either with

the Vessel Sealer® or after placing clips. Partial medial-to-lateral dissection to clearly demonstrate the ileocolic vessels is usually followed by division of the ileocolic vessels, then further medial to lateral dissection is performed prior to addressing division of the right and middle colic vessels.

It is important in the learning curve to remember that the robotic advantage is operating with three instruments and that the third arm for fixed retraction should be used to maximize operative efficiency. After dividing the ileocolic vessels, placing an open short grasper horizontally under the mesentery tents up the mesentery and facilitates medial-to-lateral and inferior-to-superior dissections of the mesentery from the retroperitoneum (Fig. 18.3). The short grasper is then used to lift the proximal transverse colon toward the liver splaying the mesentery and allowing clear visualization of the right colic and middle colic vessels. The mesentery is then divided with the Vessel Sealer® from point of transection of the ileocolic vessels to the proposed point of transverse colon transection.

It is important to know where the pancreas is located, and this is typically determined during medial-to-lateral dissection. If visualization of the ventral aspect of the mesentery is too difficult even with proper third arm tenting retraction under the mesentery, or after third arm retraction of the proximal transverse colon above the liver,

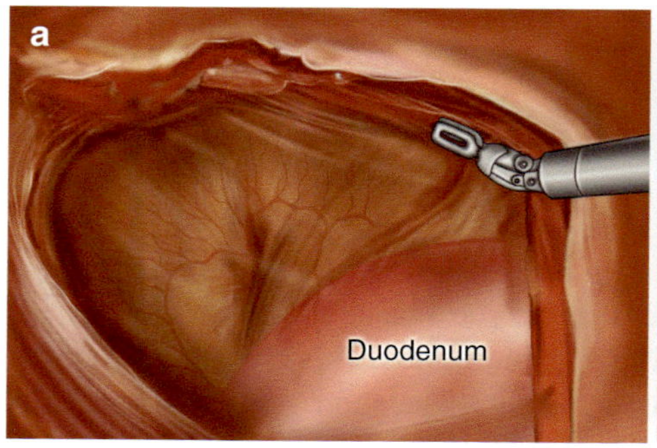
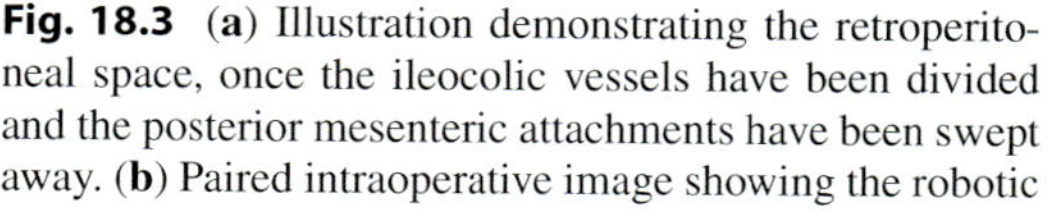

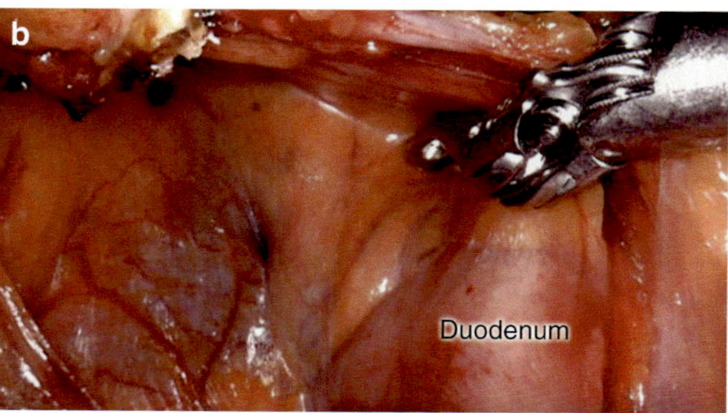

Fig. 18.3 (**a**) Illustration demonstrating the retroperitoneal space, once the ileocolic vessels have been divided and the posterior mesenteric attachments have been swept away. (**b**) Paired intraoperative image showing the robotic forceps lifting the mesentery away from the retroperitoneum after medial to lateral and inferior to superior dissection

the third arm short grasper can be used to retract the proximal transverse colon toward the left lower quadrant underneath the other operating instruments, exposing the dorsal surface of the mesentery. If enough medial to lateral dissection is performed prior to this maneuver, dissection of the right and middle colic vessels should be safe from the dorsal angle. An experienced assistant may serve as a fourth arm and help with any of these maneuvers as instructed by the operating console surgeon. The omentum is retracted cephalad above the liver with the third arm and detached from the hepatic flexure and proximal transverse colon with hot scissors and the Vessel Sealer®. Assistant retraction of the transverse colon toward the left lower quadrant facilitates this dissection.

For most surgeons performing an extracorporeal anastomosis, mobilization of the colon and mesentery and vessel division concludes the robotic part of the operation. Prior to undocking the robot and making the extraction site incision, viability of the proposed points of transection of the ileum and transverse colon may be confirmed using immunofluorescence with intravenous injection of 3 ml of indocyanine green. Alternatively, immunofluorescence may be done extracorporeal prior to the anastomosis using the robotic camera. Details on extracorporeal anastomosis can be found elsewhere.

Intracorporeal Anastomosis

For those constructing an intracorporeal anastomosis, all mesenteric attachments to the retroperitoneum are divided by medial-to-lateral, inferior-to-superior, and lateral-to-medial dissections. The mesentery is taken from the point of transection of the ileocolic vessels to the terminal ileum using the Vessel Sealer®. The mesentery to the mid-transverse colon is divided from the point of transection of the ileocolic vessels. The right colic and right branch of the middle colic or main middle colic vessels are divided after the application of clips or with the Vessel Sealer®. Immunofluorescence is then performed by intravenous injection of 3 ml of indocyanine green to

confirm viability of the proposed point of transection of the terminal ileum and transverse colon. The terminal ileum and mid-transverse colon are then divided with blue loads of the 45 mm robotic stapler. The completely detached specimen is placed in the right upper quadrant using the "roll" technique, confirming that all retroperitoneal attachments have been divided. The terminal ileum is then placed next to the mid-transverse colon in either isoperistaltic or anti-peristaltic configuration (Fig. 18.4).

Seromuscular 3-0 Vicryl or silk sutures are placed to align the ileum and colon. The third arm (prograsp or Vessel Sealer®) in subcostal D3 raises the cut end of the seromuscular suture toward the right abdominal sidewall, facilitating exposure and construction of the anastomosis. Ileal enterotomy and transverse colotomy are made with hot scissors. The robotic stapler with blue load is placed through the openings, clamped, and fired, thereby creating the anastomosis. Another seromuscular 3-0 Vicryl stay suture is placed at the end of the staple line near the common enterotomy. This allows the prograsp or Vessel Sealer® to be repositioned to retract the cut end of this stay suture toward the right abdominal side wall, allowing clear visualization of the common enterotomy in preparation for suture closure. The common enterotomy created with the stapler is then either closed with a running barbed 3-0 suture in one or two layers, or another application of the stapler. It is important to sew the common enterotomy in an inferior to superior direction because the inferior limit of the common enterotomy is most difficult to visualize and can be missed, resulting in an anastomotic defect that escapes detection. The advantage of using the Vessel Sealer® for stay suture retraction prior to suturing the common enterotomy is that it can also be used to cut the suture rather than having the assistant perform this maneuver.

The omentum is draped over the anastomosis. A locking grasper is placed on the specimen staple line to allow easy specimen extraction. Specimen extraction is done in the Pfannenstiel location after extending the suprapubic trocar incision and inserting a wound protector. The

Isoperistaltic

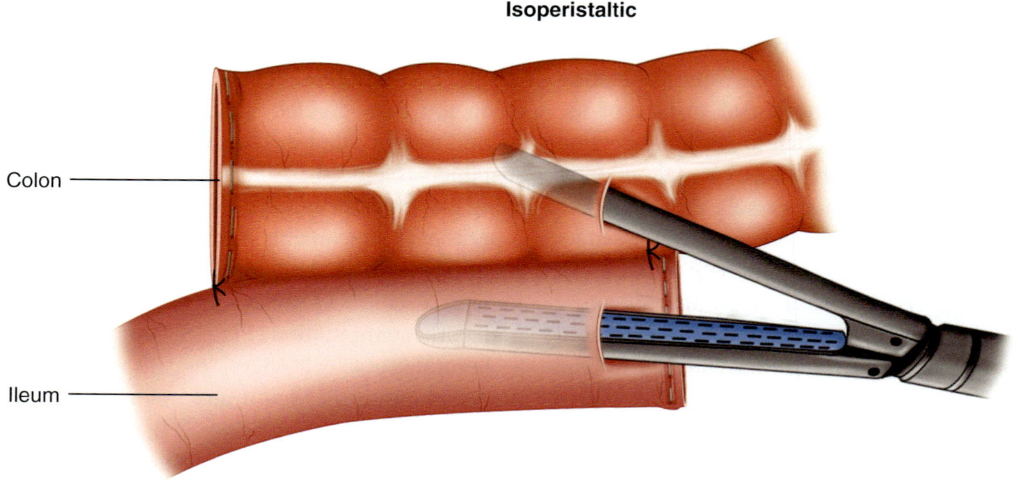

Antiperistaltic

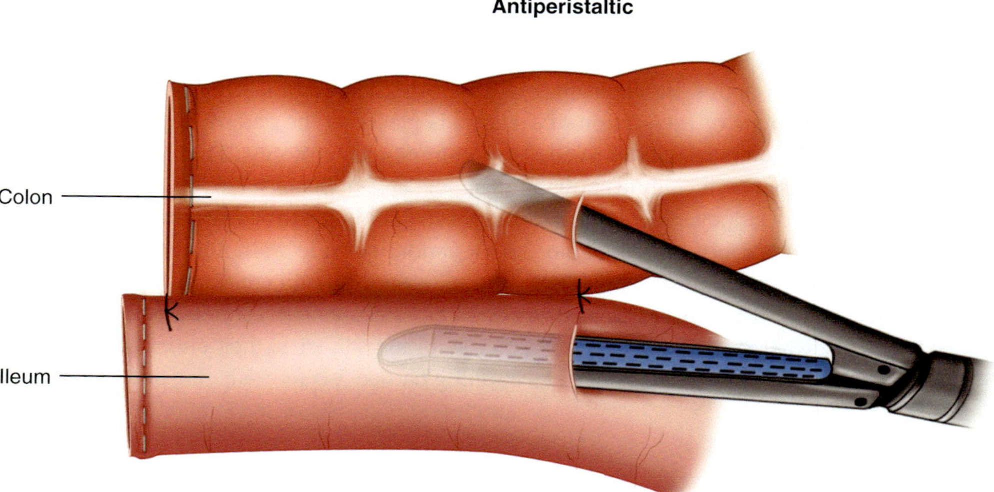

Fig. 18.4 Bowel anastomosis can be performed in an isoperistaltic or antiperistaltic fashion

13-mm D1 trocar site fascia is closed with polyglactin using the Carter-Thomason® device and the trocars are removed under direct vision. The Pfannenstiel site peritoneum and fascia are closed with running 2-0 polyglactin in separate layers. The skin is closed with running subcuticular 4-0 Monocryl®.

Da Vinci Xi System

Pneumoperitoneum and Docking the Robot

Pneumoperitoneum is established in the same way as that for the Si system using an Optiview®

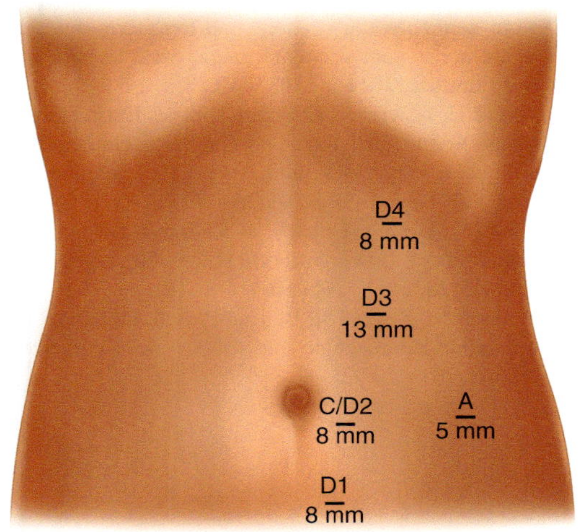

Fig. 18.5 Trocar/port placement for robotic right colectomy for Da Vinci Xi platform

trocar in the subcostal region left of the midline. An orogastric tube will keep the stomach deflated and decrease the risk of gastric injury. The Xi options for port placement are different from the Si platform because of sleeker Xi arms with additional adjustable joints that require parallel rather than angled robotic arm spatial configurations that decrease the risk for external collisions. One commonly used option is shown in Fig. 18.5.

Four trocars are placed 7–8 cm apart in a diagonal arrangement from the suprapubic region to the subcostal region, left of the midline and left of the umbilicus. The 0 ° or 30 ° down camera can be used in any of these ports but is typically started in the 8-mm D2 trocar. The 13-mm trocar is often inserted in the D3 position and used for scissors, hook, Vessel Sealer®, and stapler depending on surgeon preference. The suprapubic (D1) 8-mm trocar is for the fenestrated bipolar instrument used by the surgeon's left hand. The subcostal (D4) location also accommodates an 8-mm trocar and is the third arm for fixed retraction, typically the fenestrated "tip-up" grasper. A 5-mm assistant trocar best serves the surgeon in the left lower quadrant. The patient is placed in either slight Trendelenburg or slight reverse Trendelenburg and right side up rotation. After laparoscopic abdominal exploration and moving the small bowel mesentery to the normal

anatomic position, the robot is docked over the right side of the patient. The camera arm is attached to the camera D2 trocar and the camera is inserted for targeting the other robotic arms and instruments are passed under direct vision.

The operation is then conducted as described for the Si platform. The Xi operation is ideal for the intracorporeal anastomosis with specimen extraction through a Pfannenstiel incision created by extending the suprapubic D1 port incision, the size of which is limited only by the size of the pathology in the specimen.

Conclusions

The adoption of the robotic platform as a surgical option for right colectomy is increasing. There are outcomes advantages to the intracorporeal anastomosis and the robotic approach allows an intracorporeal anastomosis without a steep learning curve. There may be value to adopting the robotic approach for those surgeons who find the laparoscopic intracorporeal anastomosis too challenging. The value of robotic right colectomy may also relate to increasing minimally invasive surgery options that potentially decrease the prevalence of open colorectal surgery.

References

1. Halabi WJ, Kang CY, Jafari MD, et al. Robotic-assisted colorectal surgery in the United States: a nationwide analysis of trends and outcomes. World J Surg. 2013;37:2782–90.
2. Steele SR, Stein SL, Bordeianou LG, et al. American Society of Colon and Rectal Surgeons' Young Surgeons Committee. The impact of practice environment on laparoscopic colectomy utilization following colorectal residency: a survey of ASCRS Young Surgeons. Color Dis. 2012;14:374–81.
3. Moghadamyeghaneh Z, Phelan M, Smith BR, et al. Variations in laparoscopic colectomy utilization in the United States. Dis Colon Rectum. 2015;58:950–6.
4. Hollis RH, Cannon JA, Singletary BA, et al. Understanding the value of both laparoscopic and robotic approaches compared to open approach in colorectal surgery. J Laparoendosc Adv Surg Tech A. 2016;26:850–6.
5. Yeo HL, Isaacs AJ, Abelson JS, et al. Comparison of open, laparoscopic, and robotic colectomies

using a large national database: outcomes and trends related to surgery center volume. Dis Colon Rectum. 2016;59:535–42.

6. Morpurgo E, Contardo T, Molaro R, et al. Robotic-assisted intracorporeal anastomosis versus extracorporeal anastomosis in laparoscopic right hemicolectomy for cancer: a case control study. J Laparoendosc Adv Surg Tech A. 2013;23:414–7.

7. Trastulli S, Coratti A, Guarino S, et al. Robotic right colectomy with intracorporeal anastomosis compared with laparoscopic right colectomy with extracorporeal and intracorporeal anastomosis: a retrospective multicentre study. Surg Endosc. 2015;29:1512–21.

8. Milone M, Elmore U, DiSalvo E, et al. Intracorporeal versus extracorporeal anastomosis. Results from a multicenter comparative study of 512 right-sided colorectal cancers. Surg Endosc. 2015;29:2314–20.

9. Hanna MH, Hwang GS, Phelan MJ, et al. Laparoscopic right hemicolectomy: short- and long-term outcomes of intracorporeal versus extracorporeal anastomosis. Surg Endosc. 2016;30:3933–42.

10. Samia H, Lawrence J, Nobel T, et al. Extraction site location and incisional hernias after laparoscopic colorectal surgery: should we be avoiding the midline? Am J Surg. 2013;205:264–7.

11. Harr JN, Juo YY, Luka S, et al. Incisional and port-site hernias following robotic colorectal surgery. Surg Endosc. 2016;30:3505–10.

12. Widmar M, Keskin M, Beltran P, et al. Incisional hernias after laparoscopic and robotic right colectomy. Hernia. 2016;20:723–8.

Christina N. Jenkins and Elizabeth R. Raskin

Introduction

Minimally invasive surgery (MIS) has revolutionized the traditional approach to colectomy. By minimizing trauma to the abdominal wall and the field of resection, MIS colectomy has been associated with less postoperative pain, shorter return of bowel function, and reduction in hospital length of stay [1, 2]. Single-incision laparoscopy (SIL) is a derivative of traditional multiport laparoscopy, combining trocar and specimen extraction sites with the intention of reducing pain and scarring.

SIL or single-port access (SPA) surgery falls under the umbrella of natural orifice transluminal endoscopic surgery (NOTES). As implied by the name, NOTES utilizes orifices such as the stomach, vagina, anus, and umbilicus for primary instrument access and extraction of specimens. The umbilicus is considered a natural orifice from an embryologic standpoint. The first reported SIL procedures include appendectomy and cholecystectomy in the late 1990s [3, 4].

The original enthusiasm around SIL centered on the goal of minimizing the size and multiplicity of abdominal incisions for both postoperative pain and recovery, in addition to enhancing cosmesis.

As feasibility and safety were demonstrated, SIL was applied to more complex procedures, such as gastric banding, colectomy, nephrectomy, hysterectomy, and hernia repair [5–9].

In 2008, separate reports by Bucher et al. [7] and Remzi et al. [10] described the first single-incision laparoscopic surgery (SILS) for right colectomy utilizing an umbilical port site. In both reports, laparoscopic mobilization of the right colon was followed by creation of an extracorporeal ileocolic anastomosis. These successful initial forays into SILS encouraged others to apply this approach within the realm of colorectal surgery with case reports of segmental colectomy, total abdominal colectomy, and total proctocolectomy with ileoanal pouch creation [11–13].

Patient Selection and Preoperative Planning

Patients undergoing SILS right colectomy should undergo appropriate preoperative evaluation for major abdominal surgery. This should include thorough cardiopulmonary assessment to determine a patient's fitness for both general anesthesia and abdominal insufflation. In the setting of malignancy, patients should also have imaging performed for staging with careful attention to the resectability of the tumor.

The onus is on the surgeon to determine whether or not SILS is feasible and appropriate for

C. N. Jenkins · E. R. Raskin (✉)
Loma Linda University Medical Center,
Loma Linda, CA, USA
e-mail: cnjenkins@llu.edu

© Springer Nature Switzerland AG 2020
J. Kim, J. Garcia-Aguilar (eds.), *Minimally Invasive Surgical Techniques for Cancers of the Gastrointestinal Tract*, https://doi.org/10.1007/978-3-030-18740-8_19

each patient, taking into consideration the surgeon's laparoscopic experience and the complexity of the patient's condition. Early in the SILS learning curve, it is generally advisable that the surgeon select patients with lower body mass index (BMI), minor or no prior abdominal surgery, and less complicated pathology. As experience is gained, more technically challenging disease can be approached (i.e., higher BMI, larger tumor, inflammatory mass, extensive adhesive disease) according to the surgeon's comfort level.

Preoperative Care and Patient Positioning

After induction of general anesthesia and endotracheal intubation, the patient should be placed in the supine position with the left arm tucked at the side. It is important to adequately secure the patient to the bed with generous padding and straps, as the patient may require rotation into the left side down/right side up position. Urinary bladder catheterization should be performed for urine output monitoring. Lower extremity sequential compression devices should be engaged at the time of anesthesia induction. In the setting of malignancy, subcutaneous heparin (5000 units) should be administered for additional thromboembolic prophylaxis. Preoperative prophylactic antibiotics should be administered within 30 minutes of incision time. Iodophor- or chlorhexidine-based skin preparation is recommended for reduction of surgical site infection.

Port Placement

Two generally accepted port placement sites have been utilized for SILS: the umbilicus and the suprapubic location. Laparoscopically, our preferred approach is through a 2.5 cm incision at the umbilicus, which allows for a 4 cm fascial incision below (Figure 19.1a, b). Although several commercial single-incision ports are available, we typically use the Gelport™ platform by Applied Medical (Fig. 19.2) as it includes a wound protector for specimen extraction.

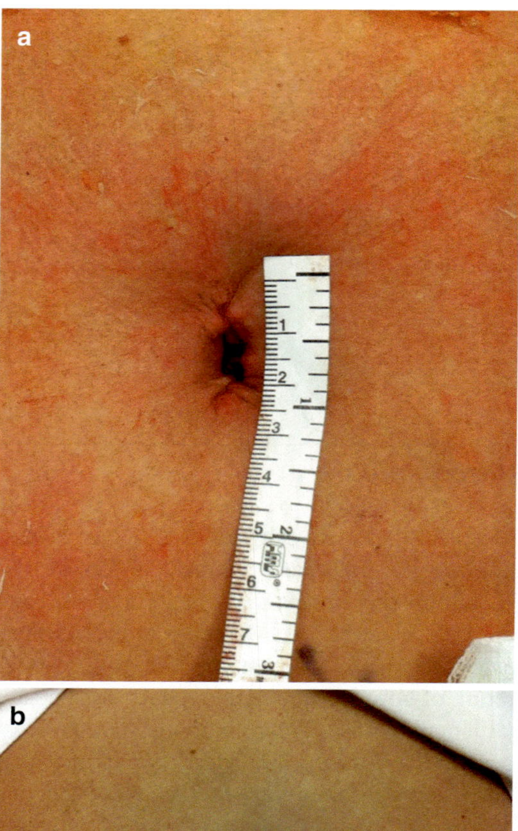

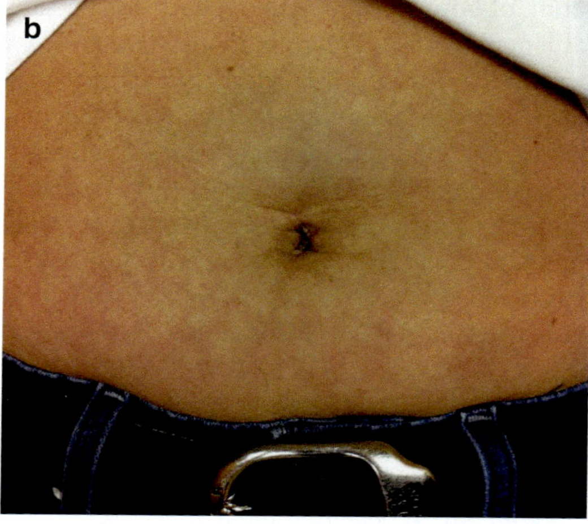

Fig. 19.1 (**a**) Measurement of the single-site incision with a ruler. Incision with ruler. (**b**) The postoperative appearance of the single-site incision

Alternatively, we have also used a wound retractor with an attached surgical glove as a single-incision port (Fig. 19.3). Insufflation can be initiated either through a port placed through the platform or through an insufflation valve on the platform. Insufflation pressure is based on distensibility of the abdominal wall but typically set at 10–15 mmHg.

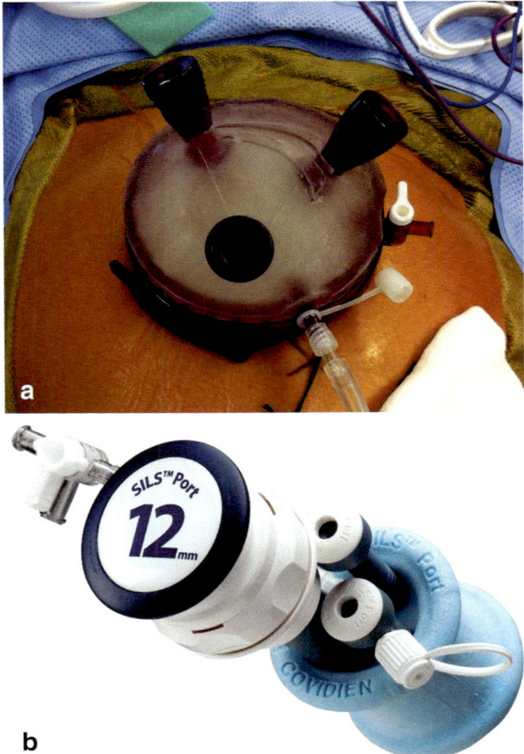

Fig. 19.2 Image of a commercially available single-site port

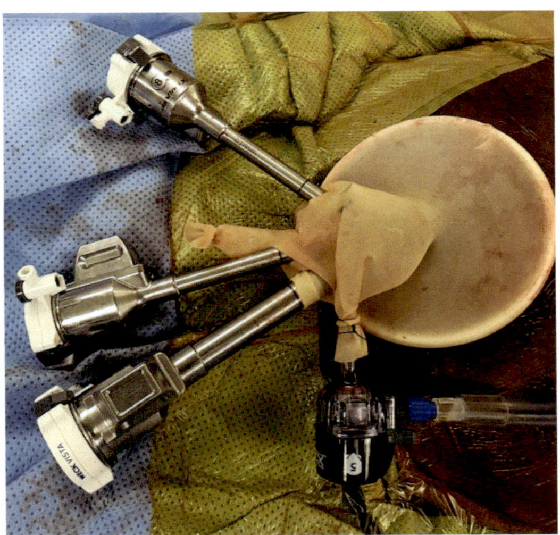

Fig. 19.3 Intraoperative image of a glove modified to serve as a single-site port

Trocars, Camera, and Instrumentation

Given spatial constraints, three ports are placed through the SILS platform: one 5/12-mm trocar for the camera and two 5-mm ports for instrumentation. It can be difficult to find room for an assistant port; however, this depends on the size of the platform and the configuration of trocar placement. Some authors report using an assistant port outside the SILS platform in a technique described as a "single-incision plus one" approach. Unlike with standard multiport laparoscopy, triangulation of the tissues can be difficult with SILS because of limited space and range of motion. Adequate exposure and traction/counter-traction can be achieved with smaller and less dramatic movements. Despite these considerations, external collisions can occur. A 30 ° bariatric length laparoscope with a right-angle light cord is recommended to allow the assistant to avoid excessive external collisions. Alternatively, a flexible tip 5 mm laparoscope can also be utilized. A grasper and energy device (monopolar or bipolar) can be used through the two working trocars.

Surgical Technique

Colonic Mobilization

Our preference is for a medial-to-lateral approach once insufflation has been achieved. It can be useful to suspend the ileocecal region using a 0-silk suture by passing a transabdominal Keith needle or by intracorporeally tacking the cecum to the anterior abdominal wall. This maneuver allows the surgeon to elevate the cecum and stretch out the ileocolic pedicle, without committing the grasper to this action. The dissection can then be carried out by carefully separating the right colonic mesentery from the retroperitoneum and, in particular, the duodenum. The lateral attachments and hepatic flexure can then be mobilized. The gastrocolic ligament should be released allowing entrance into the lesser sac. We use a 5 mm blunt-tipped LigaSure™ vessel sealing device by Covidien to ligate the ileocolic, right colic, and right branch of the middle colic vessels. The mesentery of the terminal ileum and the transverse colon can be taken with the energy device up to the edge of bowel.

Creation of the Anastomosis

Once the right colon has been completely mobilized, a resection of the bowel and creation of the anastomosis are then performed. We favor performing the anastomosis in an extracorporeal fashion, given the limited range of motion of the instruments and the technical challenge of intracorporeal anastomosis. An iso- or antiperistaltic anastomosis can be created. After reduction of the anastomosis back into the abdomen, we close the fascia with a 0-PDS and the skin with 4-0 Vicryl and Dermabond®.

Overall Outcomes

An early study by Papaconstantinou et al. [14] reported improvement in postoperative pain and decreased length of stay with SILS colectomy compared to multiport laparoscopic resection. In this case-matched study, 29 patients who underwent SILS right colectomy were matched to patients who had undergone hand-assisted laparoscopic (HAL) or standard laparoscopic right colectomy. A significant decrease in postoperative pain scores on postoperative day 1 was observed in the SILS group compared to both HAL and standard ($p < 0.05$) groups, despite similar incision length (4.5 cm, SILS vs. 5.1 cm, standard). This suggests that the addition of 5-mm ports may contribute to increased postoperative pain. However, several subsequent papers reported no difference in pain scores when comparing SILS to multiport colectomy [15]. Length of stay was decreased by 1 day in the SILS group (mean, 3 days) compared to both HAL and standard groups (mean, 4 days) ($p < 0.05$), despite

similar postoperative care. Operative times and conversion rates were similar in both groups.

Oncologic Outcomes

In addition to safety and feasibility, the maintenance of oncologic principles is critical for the adoption of new surgical techniques for colorectal malignancy. The gold standard is the achievement of negative margins combined with complete mesocolic excision with appropriate lymph node harvest. With single-incision approach, technical challenges such as instrument crowding, difficulty with triangulation, limited counter-traction, and in-line viewing are ubiquitous. Despite the lack of data to support SILS as a standard technique, several publications have demonstrated oncologic equivalency between SILS and standard multiport laparoscopic right colectomy [16–21].

Robotic-Assisted Single-Incision

To overcome some of the technical challenges posed by SILS, robotic technology has been applied to the single-incision approach. The technique involves using robotic trocars, inserted through a single-port platform, that are then docked to the surgical robot. The surgeon then controls the arms at the robotic console. Our preference is to use the da Vinci Xi® platform.

Patient Positioning

Preoperative care is identical to that mentioned above for laparoscopic SILS. We place the patient in the supine position; however, we pad and tuck both arms.

Port and Trocar Placement

We prefer to use a wound retractor with an attached glove for our platform, placed through a 3–4 cm Pfannenstiel incision. After cutting off the fingertips of the glove, the four 8-mm trocars are inserted and secured with 0-silk ties (Fig. 19.3). Through the fifth fingertip, an assistant port is secured for insufflation. Ideal insufflation pressures range from 10 to 15 mmHg, depending on the laxity of the abdominal wall.

Camera and Instrumentation

We utilize a 30 ° scope that can be rotated upward or downward during the dissection. Monopolar scissors, bipolar fenestrated grasper, and Cadiere forceps are used. Due to the small confines of the working space, it is imperative that the joints of the Xi platform are optimally spaced to allow for passage and mobilization of the instruments.

Surgical Technique

Colonic Mobilization

We begin with an inferior approach to the dissection by elevating the cecum. First, the appendix is mobilized from its lateral attachments. We enter the avascular space, carefully separating the mesocolon from the retroperitoneum. Close attention is paid to identifying and sparing the right ureter, duodenum, and pancreas. We continue this dissection all the way up to the hepatic flexure, eventually visualizing the liver parenchyma and gallbladder. The colon can then be rotated medially, allowing the lateral attachments and gastrocolic ligament to be released. We then address the ileocolic pedicle by performing a high ligation using the EndoWrist® one™ vessel sealer. The right colic and right branch of the middle colic artery are transected and sealed in a similar fashion. Lastly, the mesentery of the terminal ileum and proximal transverse colon are taken with the vessel sealer.

Creation of the Anastomosis

Upon complete release of the specimen, the right colon is placed into the left lower quadrant. We prepare for intracorporeal anastomosis by bringing the terminal ileum up to the transverse colon. A 3-0 silk suture, cut to 10 cm, is then passed through a trocar. We determine whether an anti-peristaltic or isoperistaltic anastomosis is performed by assessing the natural position of the bowel. A robotic needle driver is used to align the bowel in a side-to-side fashion.

Enterotomies are created in the aligned small bowel and colon to allow for passage of a stapler with a blue load. Once the stapler has been fired, the anastomosis is evaluated intraluminally for adequate hemostasis. The resulting enterotomy for the common channel is then closed with a 2-0 barbed suture in a running fashion.

The instruments are then removed and insufflation is terminated. After removing the glove with the attached trocars, the specimen can be brought through the wound protector. The fascia is then closed with 0-PDS suture. We irrigate the soft tissue of the wound with sterile saline and then close the skin with a running 4-0 Vicryl suture and Dermabond. Local anesthesia is then injected around the wound.

Outcomes

Spinoglio et al. reported three cases of robotic right colectomy utilizing Single-Site™ instrumentation by Intuitive Surgical, Inc. [22]. The Single-Site™ kit is comprised of a gel faceplate with curved cannulae through which semirigid robotic instruments are inserted. The instruments cross each other at the point of entry into the abdomen and are then reassigned to the surgeon's opposite hand to restore the natural alignment (Fig. 19.4). For each of the three cases, a suprapubic location was selected for platform placement. Mean operating room time was 218 ± 75.9 minutes. Intracorporeal isoperistaltic anastomoses were created in two cases with one extracorporeal anastomosis. All patients were discharged within 5 days of surgery.

Unfortunately, the lack of wristed instruments utilized in the Single-Site™ technology does not allow the surgeon to capitalize on the perceived

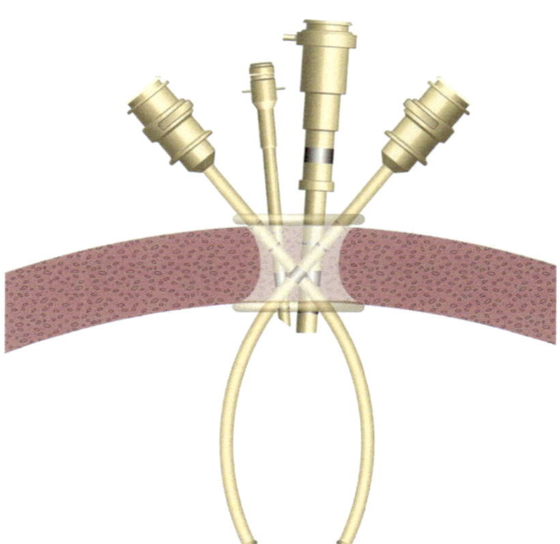

Fig. 19.4 Image of a single-site kit with cannula crossing at the level of the fascia

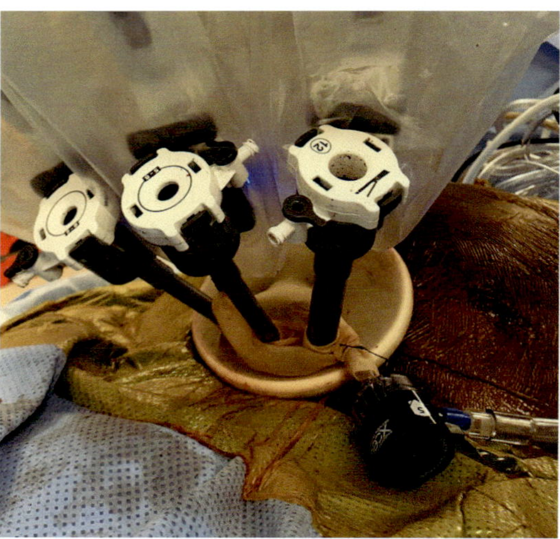

Fig. 19.5 Intraoperative image of a modified glove platform with robotic trocars

advantages of robotic surgery. Subsequent reports have largely described the use of standard wristed instruments and robotic trocars which have been inserted through a single-incision platform (Fig. 19.5).

The largest experience with single-incision robotic right colectomy to date was reported by Juo et al., describing 31 patients [23]. The da Vinci Si™ robotic system with a Gelpoint™ platform (Applied Medical) was used via an umbilical incision, employing four trocars: one 12-mm camera trocar, two 8-mm robotic trocars, and one 5-mm laparoscopic assistant port. The authors describe a "crossed-arm" technique where the two robotic arms are crossed intracorporeally to minimize instrument collisions and to improve triangulation. This technique requires the reassignment of the robotic arms to the surgeon's opposite hand (e.g., right arm assigned to surgeon's left hand). The median operating room time was 180 minutes, which is slightly longer time compared to SILS in other series [24]. Only one conversion was noted in this initial series. An incisional hernia rate of 10.2% was reported, which falls within a wide range of other reports of hernias following SILS with periumbilical extraction (4.9–12%) [24, 25].

Criticism of single-incision surgery, especially with umbilical port placement, has been centered around a focus on cosmesis at the expense of postoperative hernia formation [26]. Several papers have looked at patient preference for reduced port surgery based on size, location, visibility, and number of incisions, in addition to perceived recovery time [27, 28]. Currently, there are no studies in the literature that directly evaluate patient cosmetic satisfaction after either SILS or SILS robotic colectomy.

Conclusions

Innovation in surgery has been driven by the quest to enhance the surgical experience and improve patient outcomes. Single-incision technology has been applied to colorectal surgery with the intent of expediting recovery, enhancing cosmesis, and providing alternative laparoscopic options. While SILS has been shown to be safe, feasible, and oncologically sound, further investigation into these techniques is necessary to assess overall benefits. In addition, technological advances in platform design, optics, and instrumentation may help realize the potential advantages of the single-incision approach.

References

1. Weeks JC, Nelson H, Gelber S, et al. Short-term quality-of-life outcomes following laparoscopic-assisted colectomy vs open colectomy for colon cancer: a randomized trial. JAMA. 2002;287:321–8.
2. Chen HH, Wexner SD, Iroatulam AJ, et al. Laparoscopic colectomy compares favorably with colectomy by laparotomy for reduction of postoperative ileus. Dis Colon Rectum. 2000;43:61–5.
3. Inoue H, Takeshita K, Endo M. Single-port laparoscopy assisted appendectomy under local pneumoperitoneum condition. Surg Endosc. 1994;8:714–6.
4. Piskun G, Rajpal S. Transumbilical laparoscopic cholecystectomy utilizes no incisions outside the umbilicus. J Laparoendosc Adv Surg Tech A. 1999;9:361–4.
5. Teixeira J, McGill K, Binenbaum S, et al. Laparoscopic single-site surgery for placement of an adjustable gastric band: initial experience. Surg Endosc. 2009;23:1409–14.
6. Fader AN, Michener CM, Frasure HE, et al. Total laparoscopic hysterectomy versus laparoscopic-assisted vaginal hysterectomy in endometrial cancer: surgical and survival outcomes. J Minim Invasive Gynecol. 2009;16:333–9.
7. Bucher P, Pugin F, Morel P. Single port access laparoscopic right hemicolectomy. Int J Color Dis. 2008;23:1013–6.
8. Jacob BP, Tong W, Reiner M, et al. Single incision total extraperitoneal (one SITE) laparoscopic inguinal hernia repair using a single access port device. Hernia. 2009;13:571–2.
9. Ponsky LE, Cherullo EE, Sawyer M, et al. Single access site laparoscopic radical nephrectomy: initial clinical experience. J Endourol. 2008;22:663–6.
10. Remzi FH, Kirat HT, Kaouk JH, et al. Single-port laparoscopy in colorectal surgery. Color Dis. 2008;10:823–6.
11. Bardakcioglu O, Ahmed S. Single incision laparoscopic total abdominal colectomy with ileorectal anastomosis for synchronous colon cancer. Tech Coloproctol. 2010;14:257–61.
12. Bucher P, Pugin F, Morel P. Transumbilical single incision laparoscopic sigmoidectomy for benign disease. Color Dis. 2010;12:61–5.
13. Geisler DP, Condon ET, Remzi FH. Single incision laparoscopic total proctocolectomy with ileopouch anal anastomosis. Color Dis. 2010;12:941–3.
14. Papaconstantinou HT, Sharp N, Thomas JS. Single-incision laparoscopic right colectomy: a case-matched comparison with standard laparoscopic and hand-assisted laparoscopic techniques. J Am Coll Surg. 2011;213:72–80.
15. Chew MH, Chang MH, Tan WS, et al. Conventional laparoscopic versus single-incision laparoscopic right hemicolectomy: a case cohort comparison of short-term outcomes in 144 consecutive cases. Surg Endosc. 2013;27:471–7.
16. Waters JA, Rapp BM, Guzman MJ, et al. Single-port laparoscopic right hemicolectomy: the first 100 resections. Dis Colon Rectum. 2012;55:134–9.
17. Chen WT, Chang SC, Chiang HC, et al. Single-incision laparoscopic versus conventional laparoscopic right hemicolectomy: a comparison of short-term surgical results. Surg Endosc. 2011;25:1887–92.
18. Vettoretto N, Cirocchi R, Randolph J, et al. Single incision laparoscopic right colectomy: a systematic review and meta-analysis. Color Dis. 2014;16:O123–32.
19. Miyo M, Takemasa I, Ishihara H, et al. Long-term outcomes of single-site laparoscopic colectomy with complete mesocolic excision for colon cancer. Dis Colon Rectum. 2017;60:664–73.
20. Poon JT, Cheung CW, Fan JK, et al. Single-incision versus conventional laparoscopic colectomy for colonic neoplasm: a randomized, controlled trial. Surg Endosc. 2012;26:2729–34.
21. Huscher CG, Mingoli A, Sgarzini G, et al. Standard laparoscopic versus single-incision laparoscopic colectomy for cancer: early results of a randomized prospective study. Am J Surg. 2012;204:115–20.
22. Spinoglio G, Lenti LM, Ravazzoni F, et al. Evaluation of technical feasibility and safety of Single-Site robotic right colectomy: three case reports. Int J Med Robot. 2015;11:135–40.
23. Juo YY, Agarwal S, Luka S, et al. Single-Incision Robotic Colectomy (SIRC) case series: initial experience at a single center. Surg Endosc. 2015;29:1976–81.
24. Vestweber B, Galetin T, Lammerting K, et al. Single-incision laparoscopic surgery: outcomes from 224 colonic resections performed at a single center using SILS. Surg Endosc. 2013;27:434–42.
25. Benlice C, Stocchi L, Costedio MM, et al. Impact of the specific extraction-site location on the risk of incisional hernia after laparoscopic colorectal resection. Dis Colon Rectum. 2016;59:743–50.
26. Marks JM, Phillips MS, Tacchino R, et al. Single-incision laparoscopic cholecystectomy is associated with improved cosmesis scoring at the cost of significantly higher hernia rates: 1-year results of a prospective randomized, multicenter, single-blinded trial of traditional multiport laparoscopic cholecystectomy vs single-incision laparoscopic cholecystectomy. J Am Coll Surg. 2013;216:1037–47.
27. van den Boezem PB, Velthuis S, Lourens HJ, et al. Single-incision and NOTES cholecystectomy, are there clinical or cosmetic advantages when compared to conventional laparoscopic cholecystectomy? World J Surg. 2014;38:25–32.
28. Yeung PP Jr, Bolden CR, Westreich D, et al. Patient preferences of cosmesis for abdominal incisions in gynecologic surgery. J Minim Invasive Gynecol. 2013;20:79–84.

Alessio Pigazzi and Matthew T. Brady

Introduction

Over the past decades, advances in minimally invasive surgery have been observed in all surgical fields. Within colon and rectal surgery, the adoption of minimally invasive surgical techniques has allowed for improvements in patient care and recovery. Patients can now anticipate shorter recovery times, decreased hospital lengths of stay, less postoperative pain, and decreased risk of incisional hernia as a result of these minimally invasive approaches. Despite such advantages only 50% of annual colon resections in the USA are performed by laparoscopic techniques [1]. The low rate may be a result of the technical challenges of performing laparoscopic colon resection. This chapter aims to present a stepwise approach to laparoscopic left colectomy to aid in developing the necessary skills to master this approach. Here, we present our preferred approach as well as secondary approaches to skillfully perform laparoscopic left colectomy.

Electronic supplementary material The online version of this chapter (https://doi.org/10.1007/978-3-030-18740-8_20) contains supplementary material, which is available to authorized users.

A. Pigazzi (✉) · M. T. Brady
Department of Surgery, Division of Colon and Rectal Surgery, University of California, Irvine Medical Center, Orange, CA, USA
e-mail: apigazzi@uci.edu

Necessary Equipment

Laparoscopic left colectomy requires an adequate array of laparoscopic instruments and equipment to safely perform this procedure. Given the progress of the minimally invasive surgical era, there have been great advancements in the equipment for performing these operations. As is true for all surgical disciplines, it is important to balance the cost of equipment with its necessity. Additionally, while there are many options for equipment, it is important to use the instruments that provide the surgeon comfort and ease of use. Below is a list of equipment, categorized by its use in the operation, which we feel are important.

Positioning

To assist with colon mobilization, the operating table will be placed in a variety of positions, occasionally at steep angles. It is imperative to secure the patient to prevent sliding on the table while avoiding restriction of respiration and formation of pressure wounds. Additional positioning requirements include free access to the rectum for transanal staplers and endoscopes. Below are some available options for positioning equipment:

© Springer Nature Switzerland AG 2020
J. Kim, J. Garcia-Aguilar (eds.), *Minimally Invasive Surgical Techniques for Cancers of the Gastrointestinal Tract*, https://doi.org/10.1007/978-3-030-18740-8_20

- The Pink Pad® Advanced Trendelenburg Positioning System
- Bean bag positioners
- Lithotomy stirrups
- Split-leg operating table

Abdominal Insufflation

Numerous methods for accessing the peritoneal cavity for laparoscopic surgery have been described. We prefer to perform Veress needle insertion. This technique is safe and allows for easy placement of ports away from the umbilicus.

Mobilization

Certain equipment is necessary to safely perform laparoscopic colon mobilization. Regarding visualization, an angled laparoscope, typically 30 ° lens, is sufficient. Either a 5 mm or 10 mm lens is adequate. If visualization is poor with the 5 mm lens, it is advisable to change to a 10 mm lens. Often, laparoscopic energy devices and staplers are costly, but they remain necessary to ensure safe mobilization. Vessels can often be coagulated and transected with energy devices alone, although we prefer to apply clips prior to division. Some surgeons may prefer to staple named vessels, but this comes with increased costs compared with clips.

- High-definition angled laparoscope
- Laparoscopic energy device capable of sealing vessels (e.g., inferior mesenteric vein (IMV) and inferior mesenteric artery (IMA))
- Monopolar cautery hook
- Atraumatic graspers
- Laparoscopic scissors
- Laparoscopic suction-irrigator
- Laparoscopic clip appliers
- Laparoscopic linear staplers

Specimen Extraction

If transabdominal extraction is planned, specimen extraction is best performed through a Pfannenstiel incision given the decreased risk of hernia and improved cosmesis [2]. A wound protector should be used for specimen extraction to decrease postoperative wound complications [3].

Anastomosis

We prefer to perform the colorectal anastomosis using a transanal circular stapler. We also inspect every anastomosis using a flexible endoscope. Flexible endoscopy, as opposed to rigid proctoscopy, offers superior visualization of the anastomosis. The improved visualization allows for assessment of tissue perfusion on each side of the staple line [4], control of staple line bleeding with endoscopic clips, and identification of anastomotic disruptions.

- Transanal circular stapler for colorectal anastomosis
- Flexible endoscope

Operative Setup

Positioning

Laparoscopic left colectomy requires the patient be positioned to allow for colon mobilization both in the pelvis and upper abdomen. Patient factors such as splenic flexure position, intra-abdominal fat distribution, and prior scarring can greatly influence the ease of left colon mobilization. Importantly, mobilization is greatly aided by proper operating room table positioning during the case.

For the majority of the cases, the left side of the operating room table will be elevated to allow the small bowel to fall away from the surgical field. Both steep Trendelenburg and reverse Trendelenburg positioning are employed during pelvic and splenic flexure mobilization, respectively. Access to the rectum for transanal staplers and endoscopes require either lithotomy positioning or split-leg operating table, depending on surgeon preference and equipment access. As described above, it is imperative to have a patient positioning system that will secure the patient to the operating table to avoid patient sliding or movement. Communication with the anesthesia and nursing teams during positioning will help ensure that the patient is safely moved during the case.

Abdominal Access and Port Placement

We prefer using a Veress needle insufflation technique. The Veress needle is inserted at Palmer's point in the left upper quadrant, and the abdomen is insufflated. After gaining pneumoperitoneum the camera and working ports are placed (Fig. 20.1). The camera port is placed halfway between the xiphoid process and pubic tubercle. In the majority of cases, this position coincides with the umbilicus; if it does not, it is important not to sacrifice camera position for cosmesis. Visualization is critical to performing safe and efficient laparoscopic surgery; therefore, placing the camera port away from the umbilicus to optimize field of view supersedes cosmetic benefits. The next port is a 12-mm right lower quadrant working port that is placed approximately 8 cm from the camera port on a line connecting the camera port and the anterior superior iliac spine. This port coincides with the surgeon's right hand and the laparoscopic stapler, clip applier, energy device, and needles for suturing will be passed through this port. The remainder of the ports will be 5-mm ports. The surgeon's left hand port is placed a minimum of one handbreadth above the 12-mm port in the midclavicular line. The assistant 5-mm port is placed in the midline below the xiphoid. For the majority of the cases, the surgeon will stand below the assistant utilizing the right lower quadrant 5-mm and 12-mm ports, while the assistant will control the camera with the right hand and assist through the midline 5-mm port with the left hand (Fig. 20.2). Occasionally, when dividing the gastrocolic ligament and working toward the splenic flexure, the surgeon and assistant may switch positions, and the surgeon will work through both 5-mm ports.

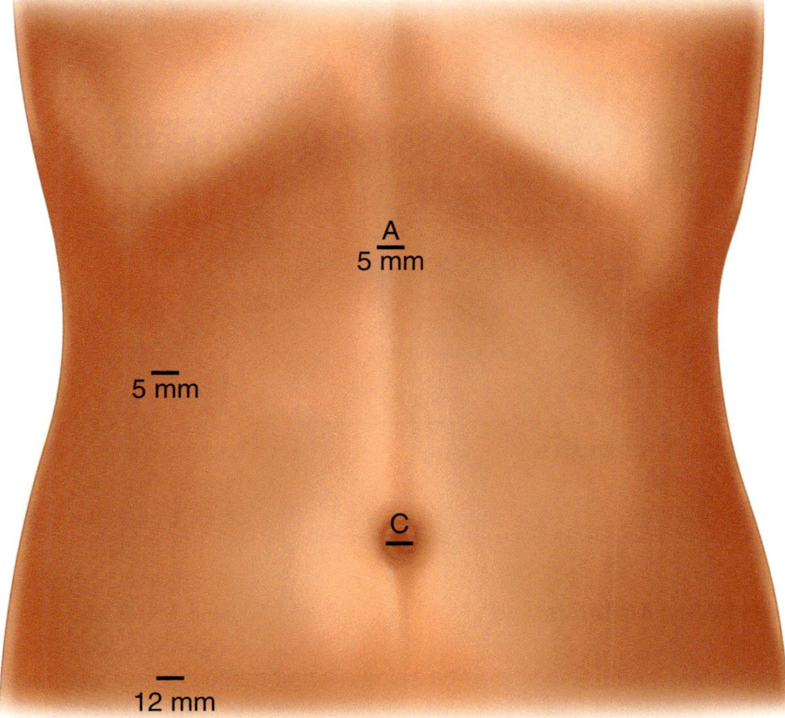

Fig. 20.1 Trocar/port placement for laparoscopic left colectomy. The camera port is placed midway between the xiphoid and pubic symphysis. The 12-mm working port is placed in the right lower quadrant on a line connecting the camera and the anterior superior iliac spine. A 5-mm port is placed in the midclavicular line in the left upper quadrant and a 5-mm port is placed below the xiphoid

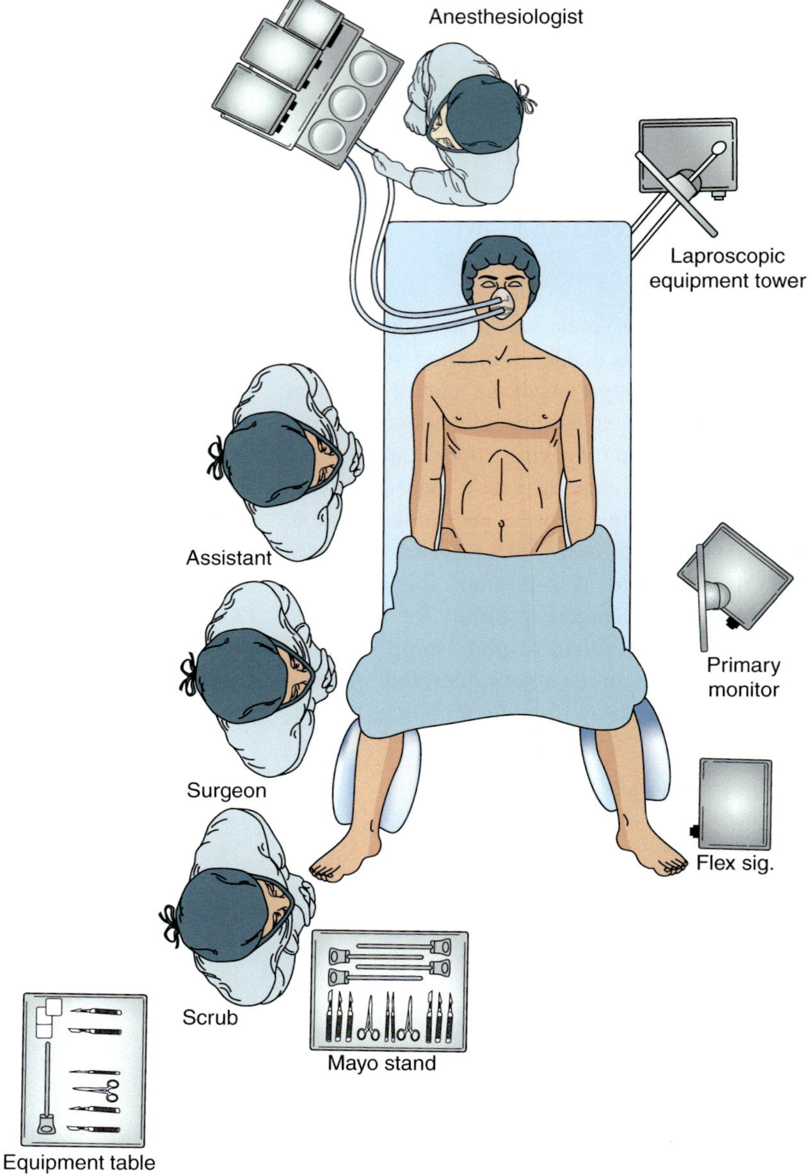

Fig. 20.2 Patient positioning and operating room setup for laparoscopic left colectomy. The patient is placed in lithotomy position with both arms tucked. The surgeon and assistant operate from the patient's right side. The laparoscopic monitor should be placed at eye level directly across from the operative field

Surgical Technique

Video 20.1

Left Colon Mobilization

The authors prefer a medial-to-lateral dissection for the majority of cases. In certain re-operative cases where the medial-to-lateral plane has already been violated, the surgeon may approach mobilization through a variety of directions. The medial-to-lateral dissection allows for early identification of critical landmarks, including the pancreas, lesser sac, ureters and gonadal vessels, and Gerota's fascia. This dissection approach also allows early identification and ligation of vascular pedicles [5]. Also, as the colon remains tethered on the abdominal sidewall at the white line of Toldt until the completion of the dissection, the medial-to-lateral approach facilitates a totally laparoscopic dissection without the need for frequent repositioning of the patient.

The medial-to-lateral dissection begins with division of the fusion plane between the left colon mesentery and the left retroperitoneum. This fusion plane forms during the 12th week of development after the colon has completed its 270 ° counter-clockwise rotation [6]. The dissection can begin either above or below the level of the inferior mesenteric artery (IMA). The authors prefer to begin the dissection above the level of the IMA at the inferior mesenteric vein (IMV). The plane between the left colon mesentery and the retroperitoneum is relatively flat in this location and facilitates both its identification and

separation. The dissection is begun by incising the peritoneum just below the IMV, which is found adjacent to the ligament of Treitz (Figs. 20.3 and 20.4). Once the peritoneum is incised, the plane is developed using blunt dissection (Fig. 20.5). In the correct fusion plane, this blunt dissection will not result in bleeding, and if bleeding is encountered, then that may likely signify that the wrong plane has been dissected and that the surgeon may need to readjust. As the dissection progresses, the IMV is clipped and divided which allows for complete mobilization of the splenic flexure. During these steps, the gonadal vein and occasionally the ureter can often be visualized at this level (Fig. 20.6).

Next, the attachments of the splenic flexure are released in a medial-to-lateral fashion as well. The mesocolic envelope is incised just above the

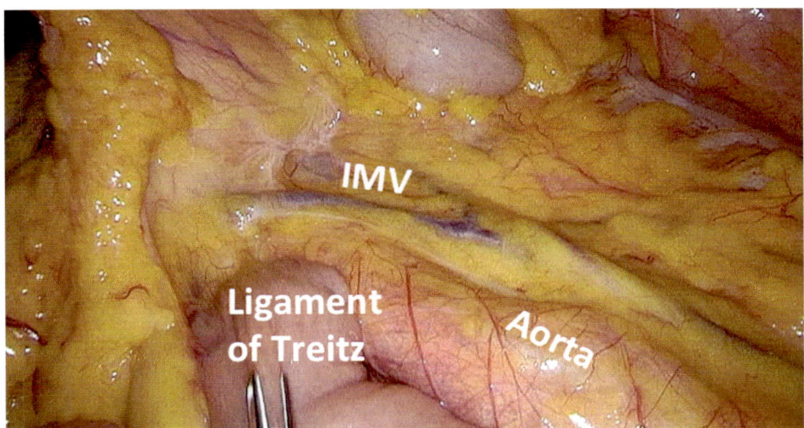

Fig. 20.3 Intraoperative images depict dissection beginning at the level of the inferior mesenteric vein (IMV), which is located adjacent to the ligament of Treitz

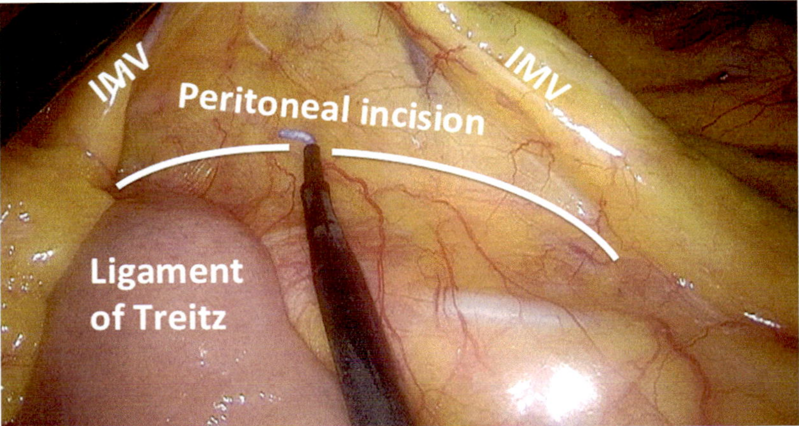

Fig. 20.4 Intraoperative image shows how the IMV is grasped and elevated and the peritoneum below is incised with electrocautery, separating the mesocolon from the retroperitoneum

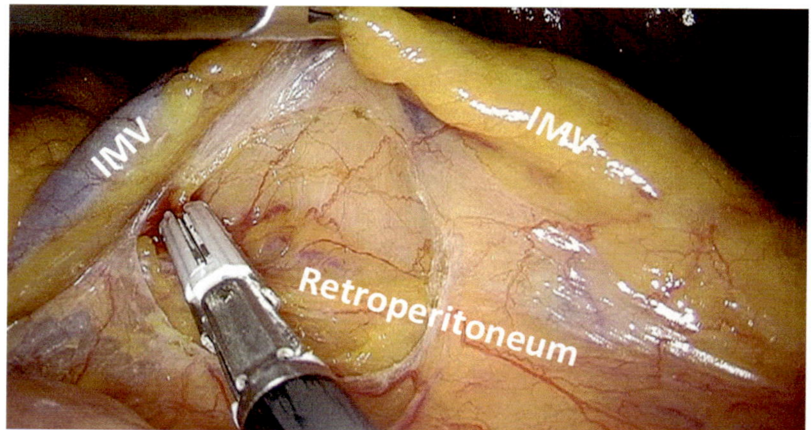

Fig. 20.5 Intraoperative image demonstrates the progression of medial-to-lateral dissection with blunt dissection of the fusion plane between the left colon mesentery and retroperitoneum

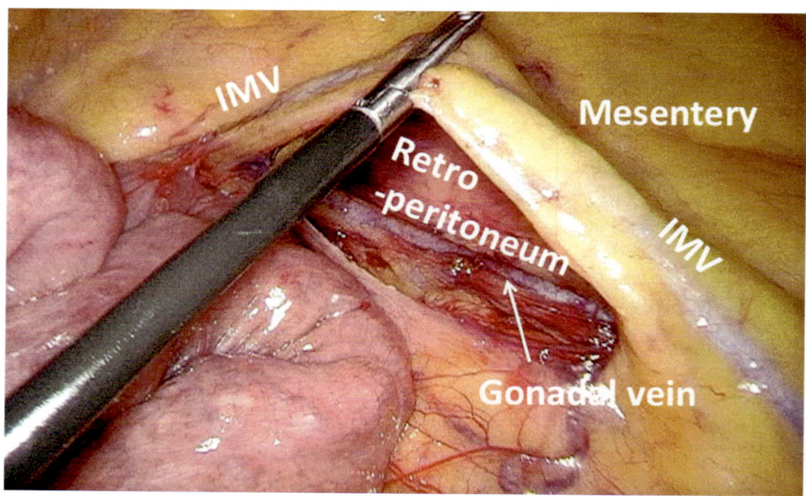

Fig. 20.6 Intraoperative image shows when the gonadal vein can be visualized during medial-to-lateral dissection

anterior surface of the pancreas and the lesser sac is entered (Fig. 20.7). It is critical to stay over the anterior surface of the pancreas. It is easy to dissect underneath the pancreas, which will lead directly to the splenic vein. Once the mesocolon is dissected off the pancreas, the inferior attachments of the mesocolon to the spleen and retroperitoneum are easily identified and divided with the energy device. The inferior splenic flexure mobilization is complete once the inferior pole of the spleen and posterior stomach are visualized and free from their attachments to the colon and mesentery.

The dissection is next moved below the level of the IMA. Again the peritoneum is incised at its base, and the mesocolon is dissected free from the retroperitoneum. Adequate elevation of the sigmoid colon by the assistant will help ensure the base of the mesentery is incised and the correct plane is entered. At this level the ureter and gonadal vessels must be identified and preserved. This dissection continues laterally to the abdominal sidewall and cephalad to join the previous dissection plane. Once this is complete, the IMA is isolated (Fig. 20.8). The IMA bifurcates into the left colic and superior hemorrhoidal arteries forming a characteristic "T"-shape configuration, which aids in its identification (Fig. 20.8). Once identified, the IMA is clipped and divided. Following division of the IMA, the white line of

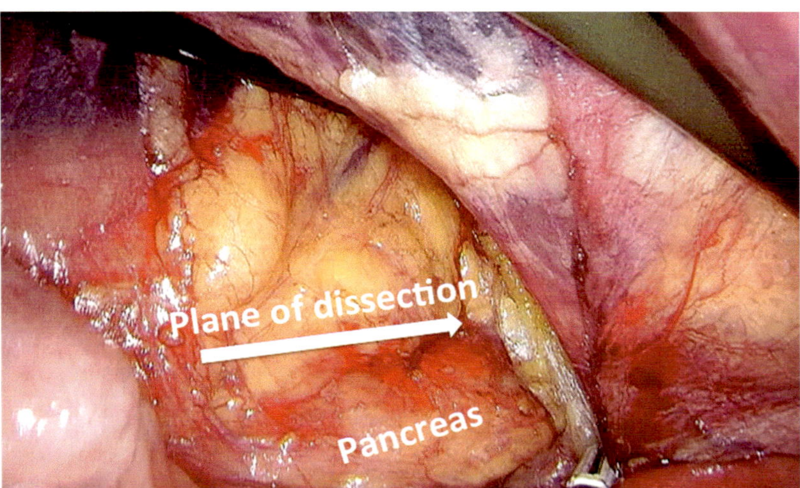

Fig. 20.7 Intraoperative images show the mobilization of the splenic flexure from beneath the left colon mesentery. The plane between the colon mesentery and pancreas is incised, and the dissection progresses over the pancreas and into the lesser sac

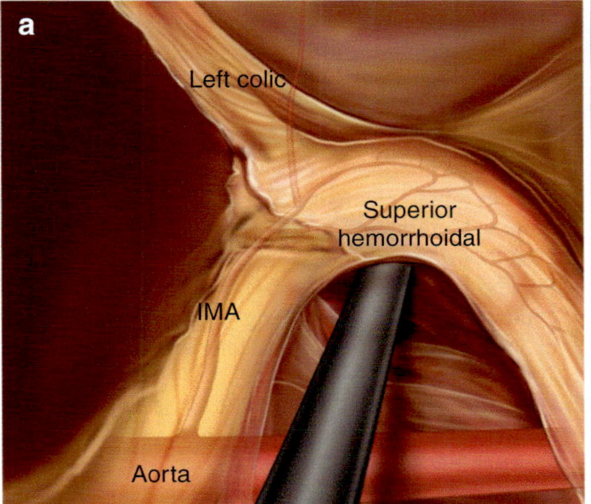

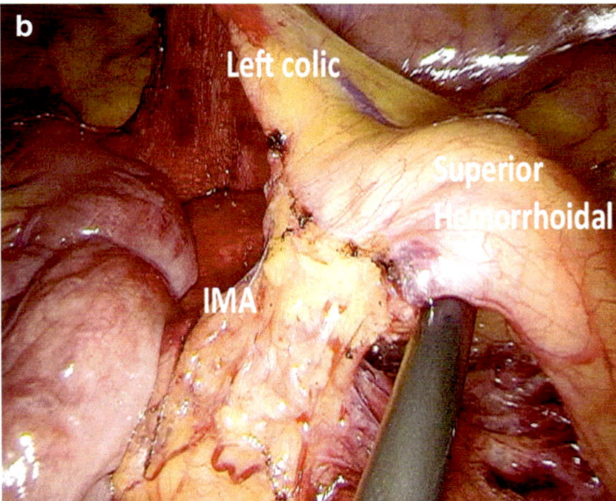

Fig. 20.8 (**a**) Illustration showing the branching of the inferior mesenteric artery (IMA) to its left colic and superior hemorrhoidal arteries. (**b**) Paired intraoperative image showing isolation of the IMA and the characteristic "T" configuration with the IMA branching into the left colic and superior hemorrhoidal arteries

Toldt is incised to release the colon from the abdominal wall. Also, the omentum is separated from the distal transverse colon to facilitate mobility.

Colon Resection and Reconstruction

Once the left colon has been fully mobilized, the next steps are division of the colon and its mesentery, specimen extraction, and reconstruction. Depending on whether the operation is performed for benign or malignant pathology, the sites of transection may vary. Once an appropriate location for transection has been selected, we proceed with intracorporeal mesocolic division at the distal resection margin. The mesocolon is grasped in the surgeon's left hand while the assistant holds the colon out toward the abdominal wall. The mesocolon is then divided with care to avoid harming the mesentery of the remaining colon. Once the wall of the colon is reached, the energy device is exchanged for a laparoscopic stapler and the colon is divided.

Next the surgeon must decide if they will perform a transabdominal extraction through a Pfannenstiel incision. In certain cases with concomitant hysterectomy or diverting ileostomy, an extraction can be performed through the vagina or stoma. In those circumstances, we perform intracorporeal division of the proximal margin. If a Pfannenstiel extraction site is selected, it is simple to extract the colon and perform extracorporeal division of the proximal margin. In this scenario, the colon is divided with electrocautery and the mesentery is divided with the energy device. A 28-mm anvil from the transanal circular stapler is inserted into the proximal colon and secured with a purse-string suture, typically a 2-0 monofilament suture. Alternatively, a side-to-end anastomosis can be performed, where the spike of the anvil is brought out the antimesenteric side of the colon and the end of the colon is stapled closed.

Once the anvil is in place and hemostasis is achieved, the colon is returned to the abdomen. The transanal stapler is then inserted and the spike deployed through the staple line of the distal margin on the rectum. The two ends are connected laparoscopically. When connecting the anvil with the stapler, it is important to move the colon with the left-handed grasper and to avoid pulling on the anvil with the right, since that may cause injury to the site of anastomosis or disrupt the purse-string. Once connected, the stapler is then closed and deployed. Care should be taken to ensure the mesentery is not twisted prior to firing the stapler. Once the anastomosis is created, it is tested by submerging it under water while insufflating with a flexible endoscope. Also, the anastomosis is inspected to ensure that viable tissue is present on both proximal and distal edges of the staple line and that there is no anastomotic hemorrhage. If brisk staple line bleeding is encountered, it can be addressed with endoscopic clips.

Conclusion

Laparoscopic left colectomy is a technically challenging operation that when it is mastered will provide the surgeon's patients with numerous advantages including shorter recovery time, decreased wound complications, and improved cosmesis. It is now a standard of care for both benign and malignant pathology [7, 8].

References

1. Fox J, Gross CP, Longo W, Reddy V. Laparoscopic colectomy for the treatment of cancer has been widely adopted in the United States. Dis Colon Rectum. 2012;55(5):501–8.
2. Shapiro R, Keler U, Segev L, et al. Laparoscopic right hemicolectomy with intracorporeal anastomosis: short- and long-term benefits in comparison with extracorporeal anastomosis. Surg Endosc. 2016;30(9):3823–9.
3. Reid K, Pockney P, Draganic B, Smith SR. Barrier wound protection decreases surgical site infection in open elective colorectal surgery: a randomized clinical trial. Dis Colon Rectum. 2010;53(10):1374–80.
4. Sujatha-Bhaskar S, Jafari MD, Hanna M, et al. An endoscopic mucosal grading system is predictive of leak in stapled rectal anastomoses. Surg Endosc. 2018;32(4):1769–75.
5. Pigazzi A, Hellan M, Ewing DR, et al. Laparoscopic medial-to-lateral colon dissection: how and why. J Gastrointest Surg. 2007;11(6):778–82.
6. Carmichael J, Mills S. Anatomy and embryology of the colon, rectum, and anus. In: Steele SR, Hull TL, Read TE, Saclarides TJ, Senagore AJ, Whitlow CB, editors. The ASCRS textbook of Colon and Rectal surgery. 3rd ed. Cham: Springer International Publishing; 2016. p. 3–26.
7. Nelson H, Sargent DJ, Wieand HS, et al. A comparison of laparoscopically assisted and open colectomy for colon cancer. N Engl J Med. 2004;350(20):2050–9.
8. Stulberg JJ, Champagne BJ, Fan Z, et al. Emergency laparoscopic colectomy: does it measure up to open? Am J Surg. 2009;197(3):296–301.

Felipe Quezada-Diaz and Emmanouil P. Pappou

Introduction

New robotic technologies are helping surgeons to overcome the limits of conventional laparoscopic surgery. Robotic colorectal surgery has been proven to be safe and provide favorable results in comparison to conventional laparoscopic techniques [1].

The concept of complete mesocolic excision with central vascular ligation for colon cancer surgery has been advocated during the past years. This technique aims to resect the entire mesocolon with central ligation of the vessels at their origin, providing a specimen with adequate margins, an intact envelope of the mesocolic fascia, and optimal lymphovascular clearance [2]. Robotic platforms may provide a suitable minimally invasive approach for a complete mesocolic excision in colon surgery due to its enhanced visualization and precise movements.

In the present chapter, we describe the operative technique for the da Vinci® Xi™ robot using a dual console, which enables an integrated teaching and supervising environment without compromising operative or patient outcomes (Video 21.1).

Indications for Robotic Left Colectomy

Left colectomy is commonly indicated for colon adenocarcinomas, as well as colonic polyps that are not amenable to endoscopic resection. A "true" left hemicolectomy is the operation of choice for tumors located in the segment of the colon between the left colic vessels and the first sigmoidal branches and involves removing the entire left colon along with the origin of the inferior mesenteric artery and its dependent lymphatic territory. Tumors in this location may also be treated with a segmental resection, requiring only the division of the left branch of the middle colic and the left colic vessels with preservation of the root of IMA and main sigmoidal vessels, without compromising oncological outcomes [3].

Multiple reports have demonstrated that robotic left colectomy is technically feasible and safe. A list of most recent retrospective studies comparing the efficacy of robotic with laparoscopic left colectomy is summarized in Table 21.1. Overall robotic left colectomy may be associated with longer operative times but shorter length of hospital stay [4–6].

Electronic supplementary material The online version of this chapter (https://doi.org/10.1007/978-3-030-18740-8_21) contains supplementary material, which is available to authorized users.

F. Quezada-Diaz
Department of Surgery Colorectal Service,
Memorial Sloan Kettering Cancer Center,
New York, NY, USA

E. P. Pappou (✉)
Department of Surgery, Memorial Sloan Kettering Cancer Center, New York, NY, USA
e-mail: pappoue@mskcc.org

Table 21.1 Summary of selected studies comparing robotic-assisted to laparoscopic left colectomy[a]

Author (Year)	Group	Patients	OR time, mean (SD), min	EBL, mean (SD), ml	Conversions, (rate, %)	Retrieved LN, mean (SD)	Complications, (rate, %)	LOS, mean (SD), d
Shin [20]	RLH	7	337 (138)	106 (80)	0	16.9 (6.6)	NS	9.1 (1.7)
	LLH	12	265 (71)	167 (62)	0	16.2 (4.7)	NS	8.9 (2.1)
Casillas et al. [4]	RLH	68	**188 (NR)**	89 (NR)	4 (5.8%)	20 (NR)	8 (11.7%)	**3.6 (NR)**
	LLH	82	**109 (NR)**	110 (NR)	9 (10.9)	17 (NR)	17 (20.7%)	**6.5 (NR)**
Miller et al. [5]	RLH	336	**254 (NR)**	NR	34 (10.1%)	NR	NR	**5.11**
	LLH	3120	**427 (NR)**	NR	427 (13.7)	NR	NR	**5.66**
Dolejs et al. [6]	RLH	418	**202.5 (106)**	NR	7.2%	NR	15.6%	**4 (2)**
	LLH	11,782	**153 (87)**	NR	8.8%	NR	19%	**4 (2)**

Items in bold are statistically significant, $p < 0.05$

OR operating room, *EBL* estimated blood loss, *LN* lymph nodes, *LOS* length of stay, *RLH* robotic left hemicolectomy, *LLH* laparoscopic left hemicolectomy, *NS* nonsignificant, *NR* not recorded

[a]Includes resections from distal transverse to sigmoid colon

Preoperative Planning

An enhanced-recovery-after-surgery protocol should be considered as standard of care postoperatively for patients undergoing a left colectomy.

In patients undergoing robotic left colectomy, we suggest the use of a mechanical bowel preparation combined with oral antibiotics because of decreased incidence of surgical site infections and anastomotic leaks [7, 8]. Thromboembolic prophylaxis and intravenous antibiotics are administered prior to surgical incision.

Operative Technique

Anatomical Considerations

Robotic left hemicolectomy requires good knowledge of the relationship of the mesentery and vascular supply of the left colon to the retroperitoneal structures. The left colon receives its blood supply from both the superior mesenteric artery (SMA) through the left branch of the middle colic artery, as well as the inferior mesenteric artery (IMA) through the left colic artery and sigmoidal branches. The inferior mesenteric vein (IMV) is formed from the union of the superior rectal veins and usually drains into the splenic vein behind the pancreas [9].

Important anatomical variations have been described for the IMA and IMV. A study using CT angiography determined that in only 45% of the patients, the left colic artery and sigmoid artery had a common trunk, whereas the left colic artery did not exist in 5% of cases. The left colic artery was located lateral to the IMV in 73% of the cases [10].

The mesentery of the left colon overlies the iliac vessels, the left ureter, the left gonadal vessels, Gerota's fascia covering the left kidney, and the distal pancreas, important structures that need to be identified and preserved during dissection. The mesentery of the left side of the transverse colon is attached to the inferior border of the pancreas. The splenic flexure of the colon is anatomically related to the lower pole of the spleen and is anchored by the splenocolic ligament.

The route of lymphatic drainage of the left colon largely mirrors that of the arterial circulation. Recent anatomical studies have showed the presence of vascular and lymphatic connections at the level of the splenic flexure between structures of the foregut (pancreas and gastrocolic ligament) and the transverse colon [11]. This path could explain the lymphatic tumor spread within the greater omentum and along the gastroepiploic vessels in transverse and left colon cancers described in some series [12, 13].

A thorough understanding the collateral circulation between SMA and IMA is of paramount importance when performing a left colectomy, as there is significant variability [9]. A recent anatomical study showed an updated description of the three most important collateral networks: the marginal artery, also known as the artery of

Drummond, which is the major collateral arcade between the SMA and IMA and runs within the mesentery of the colon and lies about 2–3 cm from the mesenteric border of the bowel; the central or Riolan's arch (18% of cases present), joining the middle colic artery with the left colic artery; and lastly the meandering mesenteric artery of Moskowitz (11% of cases present) that runs through the base of the mesocolon just above the ventral edge of the pancreas and connects the middle colic artery's proximal segment with the ascending branch of the left colic artery [14]. During medial to lateral IMV dissection, inadvertent injury of the Arc of Riolan or the meandering mesenteric artery around the IMV may result in compromised blood supply to the descending colon used for anastomosis. Preservation of these additional collateral networks can be critical in order to preserve the vascular supply of the colon conduit, as the marginal artery of Drummond may be interrupted in as many as 5–7% of individuals in the watershed area of the splenic flexure [9].

Operating Room Configuration and Patient Positioning

Robotic left colectomy is performed with a single-docking technique, with the robotic cart docked over left side of the patient (Fig. 21.1). The patient is placed in modified lithotomy position with both arms tacked and secured. A foam mattress directly under the patient and a foam pad over the patient's chest are used to prevent sliding during the operation. Pressure points are protected and a urinary catheter is placed under sterile technique. An orogastric tube is placed after induction and is removed at the end of the operation. A body warmer is used to prevent hypothermia.

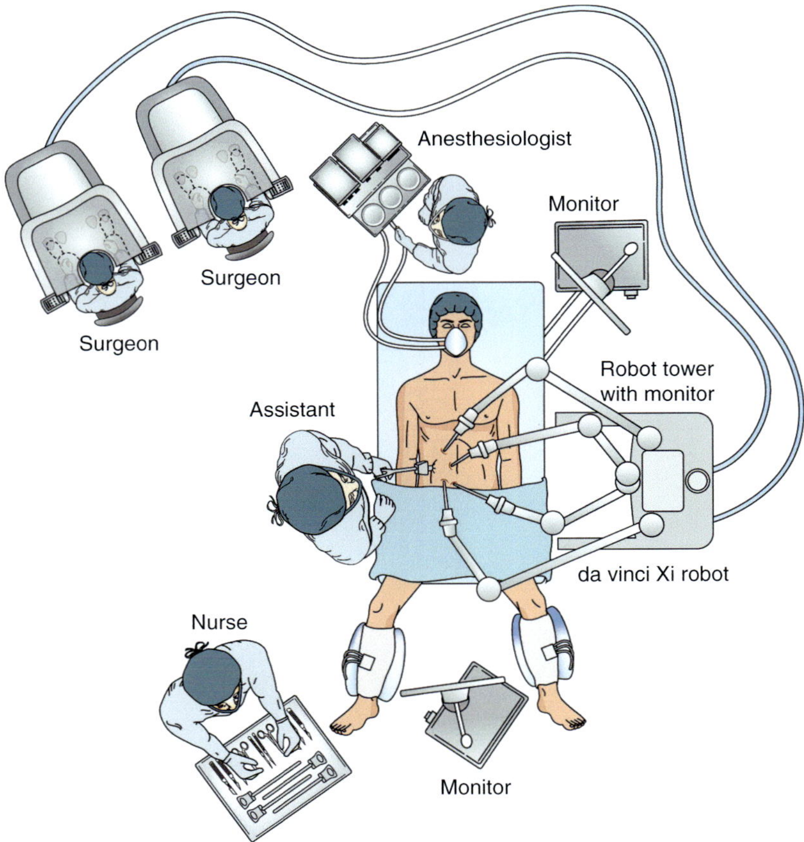

Fig. 21.1 Operating room setup for left robotic colectomy at our institution

Trocar Positioning

Pneumoperitoneum is induced with a Veress needle in the left upper quadrant (Palmer's point). Three 8-mm ports for the robot, one 12-mm robotic stapler port, and a 5-mm port for the assistant are inserted under direct visualization as shown in Fig. 21.2. The two 8-mm robotic working ports are placed at the level of the midclavicular line, and the camera port can be placed either supraumbilically at the midline or a fingerbreadth above and to the left of the umbilicus (our preferred approach). The 12-mm stapler port is placed in suprapubic position at the level of the Pfannenstiel incision used as the specimen extraction site. The patient is placed in Trendelenburg position (usually 12 degrees) and tilted right side down (usually also 12 °). Use of integrated table motion is highly recommended, as this allows to reposition the operating table in real time with the surgical robotic arms docked. A cautery hook or vessel sealer is usually used in the right working hand, a fenestrated bipolar forceps is used in the left working hand, and a ProGrasp™ or Cadiere forceps can be used via the supraumbilical port for retraction.

Surgical Field

At the start of the procedure, the abdominal cavity is examined using the robotic camera. The surface of the liver, peritoneum, and small bowel is assessed, and evidence of metastatic disease is ruled out. Next, the greater omentum is retracted cephalad, over and above the transverse colon, and the small bowel is retracted medially and on the right side of the abdominal cavity, exposing the left colon mesentery.

IMV Dissection

The surgery starts with the identification of the IMV at the level of the ligament of Treitz, which is divided. An alternative approach is to enter the mesentery of the left colon lateral to the IMV

Fig. 21.2 Trocar positioning for left robotic colectomy

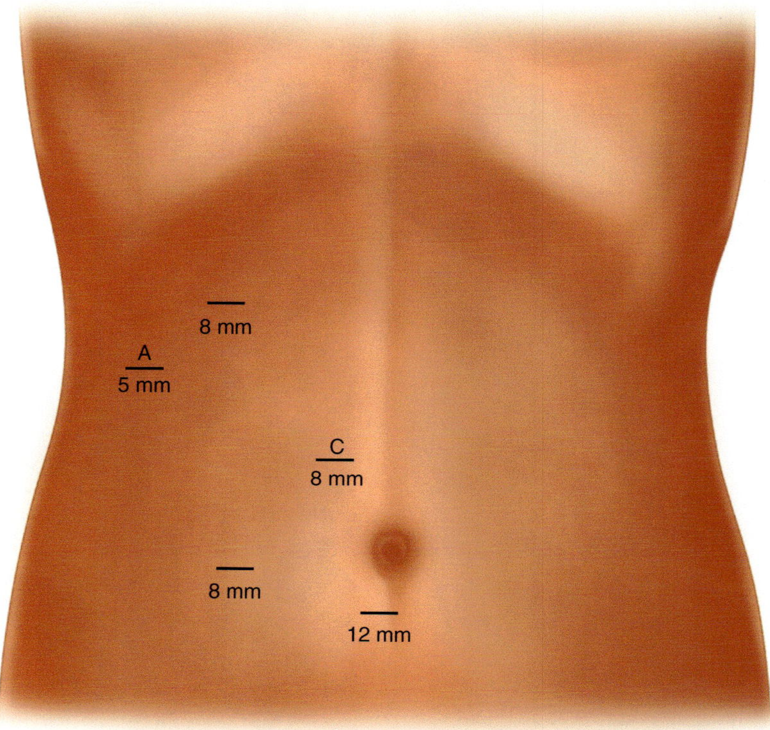

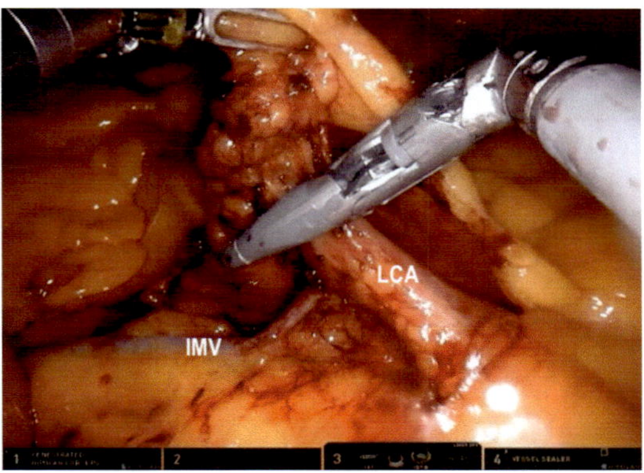

Fig. 21.3 After mobilization of small bowel, the inferior mesenteric artery is identified and the mesocolon is opened right above it. *IMV* inferior mesenteric vein

Fig. 21.4 The left colic artery is divided before it crosses the inferior mesenteric vein. *LCA* left colic artery, *IMV* inferior mesenteric vein

(Fig. 21.3), preserving the IMV for adequate venous drainage of the sigmoid colon and rectum as is the case shown in the video attached to this chapter. This IMV-first approach allows for easy and immediate identification of Toldt's fascia between the left mesocolon and retroperitoneum and allows for efficient medial to lateral dissection, as the IMV is anatomically consistent.

The medial to lateral plane is developed along the inferior border of the pancreas and Gerota's fascia in the direction of the splenic flexure. The attachments of the mesentery of the transverse colon to the inferior border of the pancreas are carefully divided, entering the lesser sac in an infra-mesocolic fashion. Next, the peritoneum along the inferior border of the IMV is incised caudally in the direction of the origin of the IMA, as the mesentery of the descending colon is lifted from the retroperitoneal structures.

IMA Dissection

The IMA is identified and dissected close to the aortic bifurcation by extending the peritoneal incision toward the sacral promontory. The mesentery of the sigmoid colon is lifted, and the space behind the superior rectal vessels is entered, exposing the left ureter, gonadal vessels, and the hypogastric plexus. The right iliac artery and the

intersigmoid fossa are landmarks commonly used during this part of the dissection [15]. The superior rectal artery is traced to the IMA. The IMA is isolated and ligated proximal to its bifurcation staying away from the aorta, in order to prevent injury to the hypogastric plexus. Large (purple color) robotic clips may be used to ligate the IMA as well. Alternatively, the main sigmoidal artery can be preserved and the left colic artery divided distal to its takeoff from the IMA (Fig. 21.4).

During robotic left colectomy for cancer, our preference is to also ligate the left branch of the middle colic vessels, which is identified at the root of the small bowel mesentery and divided at the base of the transverse mesocolon.

Splenic Flexure Mobilization

Exposure of the pancreas during IMV dissection is necessary for correct entry into the lesser sac. Dissection is carried out in a medial to lateral fashion until the splenic hilum is reached (Fig. 21.5).

The lateral attachments of the left colon are divided over Gerota's fascia for proper mobilization of the splenic flexure.

To complete splenic flexure mobilization, the omentum is released from the transverse colon beginning at the level marked by the falciform

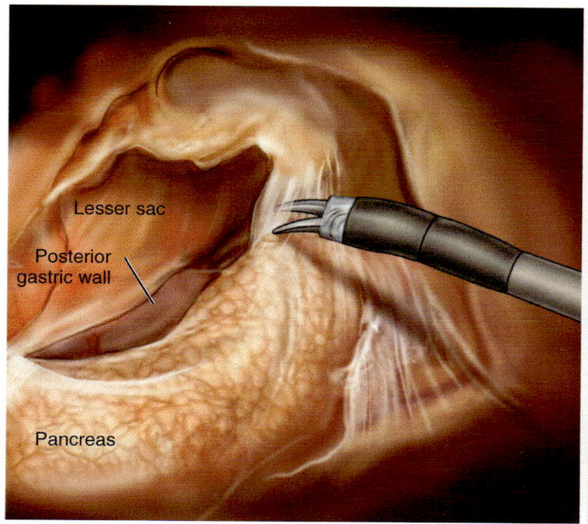

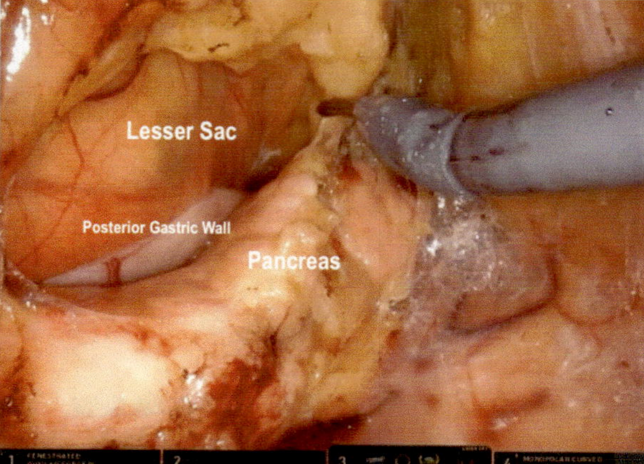

Fig. 21.5 Illustration demonstrating medial to lateral dissection over the tail of the pancreas towards the splenic hilum and paired operative image showing that after after entering the lesser sac, dissection is carried out over the surface of the tail of the pancreas in the direction of the splenic hilum

ligament, and the lesser sac is entered broadly in a supramesocolic fashion. The gastrocolic ligament is divided, and the distal transverse colon and splenic flexure are fully released to reach the pelvis. During the dissection near the splenic hilum, care must be taken to avoid injury to the short gastric vessels. En bloc resection of the colon with the left portion of the omentum can also be performed; this maneuver requires ligation of the left gastroepiploic vessels along the major curvature of the stomach.

Intracorporeal Anastomosis

The mesentery of the colon to be resected is fully divided intracorporeally using the vessel sealer. Indocyanine green can be used to assess perfusion of the remaining colon segments. The bowel wall is then transected proximally and distally using the robotic stapler.

The specimen is then extracted through a 4–5-cm Pfannenstiel incision using a wound protector, and pneumoperitoneum is reestablished in preparation for an intracorporeal anastomosis.

A tension-free, side-to-side isoperistaltic intracorporeal anastomosis is then created, making small enterotomies on the proximal and distal portions of the colon to be anastomosed using the

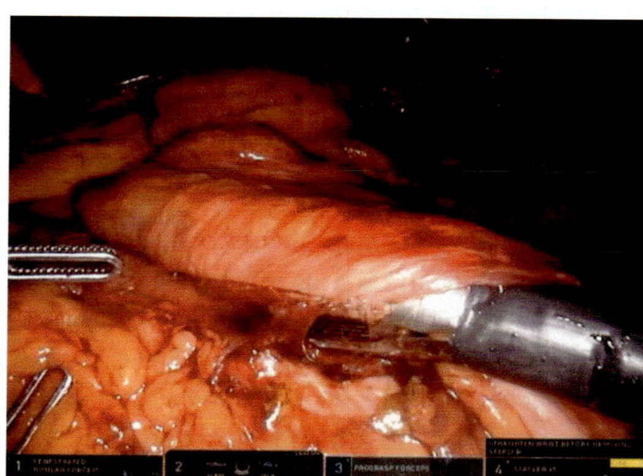

Fig. 21.6 Isoperistaltic side-to-side intracorporeal anastomosis

monopolar curved scissors. Using one or two firings of the blue loaded robotic stapler, the lumen of the anastomosis is created. The common enterotomy defect can be closed with interrupted sutures, or using self-locking sutures. A crotch stitch can be placed, and the anterior staple line can be reinforced in order to prevent tension to the anastomosis (Fig. 21.6).

Once the specimen is removed and the anastomosis completed, hemostasis is confirmed, particularly at the site of the vascular pedicles. The ports are removed under direct vision, and the Pfannenstiel incision is closed. The skin is sutured with subcuticular absorbable sutures.

Postoperative Management and Complications

Most patients undergoing robotic colectomy are managed according to enhanced recovery pathways as was previously stated [16]. Patients ambulate the day of, or the day after, surgery. We highly recommend minimizing postoperative intravenous fluids and advocate for a strictly limited use of narcotics in order to reduce postoperative ileus [17]. Patients are started on a full liquid diet on the first postoperative day and are advanced to a regular diet as tolerated. The Foley catheter is also removed on the first postoperative day.

Early reports suggest similar short-term outcomes between laparoscopic and robotic colectomies, but few studies address specifically left colectomies.

The American College of Surgeons National Surgical Quality Improvement Program database was used to compare laparoscopic and robotic approaches in 11,477 patients undergoing colorectal surgery [18]. This study demonstrated that robotic operations were associated with longer operative times, decreased hospital length of stay, and decreased rates of conversion to open.

A systematic review of laparoscopic versus robotic-assisted colectomies studies showed overall less morbidity for robotic surgery but higher associated costs and longer operative times compared to the laparoscopic approach [19]. However, these results could not be confirmed when the analysis was focused only on randomized trials.

Conclusion

Robotic left colectomy is technically safe and feasible. Although the short-term oncological and postoperative outcomes in robotic left colectomy have been reported in numerous studies, future studies assessing long-term oncologic outcomes are needed.

References

1. Pappou EP, Weiser MR. Robotic colonic resection. J Surg Oncol. 2015;112(3):315–20.
2. Bertelsen CA, Neuenschwander AU, Jansen JE, Wilhelmsen M, Kirkegaard-Klitbo A, Tenma JR, et al. Disease-free survival after complete mesocolic excision compared with conventional colon cancer surgery: a retrospective, population-based study. Lancet Oncol. 2015;16(2):161–8.
3. Rouffet F, Hay JM, Vacher B, Fingerhut A, Elhadad A, Flamant Y, et al. Curative resection for left colonic carcinoma: hemicolectomy vs. segmental colectomy. A prospective, controlled, multicenter trial. French Association for Surgical Research. Dis Colon Rectum. 1994;37(7):651–9.
4. Casillas MA, Leichtle SW, Wahl WL, Lampman RM, Welch KB, Wellock T, et al. Improved perioperative and short-term outcomes of robotic versus conventional laparoscopic colorectal operations. Am J Surg. 2014;208(1):33–40.
5. Miller PE, Dao H, Paluvoi N, Bailey M, Margolin D, Shah N, et al. Comparison of 30-day postoperative outcomes after laparoscopic vs robotic colectomy. J Am Coll Surg. 2016;223(2):369–73.
6. Dolejs SC, Waters JA, Ceppa EP, Zarzaur BL. Laparoscopic versus robotic colectomy: a national surgical quality improvement project analysis. Surg Endosc. 2017;31(6):2387–96.
7. Elnahas A, Urbach D, Lebovic G, Mamdani M, Okrainec A, Quereshy FA, et al. The effect of mechanical bowel preparation on anastomotic leaks in elective left-sided colorectal resections. Am J Surg. 2015;210(5):793–8.
8. Midura EF, Jung AD, Hanseman DJ, Dhar V, Shah SA, Rafferty JF, et al. Combination oral and mechanical bowel preparations decreases complications in both right and left colectomy. Surgery. 2018;163(3):528–34.
9. Sakorafas GH, Zouros E, Peros G. Applied vascular anatomy of the colon and rectum: clinical implications for the surgical oncologist. Surg Oncol. 2006;15(4):243–55.
10. Murono K, Kawai K, Kazama S, Ishihara S, Yamaguchi H, Sunami E, et al. Anatomy of the inferior mesenteric artery evaluated using 3-dimensional CT angiography. Dis Colon Rectum. 2015;58(2):214–9.
11. Stelzner S, Hohenberger W, Weber K, West NP, Witzigmann H, Wedel T. Anatomy of the transverse colon revisited with respect to complete mesocolic excision and possible pathways of aberrant lymphatic tumor spread. Int J Color Dis. 2016;31(2):377–84.
12. Perrakis A, Weber K, Merkel S, Matzel K, Agaimy A, Gebbert C, et al. Lymph node metastasis of carcinomas of transverse colon including flexures. Consideration of the extramesocolic lymph node stations. Int J Color Dis. 2014;29(10):1223–9.

13. Bertelsen CA, Bols B, Ingeholm P, Jansen JE, Jepsen LV, Kristensen B, et al. Lymph node metastases in the gastrocolic ligament in patients with colon cancer. Dis Colon Rectum. 2014;57(7):839–45.
14. Garcia-Granero A, Sánchez-Guillén L, Carreño O, Sancho Muriel J, Alvarez Sarrado E, Fletcher Sanfeliu D, et al. Importance of the Moskowitz artery in the laparoscopic medial approach to splenic flexure mobilization: a cadaveric study. Tech Coloproctol. 2017;21(7):567–72.
15. Somé OR, Ndoye JM, Yohann R, Nolan G, Roccia H, Dakoure WP, et al. An anatomical study of the inter-sigmoid fossa and applications for internal hernia surgery. Surg Radiol Anat. 2017;39(3):243–8.
16. Carmichael JC, Keller DS, Baldini G, Bordeianou L, Weiss E, Lee L, et al. Clinical practice guidelines for enhanced recovery after Colon and Rectal surgery from the American Society of Colon and Rectal Surgeons and Society of American Gastrointestinal and Endoscopic Surgeons. Dis Colon Rectum. 2017;60(8):761–84.
17. Lee L, Liberman S, Charlebois P, Stein B, Kaneva P, Carli F, et al. The impact of complications after elective colorectal resection within an enhanced recovery pathway. Tech Coloproctol. 2018;22(3):191–9.
18. Bhama AR, Obias V, Welch KB, Vandewarker JF, Cleary RK. A comparison of laparoscopic and robotic colorectal surgery outcomes using the American College of Surgeons National Surgical Quality Improvement Program (ACS NSQIP) database. Surg Endosc. 2016;30(4):1576–84.
19. Lorenzon L, Bini F, Balducci G, Ferri M, Salvi PF, Marinozzi F. Laparoscopic versus robotic-assisted colectomy and rectal resection: a systematic review and meta-analysis. Int J Color Dis. 2016;31(2):161–73.
20. Shin JY. Comparison of short-term surgical outcomes between a robotic colectomy and a laparoscopic colectomy during early experience. J Korean Soc Coloproctol. 2012;28(1):19–26.

Minimally Invasive Low Anterior Resection

22

Matthew Albert and Marc Dakermandji

Introduction

Laparoscopic low anterior resection (LAR) is a technically challenging operation that has two main components: complete mobilization of the hindgut followed by precise rectal dissection with precise division of the mid or distal rectum. Obtaining a completely intact mesorectal envelope (i.e., total mesorectal excision, TME) is of critical oncologic importance. As such, maintaining the rectal dissection within the proper anatomic planes has direct influence on local recurrence rates. A successful TME involves obtaining a grossly intact mesorectal envelope (grade 3), a negative circumferential resection margin (CRM ≥ 2 mm) and a negative distal resection margin (DRM) while providing sphincter preservation with adequate functional outcomes [1].

High ligation of the inferior mesenteric artery (IMA) should be performed to include routes of primary lymphatic drainage in addition to the contiguous mesorectum. Division of the IMA proximal to the ascending left colic artery as opposed to distal ligation remains an unresolved technical variation with no clear evidence supporting standardization. Surgeons also debate the necessity of routine splenic flexure mobilization, which we believe is required to provide a tension-free low pelvic anastomosis with adequate distal blood supply for surgery of the left colon and rectum [2]. While applying traditional oncologic principles for left-sided colonic cancer surgery, one must consider patient body habitus, disease status, comorbidities, as well as functional outcomes following LAR. The sigmoid colon is commonly a poor conduit, especially when narrowed and thickened with diverticular disease. Furthermore, adequate colonic mobilization to permit reconstruction with a colonic J pouch should be strongly considered and may necessitate more length. This requires complete splenic flexure mobilization to the middle colic trunk with high ligation of the IMA below the takeoff of the left colic artery; and division of the inferior mesenteric vein (IMV) at the base of the pancreas to provide maximal colonic length.

However, critics to this approach often cite routine splenic flexure mobilization as usually unnecessary and potentially detrimental to distal colonic perfusion. In our experience, for the most reproducible and standardized resection, we recommend routine splenic flexure mobilization for all patients via medial-to-lateral approach begin-

Electronic supplementary material The online version of this chapter (https://doi.org/10.1007/978-3-030-18740-8_22) contains supplementary material, which is available to authorized users.

M. Albert (✉) · M. Dakermandji
Department of Colorectal Surgery, Center for Colon & Rectal Surgery, Florida Hospital,
Orlando, FL, USA
e-mail: matthew.albert.md@adventhealth.com;
marc.dakermandji@flhosp.org

J. Kim, J. Garcia-Aguilar (eds.), *Minimally Invasive Surgical Techniques for Cancers of the Gastrointestinal Tract*, https://doi.org/10.1007/978-3-030-18740-8_22

ning at the mesoduodenal ligament. This can be achieved in multiport or reduced-port fashion with safety, efficacy, and reproducibility.

Patient Positioning

Prior to placing the patient on the bed, the controls should be interrogated to confirm proper function. The patient is placed in the modified Lloyd-Davies position using Allen stirrups, preferably on any commercially available nonslip pads. An additional strap is placed across the chest to secure the patient from slipping during steep bed movements. It is critical that the legs are abducted and placed parallel with the torso in order to prevent working collisions while operating through the lower abdominal ports. The arms are padded and tucked, gel rolls or specialized shoulder padding is placed, and a Bair Hugger

(3M, St Paul, MN) or other warming device is utilized. The patient must be placed low enough on the bed to access the anal canal for stapler placement, anticipating some degree of patient migration superiorly.

Port Placement

For laparoscopic low anterior resection, ports are most commonly utilized at the umbilicus, the suprapubic position (for easy extension to a Pfannenstiel incision), the right lower quadrant, and the right upper quadrant (Fig. 22.1a). Port placement in these positions will allow easy access to the apex of the splenic flexure with adequate length while still allowing access to the left lower quadrant for mobilization of the sigmoid colon and subsequently the pelvis. Flexibility with port placement is necessary when the splenic

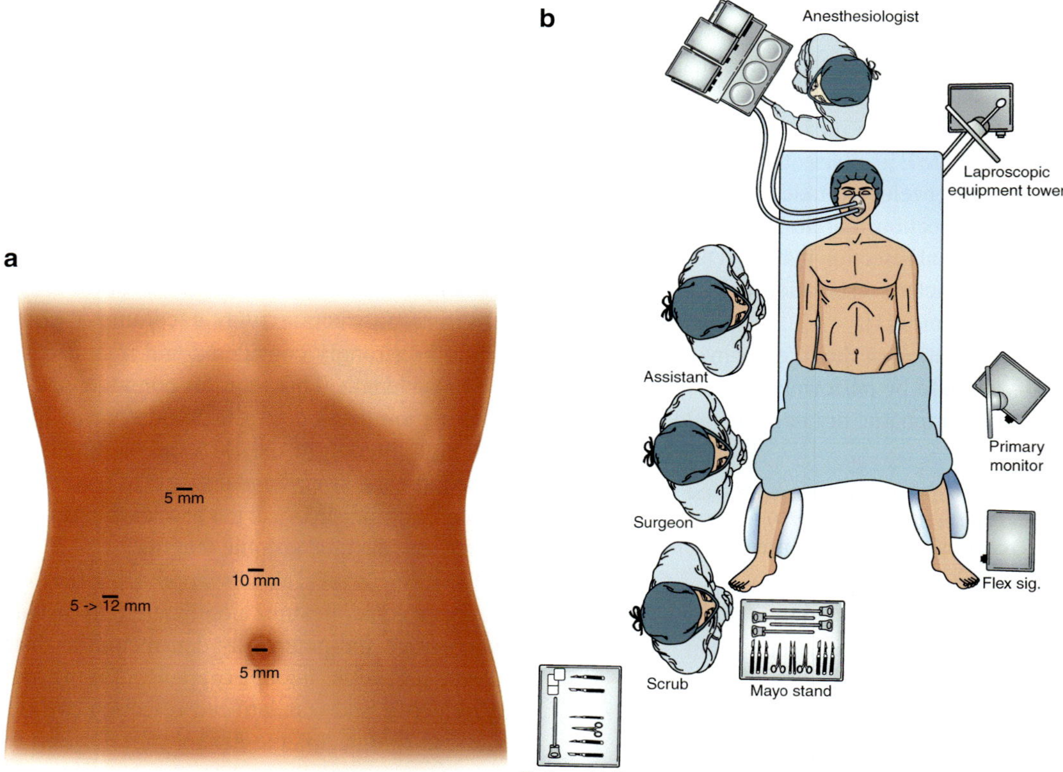

Fig. 22.1 (**a**) Trocar/port positioning for minimally invasive low anterior resection (LAR). (**b**) Patient and surgeon positioning for minimally invasive LAR

flexure is mobilized in preparation for left colon resection accompanied by high or low pelvic anastomosis. As rectal dissection begins, the addition of a left lower quadrant port is helpful for the assistant surgeon.

The benefits of utilizing a Pfannenstiel port placement are multiple, as both stapling of the rectosigmoid colon and specimen extraction can be accomplished at this location. Additionally, cosmesis is optimal here, and postoperative incisional hernia risk is extremely low. Interrogation of the anastomosis through the incision, if there is a positive leak test, is also easily performed with occasional minimal enlargement of the incision. Port placement in the right lower quadrant can be planned accordingly if a diverting stoma is anticipated, especially in patients who receive neoadjuvant chemoradiotherapy. In thin patients, specimen extraction can also be performed through the ileostomy site, and extraction can be facilitated by a wound protector. In our experience, enlarging the fascial opening to facilitate extraction is better to avoid specimen fracture or mesenteric avulsion.

Both the operating surgeon and assistant stand side by side on the right side of the table (Fig. 22.1b). The dissection is carried out by the two surgeons performing tasks from their respective vantage points and alternating between the role of assistant and camera operator. The laparoscopic monitors are positioned opposite the operating surgeon over the left shoulder of the patient and can be easily transferred down toward the left leg as the dissection moves near the pelvis. An angled 30 ° or 45 ° camera is strongly recommended.

Lateral, Medial, Inferior, and Supramesocolic Approaches

As in open colon surgery, early attempts at laparoscopic colonic surgery were generally performed with the lateral-to-medial approach initiated anywhere along the mesosigmoid recess, sigmoid colon, or descending colon. Although it may be the most intuitive approach, the lateral approach is challenging and requires

the surgeon to continuously look over the colon. As such, the splenic flexure can be difficult to take down especially when it is quite cephalad, and critical retroperitoneal structures are not identified until later in the dissection.

In contrast, the medial approach to left colon mobilization begins along the midline at the root of the mesocolic attachments and is traditionally started with a peritoneal incision over the mesosigmoid colon beneath the trunk of the IMA and toward the sacral promontory. In our experience, the left mesocolic origin is more easily targeted at the ligament of Treitz (LOT) just below the IMV, which has been referred to as the inferior or sub IMV approach. Either location allows easy access to the retroperitoneum, early high ligation of the major colonic vascular pedicles, and prompt identification of the left ureter and gonadal vessels while keeping the colon suspended by its lateral attachments. The inferior approach has become increasingly common for the proponents of routine splenic flexure mobilization. Notably, the constancy of the location of the IMV as it courses by the ligament of Treitz enables immediate and clear identification of the initial point of dissection (Fig. 22.2). Division of the IMV at the base of the pancreas permits maximal colonic length. This approach permits division of the base of the transverse mesocolon at its origin along the pancreas, entry into the lesser sac, and division of the splenorenal ligaments posteriorly to assure complete mobilization of the splenic flexure.

In the supramesocolic approach, the dissection begins with entry into the lesser sac adjacent

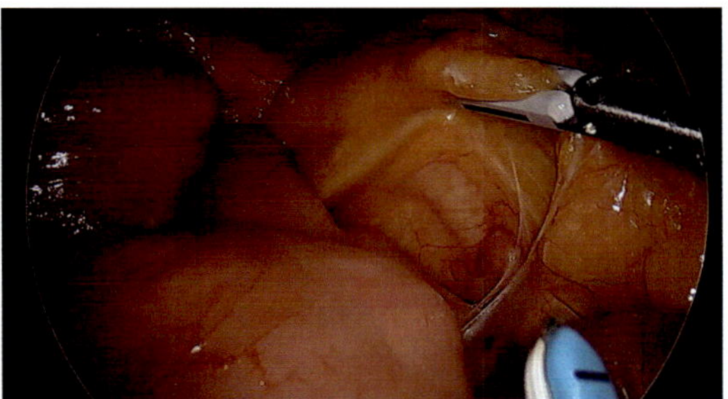

Fig. 22.2 Intraoperative image showing identification of the inferior mesenteric vein near the ligament of Treitz

to the gastroepiploic arcade and exit from the omentum attached to the colon or performing the dissection along the transverse colon wall, which will leave the omentum on the stomach. Dividing the gastrocolic and splenocolic ligaments and joining the lateral and retroperitoneal dissection will release the colon up to the middle colic pedicle. In practice, routine splenic flexure mobilization may utilize all three approaches. Performing splenic flexure mobilization in this stepwise, methodical approach allows adequate oncologic resection and identification of all critical anatomy, thus minimizing the occurrence of complications.

Operative Steps

Medial-to-Lateral Dissection

A video of the entire procedure can be seen in Video 22.1. After establishing pneumoperitoneum through an umbilical 12-mm port, the liver,

small bowel, and colon and rectum are inspected. Adequate bed positioning (right side down and moderate Trendelenburg position) is critical to displace the entire small bowel contents to the right side of the abdomen. With the IMV grasped and placed on tension toward the abdominal wall, a transverse incision is created at the base of the mesentery from just below the IMV following the contour of the left colic artery as it joins the IMA (Fig. 22.3). The correct plane between the mesocolon and retroperitoneum is easily identified, and medial-to-lateral dissection is performed on top of Gerota's and Toldt's fascias up to the inferior edge of the pancreas. It is important to dissect as far lateral as possible under the colon to the abdominal sidewall and underneath the splenic flexure (Fig. 22.4a, b).

Following the dissection superiorly along Toldt's fascia will lead the dissection posteriorly to the pancreas, quickly exposing the splenic vein first and then the splenic artery. At this point, the posterior dissection should cease, and the dissection should proceed on the anterior surface of the

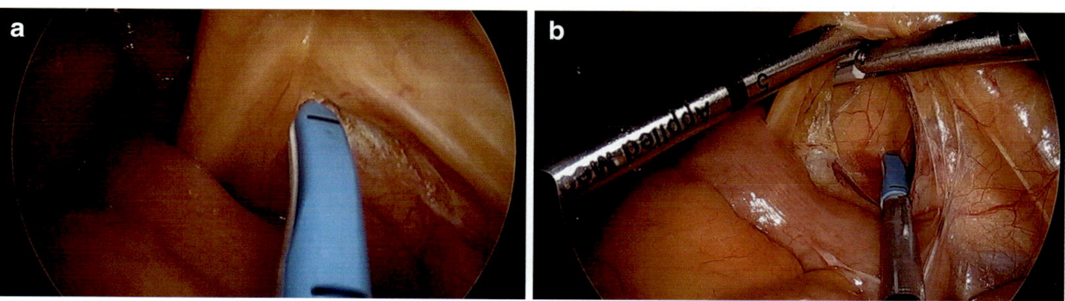

Fig. 22.3 Intraoperative image showing (**a**) incision of the mesentery directly posterior to the inferior mesenteric vein (IMV). (**b**) The space posterior to the IMV is gradually enlarged by blunt dissection with laparoscopic instruments

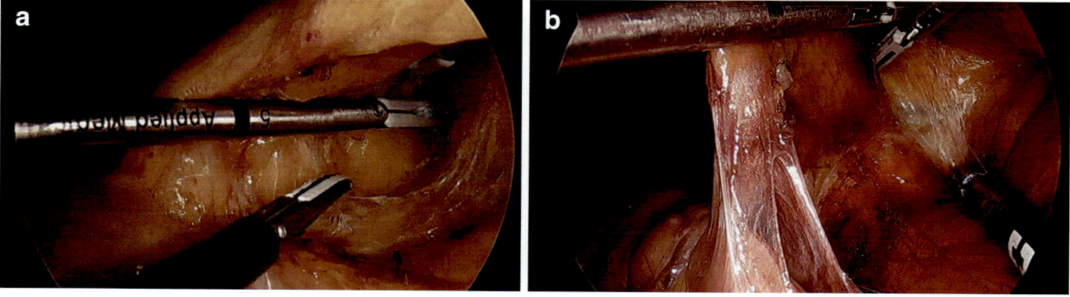

Fig. 22.4 Intraoperative images (**a**, **b**) show the medial-to-lateral dissection as it reaches the lateral abdominal wall

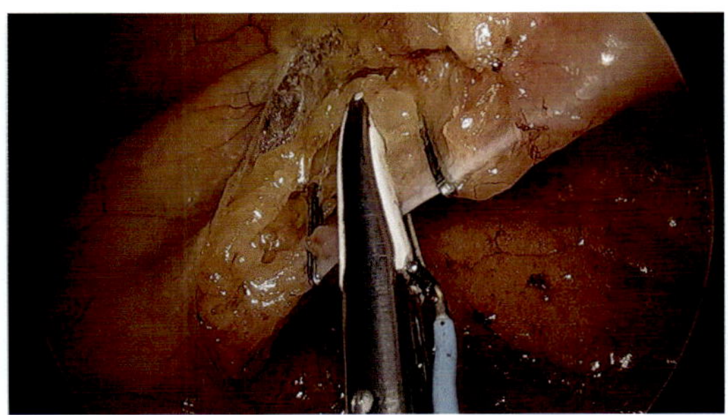

Fig. 22.5 Intraoperative image showing clipping and ligation of the inferior mesenteric vein

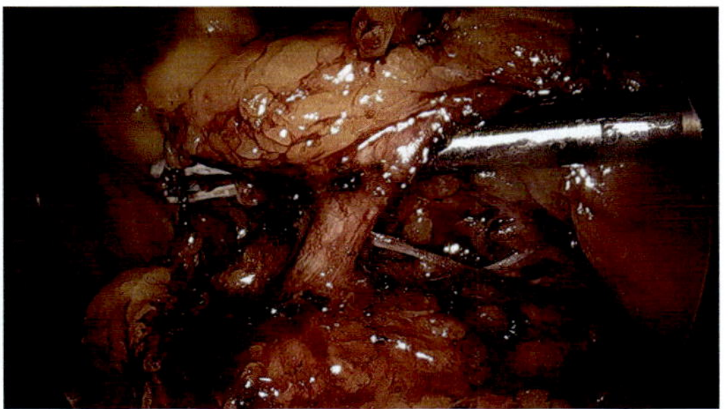

Fig. 22.6 Intraoperative image showing isolation of the inferior mesenteric artery

pancreas, making an incision at the inferior border of the pancreas at the root of the transverse mesocolon. The mesocolon is slowly divided and the lesser sac can be entered. Following lesser sac entry, the remainder of the transverse colon mesentery is divided laterally toward the tail of the pancreas.

The IMV is isolated at the base of the pancreas below the insertion of the left colic vein and is divided between clips or with an energy device (Fig. 22.5). Rarely, a meandering mesenteric artery (of Moskowitz) may run through the triangle formed by the IMV, left colic artery, and the inferior edge of the pancreas. Knowledge and preservation of this anatomic variant are critical to maintaining perfusion of the left colon.

The initial peritoneal incision is continued inferiorly over the origin of the IMA, along the origin of the mesosigmoid and mesorectum toward the pelvic inlet. From the medial-to-lateral approach, the mesocolon is mobilized off the retroperitoneum under the superior rectal artery and vein, identifying the hypogastric nerves, left ureter, and the left gonadal vessels while working toward the lateral sidewall. At this point, the instrument in the right hand can be placed below and behind the superior rectal artery, exposing the origin of the IMA proximal to the left colic branch for division with an energy device and clips (Fig. 22.6). Just prior to skeletonization of the IMA, the sigmoidal branches from the right and left splanchnic nerves are divided while preserving the lumbar splanchnic nerves. The left colic artery is also divided at this time to facilitate extraction.

The Lateral Component

With the patient in the right side down and moderate Trendelenburg position, the sigmoid colon is retracted medially using an atraumatic bowel grasper in the left hand and the peritoneal attachments in the mesosigmoid fossa can be incised over the "bruise" created from the previous retroperitoneal dissection, joining the medial and lateral dissection (Fig. 22.7a). With an instrument under the mesocolon to provide exposure while avoiding grasping the colon, the white line of Toldt can be incised along the lateral edge of the descending colon up to and occasionally cephalad to the splenic flexure (Fig. 22.7b, c). When the initial medial dissection is performed adequately and the pancreas is dropped posteriorly, the lateral dissection can be extended easily onto the transverse colon.

Supramesocolic Approach

With the patient in the right side down and moderate reverse Trendelenburg position, a third instrument (suprapubic port) is used to improve triangulation during omental dissection to retract the transverse colon toward the pelvis. With the operating surgeon facing cephalad, the greater omentum is retracted over the transverse mesocolon and grasped near the attachments of epiploic fat and transverse mesocolon. With an energy device in the right hand, the omentum is divided and the lesser sac is entered. Our preference is to divide the omentum and enter the lesser sac just

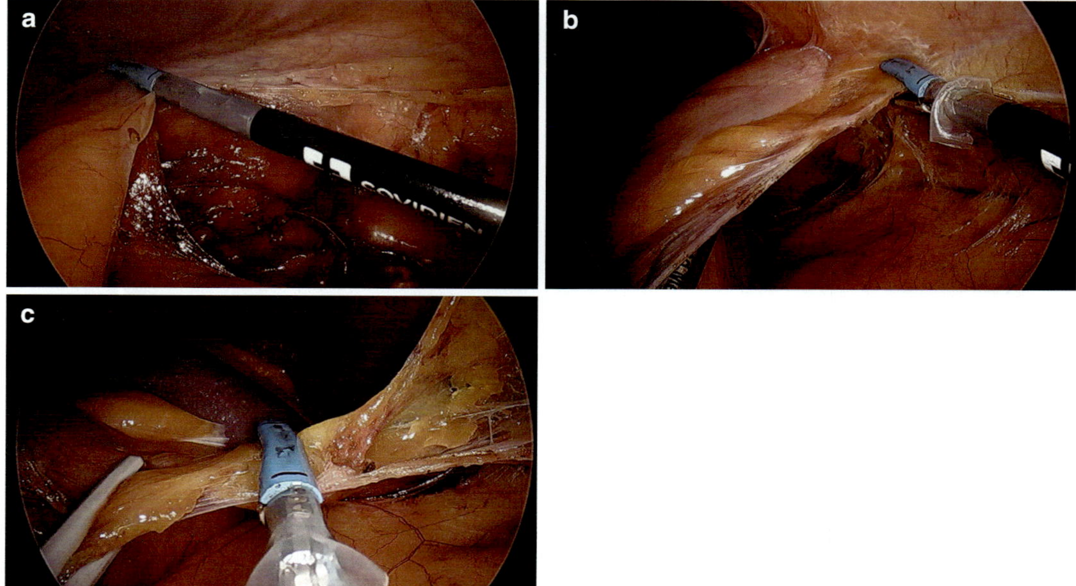

Fig. 22.7 Intraoperative images show (**a**) dissection with the lateral approach meets the medial dissection. (**b, c**) The white line of Toldt is incised cephalad to the level of the spleen

along the gastroepiploic arcade rather than along the transverse colon which is more difficult. Once lesser sac entry is established, the assistant instrument can be placed inside the lesser sac underneath the omentum and retracted caudad to protect the transverse mesocolon from accidental injury. Following division of the omentum to communicate with the lateral plane previously dissected, the mesocolic plane at the inferior edge of the pancreas is identified and incised, leading to communication with the previously established retroperitoneal plane. The final splenocolic ligaments are divided, completely releasing the splenic flexure up to the middle colic pedicle. Care must be taken when performing this approach so that the attachments to the omentum at the angle of the splenic flexure are not tethering the descending colon and hindering its mobilization into the pelvis.

Rectal Mobilization and Total Mesorectal Excision

Primary mobilization of the left mesocolon with early division of the appropriate vasculature permits safe access and exposure for initiation of the rectal dissection. At this point, critical structures including the left ureter, gonadal vessels, and superior hypogastric plexus have already been identified to guide the surgeon into the correct mesorectal planes.

The operating room setup is identical to splenic flexure mobilization but requires the main operating surgeon to use the two lateral ports while facing toward the pelvis. Cephalad and anterior traction is provided by the assistant through the suprapubic port. A camera operator stands on the left side of the abdomen. An additional left lower and/or left upper quadrant 5-mm port is required for the assistant surgeon to retract the colon out of the pelvis. An experienced assistant can provide similar retraction through the suprapubic port while standing at the patient's right hip adjacent to the operating surgeon.

The posterior dissection begins with entry into the presacral space. This can be achieved by following the mesenteric cut edge caudally and parallel to the superior rectal artery. This should be preceded by having the rectosigmoid mesocolon fully dissected off the inter-sigmoid fossa and sacral promontory and confirming the location of the left ureter laterally. The shiny visceral package of the fascia propria enveloping the mesorectum must be identified. This will allow entry into the bloodless plane between the fascia propria and presacral fascia down to the distal resection site. The innermost dissectible plane can be developed by maintaining dissection on the "yellow side of the white." An important landmark is the area where Waldeyer's fascia begins to transition anteriorly to join with the fascia propria of the rectum. One must be aware of this transition and incise Waldeyer's fascia at this location to avoid dissection deep through the presacral fascia and into the sacrum.

Of important note, pelvic exposure can be facilitated by locking the assistant's grasper (suprapubic trocar) onto the bowel just proximal to the rectosigmoid junction. This can be placed in a position which allows good clearance of the pelvic inlet from redundant bowel and mesentery while avoiding repositioning and obstructing the primary surgeon's instruments. This provides the primary surgeon with the ability to easily redirect tension to expose the right, left, and posterior working spaces with ease, often independent of the skill of the assistant.

The posterior dissection can also be facilitated by delaying the anterior and lateral rectal dissection until the distal-most extent of the posterior dissection is reached or until progress ceases. Using gauze in the main surgeon's retracting grasper can be an effective source of countertraction to better tent the fibrous tissue. This is particularly helpful when space is limited in the deeper pelvis and there is considerable fatty bulk or tissue elasticity of the mesorectum such that a grasper alone fails to achieve leverage and traction. Additionally, a laparoscopic fan retractor can be placed through the suprapubic port for both posterior retraction as well as anterior retraction in the peritoneal reflection.

The lateral dissection starts from the right side (Fig. 22.8a, b), carefully identifying and sweeping down the hypogastric nerves, which can be tented upward to the mesorectal fascia with traction. These nerves are particularly vulnerable when joining the lateral dissection with the posterior dissection. The lateral ligaments are placed under tension by drawing the rectum to the either side of the pelvis and are dissected carefully to preserve the nerve trunks that travel distally.

The anterior dissection is performed after scoring the peritoneum on either side of the rectum down the lateral rectal sulci and then continuing along the anterior surface and opening up the peritoneal reflection in the pouch of Douglas. This is continued by dissection in the cul-de-sac exposing Denonvilliers' fascia and protecting the seminal vesicles or vaginal wall separating these structures from the rectum. Denonvilliers' fascia is a key landmark, as its lateral edge is just medial to the nerves. At this location in the pelvis, the rectum acutely angulates changing course in a more horizontal fashion. Continued dissection of the extraperitoneal rectum requires constant traction, frequent changes in exposure, and continued circumferential dissection to elevate the rectum from the pelvis. Challenges in laparoscopic dissection of the distal mesorectum with variable outcomes in CRM positivity have been the impetus for evolving techniques of robotic and transanal TME (taTME) to overcome the hurdles of surgical exposure and precision.

Dynamic retraction and exposure are used to facilitate dissection of the distal mesorectum off the endopelvic fascia overlying the pelvic floor. In the posterior midline, convergence of fascial fibers forms a midline raphe which requires complete division (Fig. 22.8c). In patients with upper rectal tumors, division of the rectum 5 cm distal to the tumor is recommended (partial mesorectal excision). This approach maintains oncological principles while sparing rectum with resulting improved function compared to lower anastomoses. However, precise division of the mesorectum at its widest point is ergonomically challenging. Despite proximal transection of the rectum, complete mobilization to the pelvic floor is still necessary to allow enough mobility for mesorectal division.

Once the appropriate distal margin is identified, an endoscopic stapler is used to transect the rectum. Division of the rectum should be performed directly perpendicular to the wall to minimize the number of intersecting staple lines. Optimally, ≤ 2 firings should be used, as >2 staple lines have

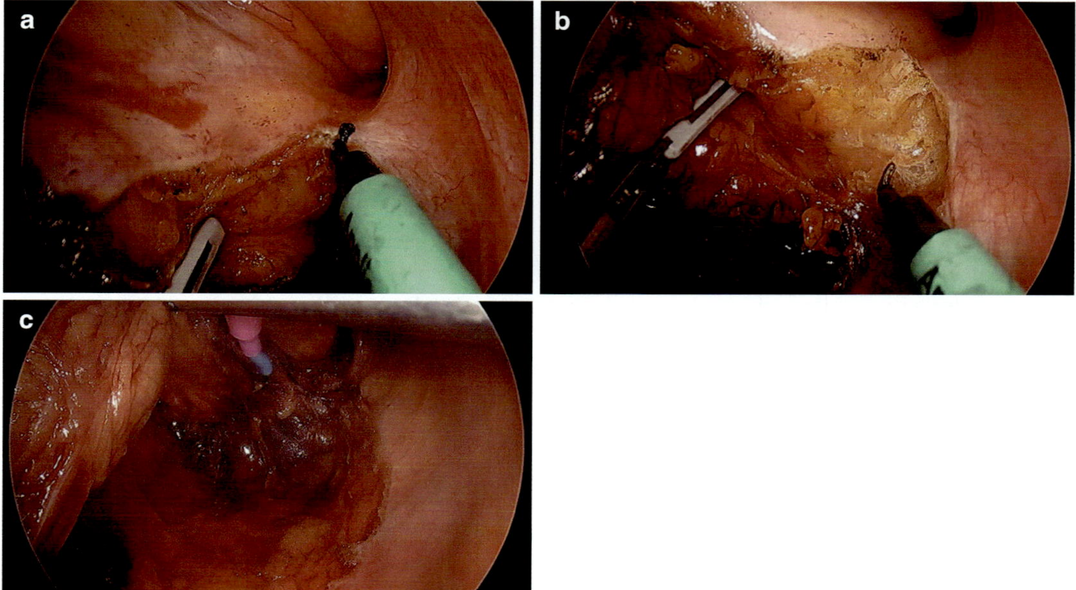

Fig. 22.8 Intraoperative images show (**a**, **b**) right lateral pelvic dissection and (**c**) deep posterior presacral rectal dissection

demonstrated increased rates of anastomotic leak. Upsizing the suprapubic or right lower quadrant port to 12 mm is necessary to introduce a traditional endoscopic linear stapler. Stapling from the right lower quadrant enables a more traditional horizontal division of the rectum. However, limitations in stapler reticulation as well as variations in port position can provide challenges. For example, inadvertent inclusion of left lateral pelvic sidewall structures at the tip of the stapler should be avoided. In addition, port site hernias through 12-mm trocar sites can occur and therefore require closure. Alternatively, introduction of the stapler through the suprapubic port can be accomplished providing a vertical transection of the rectum. With this approach, angulation of the stapler is ergonomically challenging and not possible in every pelvis. The colon is exteriorized through the Pfannenstiel incision and the IMA pedicle is identified. If it was not performed intracorporeally, the left ascending branch is divided from the IMA. The remaining mesocolon and marginal vessel are then divided up to the distal descending colon identifying the proximal colonic margin.

It is our practice to evaluate the proximal colonic transection line for adequate perfusion prior to performing an anastomosis for all left colon resections [3, 4]. The proximal transection site is chosen after intravenous injection of 2–3 ml of indocyanine green and visualization of the bowel to confirm an intact marginal vessel and mural perfusion. This perfusion assessment is used in conjunction with traditional means of assessing of conduit viability such as marginal vessel or staple line bleeding.

Reconstruction

Different methods of rectal reconstruction have been proposed. Although an end-to-end anastomosis is most simple, both colonic J pouch and end-to-side anastomosis have demonstrated superior functional outcomes. A balanced approached must be considered when striving to maximize postoperative function, as technical feasibility will frequently be the determining factor particularly when the narrow pelvis or bulky conduit may only permit an end-to-end anastomosis. A 6- to 8-cm colonic J pouch is constructed with an incision along the antimesenteric border of the colon and a single firing of a linear stapler. The anvil is then secured into the colotomy with a purse-string suture. Otherwise an end-to-side anastomosis can be fashioned by inserting the anvil portion of the stapler with its sharp spike attachment into a colotomy, which is brought out of the antimesenteric colon wall about 5 cm proximal to the blind end. The distal colon wall is then divided with a linear stapler.

The circular stapler is brought through the staple line of the rectal stump, and the anastomosis is completed with a circular stapler. Orientation of the colonic conduit should be confirmed by ensuring a straight path of the mesenteric cut edge from distal to proximal. Care must be taken to reduce herniated small bowel underneath the left mesocolon. Routine closure of the mesenteric defect to the retroperitoneum is not routinely performed as small bowel obstruction is rare.

Routine use of pelvic drains has not demonstrated reduction of pelvic sepsis and is therefore not routinely performed. Proximal fecal diversion is performed at the discretion of the surgeon, however, should be strongly considered in patients who received preoperative radiotherapy. Postoperative care includes early mobilization, resumption of solid food, and minimization of opioid pain medications consistent with Enhanced Recovery after Surgery protocols (ERAS).

patients, the mesocolon in this area is much thinner compared to other major vascular pedicles. In thin patients, lymphatic vessels that run parallel to the aorta are frequently present.

- Rarely, a meandering mesenteric artery may be encountered, and one must be familiar with this anatomic variant to avoid injury and to minimize ischemia to the left colon.
- To avoid injury to the pancreas, it is critical to identify Toldt's fascia posterior to the pancreas, since this is the stopping point for the inferior dissection. The dissection is then continued at the level of the pancreas to divide the origin of the transverse colon and to enter the lesser sac.
- Incising the transverse mesocolon from the base of the pancreas can be challenging for surgeons early in their learning curve. The lesser sac can often be more easily entered along the distal pancreas where gastropancreatic attachments are less common. Even if the lesser sac is not completely entered, it will facilitate identification of the correct plane once the lesser sac is entered through the gastrocolic ligament and the "bruise" along the pancreas is visualized.

Tips and Tricks

- Optimal exposure of the left mesocolon is ensured by appropriate patient positioning at the beginning of the operation. Correct positioning will also serve to prevent the patient from slipping during extreme steep table positions.
- Caution must be taken when dissecting below the inferior mesenteric vein after dividing the mesoduodenal ligament to avoid going into the retroperitoneum where the left gonadal vein, ureter, and left renal vein are exposed and are vulnerable to injury. Even in obese

References

1. Monson JR, Weiser MR, Buie WD, Chang GJ, Rafferty JF, Buie WD, Rafferty J. Standards Practice Task Force of the American Society of Colon and Rectal Surgeons Practice Parameters for the Management of Rectal Cancer (Revised). Dis Colon Rectum. 2013;56:535–50.
2. Ludwig, Kirk, Kosinski, Lauren. Is Splenic Flexure Mobilization Necessary in Laparoscopic Anterior Resection? Another View Diseases of the Colon & Rectum, 2012, Vol. 5, 1198–1200.
3. Foppa C, Denoya P, Tarta C, et al. Indocyanine green fluorescent dye during bowel surgery: are the blood supply "guessing days" over? Tech Coloproctol. 2014;18:753–8.
4. Wada T, Kawada K, Takahashi R, et al. ICG fluorescence imaging for quantitative evaluation of colonic perfusion in laparoscopic colorectal surgery. Surg Endosc. 2017;31:4184.

Robotic Low Anterior Resection with Double-Staple Technique

Steven J. Nurkin, Julia H. Terhune, and Sumana Narayanan

Introduction: Robotics for Rectal Surgery

The adoption of minimally invasive techniques in oncologic surgery has been slower than many other general surgery procedures, as surgeons have awaited for assurances that oncologic outcomes are equivalent between minimally invasive and open approaches. In rectal cancer, this has required the demonstration that an adequate total mesorectal excision (TME) is attainable through the use of laparoscopy or, more recently, robotics. A well-executed TME is critical in rectal cancer surgery, as it is well established that an intact TME specimen is an independent predictor of rectal cancer recurrence [1]. A properly performed TME should result in a single-digit recurrence rate.

Laparoscopy has been used for several decades for rectal surgery, but debate still remains whether it provides equivalent oncologic outcomes, even in the hands of experienced surgeons. In recent years several studies examining this point have yielded contradictory conclusions [2–4].

The COLOR II trial asserted that laparoscopy was equivalent to open surgery based on the rates of local recurrence and disease-free survival, whereas the ACOSOG Z6051 and ALaCaRT studies found lower rates of negative circumferential radial margins (CRM) and completeness of TME, and thus these studies could not demonstrate "non-inferior" short-term oncologic outcomes with laparoscopy [2, 3]. Robotic surgery has been increasing in popularity among colorectal surgeons with the demonstration of favorable oncologic outcomes and low rates of conversion to open surgery while also providing the benefits of minimally invasive surgery [5]. At our institution, we routinely perform robotic low anterior resections (LAR) and have observed distinct advantages with this technique, despite an initial steep learning curve.

Preoperative Considerations/ERAS

All patients with rectal cancer at our institution undergo multidisciplinary evaluation to determine optimal treatment. At the time of surgical evaluation, patients have a standard oncologic work-up that involves physical exam with digital rectal exam (DRE), and if the lesion is palpable, the work-up should include particular attention to the distance from the anorectal ring and whether the lesion is fixed or mobile. After multidisciplinary review, most patients will undergo

Electronic supplementary material The online version of this chapter (https://doi.org/10.1007/978-3-030-18740-8_23) contains supplementary material, which is available to authorized users.

S. J. Nurkin (✉) · J. H. Terhune · S. Narayanan
Department of Surgical Oncology, Roswell Park
Comprehensive Cancer Center, Buffalo, NY, USA
e-mail: Steven.Nurkin@RoswellPark.org

© Springer Nature Switzerland AG 2020
J. Kim, J. Garcia-Aguilar (eds.), *Minimally Invasive Surgical Techniques for Cancers of the Gastrointestinal Tract*, https://doi.org/10.1007/978-3-030-18740-8_23

neoadjuvant therapy and complete treatment at least 8–10 weeks prior to resection [6, 7]. Consistent with recent literature, we have observed that magnetic resonance imaging (MRI) of the pelvis (both pre- and post-neoadjuvant therapy) is particularly helpful when planning for surgery, as it provides a reliable evaluation of the CRM and involvement of any surrounding structures [8]. As part of the multidisciplinary approach, patients meet with a member of the enterostomal therapy team for ileostomy site marking and are provided with educational materials at least 1 week prior to surgery.

The day prior to surgery, our patients start a "Nichols prep" with oral antibiotics and mechanical bowel preparation. We have an established enhanced recovery after surgery (ERAS) protocol, which instructs patients to drink clear liquids until 2 hours prior to their procedure. Given the small incisions anticipated for this operation, we do not routinely use epidurals. Instead, we combine a preoperative oral "pain cocktail" (acetaminophen, celecoxib, and gabapentin) with other regional techniques such as bilateral transversus abdominis plane blocks, intrathecal morphine, or local infiltration of liposomal bupivacaine as part of a multimodal pain regimen.

Patient Positioning and Room Setup

Proper arrangement of the room prior to the start of the case is necessary for efficient workflow. The robot can be located on the patient's left side, and the surgeon should be able to visualize the robot, arms, and patient from the console.

Patients are secured to the bed with straps and care is taken to cushion the pressure points. To prevent sliding, we advocate the use of nonslip pads or egg crate foam (Fig. 23.1). The patient is positioned in Lloyd-Davies or split-leg position with both arms tucked; and the robot is brought into the field on the patient's left side (Fig. 23.2). This position allows access to the anus for DRE or sigmoidoscopy during the procedure to facilitate adequate distal transection margin and to evaluate the anastomosis.

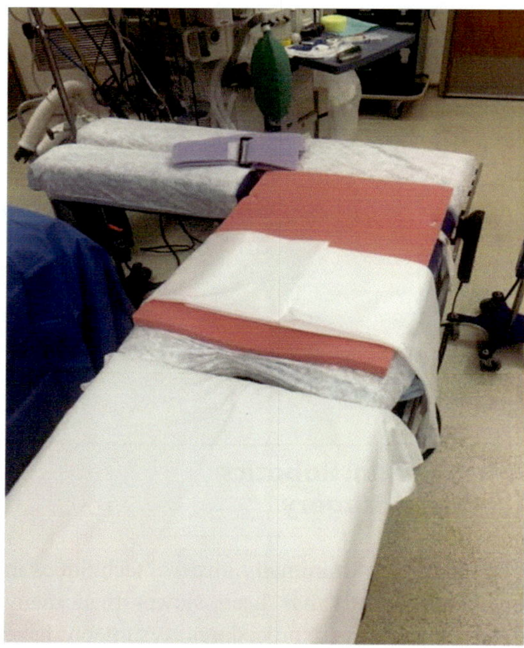

Fig. 23.1 Placement of nonslip pads for robotic low anterior resection

Abdominal Portion

Video 23.1

At our institution, we start robotic proctectomy with laparoscopy as this allows exploration of the abdomen and any dissection or mobilization in the upper abdomen to be completed prior to docking the robotic instruments. Depending on the robotic platform (Si or Xi), mobilization of the splenic flexure may require re-docking the robot, or some may prefer splenic flexure mobilization laparoscopically as it is more efficient than re-docking the robot. At our institution we use the Xi platform that allows for multi-quadrant directionality with a single docking.

The initial access to the abdomen is through insertion of a left upper quadrant (LUQ) Veress needle, and then the abdomen is insufflated. The camera port is inserted in this left upper quadrant position using OptiView entry. The abdomen is then explored for any evidence of metastatic disease with particular attention to the liver and peritoneal surfaces. Port placement should follow basic robotic principles to minimize risk of arm

Fig. 23.2 Patient positioning and robotic setup for low anterior resection

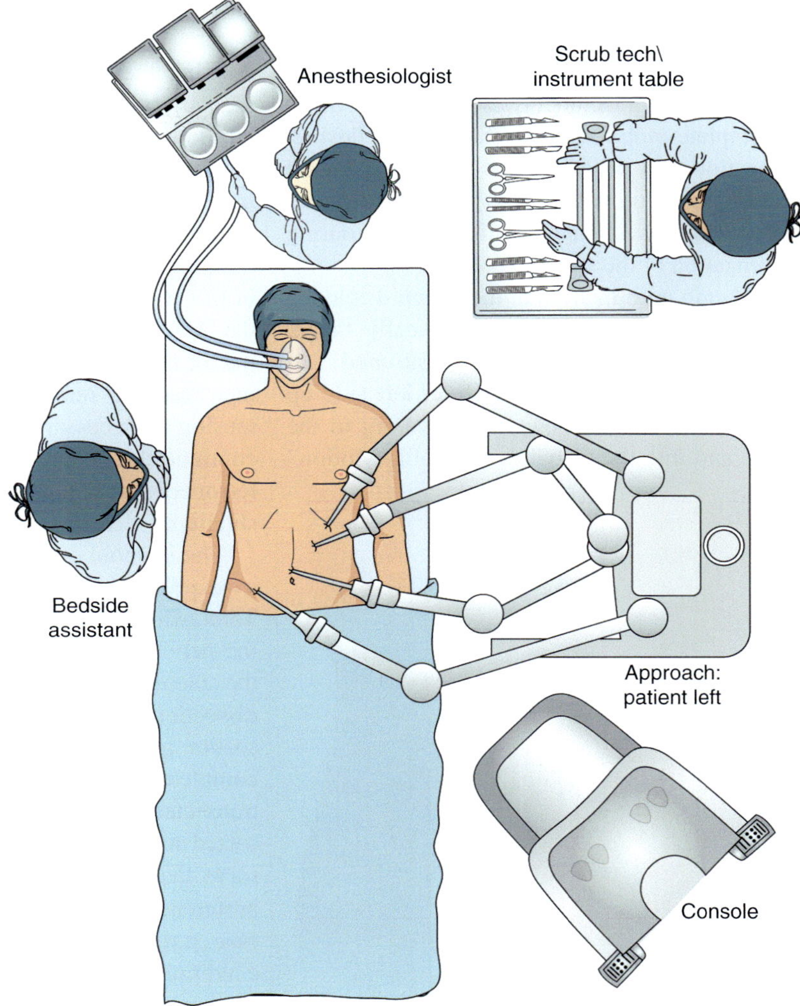

collisions, typically in a diagonal line from right lower to left upper quadrants. A port is placed in supraumbilical position, just to the right of midline, and the camera is moved to this location. Typically, one large robotic stapler port is placed on the right side of the abdomen, just at or below the level of the umbilicus. The initial LUQ camera insertion site is converted into a robotic port, and an additional robotic port is placed along the left anterior axillary line in the LUQ. Finally, one 5-mm and one 10-mm (AirSeal) assistant ports are placed in the right subxiphoid and right upper quadrant, respectively (Fig. 23.3).

The patient is placed into reverse Trendelenburg position, the omentum is moved into the upper abdomen, and the small bowel is swept to the right side of the abdomen. If the patient has had prior abdominal surgery, there may be adhesions to the omentum. If present, the adhesions are divided sharply. A medial-to-lateral mobilization of the splenic flexure is performed. This begins by identification of the ligament of Treitz (LOT) and inferior mesenteric vein (IMV), which is just lateral to the LOT. The IMV is lifted and the peritoneum just below it is incised. This plane is taken toward the origin of the inferior mesenteric artery (IMA) from the aorta and also toward the spleen and out toward the abdominal wall. The IMV is transected with care to avoid injury to collateral vessels to the region of colon supplied by the superior mesenteric artery (SMA). Then, we enter the lesser sac through the gastrocolic omentum and divide the remaining retroperitoneal attachments, which should result in complete mobilization of the splenic flexure. Dissection can be completed along the lateral descending colon at this point; or it can be completed with dissection of the line of Toldt during mobilization of the sigmoid colon.

To begin mobilization of the sigmoid colon, a medial to lateral approach is typically taken. The patient should be positioned in Trendelenburg position with slight left side up to prevent the small bowel from falling to the pelvis and into the visual field. "Table Motion"

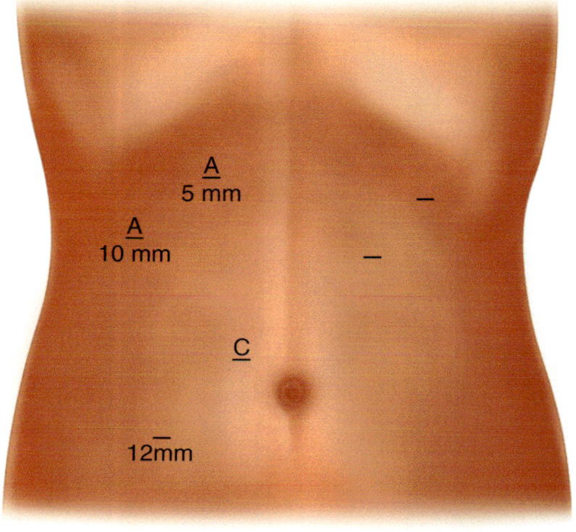

Fig. 23.3 Trocar/port placement for robotic low anterior resection

technology can help facilitate this table positioning, without the need for undocking and redocking the robot. We first identify the right iliac artery and incise the peritoneum just medially to enter the mesorectal plane; at this point, the pneumoperitoneum can facilitate dissection in this plane. We use robotic monopolar cautery or scissors to develop this plane sharply to reach the aorta near the origin of the IMA. Dissection in this area should result in harvesting fat from the IMA up to its point of transection and retaining all the lymph nodes so that the entire specimen can be removed en bloc. We readjust tension as necessary on the sigmoid colon and continue the medial-to-lateral dissection in the retroperitoneal plane where the left ureter should be identified.

The sigmoid colon is then retracted medially to expose the lateral attachments and line of Toldt, which is divided sharply both caudally into the pelvis and cranially to meet the plane from the splenic flexure mobilization. Once the lateral dissection is complete, the medial and lateral dissection planes should meet. The IMA should be completely isolated at this point and, if so, can be transected (Fig. 23.4). Whether the IMA is transected at its origin or taken further distally to preserve the left colic branch is based on surgeon preference and operative factors unique to the case. It may not be necessary oncologically in all conditions to transect the IMA at its origin, but it is often needed to have sufficient length on the colon to perform a tension-free anastomosis.

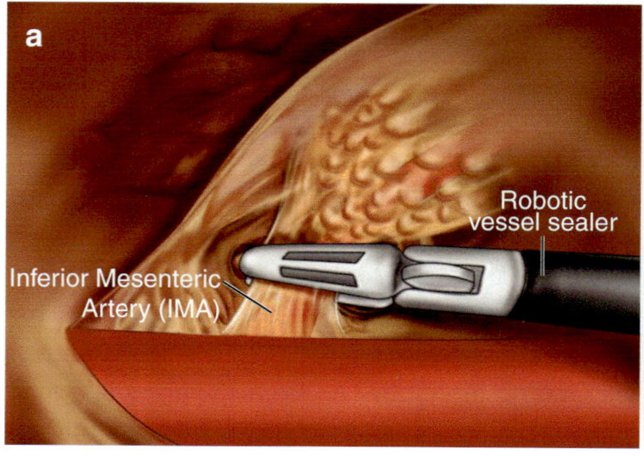

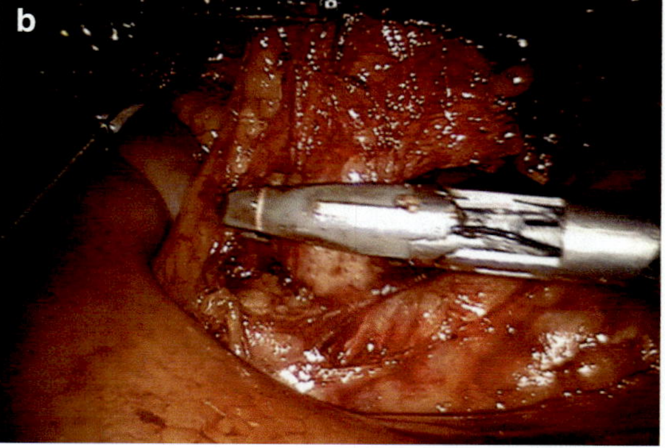

Fig. 23.4 (**a**) Illustration showing high ligation of the inferior mesenteric artery. (**b**) Paired intraoperative image demonstrating dissection and transection of the inferior mesenteric artery with the robotic vessel sealer

Once the blood supply is divided, the descending colon will be mobile and can be divided. Select the area of the descending colon to be transected, and clear off mesentery that remains in this area. A reasonable point of transection is just proximal to the location where the vascular pedicle was divided as this usually ensures adequate perfusion to the proximal margin. The colon is then divided at the desired location using an endo-GIA or a robotic stapling device.

Pelvic Dissection/TME

The dissection completed thus far has begun to expose the proper plane for posterior TME. Proper retraction of the bowel is critical to maintain this plane and adequate visualization. Retraction should involve three points: the bedside assistant retracts the specimen out of the pelvis cranially, and the third working arm provides anterior retraction leaving both the first and second arm available for direct retraction and dissection in the working space.

Before dissection begins in a new space, we ensure that the correct avascular plane is visible. Starting with the posterior TME, we place continuous anterior and superior retraction with our left hand (arm 2), to visualize the avascular plane and use the monopolar hook cautery or scissors to divide the plane. The dissection should extend laterally on both sides and can take the appearance of a "smile." This plane must continue below the level of the tumor and off the levators (if the tumor requires low dissection). Then we begin the lateral dissection down the right and left sides of the rectum. At this point, the third arm switches to retract laterally, while the assistant continues to retract anteriorly and in the opposite direction to facilitate visualization into pelvis.

The anterior dissection is the most difficult to visualize; and in females, this can be further hampered by the uterus. The third arm moves to retract cranial and posterior, while the assistant and second arms remain in their location with subtle adjustments as necessary to maintain optimal visualization. If the uterus is obstructing the view of the pelvis, a Keith needle can be used to pull up on the round ligament through the abdominal wall for retraction. Once this view is adequate, we divide the anterior plane to below the peritoneal reflection. In males, a landmark in this area is the seminal vesicles to which the dissection plane remains close. As long as the tumor is not anterior, then remaining in the anterior fat plane is adequate because the prostate is quite close to the rectal wall in this plane. If the tumor is anterior, Denonvilliers' fascia between the prostate and rectal wall will often need to be included with the specimen.

Finally, we clean off the mesorectum as much as possible to confirm that dissection has been performed below the level of the tumor. This step can be accomplished in a number of ways: using flexible sigmoidoscope, DRE, or visualization of a localizing tattoo. Robotic Tile Pro technology allows for direct visualization of both the pelvis and bedside sigmoidoscopy at the console. Any remaining mesorectum can be transected perpendicularly with a robotic vessel sealer or the monopolar hook using caution not to damage the rectal wall.

Stapling the rectum is facilitated by the use of a robotic stapler (45-mm green load), as it provides angulation/reticulation that is often superior compared to laparoscopic staplers. Proper stapler use is vital, as increased number of stapler firings has been associated with higher risk of leak [9, 10]. Ideally one or two 45-mm loads should be used. After dividing the rectum, we confirm that the colon will reach into the pelvis without tension before undocking the robot.

Specimen Extraction, Anastomosis, and Closure

There are several options for specimen extraction: a lower midline incision, at the site of ileostomy, or the Pfannenstiel incision (our preference). Regardless of the site, the use of a wound protector is advised. After extraction, the specimen should be assessed and oriented for the pathologist. To assess vascular perfusion of the descending colon, fluorescence imaging (utilizing indocyanine green, ICG) can be used prior to and after the anastomosis is performed.

For the anastomosis, the proximal colon margin is exteriorized, and the anvil is introduced into the colon in an end-to-end or an end-to-side (Baker's technique) fashion. A purse-string stitch is placed around the anvil site. The colon is dropped back into the abdomen, and pneumoperitoneum is re-established. The stapler is introduced into the rectum, and with the assistance of laparoscopic (or robotic) instruments, the anvil is mated with the stapler under direction visualization. After the mesentery is checked to ensure that it is straight and without tension, the stapler is fired and gently removed from the rectum. Anastomotic "donuts" are evaluated for completeness. A flexible sigmoidoscopy is performed to evaluate the mucosa at the anastomosis, and a "bubble test" can be performed to evaluate for leak. The decision to perform a diverting ileostomy is individually based on patient risk factors and on how "low" the anastomosis will be performed. If diversion is necessary, the location on the terminal ileum is selected, and the bowel is brought through the preselected site on the anterior abdominal wall. The fascia is then closed followed by skin closure and Dermabond placement. If an ileostomy has been created, it would be matured at this point.

Complications

Complications that occur after robotic LAR are not unique to robotic surgery. Established complications such as nerve damage or anastomotic leak may still occur. Symptoms of pelvic nerve injury typically include genitourinary dysfunction and depend on the exact location of the injury. If high ligation of the IMA was performed, an injury may result in retrograde ejaculation. If the injury occurred more distally, the risk becomes impotence; and/or other sexual dysfunction and damage at the level of the prostate or lower in women result in urinary incontinence. Not all injuries result in permanent damage, and patients may transiently develop short-term urinary retention or

incontinence requiring catheterization without long-term sequelae. Anastomotic leakage is a complication that leads to significant morbidity and even mortality for patients.

Conclusions

Robotic LAR with double staple is a safe and effective technique for resection of rectal cancer. The robot provides excellent visualization as well as the ability to easily maneuver the instruments to allow for more careful dissection in the TME plane (especially in the narrow pelvis). We feel that this can allow for equivalent oncologic outcomes to open surgery and preservation of genitourinary function. This technique also allows for the benefits of minimally invasive surgery including shorter lengths of stay in combination with ERAS protocols and diminished wound complication rates.

References

1. Heald RJ, Ryall RDH. Recurrence and survival after total mesorectal excision for rectal cancer. Lancet. 1986;1:1479–82.
2. Bonjer HJ, Deijin CL, Haglind E, et al. A randomized trial of laparoscopic versus open surgery for rectal cancer. NEJM. 2015;372:1324–32.
3. Stevenson ARL, Solomon MJ, Simes J, et al. Effect of laparoscopic-assisted resection vs open resection on pathological outcomes in rectal cancer: the ALaCaRT randomized clinical trial. JAMA. 2015;314:1456–363.
4. Fleshman J, Branda M, Nelson H, et al. Effect of laparoscopic-assisted resection vs open resection of stage II or III rectal cancer on pathologic outcomes: the ACOSOG Z6051 randomized clinical trial. JAMA. 2015;314:1346–55.
5. Sammour T, Malakorn S, Chang GJ, et al. Oncologic outcomes after robotic proctectomy for rectal cancer: analysis of a prospective database. Ann Surg. 2016;267:521–6.
6. Rodel C, Graeven U, Liersch T, et al. Oxaliplatin added to fluorouracil-based preoperative chemoradiotherapy and postoperative chemotherapy of locally advanced rectal cancer (the German CAO/ARO/AIO-04 study): final results of the multicentre, open-label, randomised, phase 3 trial. Lancet Oncol. 2015;16:979–89.

7. Probst CP, Becerra AZ, Fleming FJ, et al. Extended intervals after neoadjuvant therapy in locally advanced rectal cancer: the key to improved tumor response and potential organ preservation. J Am Coll Surg. 2015;221:430–40.

8. Taylor FG, Quirke R, Brown G, et al. Preoperative magnetic resonance imaging assessment of circumferential resection margin predicts disease-free survival and local recurrence: 5-year follow-up results of the MERCURY study. J Clin Oncol. 2014;32:34–43.

9. Kim JS, Cho SY, Kim NK, et al. Risk factors for anastomotic leakage after laparoscopic intracorporeal colorectal anastomosis with a double stapling technique. J Am Coll Surg. 2009;209:694–701.

10. Braunschmid T, Hartig N, Herbst F, et al. Influence of multiple stapler firings used for rectal division on colorectal anastomotic leak rate. Surg Endosc. 2017;31:5318–26.

Laparoscopic Total Abdominal Colectomy

24

Wolfgang B. Gaertner

Introduction

Laparoscopic colectomy is a widely accepted and safe operation that has shown to be cost effective in selective patients with diseases of the colon and rectum. The indications for total abdominal colectomy are typically divided into urgent and elective (Table 24.1). These indications typically involve diagnoses including inflammatory bowel disease (IBD), synchronous colon neoplasia, large bowel obstruction with megacolon, and inherited or familial polyposis syndromes. The operative approach relies largely on surgeon experience, the patient's disease process with the acuity of presentation being a significant factor, and patient-related factors such as obesity and previous abdominal operations. In the case of synchronous neoplasia, removal of the entire colon is often compared to two separate segmental colon resections or staged segmental colon resections, and largely depends on the underlying disease process. The risks and benefits of these

comparisons must be discussed with the patient preoperatively, as well as long-term sequelae such as functional disorders, need for more frequent endoscopic surveillance, and the potential need for additional colon resection. Patients with Lynch syndrome are at a significantly increased risk for synchronous and metachronous colorectal cancer [1, 2]. Although extended colectomy has shown to reduce the risk of metachronous colorectal cancer, it has not shown to provide significant survival benefit when appropriate endoscopic surveillance is performed [3, 4]. Similarly,

Table 24.1 Indications for total abdominal colectomy

Urgent	Elective
Toxic megacolon:	Inflammatory bowel disease:
Acute inflammatory bowel disease flare refractory to maximal medical therapy	Refractory to medical therapy
Clostridium difficile colitis	Dysplasia or dysplasia-associated lesion or mass
Large bowel obstruction	
Colonic pseudo-obstruction (Ogilvie's syndrome)	Large pseudopolyp burden or inability to perform appropriate endoscopic surveillance
Ischemic colitis	
Sigmoid volvulus with megacolon	
	Synchronous or metachronous colonic neoplasia
	Polyposis syndromes
	Repeat colectomy
	Functional disorders of the colon (*i.e.* colonic inertia)

Electronic supplementary material The online version of this chapter (https://doi.org/10.1007/978-3-030-18740-8_24) contains supplementary material, which is available to authorized users.

W. B. Gaertner (✉)
Division of Colon and Rectal Surgery, Department of Surgery, University of Minnesota,
Minneapolis, MN, USA
e-mail: gaert015@umn.edu

the risk of metachronous dysplastic lesions or worsening disease after segmental colectomy in IBD ranges from 30% to 50% [5]. Although total abdominal colectomy with ileorectal anastomosis has been shown to be safe and effective in a small and selective subset of IBD patients with rectal sparing, completion proctectomy is eventually required in a third of these patients for diverse reasons [6, 7].

Minimally invasive colectomy has been widely accepted for colorectal disorders. Compared to the open approach, laparoscopic total abdominal colectomy has been associated with faster recovery of bowel function, shorter hospital stays, and faster return to daily living activities; and in ulcerative colitis (UC) patients, sooner restorative proctectomy and ileostomy closure [8]. Although increased operating room costs and longer operative times have been associated with the laparoscopic approach, overall outcomes and costs are comparable, and many times lower with the laparoscopic approach [9–12]. Robotic colectomy will be discussed elsewhere in this work.

Preoperative Assessment

The clinical indications for minimally invasive colectomy are the same as those for traditional open colectomy. Postoperative adhesions and obesity can make the laparoscopic approach more difficult; however, obese patients have shown greater short-term benefits when the operation is successfully completed laparoscopically. Contraindications of total abdominal colectomy include medically unfit patients and unresectable metastatic disease (in the case of malignancy). Patients with poor cardiopulmonary function tolerate prolonged pneumoperitoneum poorly and should be evaluated preoperatively by an experienced anesthesia team. All patients are counseled on potential gastrointestinal and genitourinary functional disorders that may occur postoperatively. These may include chronic diarrhea, fecal

urgency, accidental bowel leakage, chronic electrolyte and fluid imbalances; and in the case of pelvic dissection for rectal resection, retrograde ejaculation, as well as urinary retention, frequency, and incontinence.

All patients who may require fecal diversion receive preoperative teaching and undergo stoma marking by a wound-ostomy-continence (WOC) nurse. Additional preoperative interventions at our institution include selective assessment of nutritional laboratory values (albumin, prealbumin, and transferrin), routine mechanical bowel preparation with oral antibiotics, and additional postoperative teaching pertaining to an enhanced recovery after surgery (ERAS) protocol. Immediately preoperative, all patients receive appropriate parenteral antibiotic prophylaxis, as well as mechanical and chemical venous thromboembolism (VTE) prophylaxis. The use of transversus abdominis plane or quadratus lumborum blocks with a long-acting anesthetic (bupivacaine liposome injectable suspension [Exparel®]) has become a routine intervention of our ERAS protocol, as well as the preoperative administration of an anti-inflammatory agent (acetaminophen or Celecoxib), gabapentin, and alvimopan (Entereg®). Parenteral antibiotics are given preoperatively and stopped at 24 h postoperation.

Positioning and Operating Room Setup

Patients are placed in modified lithotomy position with yellofin® stirrups (Allen Medical, Acton, MA) and both arms are padded and secured at the patient sides (Fig. 24.1). This allows for improved access to all abdominal quadrants and dynamic positioning of the operating surgeon and assistants. The laparoscopic equipment or tower should be placed off either shoulder with mobile video monitors placed on either side of the patient. A Foley catheter and orogastric tube are placed in all cases.

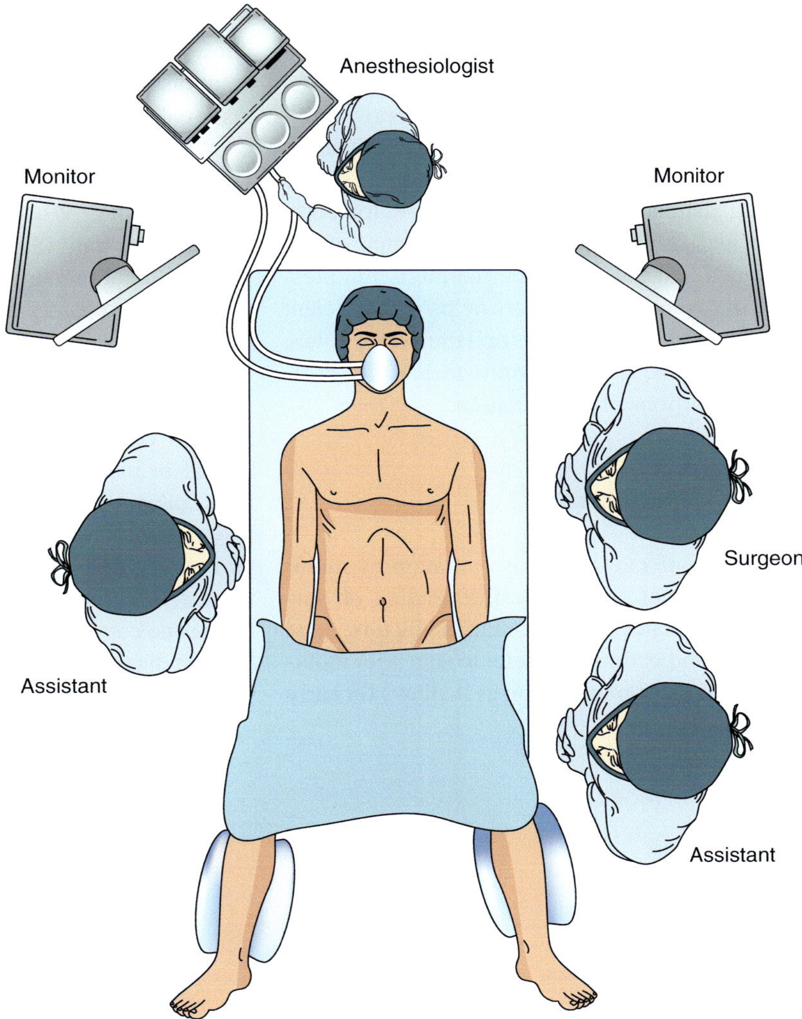

Fig. 24.1 Patient position for laparoscopic total abdominal colectomy

Operative Steps

Abdominal Access and Trocar Placement

Access to the peritoneal cavity to establish pneumoperitoneum can be performed using an open (Hassan) or closed (Veress needle or integrated camera trocar) technique. We prefer an open technique, especially in patients with previous abdominal operations or abdominal distension. The closed technique is typically performed via a periumbilical or left upper quadrant incision.

Correct trocar placement is imperative to the progress of the operation (Video 24.1). Although our description of port placement is quite standard, different anatomic circumstances may lead to variations or additions in trocar placement. In our practice, we have a low threshold for adding a 5-mm trocar to assist with improved retraction or suction when the dissection is difficult or intraoperative variations or complications are encountered. Our preference is to place a 10-mm supraumbilical trocar using an open (Hassan) technique. This port is used as the camera port. The operative team must be aware that both

10-mm and 5-mm 30 degree angled laparoscopes may be needed. After assessing the peritoneal cavity, additional trocars are placed at the mid right abdomen (12-mm), suprapubic area (5-mm), lower left abdomen (5-mm), and upper left abdomen (5-mm) (Fig. 24.2). This variation of the typical diamond configuration allows for complete and facile access to all quadrants of the abdomen and the pelvis. Furthermore, the presence of two left-sided trocars helps with efficient mobilization of the flexures and transverse colon, which are frequently the most technically challenging portions of the operation.

Sigmoid Mobilization

Although one may start this operation by mobilizing the right or left colon depending on surgeon preference, patient-related factors, and operative indication, we prefer to start with mobilization of the sigmoid colon as it allows for early transection of the rectosigmoid junction, which allows for facile mesenteric transection, and efficient dissection of the splenic flexure and transverse colon. We must disclose that total abdominal colectomy with concomitant proctectomy is rarely performed at out institution, for both IBD or malignancy. When total abdominal proctocolectomy is indicated, our current practice is to perform total abdominal colectomy first and return approximately 2 months later for proctectomy with or without anastomosis.

This step is performed with the patient in Trendelenburg position with right-side down. The sigmoid colon is mobilized using a lateral-to-medial or medial-to-lateral approach. For oncologic patients, we prefer the medial-to-lateral approach with high ligation of the inferior mesenteric artery and vein as it allows for improved mesenteric harvesting in our experience. However, there is no convincing evidence that high vascular ligation has been associated with significantly improved oncologic outcomes in colorectal cancer.

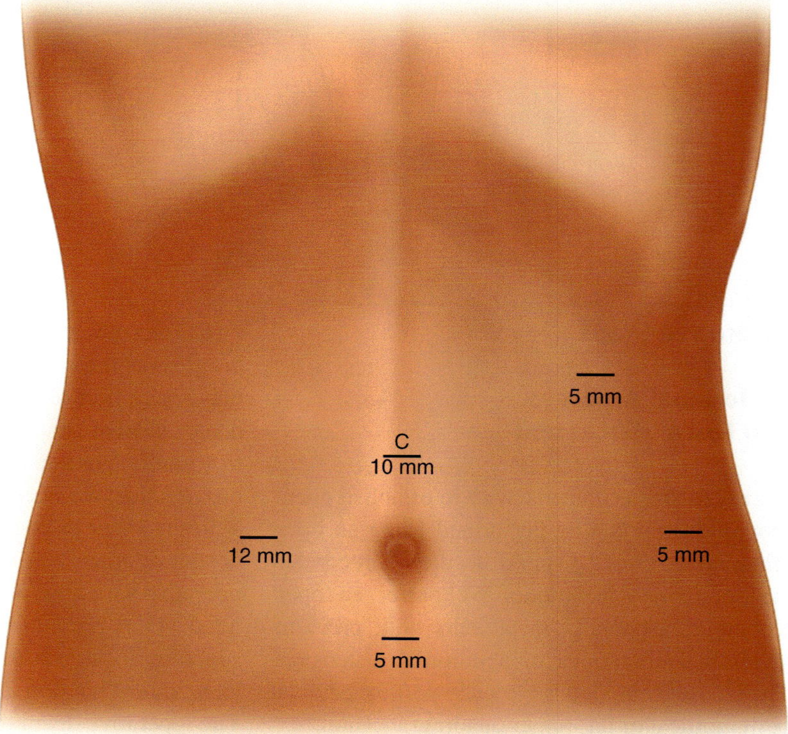

Fig. 24.2 Trocar placement and specimen extraction for laparoscopic total abdominal colectomy with end ileostomy

In our practice, the lateral-to-medial approach is typically preferred in IBD patients. The left abdominopelvic side-wall structures including the left ureter and left gonadal vein must be identified during this step. In patients with a past history of previous pelvic surgery or radiation, previous genitourinary or retroperitoneal surgery, or inflammation involving the pelvic side walls, we have a low threshold to place lighted ureteral stents in order to identify both ureters.

Rectosigmoid Transection

Next, a mesenteric window is dissected at the rectosigmoid junction, which anatomically correlates with the sacral promontory, typically where the tenia of the colon splay open. We prefer to perform transection of the rectosigmoid colon intracorporeally with an endoscopic stapler as it allows for improved specimen manipulation during the remainder of the colon dissection and specimen extraction via the ileostomy site; however, one can omit rectosigmoid transection if specimen extraction is planned through a lower midline or Pfannenstiel incision. We typically prefer this approach when an ileo-sigmoid or ileorectal anastomosis is to be performed during the same operation. For endoscopic stapling, we prefer to use a 60-mm long stapler to avoid multiple staple lines at the rectosigmoid junction.

Once the rectosigmoid junction has been transected, the mesentery of the sigmoid colon is divided with a vessel-sealing device. In patients with mesenteric atherosclerosis or in those who are undergoing high ligation of the vascular pedicles, we prefer to use an endoscopic stapler with a vascular staple load. The level of division will depend on the underlying pathology. For IBD patients, we prefer to stay relatively close to the bowel; however, in the setting of malignancy, it is important to transect the mesentery close to its origin for adequate lymphadenectomy.

Mobilization of the Left Colon

The entire left colon is mobilized using a lateral-to-medial approach. All lateral attachments are transected with a vessel-sealing device. The retroperitoneal dissection plane is used to identify the splenic flexure attachments (Fig. 24.3). Frequently, the greater omentum is attached to this segment of colon. Early dissection of the omentum from the distal transverse and descending colon is recommended for adequate visualization. Care must be taken to avoid excessive retroperitoneal dissection at the level of the splenic flexure to prevent dissecting behind the tail of the pancreas, as well as excessive retraction to prevent splenic capsule tears.

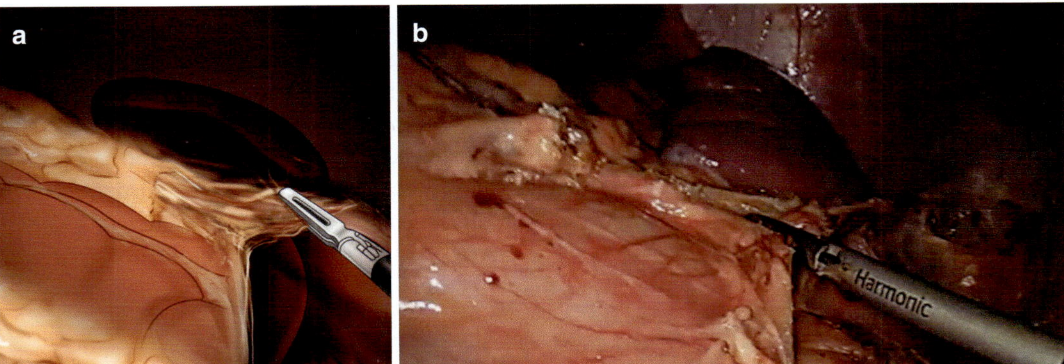

Fig. 24.3 (**a**) Illustration providing a lateral to medial takedown of the splenic flexure. (**b**) Paired operative image demonstrating the lateral to medial approach for mobilization of the left colon

Mobilization of the Transverse Colon

This step is performed in reverse Trendelenburg position, initially with right-side down, and subsequently with left-side down. As the splenic flexure is taken down and the greater omentum is dissected off of the distal transverse colon, the lesser sac is entered and the posterior aspect of the stomach is identified. Care must be taken to avoid injury to the stomach and short gastric vessels during this dissection. In cases involving neoplasia or when the omentum appears devascularized or unhealthy-appearing, we prefer to perform an infracolic omentectomy with a vessel-sealing device during this step. After transecting the gastrocolic attachments, the mesentery of the transverse colon is transected with a vessel-sealing device. Identification of the middle colic artery is crucial to prevent inadvertent injury or bleeding, and to perform high ligation with adequate lymphadenectomy in selective cases. Transection of the transverse mesocolon is the most time-consuming and meticulous portion of this operation in our experience, mainly because of the extent of omental dissection, bi-leaflet and often thickened mesentery, and proximity of the spleen, pancreas, stomach, duodenum, and gallbladder. Precise dissection and counter-traction is essential during this step; therefore, if lack of progress occurs, placement of a periumbilical or Pfannenstiel hand port is highly recommended. A key step during this portion of the operation is to completely mobilize the mid and proximal transverse colon and dissect the retroperitoneal attachments off of the duodenum before transecting the mesentery. This provides confidence at the time of mesenteric transection and avoids potential duodenal injuries. After this, the entire hepatic flexure is taken down in a top-to-bottom manner.

Mobilization of the Ascending Colon and Terminal Ileum

Most lateral attachments of the mid and distal ascending colon are dissected in continuum after taking down the hepatic flexure. The patient is then replaced in the Trendelenburg position with left-side down. It is our preference to not dissect the lateral cecal attachments in order to mobilize and transect the right colon mesentery using a medial-to-lateral approach. This allows for early identification and transection of the ileocolic vessels. Conversely, the right colon mesentery can also be transected continuing the top-to-bottom transection of the proximal transverse colon mesentery. Proper dissection of the lateral attachments of the terminal ileum as well as the mesentery of the terminal ileum from the retroperitoneum is crucial for both fashioning an end ileostomy or performing an ileorectal anastomosis. Identification of the right ureter is also key during this step of the operation. For patients who will likely undergo an ileal J-pouch in the future, it is our preference to dissect the entire ileal mesentery up to the duodenum in order to achieve adequate intestinal length, in preparation for a minimally invasive J-pouch procedure. Care must be taken to not injure the mesentery in these patients as well, in order to preserve valuable blood supply to the terminal ileum.

Specimen Extraction

After corroborating that the entire colon is mobilized and hemostasis has been achieved, the proximal rectosigmoid staple-line is grasped with a locking laparoscopic grasper. Pneumoperitoneum is desufflated and an extraction incision is planned. It is our preference to extract the specimen through a previously marked right-sided abdominal incision (typically the 12-mm trocar site). If a hand-sewn ileorectal anastomosis is to be performed or the specimen is too large for a 3–4 cm circular incision, a Pfannenstiel or lower midline incision is placed. Commercially available wound protectors are helpful for specimen extraction.

End Ileostomy or Ileorectal Anastomosis

After dissecting the ileocecal fold or ligament of Treves, the terminal ileum is transected proximal to the ileocecal valve. This can be performed with a surgical stapler if an end ileostomy is to be performed, or sharply if an ileorectal anastomosis is planned. End ileostomy is constructed in a Brooke fashion pointing downwards to facilitate stoma pouching. Ileorectal anastomosis is typically performed by securing an EEA (circular stapler) anvil into the terminal ileum with a purse-string suture, re-insufflating pneumoperitoneum, and performing the anastomosis laparoscopically in an end-to-end fashion with an EEA stapler.

Postoperative Cares

All patients are started on a liquid diet the day of the operation and progressed as tolerated to a low residue diet on postoperative day 1. Postoperative analgesia with a narcotic-limiting strategy is highly encouraged. Parenteral antibiotics are limited to 24 h postoperative, and the urinary catheter is removed on postoperative day 1. Ileostomy patients must show proficiency in stoma cares before discharge to home.

Postoperative Sequelae

Common postoperative sequelae after total abdominal colectomy include chronic diarrhea, fecal urgency, and accidental bowel leakage. After ruling out infectious, inflammatory, and dietary etiologies; helpful interventions include bulking agents such as fiber supplements, as well as anti-diarrheal agents including loperamide, diphenoxylate/atropine, and tincture of opium. Cholestyramine is typically helpful in patients with prior cholecystectomy. For patients with IBD, endoscopic evaluation of the rectum is imperative and will dictate the need for completion proctectomy with end ileostomy or ileal pouch-anal anastomosis.

Infertility after total abdominal colectomy, especially in women, is typically not discussed preoperatively. Although female fertility has been reported to be lower than the average population in both UC and familial adenomatous polyposis (FAP) after colorectal resection [13–15], fertility has been reported to be preserved after

total abdominal colectomy with ileorectal anastomosis in UC patients [16].

The risk of rectal neoplasia and persistent inflammation is another major concern after ileorectal anastomosis and requires frequent endoscopic surveillance with biopsies, as well as regular multidisciplinary discussions.

Discussion

Laparoscopic total abdominal colectomy with or without restoration of bowel continuity is a safe and effective operation that has significant benefits over the open approach without significantly compromising functional or oncologic outcomes. This operation often requires upfront and diligent discussions with patients and a multidisciplinary team in order to optimize postoperative outcomes. Preparation with regards to the operative technique is crucial for success.

References

1. Win AK, Parry S, Parry B, Kalady MF, Macrae FA, Ahnen DJ, Young GP, Lipton L, Winship I, Boussioutas A, Young JP, Buchanan DD, Arnold J, Le Marchand L, Newcomb PA, Haile RW, Lindor NM, Gallinger S, Hopper JL, Jenkins MA. Risk of metachronous colon cancer following surgery for rectal cancer in mismatch repair gene mutation carriers. Ann Surg Oncol. 2013;20(6):1829–36.
2. Parry S, Win AK, Parry B, Macrae FA, Gurrin LC, Church JM, Baron JA, Giles GG, Leggett BA, Winship I, Lipton L, Young GP, Young JP, Lodge CJ, Southey MC, Newcomb PA, Le Marchand L, Haile RW, Lindor NM, Gallinger S, Hopper JL, Jenkins MA. Metachronous colorectal cancer risk for mismatch repair gene mutation carriers: the advantage of more extensive colon surgery. Gut. 2011;60(7):950–7.
3. Anele CC, Adegbola SO, Askari A, Rajendran A, Clark SK, Latchford A, Faiz OD. Risk of metachronous colorectal cancer following colectomy in lynch syndrome: a systematic review and meta-analysis. Color Dis. 2017;19(6):528–36.
4. Renkonen-Sinisalo L, Seppälä TT, Järvinen HJ, Mecklin JP. Subtotal colectomy for colon cancer reduces the need for subsequent surgery in lynch syndrome. Dis Colon Rectum. 2017;60(8):792–9.
5. Maser EA, Sachar DB, Kruse D, Harpaz N, Ullman T, Bauer JJ. High rates of metachronous colon cancer or dysplasia after segmental resection or subtotal colectomy in Crohn's colitis. Inflamm Bowel Dis. 2013;19(9):1827–32.

6. Pastore RL, Wolff BG, Hodge D. Total abdominal colectomy and ileorectal anastomosis for inflammatory bowel disease. Dis Colon Rectum. 1997;40(12):1455–64.
7. O'Riordan JM, O'Connor BI, Huang H, Victor JC, Gryfe R, MacRae HM, Cohen Z, McLeod RS. Long-term outcome of colectomy and ileorectal anastomosis for Crohn's colitis. Dis Colon Rectum. 2011;54(11):1347–54.
8. Chung TP, Fleshman JW, Birnbaum EH, Hunt SR, Dietz DW, Read TE, Mutch MG. Laparoscopic vs. open total abdominal colectomy for severe colitis: impact on recovery and subsequent completion restorative proctectomy. Dis Colon Rectum. 2009;52(1):4–10.
9. Onder A, Benlice C, Church J, Kessler H, Gorgun E. Short-term outcomes of laparoscopic versus open total colectomy with ileorectal anastomosis: a case-matched analysis from a nationwide database. Tech Coloproctol. 2016;20(11):767–73.
10. Pokala N, Delaney CP, Senagore AJ, Brady KM, Fazio VW. Laparoscopic vs open total colectomy: a case-matched comparative study. Surg Endosc. 2005;19(4):531–5.
11. Keller DS, Delaney CP, Hashemi L, Haas EM. A national evaluation of clinical and economic outcomes in open versus laparoscopic colorectal surgery. Surg Endosc. 2016;30(10):4220–8.
12. Noblett SE, Horgan AF. A prospective case-matched comparison of clinical and financial outcomes of open versus laparoscopic colorectal resection. Surg Endosc. 2007;21(3):404–8.
13. Ørding Olsen K, Juul S, Berndtsson I, Oresland T, Laurberg S. Ulcerative colitis: female fecundity before diagnosis, during disease, and after surgery compared with a population sample. Gastroenterology. 2002;122(1):15–9.
14. Olsen KO, Joelsson M, Laurberg S, Oresland T. Fertility after ileal pouch-anal anastomosis in women with ulcerative colitis. Br J Surg. 1999;86(4):493–5.
15. Olsen KØ, Juul S, Bülow S, Järvinen HJ, Bakka A, Björk J, Oresland T, Laurberg S. Female fecundity before and after operation for familial adenomatous polyposis. Br J Surg. 2003;90(2):227–31.
16. Mortier PE, Gambiez L, Karoui M, Cortot A, Paris JC, Quandalle P, Colombel JF. Colectomy with ileorectal anastomosis preserves female fertility in ulcerative colitis. Gastroenterol Clin Biol. 2006;30(4):594–7.

Robotic Total Abdominal Colectomy: A Step-by-Step Approach

Rosa Jimenez-Rodriguez, Felipe Quezada-Diaz, and Julio Garcia-Aguilar

Introduction

The use of robotic surgery for segmental colon resection has increased worldwide due to the enhanced three-dimensional visualization and improved dexterity of the robotic platform. While the literature suggests that the robotic approach may be associated with reduced conversion rates and lower morbidity compared to laparoscopic surgery, the robotic approach seems to be associated with longer operative time and higher hospital costs [1–3].

The numbers of segmental colectomies and proctectomies performed with the robotic platform are increasing worldwide [4, 5], but the number of total colectomies performed robotically is limited due to the need to reposition the patient-side surgical cart to access both sides of the abdomen [4, 6–8]. The new da Vinci Xi system, in which all arms are anchored in a single boom, facilitates working in all four quadrants of the abdomen without the need to reposition the patient-side cart, which can be placed between the patient's legs, allowing rotation of the boom from left to right and permitting precise work on both sides of the abdomen. Placing the boom in the midline oriented towards the patient's feet facilitates access to all four quadrants of the abdomen and the pelvis.

Indications for Robotic Total Colectomy

Apart from emergency conditions, total colectomy could be indicated for familial adenomatous polyposis (FAP), Lynch syndrome, or synchronous tumors in which the conservation of small portions of the colon is not possible. Other common indications for total abdominal colectomy is inflammatory bowel disease (IBD), i.e., Crohn's or ulcerative colitis when there is no response to medical treatment or because of the development of complications.

Preoperative Planning

Total colectomy is a major surgical procedure and the patient should be informed and the consent should be obtained. Patients must be informed of possible long-term outcomes. A stoma site should be marked by a stoma nurse specialist. Antibiotics and heparin should be

Electronic supplementary material The online version of this chapter (https://doi.org/10.1007/978-3-030-18740-8_25) contains supplementary material, which is available to authorized users.

R. Jimenez-Rodriguez (✉) · F. Quezada-Diaz
Department of Surgery Colorectal Service,
Memorial Sloan Kettering Cancer Center,
New York, NY, USA

J. Garcia-Aguilar
Department of Surgery, Memorial Sloan Kettering
Cancer Center, New York, NY, USA
e-mail: garciaaj@mskcc.org

administered according to the protocol of each center.

Operative Technique

Anatomical Considerations

For total abdominal colectomy, branches of the superior mesenteric artery should be divided, with the ileocecal and right colic vessels first and then followed by the middle colic vessels. The inferior mesenteric artery could be divided at its origin or the superior rectal artery can be preserved. The mobilization of the mesentery of colon should be done through embryological planes so a central vascular tie could be performed to completely remove all apical nodes along vessels in case of oncological surgery. The removal of the mesentery with complete peritoneal fascia is also important to avoid bleeding and disruption of tumor drainage vessels.

Operation Room Configuration

One of the primary disadvantages of the da Vinci robot is the size of their components: the patient-side cart, the console, and the cart for the ERBE VIO dV platform. As such, proper configuration of the operating room is essential.

For robotic total abdominal colectomy, the patient-side cart should be placed between the legs of the patient. From there and turning the boom where the arms are anchored, the surgeon will have access to the right side first and the left side second (Fig. 25.1). When pelvic dissection is needed, the boom should be rotated to face the rectum, keeping the patient-side cart in its original place between the legs of the patient (Fig. 25.2). The assistant surgeon can be placed on the left or right side of the patient, depending on the quadrant in which the surgeon is working. The patient should be placed in lithotomy position, with the legs flexed and the arms tucked. The patient should be secured to the bed

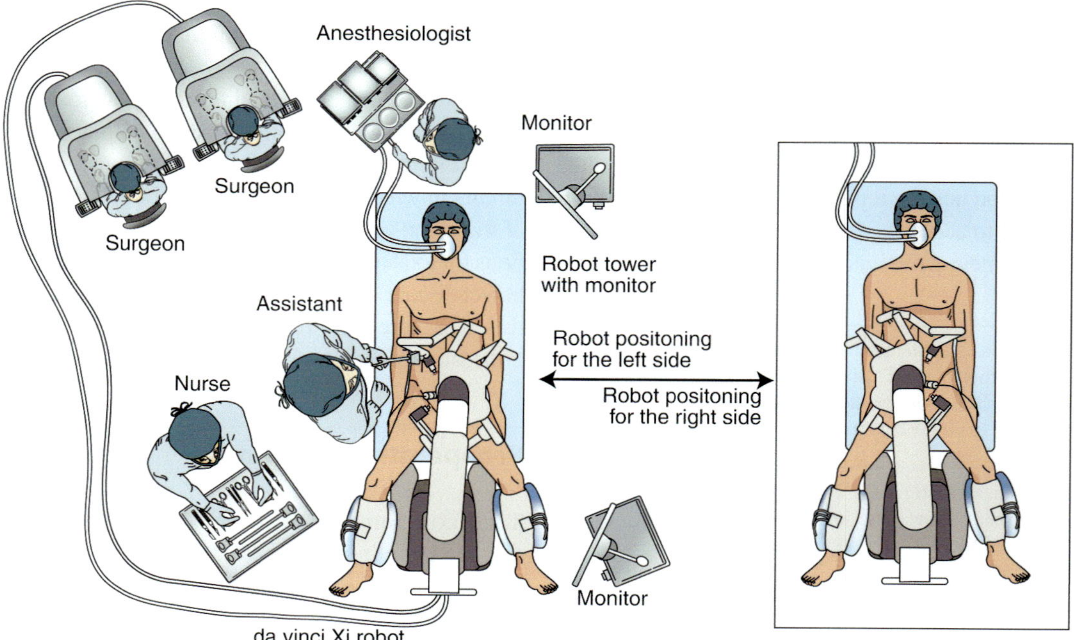

Fig. 25.1 Patient positioning and robotic setup for total colectomy. The patient-side surgical cart is placed between the patient's legs and the boom is rotated to the right or left, depending on the operative steps

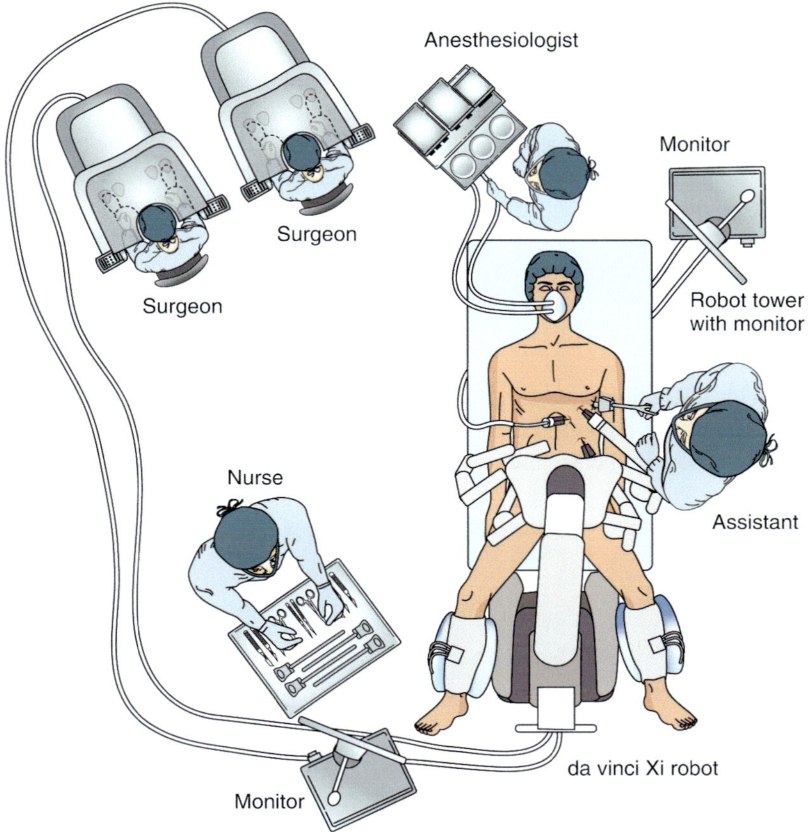

Fig. 25.2 Patient positioning and robotic setup for pelvic dissection during total colectomy. The boom is rotated to face the pelvis for this operative step

with straps around the chest and legs and shoulder pads to prevent the patient from sliding when the bed is tilted.

Trocar Positioning

For the robotic procedure, the patient is placed in modified lithotomy position with the legs in Allen stirrups. After pneumoperitoneum is created with a Veress needle in the left subcostal space, a total of seven ports are placed as shown in Fig. 25.3. A 12-mm port is placed in the right iliac fossa; 8-mm ports are placed in the umbilical region, in the left iliac fossa, and in the right and left upper quadrants; and 5-mm ports are placed in the right and left flanks. After the patient is placed in 10 ° Trendelenburg position with 15 ° right-side tilt, the patient-side surgical cart is positioned between the legs of the patient and docked.

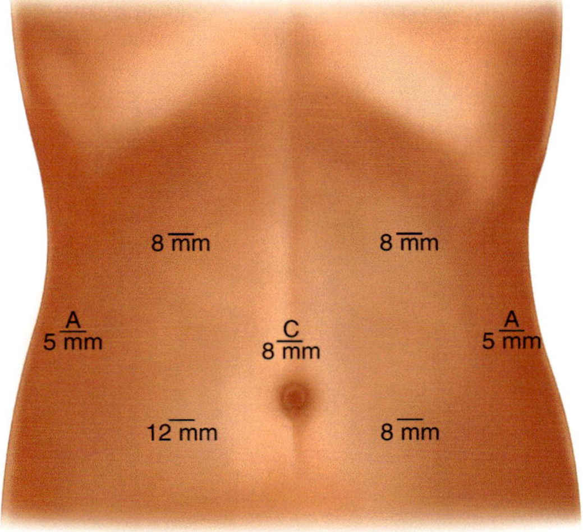

Fig. 25.3 Trocar/port position for robotic total colectomy

Surgical Field

As with many other procedures, a general view of the abdominal cavity is recommended to identify metastasis in solid organs or in the peritoneum. This diagnostic step should be completed before docking the robot.

Right Side

Video 25.1

With the patient-side surgical cart in between the legs of the patient, the procedure begins on the right side with entry into the retroperitoneum in the avascular portion of the mesentery between the superior mesenteric artery and the ileocolic vessels (Fig. 25.4). After the retroperitoneal structures including the third portion of the duodenum and the pancreas are gently pushed posteriorly (Fig. 25.5), the ileocolic vessels are isolated and divided close to their origin. Dissection proceeds along the superior mesenteric vein axis to identify the right colic artery (Fig. 25.6) and vein (when present) and the middle colic artery and vein. All vascular pedicles are controlled with either the robotic vessel sealer or Hem-o-lok clips based on surgeon preference. The mesentery of the right colon is mobilized from medial to lateral, leaving behind the pancreas, duode-

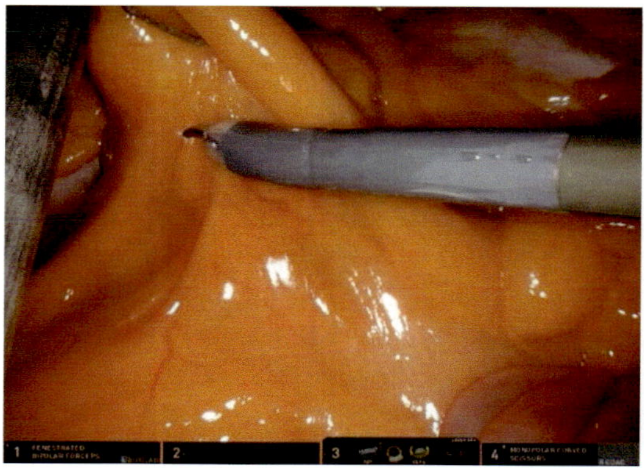

Fig. 25.4 Intraoperative image demonstrating identification of the ileocecal vessels. The dissection is performed with scissors and monopolar energy instrument

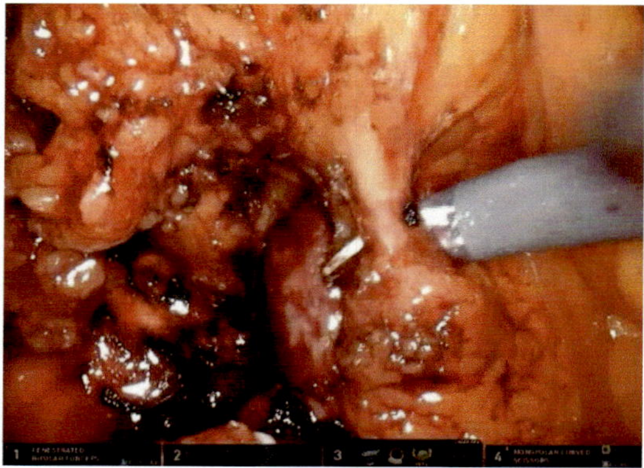

Fig. 25.6 Intraoperative image revealing dissection of the right colic artery with robotic scissors and monopolar energy instrument. The superior mesenteric vein is in the background

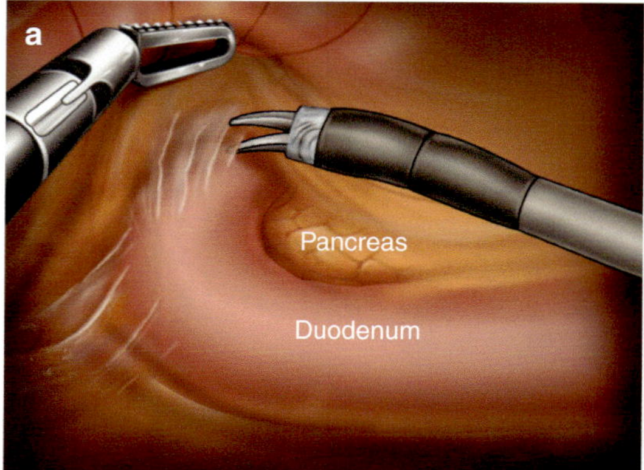

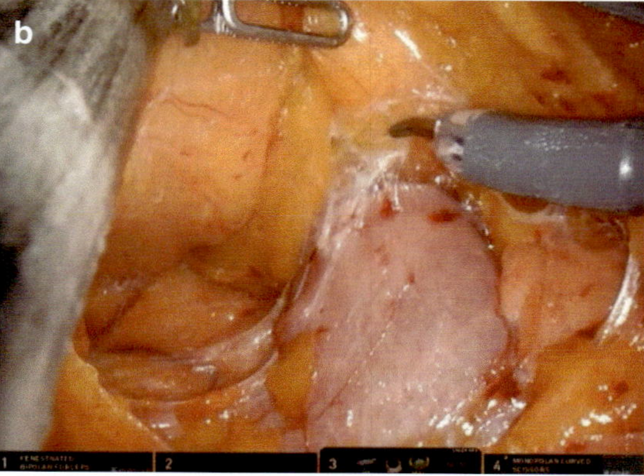

Fig. 25.5 (**a**) Illustration showing medial to lateral dissection of the right colon with identification of the duodenum and pancreas in the retroperitoneum. (**b**) Paired intraoperative image demonstrating medial to lateral dissection with identification of the duodenum and pancreas by dissection through embryological planes and maintaining the integrity of the mesentery

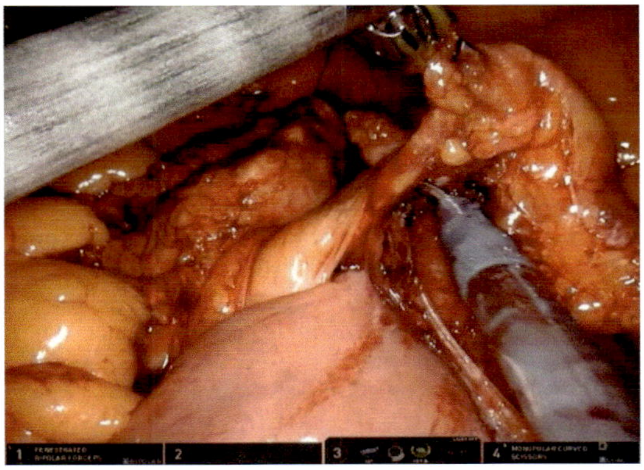

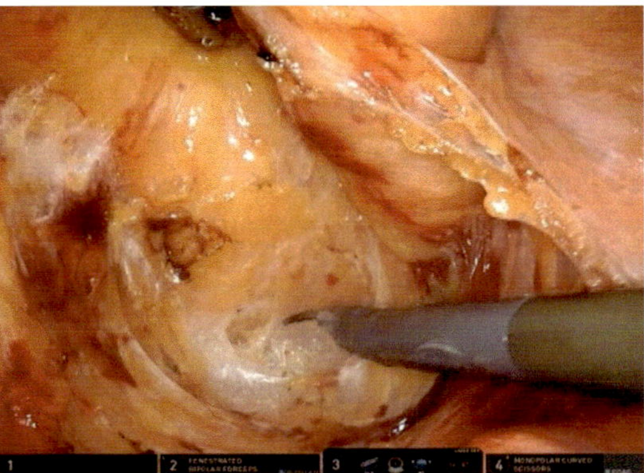

Fig. 25.7 Intraoperative image depicting dissection of the inferior mesenteric vein to mobilize the left colon and splenic flexure

Fig. 25.8 Intraoperative image showing the posterior plane of mesorectal excision

num, and retroperitoneal structures. The omentum is then opened to enter the lesser sac and complete the mobilization of the right colon. For patients receiving an end ileostomy, the terminal ileum is divided with an EndoWrist stapler.

Left Side

The arms of the robot are then detached from the trocars, the boom is rotated 180° without moving the patient-side cart (Fig. 25.1), and the patient is repositioned with maintenance of Trendelenburg position but with the left side of the patient tilted 15° upward. The robotic arms are then connected to the trocars without moving the patient-side surgical cart. The inferior mesenteric artery and vein are divided (Fig. 25.7), and a medial-to-lateral approach is used to detach the left mesocolon from the pancreas tail, the ureter, and gonadal vessels. The left paracolic gutter is opened to the splenic flexure, which is taken down. The omentum is completely disconnected from the left side of the transverse colon until the transverse colon is also completely released.

Pelvic Dissection

If proctectomy is needed at this point, the robotic arms are detached, the patient is placed in 25 ° Trendelenburg position without lateral tilt, and the boom is turned to face the pelvis (Fig. 25.2). Total mesorectal excision is carried out to the pelvic floor with sparing of sympathetic and parasympathetic nerves (Fig. 25.8). If coloanal anastomosis is performed, intersphincteric dissection starting at the intersphincteric groove is made, and the specimen is extracted through the anus. If proctectomy is not needed, the robotic stapler is used to divide the superior rectum or distal sigmoid, and a transverse incision is made to extract the specimen and prepare the ileum for anastomosis.

Postoperative Management and Complications

Postoperative care for robotic total abdominal colectomy, as well as other procedures follows a routine protocol at our hospital, Memorial Sloan Kettering Cancer Center. Patients undergo an enhanced-recovery program with early oral ingestion, ambulation, and standardized pain control strategy. The urinary catheter is removed on postoperative day 2 and the drainage is maintained until the amount of fluid is minimal. Abdominal sutures should be removed in 7–10 days after surgery. Special care should be taken regarding strenuous physical activity. In case of leakage an aggressive management of dehiscence with early intervention with or without surgical approach should be conducted.

Conclusions

The da Vinci Xi robotic platform may overcome some of the disadvantages of older-generation platforms and is associated with similar operative time for this specific complex colorectal operation.

References

1. D'Annibale A, Morpurgo E, Fiscon V, et al. Robotic and laparoscopic surgery for treatment of colorectal diseases. Dis Colon Rectum. 2004;47:2162–8.
2. Hellan M, Anderson C, Ellenhorn JD, et al. Short-term outcomes after robotic-assisted total mesorectal excision for rectal cancer. Ann Surg Oncol. 2007;14:3168–73.
3. Zhang X, Wei Z, Bie M, et al. Robot-assisted versus laparoscopic-assisted surgery for colorectal cancer: a meta-analysis. Surg Endosc. 2006;30:5601–14.
4. Moghadamyeghaneh Z, Hanna MH, Carmichael JC, et al. Comparison of open, laparoscopic, and robotic approaches for total abdominal colectomy. Surg Endosc. 2016;30:2792–8.
5. Hanai T, Maeda K, Masumori K, et al. Technique of robotic-assisted total proctocolectomy with lymphadenectomy and Ileal pouch-anal anastomosis for transverse colitic cancer of ulcerative colitis, using the single cart position. Surg Technol Int. 2015;27:86–92.
6. Baik SH, Kwon HY, Kim JS, et al. Robotic versus laparoscopic low anterior resection of rectal cancer: short-term outcome of a prospective comparative study. Ann Surg Oncol. 2009;16:1480–7.
7. Heemskerk J, de Hoog DE, van Gemert WG, et al. Robot-assisted vs. conventional laparoscopic rectopexy for rectal prolapse: a comparative study on costs and time. Dis Colon Rectum. 2007;50:1825–30.
8. Prete FP, Pezzolla A, Prete F, et al. Robotic versus laparoscopic minimally invasive surgery for rectal cancer: a systematic review and meta-analysis of randomized controlled trials. Ann Surg. 2018;267:1034–46.

Amy L. Lightner and David W. Larson

Introduction

Since its introduction in 1978 by Parks and Nicholls [1], restorative proctocolectomy with ileal pouch-anal anastomosis (IPAA) has become the procedure of choice for ulcerative colitis (UC) and familial adenomatous polyposis (FAP) [2]. The operation is traditionally performed in two or three stages by using either an open, hand-assisted laparoscopic, or totally laparoscopic approach. In the past decade, the use of laparoscopy has greatly increased due to shorter post-operative length of stay [3, 4], improved body image [5], decreased infertility rates [6, 7], and decreased intravenous narcotic use [3].

In recent years, the da Vinci robot (Intuitive Surgical, Sunnyvale, CA) has become an increasingly popular and accepted modality in colorectal surgery for both benign and malignant conditions [8, 9]. Many studies including meta-analyses

Electronic supplementary material The online version of this chapter (https://doi.org/10.1007/978-3-030-18740-8_26) contains supplementary material, which is available to authorized users.

A. L. Lightner (✉)
Cleveland Clinic, Colorectal Surgery,
Cleveland, OH, USA
e-mail: lightna@ccf.org

D. W. Larson
Mayo Clinic, Colon and Rectal Surgery,
Rochester, MN, USA
e-mail: larson.david2@mayo.edu

have now reported equivalent safety and efficacy with a robotic approach in colorectal operations as compared to conventional laparoscopy [10]. The improved dexterity, visualization, and ergonomics of the robotic platform have contributed to the surge in robotics in rectal cancer. This same surge in use may be observed in surgeons performing IPAAs in the coming years despite possible increased costs [11] and lack of hepatic feedback [12, 13]. Herein, we describe our technique for robotic IPAA and highlight steps that may require intraoperative troubleshooting.

Two- Versus Three-Stage IPAA

Traditionally, IPAA was performed as a two-stage operation. The first stage was total proctocolectomy with diverting loop ileostomy, and the second stage was reversal of the protective diverting loop ileostomy. In the era of biologic therapy, an increasing number of IPAAs are performed as a three-stage procedure due to increased patient immunosuppression, anemia, and malnutrition. In a three-stage approach, the first stage is subtotal colectomy with end ileostomy, the second stage is completion proctectomy with IPAA and diverting loop ileostomy, and the third stage is reversal of diverting ileostomy. For the purposes of our discussion, we will describe a three-stage approach with the robotic IPAA as the second stage of surgery. Thus, patients will have previously undergone subtotal colectomy with end ileostomy.

J. Kim, J. Garcia-Aguilar (eds.), *Minimally Invasive Surgical Techniques for Cancers of the Gastrointestinal Tract*, https://doi.org/10.1007/978-3-030-18740-8_26

Construction of the Pouch

After induction with general anesthesia, the patient is placed into combined lithotomy position with both arms tucked. Prior to robotic port placement, the terminal ileostomy is incised in its circumference to the peritoneum by using sharp dissection and electrocautery. Once dissected to the level of the fascia, a linear stapler is used to seal the terminal ileum. The distal ileum is exteriorized through the ileostomy site. Approximately 16–20 cm proximal from the distal ileal staple line, the bowel is opened on the antimesenteric side with electrocautery. This marks the apex of the pouch. A 15–20 cm J pouch is constructed using two firings of the 100 mm extracorporeal linear staples (GIA100, Covidien; Boulder, CO). A 2-0 nylon suture is placed as a purse-string, and the anvil to the circular stapler (EEA 25, 27 or 29 mm) is then placed into the apex (Fig. 26.1). The blind limb of the pouch and the linear staple line is then oversewn with 3-0 silk sutures. Once created, the anvil and pouch are both dropped back into the abdomen and the 15-mm balloon trocar is placed in the ileostomy site for insufflation.

Patient Positioning and Port Placement

The 15-mm balloon trocar serves as an accessory port for the assistant. A 30 ° angle camera is then placed into this port. Four robotic ports are then placed under direct visualization in a transverse fashion across the abdomen approximately 20 cm from the pubis, with each port 8–10 cm apart for the S and Si system and 6–8 cm apart for the Xi system to avoid external or internal collisions (Fig. 26.2).

Critical issues to consider when placing ports are the distance to the target anatomy, and the potential for bony aspects of the pelvic sidewall and sacral promontory to impede surgical dissection. For example, the robotic monopolar scissors is 57 cm in length with a working length of 27 cm from the remote center to the tip. Therefore, trocars that are placed too far cephalad in a patient with a long torso will increase the difficulty of the presacral dissection because of the lack of reach toward the pelvic floor. Likewise, the sacral promontory can act as a fulcrum and lead to poor angles of dissection in the presacral space. Finally, trocars placed too far laterally (particularly in male patients)

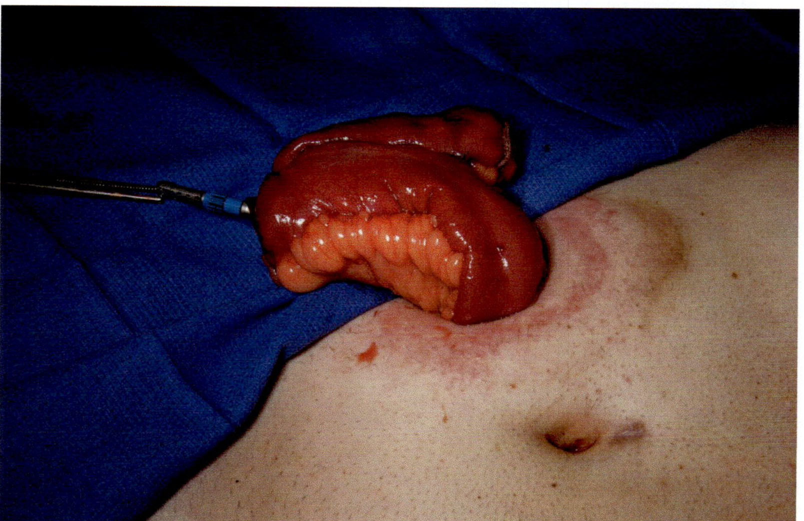

Fig. 26.1 Construction of the ileal pouch through the previous ileostomy site

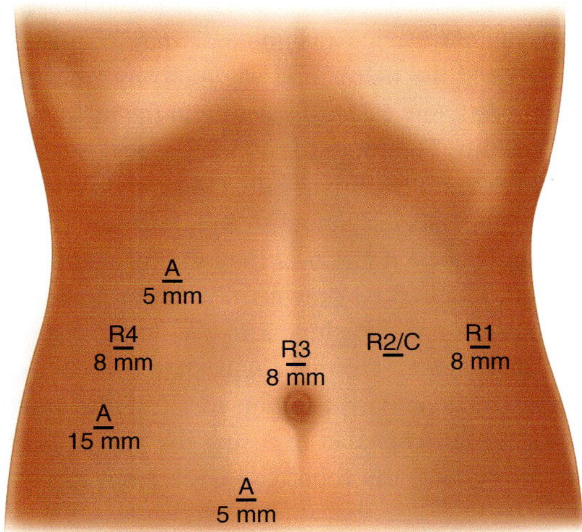

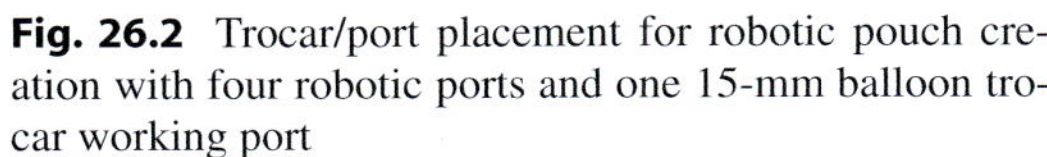

Fig. 26.2 Trocar/port placement for robotic pouch creation with four robotic ports and one 15-mm balloon trocar working port

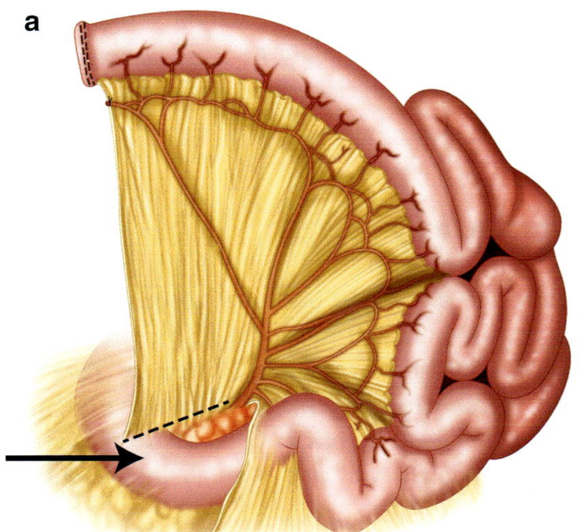

will increase the difficulty of the low pelvic dissection secondary to collisions with the lateral pelvic sidewall.

Surgical Technique

Mobilization of the Mesentery

The length of the mesentery will determine the ability to construct a pouch. Inability to construct a pouch is associated with increased body mass index (BMI), likely due to the foreshortening of the mesentery [14]. With mobilization and stair stepping of the mesentery, additional length can be gained and will likely be required to prevent tension on the pouch anastomosis. This portion of the operation can be performed laparoscopically through the robotic trocars with methods previously described [15–18]. The first step is mobilizing the lateral attachments in a cephalad direction until the inferior border of the duodenum and pancreas are reached (Fig. 26.3a), making sure to identify and protect the superior mesenteric artery (SMA). If reach remains inadequate, a series of stepwise incisions on the anterior and posterior mesentery can be made to increase mesenteric length (Fig. 26.3b) using

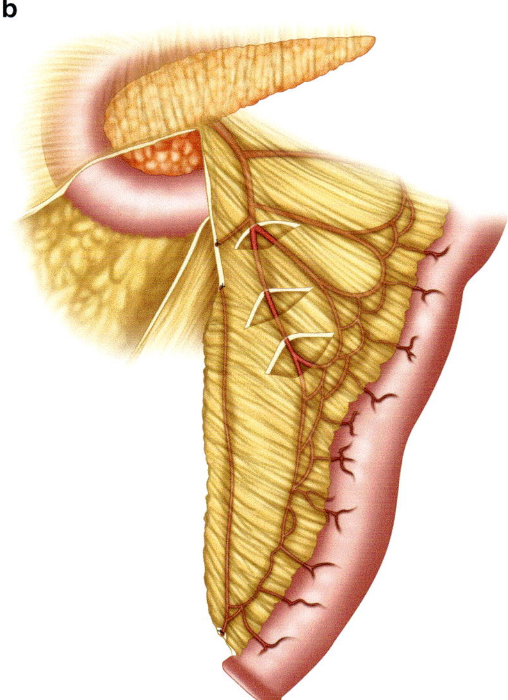

Fig. 26.3 (**a**) The first step in mesenteric mobilization is mobilizing the lateral attachments cephalad until the inferior border of the duodenum (black arrow) and pancreas are reached. (**b**) A series of stepwise incisions on the anterior and posterior mesentery can be made to increase mesenteric length

electrocautery to score the mesentery superficial to the vasculature. With this particular technique, it may be necessary for these peritoneal incisions to be made prior to pouch creation, if there is any concern that reach might be an issue (especially with male patients, increased BMI, and increased height).

Proctectomy

Once the mesentery has been adequately mobilized, the attention is turned to the proctetomy portion of the operation. In female patients, the uterus can be retracted toward the anterior abdominal wall by placing a Keith needle across the abdominal wall and through the fundus or round ligaments of the uterus. Alternatively, a transvaginal uterine manipulator may be placed to suspend the uterus and vagina away from the rectum to allow easier dissection in the rectovaginal septum. The robot (da Vinci Surgical System, Intuitive Surgical; Sunnyvale, CA) is then docked on the patient's left lateral side (Fig. 26.4). The Si system is docked just over the left hip such that a straight line can be drawn from the midpoint of the camera arm attachment to the anterior superior iliac spine. The patient is then placed into steep Trendelenburg position to allow the small bowel to fall cephalad exposing the pelvis. With the Xi system, the robot can dock from the left

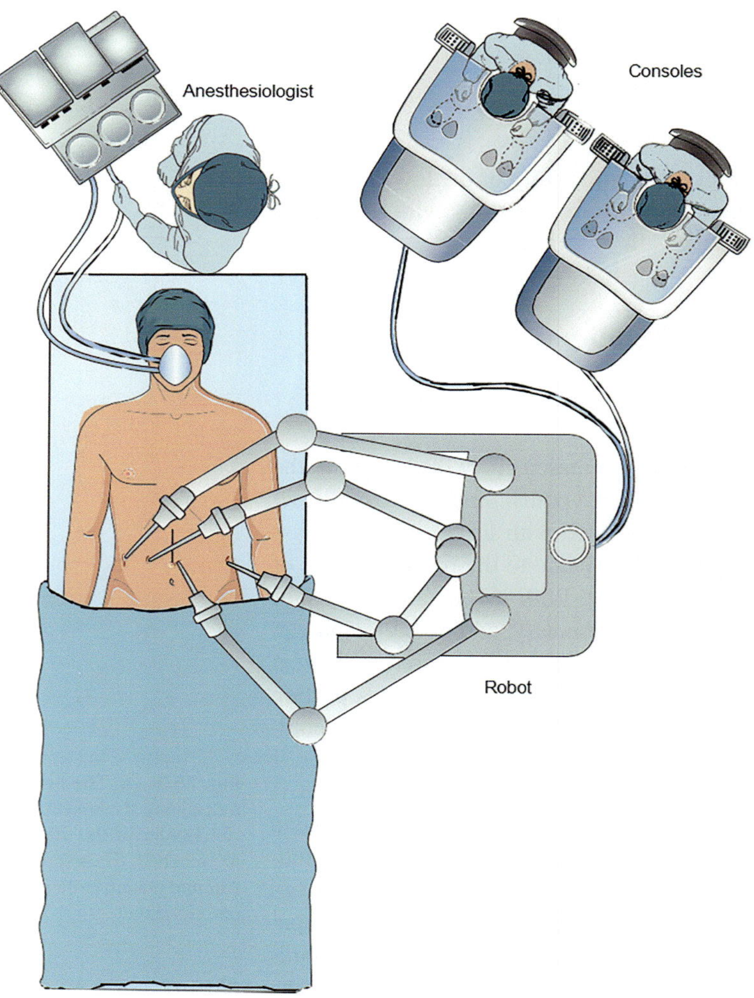

Fig. 26.4 Patient positioning and operating room setup for robotic pouch creation with the Da Vinci Xi platform

side of the patient. With the camera focused on the pelvis, the robot will automatically rotate to the proper position. The robotic scissors are placed in arm 1, the camera in arm 2, the bipolar fenestrated forceps in arm 3, and small grasper in arm 4.

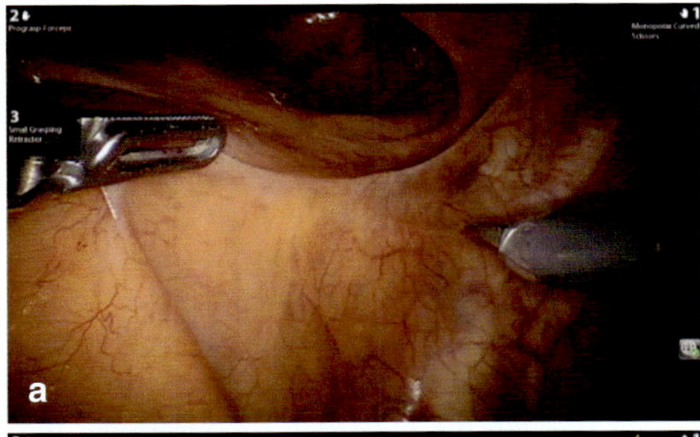

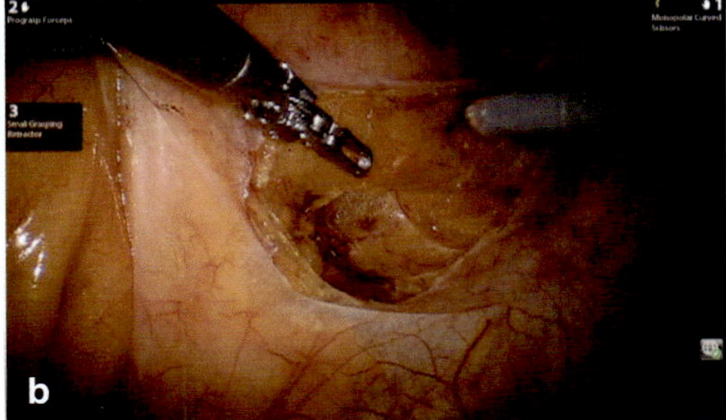

Fig. 26.5 (**a**) Robotic forceps are used to place the peritoneum overlying the right pelvic gutter on stretch to enable safe scoring of the peritoneum with robotic monopolar scissors. (**b**) An avascular plane has been developed along the right pelvic gutter using the robotic forceps and scissors

The top of the rectal stump and the sacral promontory are identified, with the ureter and iliac vessels on the patient's right side. The proctectomy begins by entering the presacral space from the right side. The dissection is initiated by lifting the rectum such that the peritoneum overlying the right pelvic gutter is placed on tension and the monopolar scissors are then used to score the peritoneum (Fig. 26.5a). A filmy, avascular plane should be revealed which can be followed posteriorly and to the contralateral side, lifting the mesentery anteriorly and keeping the retroperitoneal structures posteriorly (Fig. 26.5b). The posterior dissection is continued toward the pelvic floor and then extended to the contralateral side, identifying the left ureter, gonadal vessels, and iliac vessels. The superior hypogastric nerves are also identified during the dissection, and they are preserved by gently sweeping them posteriorly toward the sacrum. Once the posterior space has been dissected, the lateral stalks are taken while appreciating both right and left ureters. The mesentery (which includes the remaining superior rectal artery) is divided using the robotic Vessel Sealer (Intuitive Surgical).

The anterior dissection is performed last (Fig. 26.6). Arm 3 is used to pull the rectal stump out of the pelvis and with posterior retraction to provide proper tension on the anterior structures. The assistant aids the dissection by placing a suction device or grasper at the level of the seminal vesicles or posterior vagina and lifting

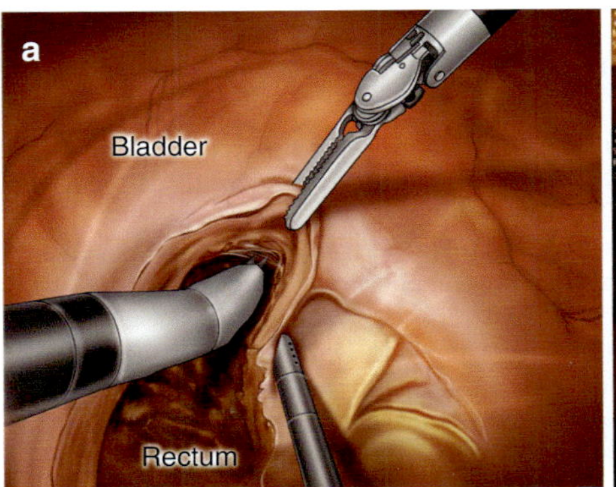

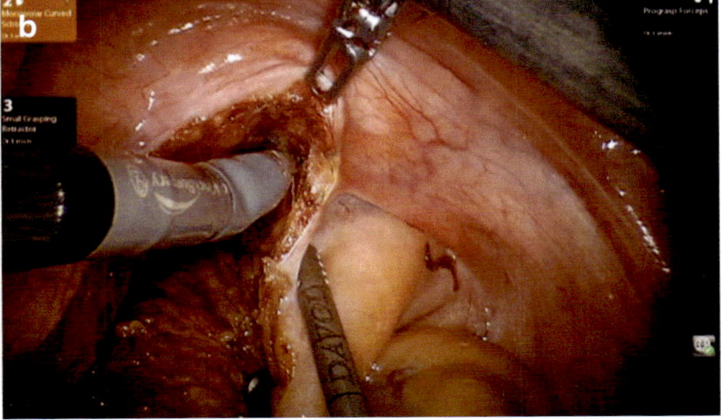

Fig. 26.6 (**a**) Illustration showing the last step of pelvic dissection. (**b**) Paired intraoperative image showing anterior dissection that is performed after the posterior and lateral dissections have been completed. This step is performed using the robotic scissors in arm 2 and forceps in arm 1

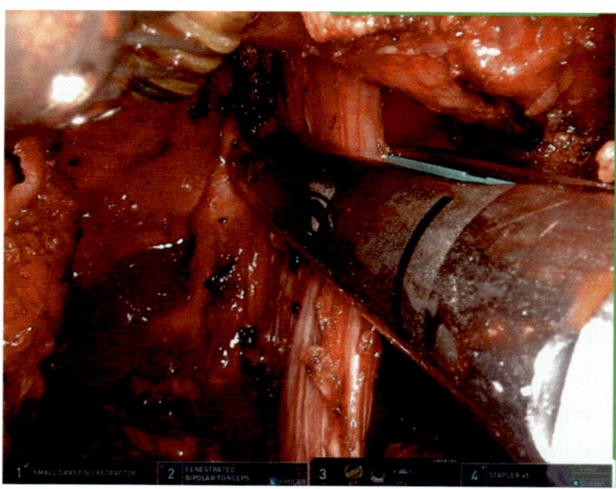

Fig. 26.7 Upon completion of dissection, the rectum is skeletonized at the pelvic floor. A robotic stapler is used to fire a 60 mm green cartridge across the lower rectum, just above the pelvic floor

anteriorly. This counter-traction anterior to the rectum allows the dissection to progress to the level of the pelvic floor. Once the pelvic floor has been identified, the rectum is digitally examined by transanal approach to assess adequate dissection and to ensure that the anastomosis will be performed approximately 1–2 cm above the dentate line. The rectum is then stapled 1–1.5 cm above the dentate line using an endoscopic stapling device (iDrive Ultra, Covidien) (Fig. 26.7). The specimen is extracted through the ileostomy site after the IPAA has been stapled to the anal canal and prior to creation of the loop ileostomy.

Construction of the Anastomosis

Moving the transected rectum out of the pelvis, the pouch is connected to the anus under robotic visualization. Under robotic control the pouch and the anvil are brought toward the pelvis. A series of rectal dilators are inserted into the anal canal followed by the EEA 29-mm stapler. The stapler pin is deployed and it is connected to the anvil under direct robotic visualization (Video 26.1). Once the pouch

has been successfully connected to the anus, the patient is placed into reverse Trendelenburg position and irrigation is placed into the pelvis. Proctoscopic visualization and insufflation of the pouch under saline may assure the surgeon that there is no leak.

Diverting Loop Ileostomy

A diverting loop ileostomy is fashioned at the previous ileostomy site to protect the IPAA. A site is picked proximal to the pouch inlet that allows no tension to be placed on the pouch. This is typically 25–50 cm proximal from the pouch inlet. A 19-Fr abdominal drainage catheter is then placed through the left-sided robotic trocar into the pelvis.

Conclusions

A robotic approach provides the additional tools for minimally invasive approach to IPAA. While there are no randomized studies comparing robotic and laparoscopic IPAA, the known advantages of the robotic platform include improved visualization of neurovascular bundles, especially in a narrow male pelvis, and improved ergonomics. In the near future, the robotic approach has the potential to become the preferred minimally invasive approach for IPAA.

References

1. Parks AG, Nicholls RJ. Proctocolectomy without ileostomy for ulcerative colitis. Br Med J. 1978;2:85–8.
2. Fazio VW, Ziv Y, Church JM, et al. Ileal pouch-anal anastomoses complications and function in 1005 patients. Ann Surg. 1995;222:120–7.
3. Larson DW, Cima RR, Dozois EJ, et al. Safety, feasibility, and short-term outcomes of laparoscopic ileal-pouch-anal anastomosis: a single institutional case-matched experience. Ann Surg. 2006;243:667–70; discussion 670–662.

4. White I, Jenkins JT, Coomber R, et al. Outcomes of laparoscopic and open restorative proctocolectomy. Br J Surg. 2014;101:1160–5.
5. Ahmed Ali U, Keus F, Heikens JT, et al. Open versus laparoscopic (assisted) ileo pouch anal anastomosis for ulcerative colitis and familial adenomatous polyposis. Cochrane Database Syst Rev. 2009;1:CD006267.
6. Bartels SA, D'Hoore A, Cuesta MA, et al. Significantly increased pregnancy rates after laparoscopic restorative proctocolectomy: a cross-sectional study. Ann Surg. 2012;256:1045–8.
7. Beyer-Berjot L, Maggiori L, Birnbaum D, et al. A total laparoscopic approach reduces the infertility rate after ileal pouch-anal anastomosis: a 2-center study. Ann Surg. 2013;258:275–82.
8. Yang Y, Wang F, Zhang P, et al. Robot-assisted versus conventional laparoscopic surgery for colorectal disease, focusing on rectal cancer: a meta-analysis. Ann Surg Oncol. 2012;19:3727–36.
9. Juo YY, Hyder O, Haider AH, et al. Is minimally invasive colon resection better than traditional approaches?: first comprehensive national examination with propensity score matching. JAMA Surg. 2014;149:177–84.
10. Trinh BB, Jackson NR, Hauch AT, et al. Robotic versus laparoscopic colorectal surgery. J Soc Laparoendosc Surg. 2014;18:816–30.
11. Tyler JA, Fox JP, Desai MM, et al. Outcomes and costs associated with robotic colectomy in the minimally invasive era. Dis Colon Rectum. 2013;56:458–66.
12. Rawlings AL, Woodland JH, Vegunta RK, et al. Robotic versus laparoscopic colectomy. Surg Endosc. 2007;21:1701–8.
13. Bertani E, Chiappa A, Biffi R, et al. Assessing appropriateness for elective colorectal cancer surgery: clinical, oncological, and quality-of-life short-term outcomes employing different treatment approaches. Int J Color Dis. 2011;26:1317–27.
14. Khasawneh MA, McKenna NP, Abdelsattar ZM, et al. Impact of BMI on ability to successfully create an IPAA. Dis Colon Rectum. 2016;59:1034–8.
15. Burnstein MJ, Schoetz DJ Jr, Coller JA, et al. Technique of mesenteric lengthening in ileal reservoir-anal anastomosis. Dis Colon Rectum. 1987;30:863–6.
16. Araki T, Parc Y, Lefevre J, et al. The effect on morbidity of mesentery lengthening techniques and the use of a covering stoma after ileoanal pouch surgery. Dis Colon Rectum. 2006;49:621–8.
17. Martel P, Majery N, Savigny B, et al. Mesenteric lengthening in ileoanal pouch anastomosis for ulcerative colitis: is high division of the superior mesenteric pedicle a safe procedure? Dis Colon Rectum. 1998;41:862–6; discussion 866–867.
18. Thirlby RC. Optimizing results and techniques of mesenteric lengthening in ileal pouch-anal anastomosis. Am J Surg. 1995;169:499–502.

Robotic Abdominoperineal Resection

Felipe Quezada-Diaz, Rosa Jimenez-Rodriguez, and Jesse Joshua Smith

Introduction

Abdominoperineal resection (APR) has been considered the operation of choice for lower rectal and anal canal tumors. First described by W. Ernest Miles in 1908 as a combined perineal and abdominal approach [1], APR has experienced many changes with the availability of minimally invasive techniques, but it follows the same key oncological principles. In this chapter, we describe robotic APR with different perineal approaches (lithotomy and prone) (Video 27.1).

Indications for Abdominoperineal Resection

APR is a standard treatment for adenocarcinomas that are fixed and/or infiltrate or about the anorectal ring. APR is usually indicated when the likelihood of obtaining an oncologically safe circumferential margin is low, rather than as a

distal negative-margin compromise. It is the procedure of choice for patients with persistent or recurrent anal squamous cell carcinoma after definitive chemoradiotherapy [2]. Rare cases of melanoma, sarcoma, or gastrointestinal stromal tumors may require APR. APR can also be necessary in cases of vulvar, vaginal, and/or prostate cancer. During the decision process, anal continence should be taken into consideration. APR can result in a better quality of life in patients after a low anterior resection (LAR) and poor previous anal sphincter function [3]. APR can be considered in some cases of benign disease such as familial adenomatous polyposis syndrome or inflammatory bowel disease, but it is not the standard of care.

Preoperative Planning

APR is associated with considerable morbidity, making a proper preoperative evaluation mandatory. A digital rectal exam is necessary to evaluate the tumor mobility and distance from the anorectal ring. MRI is an excellent modality for evaluating the relationship of the tumor to various pelvic structures and for determining the extent of the planned resection [4]. Endorectal ultrasound can also be helpful for evaluating anorectal ring infiltration when there is doubt [5].

All patients should have medical clearance prior to surgery, and a colostomy site should be

Electronic supplementary material The online version of this chapter (https://doi.org/10.1007/978-3-030-18740-8_27) contains supplementary material, which is available to authorized users.

F. Quezada-Diaz · R. Jimenez-Rodriguez
J. J. Smith (✉)
Department of Surgery Colorectal Service, Memorial Sloan Kettering Cancer Center, New York, NY, USA
e-mail: quezadaf@mskcc.org; smithj5@mskcc.org

© Springer Nature Switzerland AG 2020
J. Kim, J. Garcia-Aguilar (eds.), *Minimally Invasive Surgical Techniques for Cancers of the Gastrointestinal Tract*, https://doi.org/10.1007/978-3-030-18740-8_27

marked by a stoma therapist. Patients must be informed of possible long-term outcomes, particularly sexual and urinary dysfunction [6]. An enhanced-recovery-after-surgery protocol should be considered as standard of care postoperatively for patients undergoing APR. [7]

Operative Technique

Anatomical Considerations

The key to a successful APR is complete knowledge of the pelvic structures and pelvic floor. The pelvic floor is formed by the levator ani and coccygeus muscles, with the levator ani comprising the puborectalis, pubococcygeus, and iliococcygeus muscles. The fibers of the levator ani muscle are excised in an APR, while the coccygeus muscle is often preserved.

The rectum is usually described as the last 15 cm of the large bowel, but no clear boundaries have been defined. Internally, the rectum contains three valves, known as Houston valves, which can be used as a reference for locating rectal tumors. A more accepted and widespread method is to measure the distance of the lesion from the anal verge using a rigid or flexible scope. The anorectal junction, which is palpable at the top of the anorectal ring, is another important surgical landmark, comprising mainly the puborectalis and external sphincter muscle.

The mesorectum (mesentery of the rectum) carries all the vessels, nerves, and lymphatic drainage. It gains more prominence in the extraperitoneal portion of the rectum, becoming thick and bilobar in the posterior aspect. In its most distal part, the mesorectum narrows until it disappears at the pelvic floor. The fascia propria of the rectum varies in thickness. Anteriorly, the presence of a thin layer known as Denonvilliers' fascia separates the rectum from the urogenital structures. In the posterior aspect, a dense layer of fibrous tissue known as Waldeyer's fascia extends from the sacral vertebrae to the anorectal ring. It is very important to understand the anatomy of the posterior aspect of the rectum because

dissection should begin there and requires accurately identifying the loose connective tissue that separates the mesorectum from Waldeyer's fascia. The lateral aspects of the extraperitoneal rectum are fused with the connective tissue and nerve plexus of the pelvic sidewall, forming lateral stalks. In some patients, the accessory middle rectal vessel is located at these structures.

The arterial supply from the upper rectum comes from the superior rectal artery, which is a terminal branch of the inferior mesenteric artery (IMA). The lower rectum receives blood from the inferior rectal artery, a branch of the pudendal artery providing blood to the anal canal and anal sphincter. Venous drainage comes from the superior rectal vein, which runs with its homonymous artery and joins the left colic vein to drain into the inferior mesenteric vein (IMV). The inferior rectal vein drains directly into the internal iliac veins. The middle rectal vessels are inconsistent branches that form part of the iliac vessels.

Important factors regarding the regional nerve anatomy must be considered in planning rectal cancer surgery, because correct identification of the nerve plexus is essential for better functional outcomes. The hypogastric plexus, located at the lower aorta, contains sympathetic fibers that arise from the lumbar sympathetic trunk. At the level of the aorta bifurcation, two well-defined hypogastric nerves run over the internal iliac vessels to the pelvic sidewall [8]. At the sidewall, they merge with fibers of the parasympathetic plexus from S3 to S4, which innervates most of the pelvic urogenital structures. Pudendal nerves originate from the sacral plexus, comprising somatosensory and parasympathetic fibers that innervate the perineal region and anal sphincter.

Operating Room Configuration and Patient Positioning

One of the most important aspects to consider is operating room configuration and patient positioning. For the robotic approach, this task is

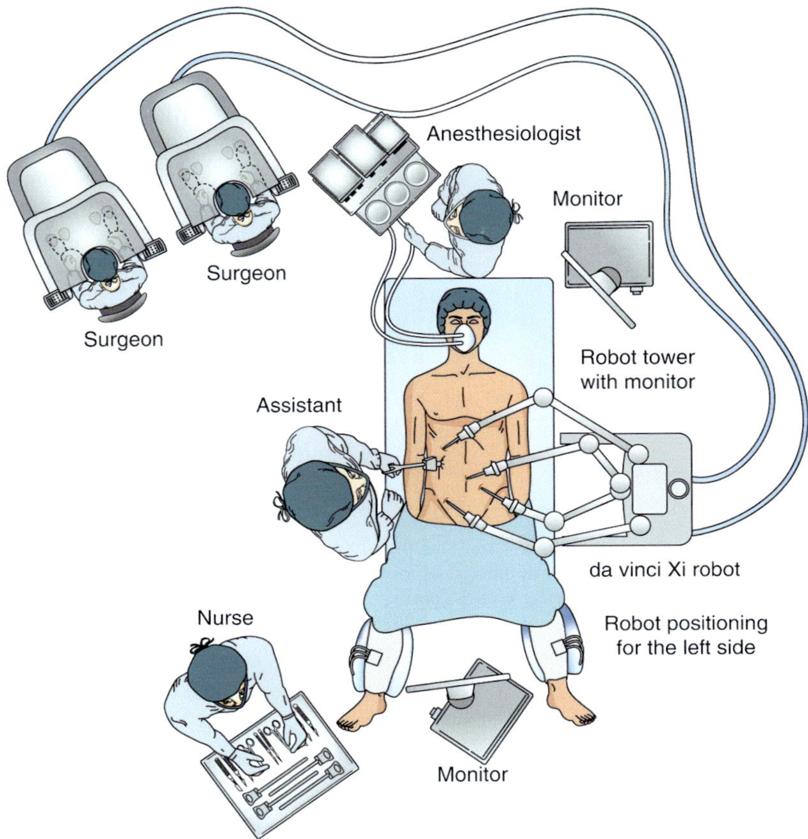

Fig. 27.1 Typical operating room setup for the abdominal portion of robotic APR at our institution

essential. The robot cart should be positioned to the left of the patient, allowing the surgeon to have direct access to the pelvis, keeping in mind that the cart should be removed before proceeding with the perineal part of the procedure (Fig. 27.1).

For the abdominal part of the surgery, the patient should be placed in the lithotomy position, with legs flexed and arms tucked in, but always ensuring easy access for the anesthesiologist. The patient should be secured to the bed with straps around the chest and legs and shoulder pads to prevent the patient from sliding when the bed is tilted. Care must be taken to protect points of pressure in order to prevent iatrogenic lesions. At Memorial Hospital, a rectal washout and closure of the anus with a silk suture are done before sterile drapes are positioned.

Trocar Positioning

Trocars should be positioned after pneumoperitoneum is established because abdominal wall distension can alter the original positioning. Once the patient is correctly positioned and anesthetized, pneumoperitoneum can be established through an open approach with a Hasson port site after a 1.5-cm midline incision or with a Veress needle in the left upper quadrant directly under the costal border. Arm 1 should be positioned in the upper right quadrant during the dissection of the IMA and superior rectal vessels. Arms 2 and 4 are used for the pelvic part of the dissection and are located as shown in Fig. 27.2. During pelvic dissection, arm 1 can be positioned in the left lower quadrant for retraction of the vagina or prostate. Trocar 3 is generally used for the camera (Fig. 27.2 C(R3)).

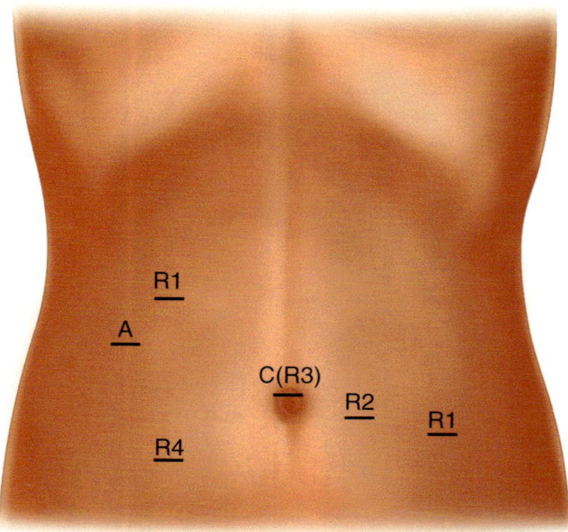

Fig. 27.2 Trocar positioning for the abdominal portion of robotic APR. Trocars are numbered according to the numbering of the robotic arms. A: assist port

Surgical Field

Once the ports are placed, a general examination is recommended to evaluate the possibility of metastatic disease in the peritoneum, liver, or any other abdominal organs. This should be done before docking the robot. Once the robot is docked and the patient positioned right side and head down, the next step is to expose the IMA, which can be found after identifying the right iliac artery and following it caudally. Proper mobilization of the small bowel from the surgical field is essential to avoid inadvertent injury/enterotomy and to facilitate IMA dissection. This occasionally requires sharp dissection and mobilization of embryologic adhesions to better expose the sacral promontory and to better visualize the target anatomy.

Inferior Mesenteric Artery Dissection

After IMA identification, one of the robotic arms should maintain tension to obtain correct exposure. A parallel incision to the right iliac artery should be done nearly perpendicular to the IMA

following the insertion into the aorta. The pneumoperitoneum will help identify the plane in which the dissection will be performed. All the periaortic and peri-mesenteric artery tissue should be removed carefully to ensure a proper oncological resection. The dissection can be done with a 0 ° camera, but a 30 ° camera can also be used. Once the plane is identified, the superior rectal artery can be elevated with an arm, and medial-to-lateral dissection can be carried out with proper identification of the ureter and gonadal vessels. This dissection can be performed with robotic scissors or with a vessel sealer although these authors prefer use of the scissors for more precise dissection. The psoas muscle should not be exposed because the ureter and gonadal structures run over this plane, and dissection here increases the risk of injury, although in very thin patients with scarce intra-abdominal fat tissue, it can be difficult to find the correct plane.

The IMA can then be divided using a conventional linear endostapler through assistant port sites, a robotic linear stapler, a vessel sealing device, or the Hem-o-lok system. Using a stapler helps avoid extreme dissection of the artery, while using Hem-o-lok facilitates identification of the artery, although more time is required for the dissection. A selective dissection of the superior rectal artery and sigmoid branches can be performed (Fig. 27.3), but a proper lymphadenectomy should be done if there is suspicious preoperative lymphadenopathy to reduce the risk of recurrence [9].

Medial-to-Lateral Dissection

After the artery is divided, the stump should be gently lifted to complete the medial-to-lateral dissection. Correct dissection here is important in order to protect autonomic nerve function. When the wall of the colon is reached, the dissection should end. The third arm, which was used to lift the colon and then the stump of the artery, should now retract the colon from the abdominal wall to expose Toldt's fascia, which should be opened to

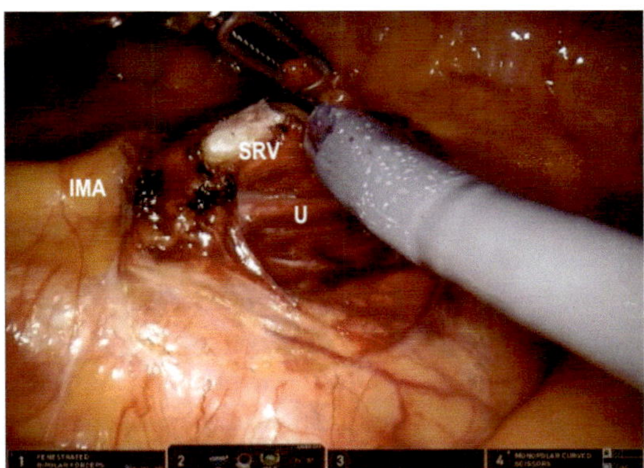

Fig. 27.3 A selective section of superior rectal vessels (SRV) can be performed, but a proper lymphadenectomy should be done if there is suspicious preoperative lymphadenopathy at the root of the inferior mesenteric artery (IMA). Clear visualization of the left ureter (U) before vascular section is essential

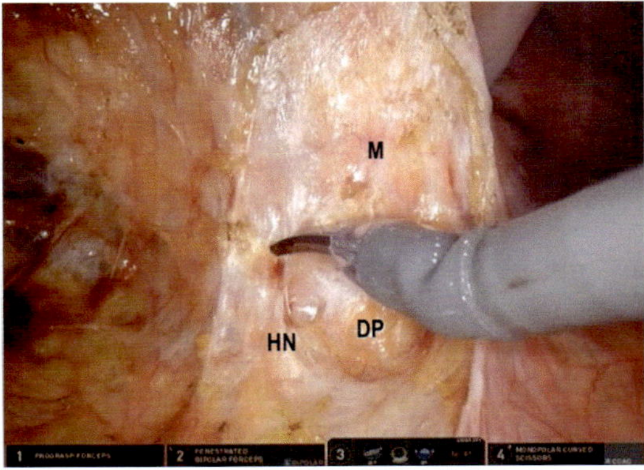

Fig. 27.4 Posterior dissection in the areolar space between the mesorectal fascia and presacral fascia. M, mesorectum; HN, hypogastric nerve; DP, dissection plane

meet the retromesocolic dissection plane. When the medial-to-lateral dissection is not done to completion, the risk to the ureter or gonadal vessels is further increased, and special attention to this step is necessary to avoid harm.

Pelvic Dissection

For dissection of the mesorectum, the importance of the third robotic arm is greater than in previous steps because this arm is used to retract the rectum and provide a correct view of the pelvis, first of the posterior mesorectal plane from the promontory to the pelvic floor and second of the lateral and anterior planes (Fig. 27.4). Pelvic peritoneum should be opened on both sides, and a sharp posterior dissection should be performed with robotic scissors. Care must be taken to avoid bleeding from the posterior venous sacral plexus and potential injury to the hypogastric nerves and lateral pelvic plexus. This plane should be dissected to the pelvic floor to avoid a cylindrical resection. Lateral mesorectal dissection can be particularly challenging, and special attention should be paid to avoid damage to neurovascular structures.

The anterior plane should be the last part of the mesorectal excision. The third arm can now be used to first lift the bladder and then the prostate or the vagina. With the anterior pelvic peritoneum now open, the dissection is extended just inferior to the cervix or the seminal vesicles. Careful dissection should be carried out with meticulous hemostasis to avoid unnecessary bleeding in the lower pelvis.

Division of the Colon and Creation of a Colostomy

Once the mesorectal excision is completed, the mesocolon and the colon should be divided. The artery stump and all the lymphovascular tissue excised should be included in the specimen. The colon should be divided with an endostapler, and tension of the proximal colon must be evaluated for the creation of a proper terminal colostomy. The surgical specimen is then abandoned in situ for extraction during the perineal phase. Pelvic drains should be secured before placing the patient in the prone position. The drains should be secured to the specimen. After examination of the abdominal cavity, with careful attention paid to dissection planes, the ports are closed and a colostomy is created at a previously marked location.

Perineal Dissection

The perineal dissection in a robotic APR can be performed with the patient in either the classic lithotomy position or a prone position. Both approaches have pros and cons, but they share the same oncological principle of exposing and sectioning the levator muscle from below. There has been some discussion regarding the degree of sectioning of the levators in the context of a standard APR. An intralevator dissection entails more medial sectioning of the levator muscles, sometimes resulting in a surgical specimen in the shape of an hourglass and increasing the risk of circumferential resection margin positivity and intraoperative perforation [10]. This technique can be the definitive treatment for smaller T1/T2 tumors, helping to preserve tissue for more effective closure of the perineal wound. For bigger tumors, a wider dissection known as extralevator APR is more appropriate. An extralevator APR produces a truly cylindrical specimen, diminishing the risk of a positive resection margin [11]. This procedure is usually associated with wider perineal defects requiring flaps and/or mesh for closure.

Perineal Lithotomy Dissection

For perineal dissection, a second tray is used in order to reduce potential contamination between surgical fields. As the patient is placed in a supine position, care should be taken to ensure that the patient's buttocks are at the very end of the table, providing good exposure of the perineum. A high lithotomy position is recommended for visualization of the levator muscles during dissection. Usually, two surgeons are needed, with an assistant helping with retraction in the anterior perineum.

An elliptical incision is made around the anus, and the dissection is carried out through the ischiorectal fat just outside the sphincter complex. Anteriorly, the dissection proceeds until the perineal body is reached. The anococcygeal ligament is used as an anatomical landmark in the posterior dissection to facilitate exposure of the levator muscles lateral to it.

One of the main advantages of the perineal approach is that it allows abdominal visualization via the robotic camera to guide dissection. Usually, the levator muscles are initially sectioned in the posterior aspect above or with the coccyx, with sectioning continuing bilaterally, creating an opening in the posterior aspect.

Anterior dissection can be difficult, especially in men with a narrow pelvis, elevating the risk of lesion in the membranous urethra and prostate. Partial extraction and eversion of the surgical specimen can facilitate the dissection, but care must be taken during manipulation not to tear or expose the tumor. In women, dissection can be completed with intermittent palpation of the posterior vaginal wall.

The use of the lithotomy position for APR also offers the advantages of shorter operative time, if two surgical teams are used, and safer access in case of major bleeding.

Perineal Prone Dissection

The use of a second operating table is ideal for minimizing the time required for patient repositioning. This table is secured and all equipment required for this portion is obtained while beginning the first portion of the operation. A large hip roll is used at the break in the table, and secondary rolls are used to support the patient's chest in order to avoid brachial nerve plexus injury (Fig. 27.5). The patient should be secured at the level of the legs and trunk. The patient's legs can be separated if a split table is used, allowing the surgeon to face the surgical site directly.

An elliptical incision is made immediately outside the lateral edge of the external sphincter and medial to the ischial tuberosity. Once the skin is open, the use of a Lone Star retractor (Cooper Surgical, Inc.) can be helpful. Anteriorly, the perineal body should be sectioned, and in the posterior dissection, the incision should be made at the midline between the coccyx and anus. For tumors that do not involve the sphincter or the levator ani muscle, a narrower incision can be made, sparing the ischiorectal fascia and facilitating wound closure. Wider resections may be necessary in cases of recurrent disease or minimal response to multimodal therapy with a bulky tumor. The dissection is made with electrocautery. A helpful maneuver is to palpate the coccyx

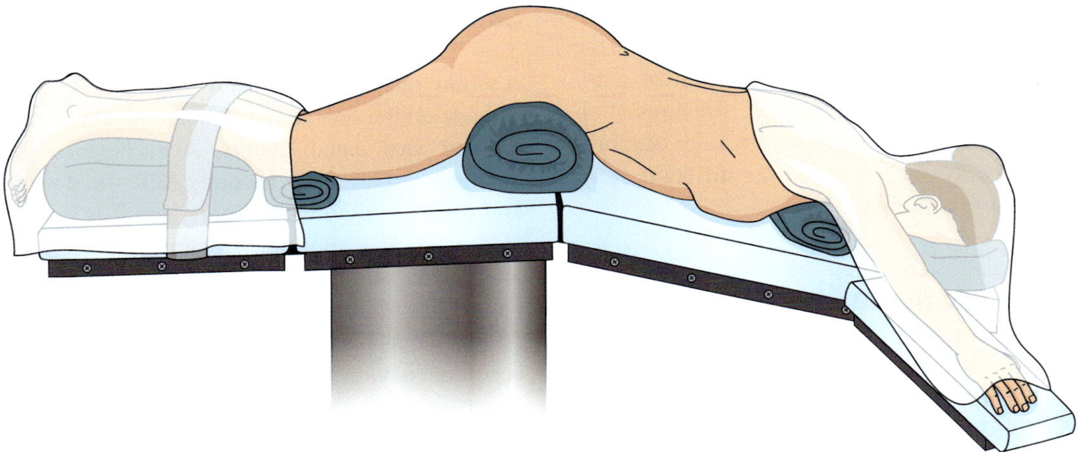

Fig. 27.5 Prone jackknife position for perineal dissection. Padding is used under the chest, hips, knees, and feet

posteriorly and aim in a plane directly anterior to it. The coccyx can be removed, but we do it only if it is compromised by the tumor or if necessary to remove a large, bulky tumor. A key point is to divide the anococcygeal ligament at the tip of the coccyx, connecting the perineal surgical field with the posterior mesorectal dissection. The levator ani muscle should be sectioned bilaterally, beginning at the apex of the ischiorectal fossa and close to the obturator internus muscle (Fig. 27.6). The puborectalis muscle should be sectioned anteriorly before reaching the transverse perineal muscle.

The complete specimen is then extracted (note that the drain from above should be attached), and the dissection is continued proximal to distal and medial to lateral rather than from the bottom. The prone position facilitates exposure of the neurovascular bundle and can help prevent injury to the urethra, especially in men.

Perineal Defect Closure

Once the specimen is removed, copious irrigation of the surgical site is performed. The pelvic drains are now secured in the final position before wound closure. In a primary closure, large absorbable sutures are used in a multilayer fashion to close the ischiorectal fat. Discontinuous nylon sutures are used to close the skin, and we

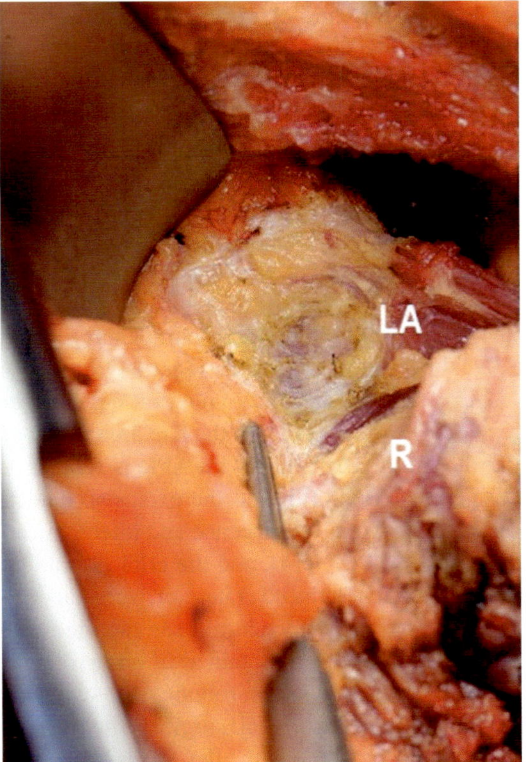

Fig. 27.6 Exposure of levator ani (LA) muscles for proper division. R: rectum

prefer a vertical mattress method. It is the authors' preference to use a negative-pressure surface dressing over an antibiotic impregnated dressing for the first 3 days to keep the wound clean and dry. To prevent surgical site infection and perineal hernia, especially in wider resections, a biological absorbable mesh or autologous tissue flaps can be used. Previous studies have shown no difference in the rates of morbidity or dehiscence between the different options of reconstruction [12, 13].

Postoperative Management and Complications

Postoperative care for APR follows a routine pathway at Memorial Hospital. We advocate the use of an enhanced-recovery-after-surgery protocol with early oral ingestion of fluids, early ambulation, and a standardized pain-control strategy minimizing or avoiding use of opiates. The urinary catheter is removed on post operative day (POD) 3 after an extensive pelvic dissection and on POD 2 on a standard dissection. Drainage continues for some time due to the excessive amount of fluid. If a flap was used, drainage may continue after hospital discharge. The perineal wound should be protected, and strenuous physical activity and direct pressure with sitting must be restricted. Perineal sutures remain in place for 3–4 weeks, until the wound is completely closed. Special care should be taken regarding activities like excess bending or prolonged sitting, in order to avoid shear or tension in the flap area. Most of the morbidity associated with APR is related to the perineal wound due to the extensive defect. The rates of wound dehiscence and infection can be as high as 30% [14], and the etiology can be multifactorial. Reduced rates of surgical site infection and recurrence have been reported [15, 16], but the data were obtained in observational studies. In our local series, robotic APR is associated with less abdominal surgical site rate of infection compared with the open approach (unpublished data). Aggressive management of dehiscence with early intervention, local wound care, and negative-pressure dressings can salvage most wounds with a good outcome.

Conclusion

Abdominoperineal resection (APR) has been considered the operation of choice for lower rectal and anal canal tumors. According to the authors' experience, robotic APR is a safe approach for low rectal tumors, and it is associated with less morbidity mainly due to less abdominal surgical site infection rates. Prone patient positioning for the perineal portion of APR is a feasible approach and should be used in accordance with the surgeon's preference and expertise.

References

1. Lange MM, Rutten HJ, van de Velde CJ. One hundred years of curative surgery for rectal cancer: 1908–2008. Eur J Surg Oncol. 2009;35:456–63. https://doi.org/10.1016/j.ejso.2008.09.012.
2. Mullen JT, Rodriguez-Bigas MA, Chang GJ, Barcenas CH, Crane CH, Skibber JM, et al. Results of surgical salvage after failed chemoradiation therapy for epidermoid carcinoma of the anal canal. Ann Surg Oncol. 2007;14:478–83. https://doi.org/10.1245/s10434-006-9221-7.
3. Pachler J, Wille-Jörgensen P. Quality of life after rectal resection for cancer, with or without permanent colostomy. Cochrane Database Syst Rev. 2012;12. Art. No.: CD004323. https://doi.org/10.1002/14651858.CD004323.pub4.
4. Torkzad MR, Kamel I, Halappa VG, Beets-Tan RG. Magnetic resonance imaging of rectal and anal cancer. Magn Reson Imaging Clin N Am. 2014;22(1):85–112. https://doi.org/10.1016/j.mric.2013.07.007.
5. Zhou Y, Shao W, Lu W. Diagnostic value of endorectal ultrasonography for rectal carcinoma: a meta-analysis. J Cancer Res Ther. 2014;10(Suppl):319–22. https://doi.org/10.4103/0973-1482.151542.
6. Kasparek MS, Hassan I, Cima RR, Larson DR, Gullerud RE, Wolff BG. Long-term quality of life and sexual and urinary function after abdominoperineal resection for distal rectal cancer. Dis Colon Rectum. 2012;55:147–54. https://doi.org/10.1097/DCR.0b013e31823d2606.
7. Carmichael JC, Keller DS, Baldini G, Bordeianou L, Weiss E, Lee L, et al. Clinical practice guideline for enhanced recovery after colon and rectal surgery from the American Society of Colon and Rectal Surgeons (ASCRS) and Society of American Gastrointestinal

and Endoscopic Surgeons (SAGES). Surg Endosc. 2017; https://doi.org/10.1007/s00464-017-5722.

8. Guillem JG, Lee-Kong SA. Autonomic nerve preservation during rectal cancer resection. J Gastrointest Surg. 2010;14:416–22. https://doi.org/10.1007/s11605-009-0941-4.

9. Titu LV, Tweedle E, Rooney PS. High tie of the inferior mesenteric artery in curative surgery for left colonic and rectal cancers: a systematic review. Dig Surg. 2008;25:148–57. https://doi.org/10.1159/000128172.

10. Nagtegaal ID, van de Velde CJ, Marijnen CA, van Krieken JH, Quirke P, Dutch Colorectal Cancer Group, Pathology Review Committee. Low rectal cancer: a call for a change of approach in abdominoperineal resection. J Clin Oncol. 2005;23:9257–64.

11. West NP, Anderin C, Smith KJ, Holm T, Quirke P, European Extralevator Abdominoperineal Excision Study Group. Multicentre experience with extralevator abdominoperineal excision for low rectal cancer. Br J Surg. 2010;97:588–99.

12. Foster JD, Pathak S, Smart NJ, Branagan G, Longman RJ, Thomas MG, et al. Reconstruction of the perineum following extralevator abdominoperineal excision for carcinoma of the lower rectum: a systematic review. Color Dis. 2012;14:1052–9. https://doi.org/10.1111/j.1463-1318.2012.03169.x.

13. Butt HZ, Salem MK, Vijaynagar B, Chaudhri S, Singh B. Perineal reconstruction after extra-levator abdominoperineal excision (eLAPE): a systematic review. Int J Color Dis. 2013;28:1459–68. https://doi.org/10.1007/s00384-013-1660.6.

14. Althumairi A, Canner J, Gearhart S, Safar B, Sacks J, Efron J. Predictors of perineal wound complications and prolonged time to perineal wound healing after abdominoperineal resection. World J Surg. 2016;40:1755–62.

15. Dinaux AM, Amri R, Berger DL. Prone positioning reduces perineal infections when performing the miles procedure. Am J Surg. 2017;214:217–21. https://doi.org/10.1016/j.amjsurg.2017.05.021.

16. Anderin C, Granath F, Martling A, Holm T. Local recurrence after prone vs supine abdominoperineal excision for low rectal cancer. Color Dis. 2013;15:812–5. https://doi.org/10.1111/codi.12148.

Tsuyoshi Konishi

Introduction

Pelvic exenteration is one of the most challenging procedures in gastrointestinal surgery. First, extended resection outside of total mesorectal excision (TME) often encounters massive bleeding from internal iliac vessels [1]. Second, the surgical view in the pelvis is often limited by fixed bulky T4 tumors. Third, transection of Santorini's dorsal venous complex and urethra is an uncommon but risky procedure which could lead to uncontrolled venous bleeding. A minimally invasive approach to pelvic exenteration could overcome these difficulties [2, 3]. Pneumoperitoneum under Trendelenburg position minimizes venous bleeding within the pelvis. Additionally, magnified laparoscopic views may provide better identification of vessels in the narrow pelvis occupied by large tumors, which may further reduce bleeding with meticulous dissection. When transecting Santorini's dorsal venous complex and urethra, bipolar forceps or vascular staplers under higher

Electronic supplementary material The online version of this chapter (https://doi.org/10.1007/978-3-030-18740-8_28) contains supplementary material, which is available to authorized users.

T. Konishi (✉)
Department of Gastroenterological Surgery, Colorectal Division, Cancer Institute Hospital of the Japanese Foundation for Cancer Research, Tokyo, Japan
e-mail: tkonishi-tky@umin.ac.jp

pneumoperitoneal pressure are useful in reducing the risk of bleeding. Understanding the anatomy outside of TME is mandatory to perform laparoscopic pelvic exenteration.

Outcomes of Laparoscopic Pelvic Exenteration in Literature

Although there have been some reports on the safety and feasibility of laparoscopic pelvic exenteration in the fields of urology and gynecology [4–6], data on colorectal malignancies are very limited (Table 28.1) and mainly from Japan where laparoscopic lateral pelvic lymph node dissection is commonly performed [7–10]. A case series that compared short-term outcomes of laparoscopic ($n = 9$) and open ($n = 58$) pelvic exenteration for colorectal pelvic malignancies [2] showed less blood loss (830 mL vs. 2769 mL), similar operative time (935 min vs. 883 min), and similar R0 resection rate (77.8% vs. 75.9%) in laparoscopic pelvic exenteration. Postoperative overall complication rate (66.7% vs. 89.7%) and major complication rate (0% vs. 32.8%) were lower in laparoscopic pelvic exenteration although the differences were not statistically significant. A larger series that compared laparoscopic ($n = 13$) and open ($n = 18$) pelvic exenteration for primary and recurrent colorectal malignancies [3] reported similar results, showing less blood loss (930 mL vs. 3003 mL),

Table 28.1 Published series of pelvic exenterations on colorectal malignancies

Author	Year	N	Operation time, min	Blood loss, mL	R0 resection rate	Overall complications	Major complications
Uehara K	2016	9	935	830	78	67%	0%
Ogura A	2016	13	829	930	100	62%	23%
Yang K	2015	11	565	547	N/A	36%	N/A

N/A not available

similar operative time (829 min vs. 875 min), and similar R0 resection rate (100% vs. 100%) in laparoscopic pelvic exenteration. Postoperative overall complication rate (61.5% vs. 83.3%) and major complication rate (23.1% vs. 44.4%) were again lower in laparoscopic pelvic exenteration although the differences were not significant. Although these studies are limited by selection bias due to the retrospective nature of the studies, the data supports safety and feasibility of laparoscopic pelvic exenteration with possible advantage in reducing intraoperative bleeding.

Anatomy of Pelvic Exenteration

Posterior Dissection

Posterior landmarks for pelvic exenteration are the same as TME, dissecting the avascular layer between the fascia propria of the rectum and sacral bone. If sacrectomy is required, then the proposed transection line of the sacral bone should be carefully determined on preoperative magnetic resonance imaging (MRI). The distance from the sacral promontory to the transection line should be measured, since it is the only landmark to determine the transection line during laparoscopic surgery.

Lateral Dissection

Lateral landmarks for pelvic exenteration are the lateral pelvic wall muscles, i.e., psoas, piriformis, and internal obturator muscles (Fig. 28.1). Simply, the steps of lateral dissection result in exposure of these muscles. Additionally, the

internal iliac artery and vein are good landmarks to identify the visceral vessels that should be ligated. More anatomic details are available in the chapter on laparoscopic lateral pelvic lymph node dissection (LPLND).

Anterior Dissection

Anterior landmarks include the bladder, prostate, Santorini's dorsal venous complex, and urethra (Fig. 28.2). These landmarks should be exposed before dividing Santorini's dorsal venous complex and urethra.

Levator Muscle and Tendinous Arch

The levator muscles laterally attach to the internal obturator muscle, forming a tendinous whitish line named the tendinous arch (Fig. 28.2). If the tumor invades the levator muscle, extended wide resection of the levator muscle is needed, requiring dissection close to or on the tendinous arch (Fig. 28.3).

Patient Positioning and Port Placement

Patient position is essentially the same as that used in TME. Typically, the patient is placed in Trendelenburg position so that the small bowel, colon, and omentum are moved out of the pelvic surgical field by gravity. The degree of Trendelenburg position should be minimized because of long operative times.

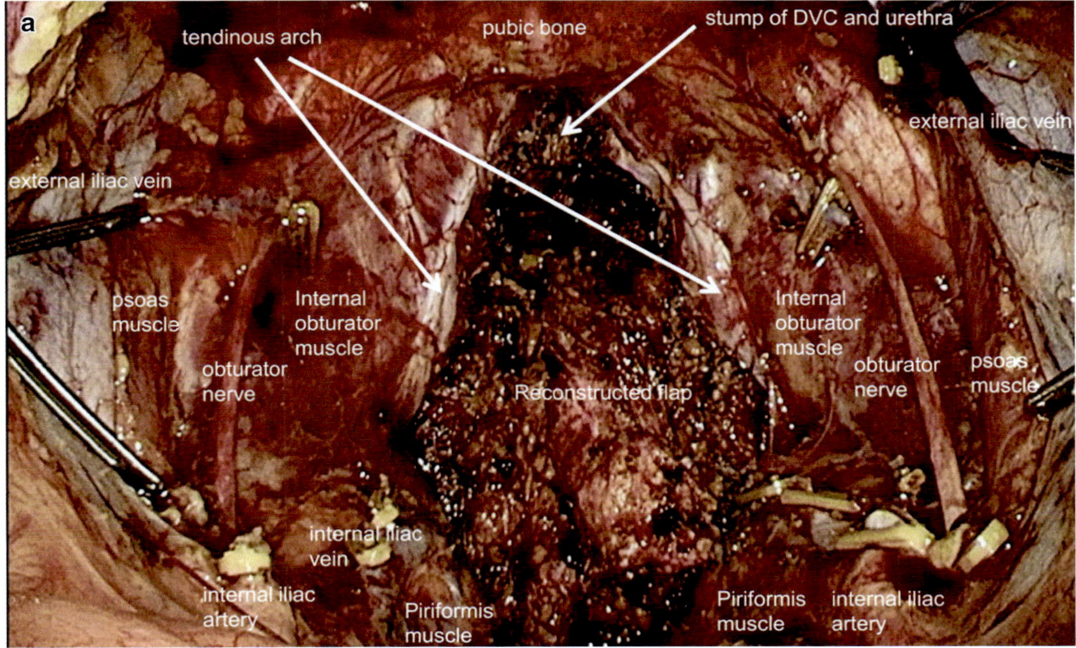

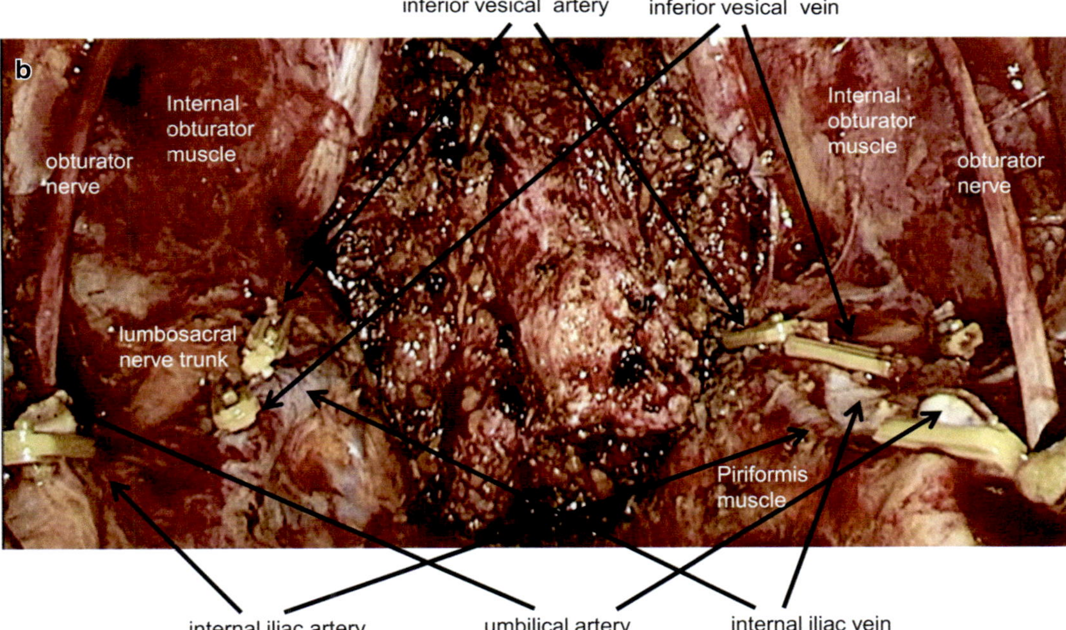

Fig. 28.1 Laparoscopic views (**a**) distant view of pelvis; (**b**) magnified view of ligated vessels after completion of pelvic exenteration. The patient underwent V-Y flap reconstruction using the gluteus maximus muscle. All the visceral branches from the internal iliac vessels were ligated at the root. DVC, dorsal venous complex

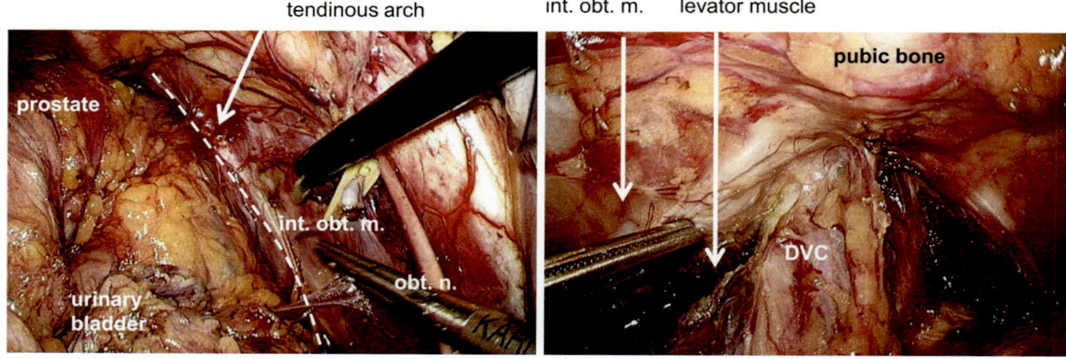

Fig. 28.2 Anterior anatomy around the prostate. Left, intraoperative view after exposure of levator muscle lateral to the prostate. Right, intraoperative view after exposure of Santorini's dorsal venous complex

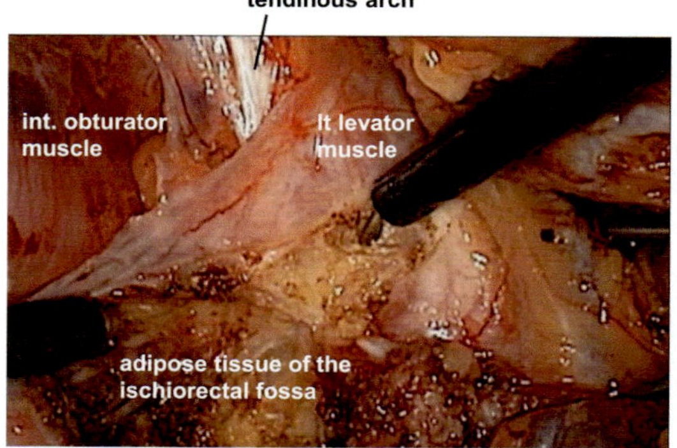

Fig. 28.3 Laparoscopic dissection of the levator muscle. If the tumor invades the levator muscle, extended wide resection of the levator muscle is needed, dissecting close to the tendinous arch. Adipose tissue of the ischiorectal fossa is exposed after dissecting the levator muscle

Typical port placement is described in Fig. 28.4. We typically place one 12-mm camera port at the umbilicus, one 12-mm port in the right lower quadrant, and three 5-mm ports in the right middle, left lower, and left middle quadrants. An additional port may be placed in the lower midline for handling a large fixed tumor or to use linear staplers to divide Santorini's dorsal venous complex and urethra. At least one 12-mm port is to be used so that gauze can be quickly inserted in case of bleeding.

For most of the procedure, the surgeon operates from the right side of the patient. The surgeon may operate from the left side when dissecting the right pelvic sidewalls, including the psoas muscle, internal obturator muscles, and obturator canal.

Step-by-Step Procedures of Pelvic Exenteration (Video 28.1)

In this chapter, the procedures are described for the pelvic phase after mobilization of the sigmoid colon and ligation of the inferior mesenteric vessels have been completed.

Posterior Dissection

The presacral avascular space is widely opened and sharply dissected caudally to reach the levator muscle in the same manner as that with TME.

Isolation and Division of the Left Ureter

The left ureter is identified and taped and isolated distally. Connective tissue and small vessels that envelop the ureter should be carefully preserved to prevent postoperative ischemic stricture and hydroureter. At its entry point to the bladder, the ureter is ligated with a clip and divided (Fig. 28.5). Note that length of the left ureter should be maintained long enough to reach the right-sided ileal conduit.

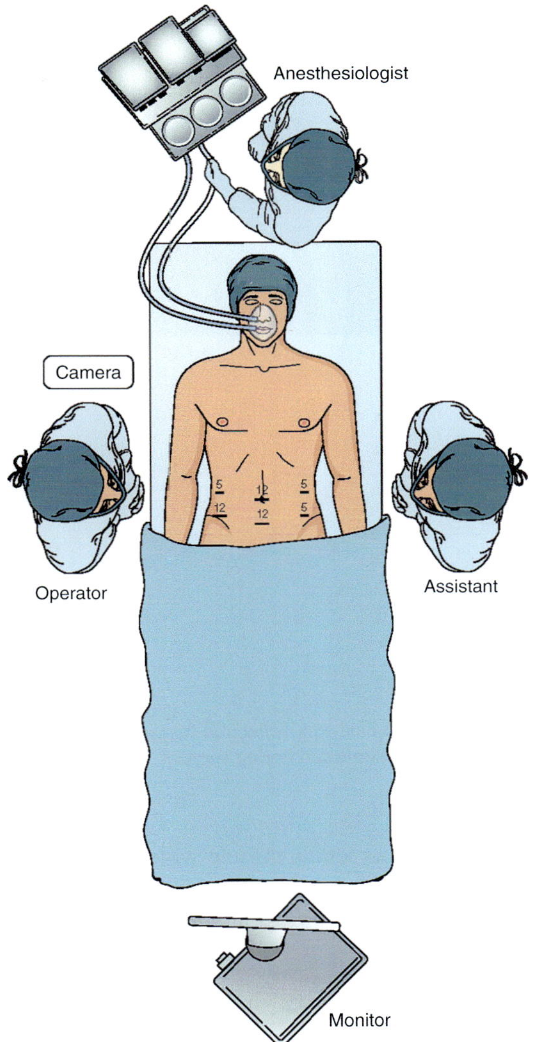

Fig. 28.4 Trocar/port positions and operating room setup for laparoscopic pelvic exenteration. Trocar positions are similar to the positions for total mesorectal excision. The lower midline 12-mm port is optional for handling large, fixed tumors or for using staplers when dividing Santorini's dorsal venous complex and urethra

Insertion of a Ureteral Catheter

The distal end of the left ureter is extracted from the left lower port and a ureteral catheter is inserted under direct vision (Fig. 28.5). The catheter is connected to a bag and kept out of the abdominal cavity during the procedure so that the urine volume for the left kidney can be monitored.

Lateral Pelvic Wall Dissection

The lateral dissection plane is essentially the same as laparoscopic LPLND [11, 12]. The peritoneum is widely opened toward the anterior of the bladder. The psoas muscle is identified behind the internal border of the external iliac vein. Dissection follows on the surface of the psoas muscle followed by the internal obturator muscle (Fig. 28.1a). The surface of these pelvic wall muscles is avascular and has minimal risk for bleeding. Anteriorly, the distal aspects of both umbilical artery and vas deferens are ligated and divided so that the lateral space is widely opened. The lymphatic chain from the inguinal nodes to obturator nodes is ligated behind the distal external iliac vein to prevent postoperative lymphorrhea. The obturator nerve is identified and isolated from obturator vessels and is preserved. Obturator vessels are ligated at the entry point into the obturator canal. Dissection continues on the surface of the internal obturator muscle down to reach the tendinous arch where the levator muscle attaches to the internal obturator muscle. Dissection proceeds anteriorly to expose the internal obturator muscle and tendinous arch, opening the paravesical (Retzius) space.

Dissection of the Dorsal Plane and Ligation of Visceral Branches

Before approaching the internal iliac vessels, the proximal sigmoid colon is retracted cephalad using a cotton tape tied around the sigmoid colon or an organ retractor to provide better working space in the pelvis. Thereafter, dissection follows the surface of the internal iliac artery and vein. Division of the visceral branches from the internal iliac vessels in laparoscopic pelvic exenteration is essentially the same as that in laparoscopic LPLND [11, 12]. Visceral branches are ligated and divided at the root, including the umbilical artery and vesical vessels (Fig. 28.1b). The proximal obturator vessels are also ligated and dissection follows the surface of the lumbosacral nerve trunk.

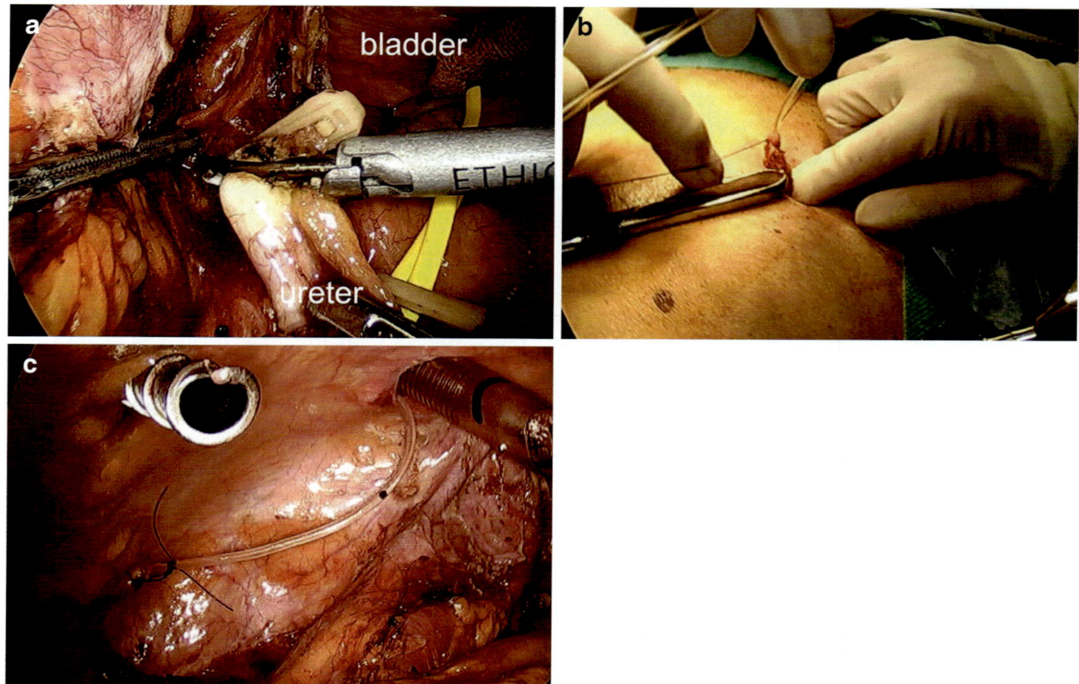

Fig. 28.5 (**a**) The ureter is ligated at the entry point to the bladder. (**b**) After extracting the ureter from a port site, a ureteral catheter is inserted under direct vision. (**c**) The catheter is connected to a collection bag so that the urine volume can be monitored during surgery

Dissection of Autonomic Nerves

The dorsal plane of the lateral compartment is demarcated from the presacral space behind the mesorectum by the hypogastric nerve and pelvic nerve plexus. The nerves are divided by electro-cautery, exposing the piriformis muscle. After dividing the S4 pelvic splanchnic nerve, the dissection reaches the levator muscle.

Dissection of the Levator Muscle

The levator muscle is incised and dissected from the abdominal cavity, and ischiorectal adipose tissue is exposed. The dissection line of the levator muscle is determined by the extent of tumor invasion. If wide resection of the levator muscle is required, the incision follows the tendinous arch without dissecting between the levator muscle and the mesorectum (Fig. 28.3). Anteriorly, the incision on the levator muscle can be either along the puborectalis muscle which attaches to the prostate (inside) or the tendinous arch (outside) according to the extent of tumor invasion.

Takedown of the Bladder and Anterior Division

The peritoneum is opened anteriorly to the bladder, and the paravesical space is opened from lateral to anterior, taking down the bladder. Takedown of the bladder should be awaited until this step to avoid having it interfere with the surgical view in the pelvis. At this point, Santorini's dorsal venous complex is exposed by incising the endopelvic fascia laterally to the prostate and dividing the anterior peri-prostatic adipose tissues using a thermal coagulation device. When dividing the dorsal venous complex, the pneumoperitoneum pressure is increased to 15 mmHg to compress the venous complex and minimize bleeding, and the urethral catheter is withdrawn.

Transection of the venous complex and urethra can be done using a thermal coagulation device, a linear stapler, or suturing method (bunching method). Pre-coagulation of the dorsal venous complex using the soft coagulation mode of the VIO system (Erbe) is useful to minimize venous bleeding before transecting the venous complex with a thermal coagulation device. After transection of the urethra, the anterior perirectal fat is exposed, and dissection continues anteriorly to the rectum.

Perineal Approach

The proximal sigmoid colon is divided using a linear stapler, and then the procedure proceeds to the perineal approach. We usually perform perineal dissection in the lithotomy position. After closing the anal canal with purse-string sutures, the perianal skin is incised and ischiorectal fat is dissected away to reach the dissection line from the abdominal cavity. From posterior to lateral to anterior, dissection continues guided by the fingers and a laparoscopic view from within the abdomen. After completion of this step, the specimen is removed through the perineal wound. The wound is washed with saline and closed primarily. Occasionally, the jackknife position is useful, e.g., in case of sacrectomy or flap construction using the gluteus maximus muscle.

Urinary Reconstruction and Ostomy

After restarting pneumoperitoneum following closure of the perineum, the right colon is mobilized and extracted from the urostomy marking site at the right lower quadrant or umbilical incision. An ileal conduit that is 20 cm in length and approximately 20–40 cm from the ileocecal valve is resected while preserving the blood supply. Ureters are guided to the urostomy site and anastomosed to the ileal conduit under direct vision. Finally, the urostomy is matured at the right lower quadrant, and the sigmoid colostomy is matured at the left lower quadrant. Finally, a drain catheter is placed in the pelvis.

Pros and Cons of Laparoscopic Pelvic Exenteration

The strengths of the laparoscopic approach for pelvic exenteration include reduced bleeding, better surgical views in the deep pelvis, and possibly decreased postoperative complications. Although laparoscopic surgery for bulky tumors may require big incisions to retrieve large surgical specimens, the advantages of the laparoscopic approach outweigh the cosmetic benefits. On the other hand, there are limitations to the laparoscopic approach. Manipulation using laparoscopic straight forceps is often difficult with a bulky, fixed tumor, occasionally requiring additional trocars to help access the deep pelvis with straight forceps.

Another limitation is the management of major bleeding. The internal iliac vessels, presacral venous complex, and Santorini's dorsal venous complex may cause massive bleeding if injured. Increasing pneumoperitoneum pressure to 15 mmHg can compress the vein and reduce venous bleeding. Thermal coagulation devices are also useful for hemostasis in case of venous bleeding. Use of a laparoscopic linear stapler for dividing major vessels or the dorsal venous complex can also minimize bleeding.

Currently, laparoscopic pelvic exenteration is indicated for very select patients by a small number of surgeons. However, with more advanced knowledge of pelvic anatomy through laparoscopic extended resections, the procedure will be more commonly performed and accepted by laparoscopic colorectal surgeons. Further studies are needed to assess the long-term oncologic safety of this procedure.

References

1. Ike H, Shimada H, Yamaguchi S, et al. Outcome of total pelvic exenteration for primary rectal cancer. Dis Colon Rectum. 2003;46:474–80.
2. Uehara K, Nakamura H, Yoshino Y, et al. Initial experience of laparoscopic pelvic exenteration and comparison with conventional open surgery. Surg Endosc. 2016;30:132–8.
3. Ogura A, Akiyoshi T, Konishi T, et al. Safety of laparoscopic pelvic exenteration with urinary diver-

sion for colorectal malignancies. World J Surg. 2016;40:1236–43.

4. Kanao H, Aoki Y, Hisa T, Takeshima N. Total laparoscopic pelvic exenteration for a laterally recurrent cervical carcinoma with a vesicovaginal fistula that developed after concurrent chemoradiotherapy. Gynecol Oncol. 2017;146(2):438–9.

5. Kaufmann OG, Young JL, Sountoulides P, Kaplan AG, Dash A, Ornstein DK. Robotic radical anterior pelvic exenteration: the UCI experience. Minim Invasive Ther Allied Technol. 2011;20(4):240–6.

6. Martínez A, Filleron T, Vitse L, Querleu D, Mery E, Balague G, Delannes M, Soulie M, Pomel C, Ferron G. Laparoscopic pelvic exenteration for gynaecological malignancy: is there any advantage? Gynecol Oncol. 2011;120(3):374–9.

7. Akiyoshi T, Nagasaki T, Ueno M. Laparoscopic total pelvic exenteration for locally recurrent rectal Cancer. Ann Surg Oncol. 2015;22(12):3896.

8. Mukai T, Akiyoshi T, Ueno M, Fukunaga Y, Nagayama S, Fujimoto Y, Konishi T, Ikeda A, Yamaguchi T. Laparoscopic total pelvic exenteration with en bloc lateral lymph node dissection after neoadjuvant chemoradiotherapy for advanced primary rectal cancer. Asian J Endosc Surg. 2013;6(4):314–7.

9. Nagasaki T, Akiyoshi T, Ueno M, Fukunaga Y, Nagayama S, Fujimoto Y, Konishi T, Yamaguchi T. Laparoscopic abdominosacral resection for locally advanced primary rectal cancer after treatment with mFOLFOX6 plus bevacizumab, followed by preoperative chemoradiotherapy. Asian J Endosc Surg. 2014;7(1):52–5.

10. Yang K, Cai L, Yao L, Zhang Z, Zhang C, Wang X, Tang J, Li X, He Z, Zhou L. Laparoscopic total pelvic exenteration for pelvic malignancies: the technique and short-time outcome of 11 cases. World J Surg Oncol. 2015;13(1):301.

11. Konishi T, Kuroyanagi H, Oya M, Ueno M, Fujimoto Y, Akiyoshi T, Yoshimatsu H, Watanabe T, Yamaguchi T, Muto T. Lateral lymph node dissection with preoperative chemoradiation for locally advanced lower rectal cancer through a laparoscopic approach. Surg Endosc. 2011;25(7):2358–9.

12. Konishi T, Kuroyanagi H, Watanabe T. Combined resection of the iliac vessels for lateral pelvic lymph node dissection can be safely performed through laparoscopic approach. Ann Surg Oncol. 2011;18(S3):237.

Songphol Malakorn, Tarik Sammour,
and George J. Chang

Introduction

Colorectal cancer is one of the most common causes of cancer death in the USA [1]. In addition, 15–20% of colorectal cancers present with adherence to or invasion of adjacent organs [2]. This is especially true for rectal cancer, since pelvic organs occupy the relatively narrow pelvic space around the rectum (e.g., anteriorly, urinary bladder, seminal vesicles, prostate, uterus, and vagina; posteriorly, sacrum, coccyx, sacral nerve roots, and piriformis muscle; and laterally, ureters, iliac vessels, obturator nerve, sacral plexus, sciatic nerve, and acetabulum (Fig. 29.1a, b)).

Locally advanced rectal cancers with local invasion of adjacent organs (T4) have significantly higher risk for positive resection margins and poorer oncologic outcomes [3, 4]. However, in selected patients, a curative intent treatment strategy can provide a chance for cure, better long-term oncologic outcomes, acceptable postoperative morbidity and mortality, and better quality of life [5, 6]. The curative intent treatment strategy includes two essential components: first, tailored pre-, intra-, and postoperative multimodality therapy including induction/consolidation chemotherapy, neoadjuvant long-course chemoradiation therapy, intraoperative radiation therapy, and adjuvant chemotherapy; second, oncologic surgical resection to achieve histologically negative resection margins (R0) and adequate lymph node removal. To this end, en bloc multivisceral organ resection or pelvic exenteration is usually needed for T4 rectal cancers [7, 8]. Pelvic exenteration is a technically demanding procedure, in which the dissection planes are wider than that for standard total mesorectal excision (TME) (Fig. 29.2). However, exenteration

Electronic supplementary material The online version of this chapter (https://doi.org/10.1007/978-3-030-18740-8_29) contains supplementary material, which is available to authorized users.

S. Malakorn
Department of Colorectal Surgery, Faculty of Medicine, Chulalongkorn University, Bangkok, Thailand

Department of Surgical Oncology, The University of Texas MD Anderson Cancer Center, Houston, TX, USA

T. Sammour
Department of Surgical Oncology, The University of Texas MD Anderson Cancer Center, Houston, TX, USA

Colorectal Unit, Department of Surgery, Royal Adelaide Hospital, University of Adelaide, Adelaide, SA, Australia

G. J. Chang (✉)
Department of Surgical Oncology, The University of Texas MD Anderson Cancer Center, Houston, TX, USA
e-mail: gchang@mdanderson.org

© Springer Nature Switzerland AG 2020
J. Kim, J. Garcia-Aguilar (eds.), *Minimally Invasive Surgical Techniques for Cancers of the Gastrointestinal Tract*, https://doi.org/10.1007/978-3-030-18740-8_29

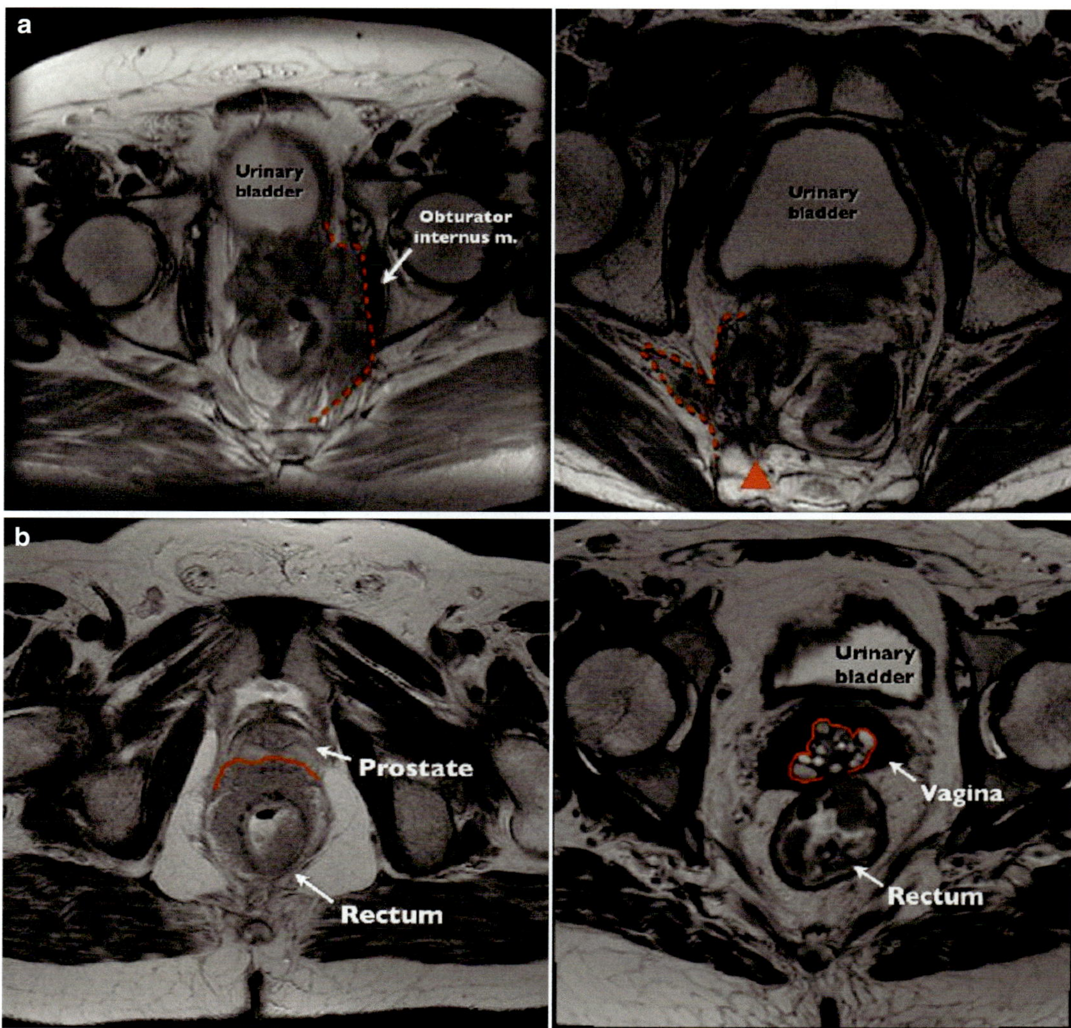

Fig. 29.1 (**a**) Examples of magnetic resonance imaging (MRI) demonstrate tumors that are not suitable for the robotic approach with regard to invasion into the lateral compartment (red broken line) and sacral nerve root (red arrow head). (**b**) Examples of MRI demonstrate tumors that are suitable for the robotic approach. The solid red line indicates location of central invasion to the prostate and vagina

can be accomplished successfully with acceptable outcomes in selected patients using a multidisciplinary team approach (including colorectal surgical oncologists, urologists, plastic surgeons, vascular surgeons, and neurosurgery/orthopedics) [9–11].

Although the feasibility of a laparoscopic approach for T4 rectal cancers has been recently reported [12–15], some studies have also demonstrated a significantly higher positive circumferential resection margin rate for laparoscopic surgery when compared to open surgery for locally advanced rectal cancer [16]. In fact, extension of rectal cancer beyond the TME plane is a major reason for conversion from laparoscopic to open surgery [17–19]. The higher conversion rate is also associated with poorer short-term and long-term oncologic outcomes [20, 21]. Therefore, the applicability of laparoscopic surgery for T4 rectal cancer remains controversial [22]. The potential benefits from a minimally invasive approach have to be weighed against the risk of having positive resection margins that compromise oncologic outcomes.

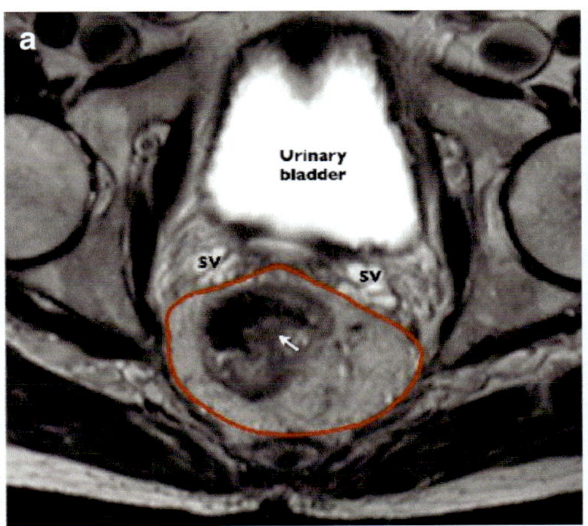

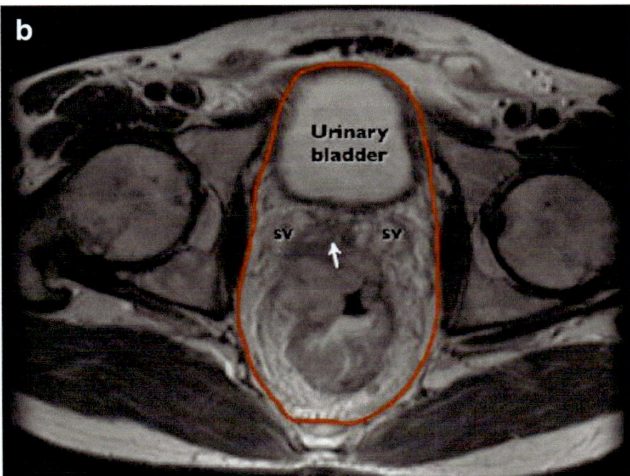

Fig. 29.2 (**a**) Magnetic resonance imaging demonstrates the standard total mesorectal excision (TME) plane. The red line shows the standard TME plane around the fascia propia of the rectum. The arrow points to the tumor that is confined within the TME plane. (**b**) MRI demonstrates extension beyond the standard TME plane (red line) with the arrow showing anterior invasion to the seminal vesicle. SV, seminal vesicle

There has been significant growth in the use of robotic surgery for rectal cancer worldwide. Emerging data appears to support the feasibility of robotic surgery for T4 rectal cancers with comparable short-term oncologic outcomes [23–26]. The advantages of robotic surgery over conventional laparoscopic surgery include better pelvic visualization by 3-D adjustable cameras and more degrees of freedom with wrist-articulated instrumentation, thus achieving more precise dissections. These benefits may compensate for some of the limitations of conventional laparoscopic surgery, especially during complex pelvic dissection. In carefully selected cases, the robotic approach may expand our ability to offer minimally invasive surgery to this subset of locally advanced rectal cancer patients. In this chapter, we clarify a step-by-step approach of robotic pelvic exenteration for T4 rectal cancers.

Patient Selection and Preoperative Preparation

This is a crucial step for any surgical procedure, but it is particularly important when extending the indications for this procedure. As a matter of principle, the indications for pelvic exenteration must be met before considering a robotic approach. Relative contraindications for pelvic exenteration for rectal cancer include high sacral/lateral bone involvement, distant/peritoneal metastasis, sciatic nerve or lateral compartment involvement beyond the vascular plane, encasement of common or external iliac vessels, common iliac or retroperitoneal lymph node metastases, and multifocal disease. Once the indication for pelvic exenteration has been established, three factors should be carefully examined when considering the robotic approach for pelvic exenteration.

Patient Factors

Beyond the common assessments of patient fitness for surgery and extent of previous abdominal surgery, specific anatomic considerations for these procedures must be evaluated. For example, flap closure of an exenteration defect may necessitate extensive abdominal wall tissue harvest, which would negate any potential benefit from smaller incisions for dissection. This can depend on patient body size and availability of other sites for tissue harvest and should be discussed with the involved plastic surgery service. In addition, the primary surgeon should thoroughly explain to the patient (as part of the informed consent process) the evidence for the robotic approach and potential benefits and limitations of this approach. Both patient and family expectations should be clarified.

Tumor Factors

The presence of distant disease should be ruled out with cross-sectional imaging with computed tomography (CT) and positron emission tomography (PET) scans as needed, and high-resolution magnetic resonance imaging (MRI) is needed to assess local resectability. The most appropriate tumors are those with central pelvic extension (e.g., prostate, vagina, uterus, urinary bladder, or limited lateral extension) and those with a single direction of extension. In contrast, very bulky tumors will limit the ability to retract and provide exposure around the tumor and are not good candidates for the robotic approach (Table 29.1, Fig. 29.1). However, the need for an extravascular approach is not an absolute contraindication.

Surgeon Factors

The primary rectal surgeon should have abundant experience with robotic rectal surgery prior to attempting robotic pelvic exenteration. In addition, every surgeon in the multi-surgical specialist team should be consulted with

Table 29.1 Favorable and unfavorable factors for robotic exenteration

Favorable factors for robotic approach	Unfavorable factors for robotic approach
Central pelvic extension	Lateral compartment involvement beyond the vascular plane
Anterior invasion (e.g., prostate, vagina, uterus, or urinary bladder) Limited lateral/posterior extension	Encasement of iliac vessels High sacral bone involvement
Tumor with one direction of extension	Tumor with more than one direction of extension
Less bulky, mobile tumor	Bulky tumor with limited mobility
Good response to preoperative treatment	

advanced notice to ensure that the indication is acceptable and the required expertise is available.

Operating Room Setting

Setting up the operating room to allow sufficient free space between the robotic system and surrounding instruments is important. As with any robotic procedure, interference between the operating table, consoles, patient cart, and monitors should be avoided, as contamination or prolonged docking times may occur. In fact, a well-trained scrub nurse and assistant surgeon share critical roles in facilitating the operation and providing them a comfortable working space will facilitate surgical work flow. Figure 29.3a demonstrates the example of a room setting for robotic pelvic exenteration.

Because of the procedure's length and complexity, anesthesia setup is another core requirement to ensure patient safety. The anesthesiologist needs to participate in decisions around patient positioning and access during the operation. This is particularly true for robotic cases without a synchronized moveable table, as patient position is difficult to change during surgery unless the robotic system is undocked. Arterial lines, intravenous access, and noninvasive monitoring devices should be protected from dislodgement or blockage and tested for function prior to robotic cart docking.

Patient Position

Patient position should be optimized before the docking process is undertaken. First, the patient should be positioned in lithotomy on a nonslip surface with the pelvis low enough on the table to provide coccyx accessibility. Both arms should be wrapped by the patient's side, while placing adequate padding around weight-bearing or prominent areas to avoid compression and nerve injury (Fig. 29.3b) [27]. Further strapping is required to secure the patient on the table because any accidental movement after docking could result in injury since the robotic arms are relatively fixed. Once the above is confirmed, right-side down Trendelenburg position is the position of choice, aiming to clear the small bowel out of the pelvis and retroperitoneal vascular pedicles. Only enough tilt as needed for exposure should be applied, taking care to avoid any extremes in positioning, particularly given the potential for prolonged surgery. Once enough exposure is obtained, the steepness of right-side down and Trendelenburg tilt should be reduced as much as possible.

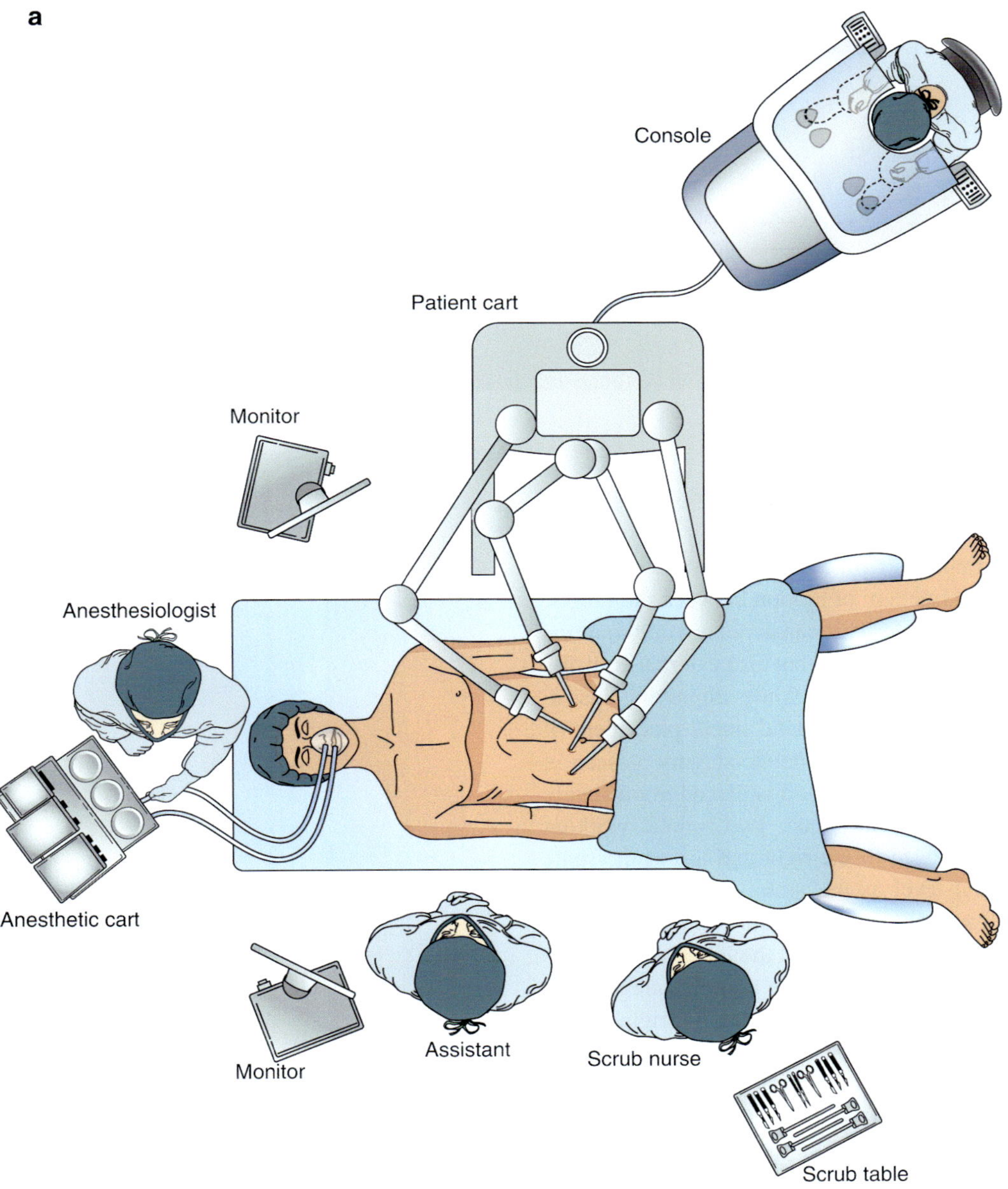

Fig. 29.3 (**a**) Robotic setup (daVinci Xi platform) for pelvic exenteration. The boom is rotated and robotic arms are set up oriented for pelvic surgery. (**b**) Patient positioning with adequate padding around weight-bearing and prominent areas to avoid compression and nerve injury

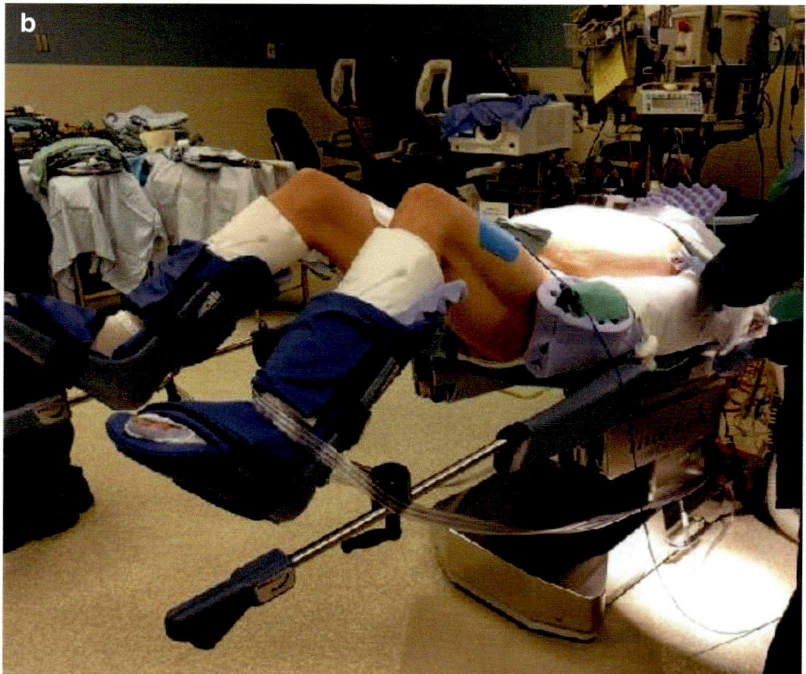

Fig. 29.3 (continued)

Port Placement

Appropriate port placement aimed to maximize space and freedom of motion between the robotic arms is desirable. This can avoid not only internal collision of instruments but also external collision of bulky robotic arms, while improving instrument reach. We recommend linear placement of the ports optimized for pelvic surgery as seen in Fig. 29.4. The camera port is placed immediately superior to the umbilicus. Two robotic working ports are placed to the right and left at the same horizontal level as the umbilicus, at least 8 cm away from camera port. A third robotic arm port is placed supero-medial to the left anterior-superior iliac spine (ASIS). One conventional laparoscopic assistant port is placed at the right lateral abdomen, and one 5-mm port in the right upper quadrant may facilitate retraction and suction by the surgical assistant. Port placement should be subtly adjusted depending on the patient's body

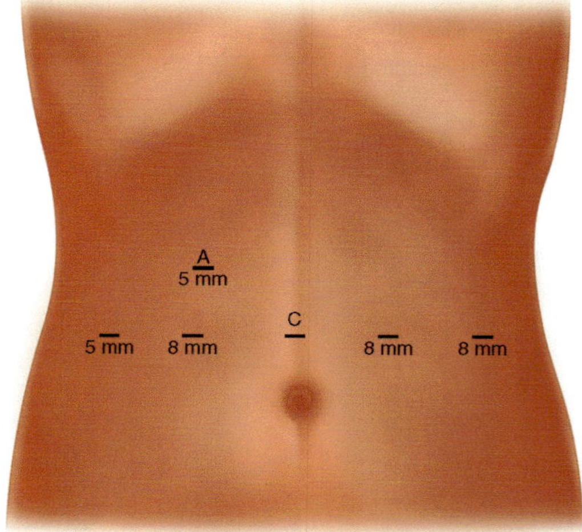

Fig. 29.4 Trocar/port placement for robotic total pelvic exenteration with the Xi platform. C, camera; 8-mm robotic ports; 5-mm laparoscopic assistant port to facilitate retraction and suction

habitus but should consider principles to maximize instrument clearance while optimally positioning for the primary target.

Robot and Assistants

The daVinci Xi robot is docked from the patient's left hip with the boom rotated to target the pelvis with the main robot tower and screen over the patient's left shoulder. The daVinci Si robot is docked with the cart between the legs. Both the scrub nurse and surgical bedside assistant stand on the patient's right side for the duration of the robotic dissection.

Surgical Approach

First Steps

Any oncological abdominal operation begins with diagnostic exploration. In this setting, careful inspection is performed to assess the resectability of the disease, as well as contraindications for pelvic exenteration. In particular, peritoneal carcinomatosis or small-volume distant metastatic disease that could not be detected on preoperative imaging studies should be actively sought. If the decision is made to proceed, optimizing the surgical exposure by elevating the omentum and transverse colon over the liver to uncover the small bowel is performed. The small bowel is then subsequently reflected to the right upper abdominal quadrant and out of the pelvis. Gravity is used to hold the small bowel in place often with the assistance of a small gauze sponge which is carefully positioned at the right lower quadrant along the ileal mesentery. The bedside assistant can gently press down on the gauze sponge with a laparoscopic instrument to stop the small bowel from falling down into the pelvic cavity.

Medial Colonic Dissection

Dissection begins by using the assistant robotic arm (arm #4) to retract the rectosigmoid colon laterally and out of the pelvis and by using the left working robotic arm (arm #3) to tent the peritoneum and create appropriate tension at the base of the superior rectal artery (Fig. 29.5a). Then, the peritoneum is scored along the right side of the base of the mesosigmoid over the sacral promontory (Fig. 29.5b, c). At this point, the assistant can help to tent the mesocolon up, providing a triangular force vector as needed to aid exposure of the dissection plane. The dissection will be subsequently performed along the retrovascular mesocolic plane in a medial to lateral fashion (Fig. 29.5d) until the lateral peritoneal reflection is reached. The hypogastric nerve plexus, ureter, and gonadal vessel are identified and preserved (Fig. 29.5e).

Division of the Inferior Mesenteric Artery

There are multiple options available to manage the inferior mesenteric artery (IMA). Routine low ligation of the superior rectal artery (ligation below the left colic artery take-off) with complete D3 IMA lymph node dissection is our standard approach [28]. The high ligation technique (ligation proximal to the left colic artery take off) provides better length for colorectal or colo-anal anastomosis, but this is usually not required in exenteration surgery. To identify the origin of the IMA, the dissection should continue proximally in the same plane as the medial to lateral dissection until the junction with the aorta is identified. Our preference is to divide between locking clips.

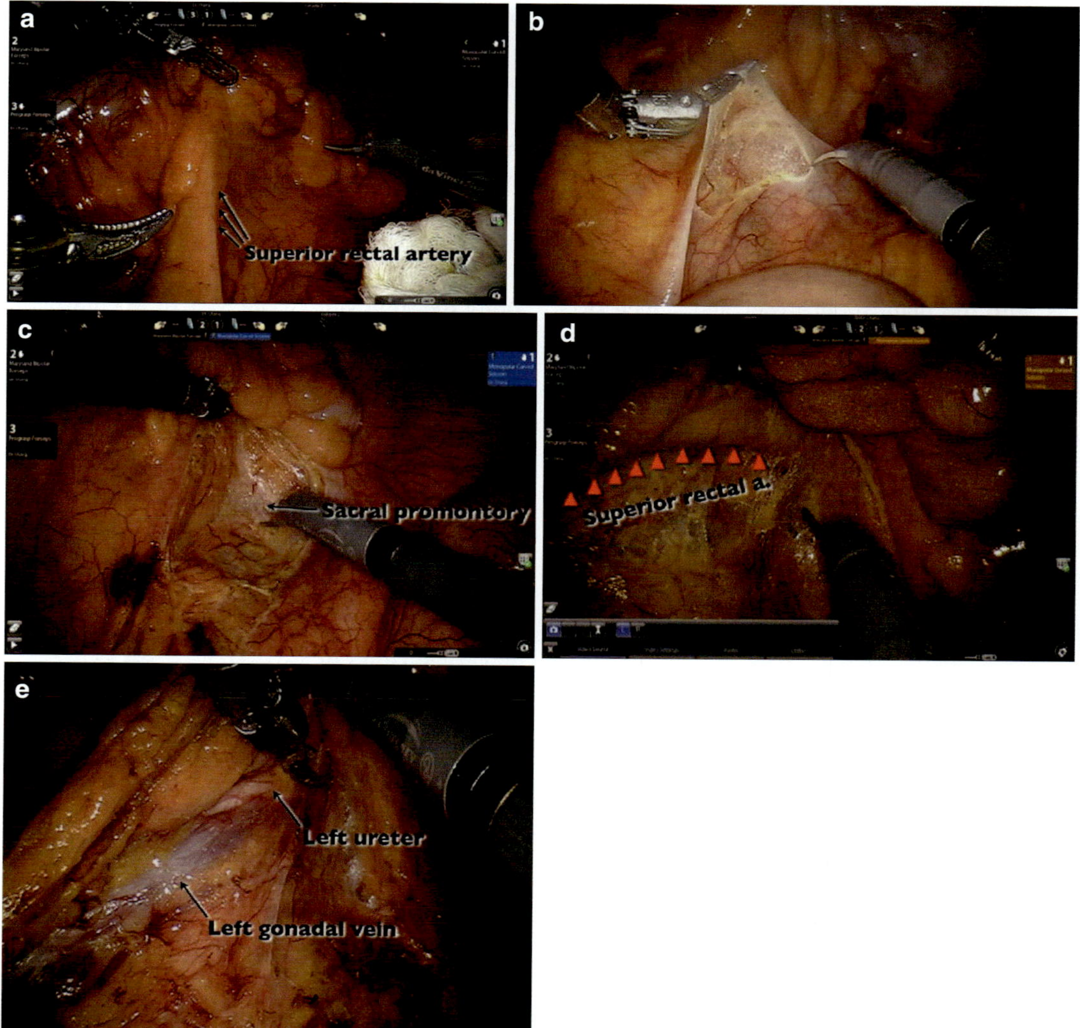

Fig. 29.5 (**a**) Intraoperative image demonstrating the left working robotic arm tenting the peritoneum and creating appropriate tension at the base of the superior rectal artery to expose its vascular pedicle. The arrows indicated the tented peritoneum at the base of the superior rectal artery. (**b**) Image showing the peritoneum dissected along the right side of the base of the mesosigmoid over the sacral promontory. (**c**) Image showing dissection over the sacral promontory. The arrow indicates the sacral promontory. (**d**) Image shows the dissection performed along the avascular plane just below the superior rectal artery. The red arrowheads indicate the inferior border of the superior rectal artery. (**e**) Image shows the dissection performed along the retrovascular mesocolic plane in a medial to lateral fashion, until the lateral peritoneal reflection is reached. The arrows indicate the ureter and gonadal vessel which are identified and preserved

Division of the Inferior Mesenteric Vein

Since most patients will undergo end colostomy formation, the inferior mesenteric vein (IMV) can be divided at the same level as the IMA or superior rectal artery. If a modified exenteration with sphincter-preserving reconstruction is performed, high ligation of the IMV at the inferior border of the pancreas aiming for colonic lengthening may be required. This sometimes requires re-docking the robot with orientation cephalad to mobilize the splenic flexure (see below).

Lateral Colonic Dissection

Lateral dissection is performed to mobilize the sigmoid and descending colon attachments, ultimately meeting the previously completed medial dissection plane along the mesocolon. Mobilization of the splenic flexure is not necessary unless sphincter preservation is planned, but can be performed after robotic re-docking as described above.

Posterior Pelvic Dissection

It is very important to assess tumor location on preoperative imaging and correlate anatomic landmarks with the area of tumor invasion to determine the extent of dissection and to avoid inadvertent tumor violation or unnecessary organ injury. It is appropriate to begin the posterior dissection at the sacral promontory which is the easiest location to find the plane. The conventional posterior dissection plane is between the fascia propria of the rectum and presacral fascia. However, if the tumor is close to the posterior surgical margin, the dissection plane should be taken deeper (between the presacral fascia and sacral periosteum/presacral veins) (Fig. 29.6).

For tumors that directly invade the sacral bone, the posterior dissection has to be stopped before reaching the invasion area, and well-planned sacrectomy should be performed to remove the tumor *en bloc*.

Lateral Pelvic Dissection

The lateral pelvic dissection plane for pelvic exenteration may be wider than the usual TME plane depending on the clearance required (Fig. 29.2). Detailed understanding of lateral pelvic compartment anatomy is crucial. In particular, the relationship between the internal iliac vessels, obturator nerve, sacral nerve root, piriformis muscle, spinous process, and the sciatic notch should be clear. Large bulky tumors with significant lateral extension can pose significant difficulty for exposure and are not good candidates for the robotic approach.

In order to facilitate rectal retraction, a gauze is tied around the rectosigmoid junction, and this is retracted cephalad and laterally using the assistant's locking grasper. Next, the right lateral pelvic parietal peritoneum is opened just proximal to the sacral promontory area (Fig. 29.7), and the right ureter is identified

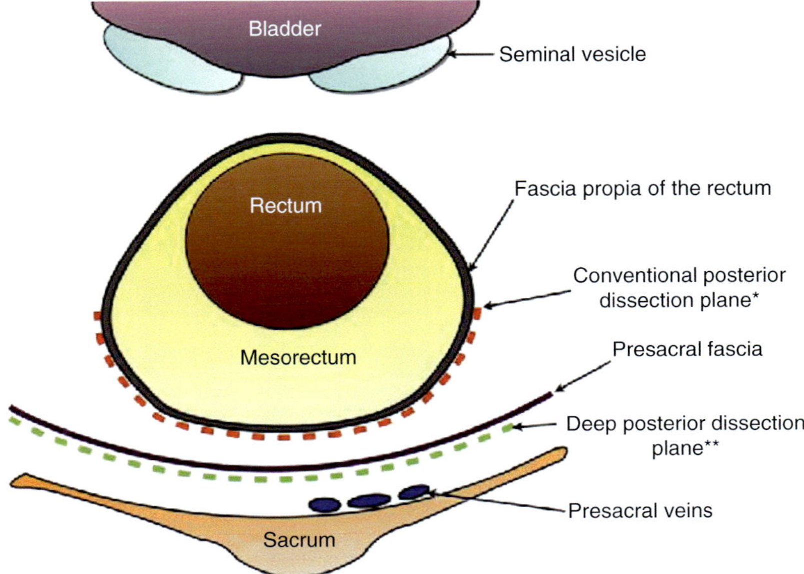

Fig. 29.6 Illustration of the posterior dissection plane. The red broken line shows the conventional posterior dissection plane or total mesorectal excision plane, which is between the fascia propria of the rectum and presacral fascia. The green broken line shows the deep posterior dissection plane. If the tumor is close to the posterior surgical margin, the dissection plane should be taken deeper between presacral fascia and sacral periosteum/presacral veins

underneath. When scoring the lateral pelvic parietal peritoneum laterally, the vas deferens or round ligament is identified, ligated, and divided (Fig. 29.8). The ureter accompanied with meso-ureter is then isolated and mobilized distally until the ureterovesical junction is reached (or as far distal as possible). If there is direct tumor invasion into the ureter, ureteric isolation should be stopped proximal to the area of invasion in order to preserve an adequate resection margin.

Next, robotic arm 4 is used to retract the ureter medially, while at the same time, the assistant's grasper or suction instrument is used to gently push on the external iliac vessels laterally. This facilitates opening the lateral pelvic dissection plane. The dissection continues into this plane, and if required, internal iliac artery branches can be individually identified and selectively ligated and divided (Fig. 29.9a). If the tumor invades the central pelvic compartment in isolation, then only distal branches of the internal iliac artery are ligated (superior vesicle branches, posterior vesicle branches, middle rectal artery, and uterine vessels) (Fig. 29.9b). In contrast, if the tumors invade the lateral compartment, more proximal internal iliac branches may need to be ligated (origin of internal iliac artery, origin of anterior/posterior division, and superior/inferior gluteal artery) (Fig. 29.9c). However, lateral compartment invasion with a bulky tumor will limit adequate exposure for distal dissection and may be a contraindication for the minimally invasive approach.

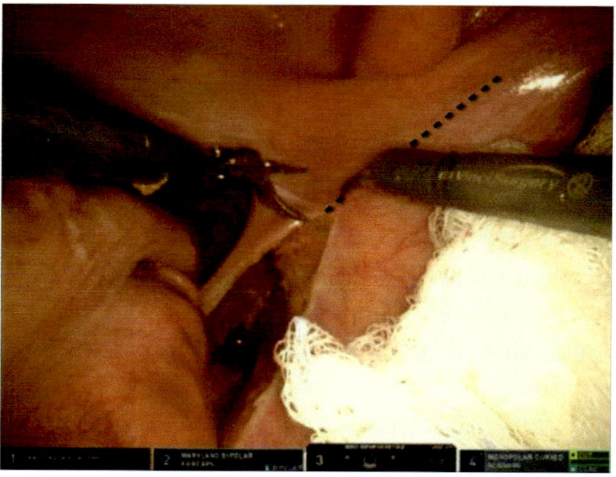

Fig. 29.7 Intraoperative image showing right lateral pelvic parietal peritoneum is opened just proximal to the sacral promontory area. Then the right ureter and vas deferens or round ligament will be identified underneath. The broken line indicates the scored line of the lateral pelvic parietal peritoneum laterally

Fig. 29.8 Intraoperative image demonstrating identification of the vas deferens during scoring of the lateral pelvic parietal peritoneum

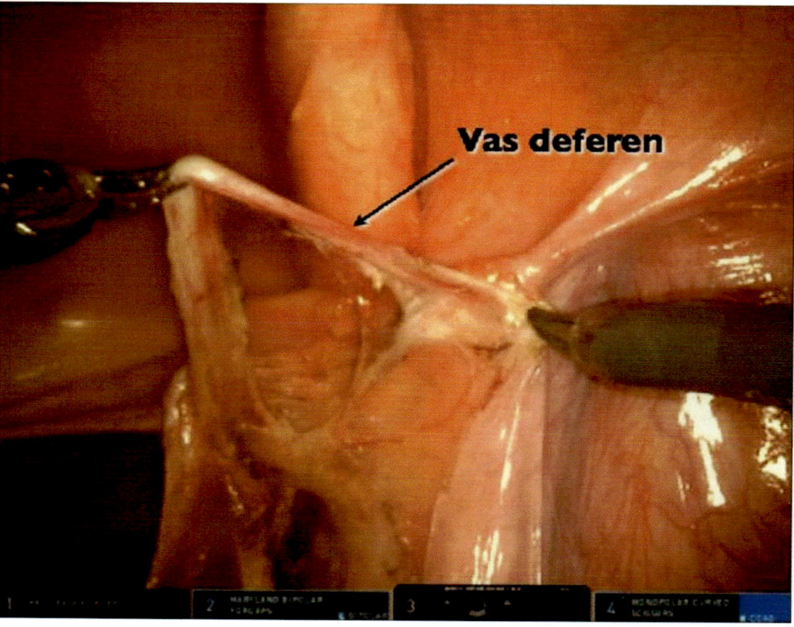

a

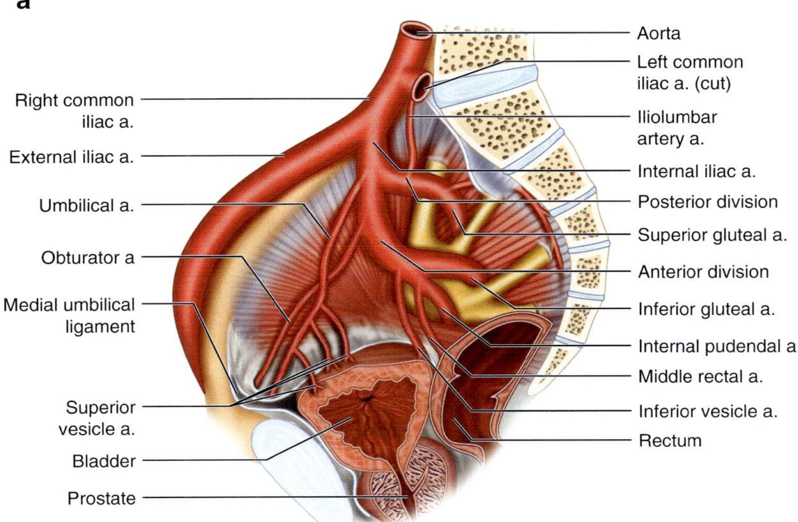

b

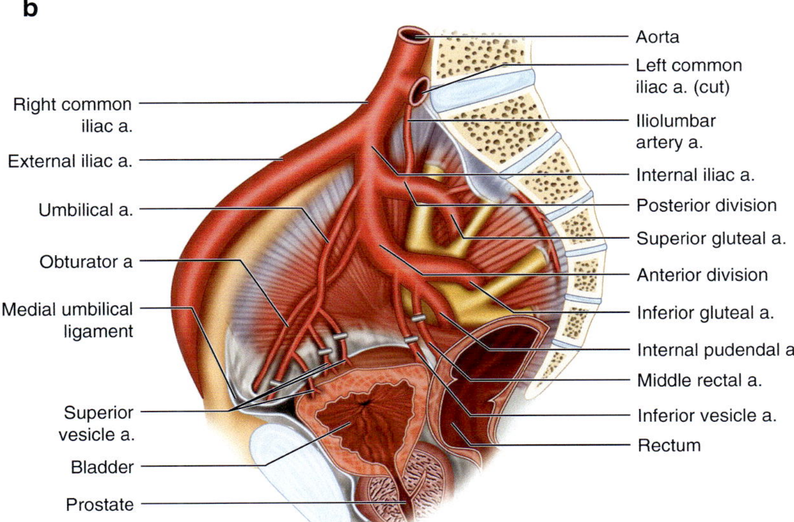

Fig. 29.9 (**a**) Illustration showing the branches of the internal iliac artery. During dissection into the lateral pelvic dissection plane, internal iliac artery branches can be individually identified, and selectively ligated, if required. (**b**) Illustration showing ligation of individual branches of the internal iliac artery in the event of tumor in the central compartment. The white lines indicate ligation of the distal branches of the internal iliac artery (i.e., superior vesicle branches, posterior vesicle branches, middle rectal artery, and uterine vessels). (**c**) Illustration showing ligation of the individual branches of the internal iliac artery in the event that tumor invades the lateral compartment. The white lines indicate ligation of more proximal internal iliac branches (i.e., origin of internal iliac artery, origin of anterior/posterior division, and superior/inferior gluteal artery)

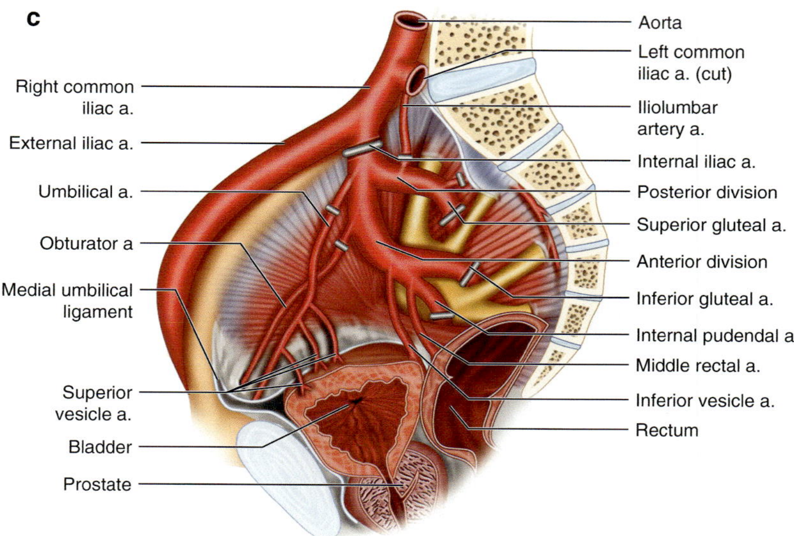

Fig. 29.3 (continued)

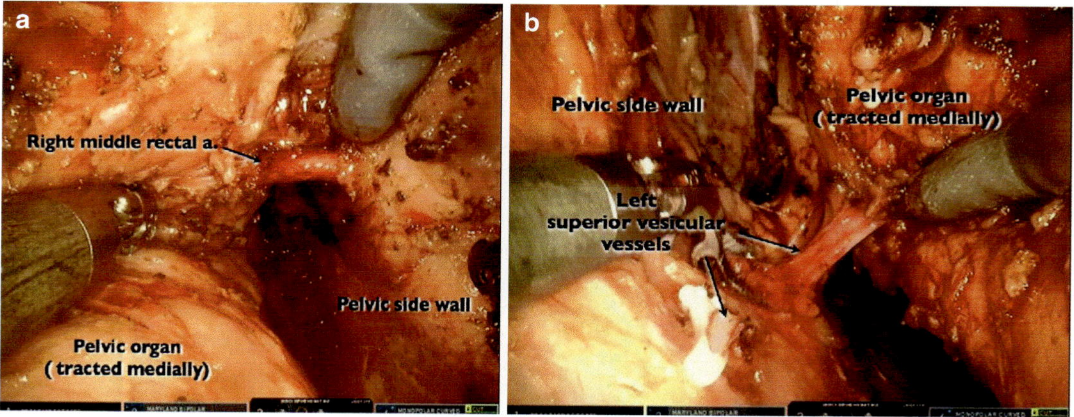

Fig. 29.10 (**a**) Intraoperative image shows individual ligation of the right internal iliac vessel branch. To open the right lateral pelvic dissection plane, the assistant's grasper or suction instrument retracts the pelvic side wall laterally and robotic arm 4 retracts the pelvic organ medially. The arrow indicates the right middle rectal artery. (**b**) Intraoperative image shows individual ligation of the left internal iliac vessel branches. To open the left lateral pelvic dissection plane, the assistant's grasper retracts the pelvic organ medially and robotic arm 4 retracts the pelvic side wall laterally. The arrow indicates superior vesicular vessels

Individual ligation of internal iliac venous tributaries can also be performed. These venous tributaries exhibit significant variation, low pressure, and high flow and are easily disrupted. Thus, slow meticulous dissection is very important at this step, otherwise massive bleeding can ensue obscuring the view for further dissection. The obturator nerve and vessels should be identified laterally and preserved unless invaded by tumor.

Completing as much dissection as possible from the right side facilitates not only the dissection on the left side but also deep posterior dissection. Left side dissection is then performed in the same fashion as the right side dissection (Fig. 29.10a, b). The dissection continues circumferentially until the pelvic floor is reached posteriorly and bilaterally. At this point, the pelvic floor can be divided to enter the ischioanal fossa.

Retzius Space Dissection

Once the deep posterior and lateral dissections are complete, dissection is then performed in the plane anterior to the bladder. Cephalad-midline rectal traction by the assistant's grasper will again facilitate this dissection. The dissection continues down into the space of Retzius, after which the urethra is identified and transected. Suture ligature of the dorsal venous complex using a barbed suture can facilitate hemostasis during this step. The Foley catheter is then removed. In select supra-levator exenteration cases, rectal transection can be performed using an articulated laparoscopic stapler and colorectal or coloanal anastomosis can be performed at a later step. Then, the mesentery of the proximal colon is divided, and the proximal colon is transected by a laparoscopic or robotic stapler.

Perineal Dissection

In cases where an anastomosis is not possible, the perineal dissection can be performed in either lithotomy or prone jack-knife position. However, in patients who need additional sacrectomy x, prone jack-knife position may be required. The anus is closed by a purse-string suture to prevent perineal wound contamination. Perineal skin incision, as well as the ischioanal fat and pelvic floor dissection, is performed in the same fashion as abdominoperineal resection. However, in patients who need additional sacrectomy, the incision can be extended over the sacral area. The specimen is then retrieved through the perineal wound. A sponge is inserted to occlude the defect and pneumoperitoneum can then be re-established.

Pelvic Floor and Perineal Reconstruction

The residual pelvic cavity is a fixed space generally within an irradiated field, and there are three main issues that need to be addressed after specimen removal. First, to prevent perineal herniation (especially after additional sacrectomy) and potential small bowel obstruction, the pelvic inlet needs to be occluded. Second, the pelvic space beneath this area must be filled to guard against pelvic collections above the perineal skin repair. Third, reconstruction of the large perineal or vaginal defect is required recognizing that most of these patients have irradiated soft tissues that are prone to delayed wound healing.

There are several options available to deal with these three issues with inherent advantages and disadvantages. Detailed discussion of these issues is beyond the scope of this chapter. Briefly, an omental flap can be used to partially fill pelvic dead space and close the pelvic inlet but cannot restore the perineal defect. In low body mass index patients, the omentum is usually short and not sufficient. The vertical rectus abdominis muscle (VRAM) flap is able to fill the pelvic dead space and reconstruct the large perineal defect. However, the VRAM flap requires a large abdominal wall incision which needs to be reconstructed, with careful siting of the colostomy or the ileal conduit stoma. We generally prefer robotic-assisted VRAM flap or gluteal advancement flap in combination with omental flap support owing to its robustness and minimally invasive benefits [29]. Gluteal myocutaneous flaps, gracilis flaps, and posterior and anterior thigh flaps are helpful for perineal reconstruction but cannot close the pelvic inlet or fill the pelvic dead space. Nevertheless, they can be vitally useful in cases with larger perineal skin defects where additional skin is required. Free flaps are rarely needed but should be available in the armamentarium of the team.

Urinary and Colonic Reconstruction

An ileal conduit can be constructed intracorporeally by the robotic approach or extracorporeally via Pfannenstiel or low midline incision. Finally, an end colostomy is performed.

Complications

Complication rates of open pelvic exenteration have been consistently reported to be around 40% [30]. While there may be some potential gains from the robotic approach in terms of abdominal wound morbidity, this remains to be demonstrated and it is likely that major complication rates will not be influenced. Regardless of the approach, earlier detection of major complications with prompt rescue in an experienced unit is a vital component of the postoperative care of these patients.

Intraoperatively, major hemorrhage, while rare, is the most immediate life-threatening complication. The lateral pelvic sidewall vasculature and dorsal venous complex are the most common sites of troublesome bleeding during surgery. Prevention is the goal, and a detailed understanding of the anatomy of internal iliac branches and their possible variations is important. Meticulous dissection and utilization of appropriate energy devices, vascular clips, and adherence to vascular principles are key. Early conversion to open surgery while maintaining pressure on bleeding vessels should be performed in the event bleeding cannot be controlled robotically. However, the pneumoperitoneum should be maintained as long as possible during conversion to reduce bleeding complications. Bleeding from the dorsal venous complex during anterior dissection can be reduced by dissection close to the periosteum of pubic bone, as well as prophylactic suturing prior to division.

Postoperative complications such as anastomotic leak, urine leak, infected pelvic collection, and wound or flap failures are all possible as they are with open surgery. This is particularly true in patients who have some degree of underlying malnutrition which may affect wound healing. Appropriate pelvic drain placement be helpful in early control of urine leak issues and prevention of perineal wound failure due to serous fluid discharge. Early detection of urine leakage can be achieved by examining the creatinine level from the drainage fluid. Prompt management such as nephrostomy, ureteric stent, adequate drainage, or reoperation is required. A variety of operations exist for perineal wound complications such as vacuum-assisted suction dressing and debridement as required. The main aim of complication management is to facilitate patient recovery and to avoid potential delays to adjuvant therapy.

Conclusions

In highly selected patients, robotic pelvic exenteration is a feasible procedure which may provide some short-term benefits in eligible patients with locally advanced pelvic tumors. The principles of dissection, vascular control, reconstruction, and recovery are very similar to the open approach. This procedure should only be undertaken in centers experienced with both exenterative and robotic surgery.

References

1. Jemal A, Ward EM, Johnson CJ, et al. Annual report to the nation on the status of cancer, 1975–2014, featuring survival. J Natl Cancer Inst. 2017;109(9). https://doi.org/10.1093/jnci/djx030.
2. O'Connell JB, Maggard MA, Liu JH, et al. Are survival rates different for young and older patients with rectal cancer? Dis Colon Rectum. 2004;47:2064–9.
3. Russell MC, You YN, Hu CY, et al. A novel risk-adjusted nomogram for rectal cancer surgery outcomes. JAMA Surg. 2013;148:769–77.
4. Govindarajan A, Coburn NG, Kiss A, et al. Population-based assessment of the surgical management of locally advanced colorectal cancer. J Natl Cancer Inst. 2006;98:1474–81.
5. Gannon CJ, Zager JS, Chang GJ, et al. Pelvic exenteration affords safe and durable treatment for locally advanced rectal carcinoma. Ann Surg Oncol. 2007;14:1870–7.
6. Levy M, Lipska L, Visokai V, et al. Quality of life after extensive pelvic surgery. Rozhledy v chirurgii: mesicnik Ceskoslovenske chirurgicke spolecnosti. 2016;95:358–462.
7. Beyond TME Collaborative. Consensus statement on the multidisciplinary management of patients with recurrent and primary rectal cancer beyond total mesorectal excision planes. Br J Surg. 2013;100:1009–14.
8. Valentini V, Coco C, Rizzo G, et al. Outcomes of clinical T4M0 extra-peritoneal rectal cancer treated with preoperative radiochemotherapy and surgery: a prospective evaluation of a single institutional experience. Surgery. 2009;145:486–94.
9. Smith JD, Nash GM, Weiser MR, et al. Multivisceral resections for rectal cancer. Br J Surg. 2012;99:1137–43.
10. Monson JR, Weiser MR, Buie WD, et al. Practice parameters for the management of rectal cancer (revised). Dis Colon Rectum. 2013;56:535–50.
11. Lehnert T, Methner M, Pollok A, et al. Multivisceral resection for locally advanced primary colon and rectal cancer: an analysis of prognostic factors in 201 patients. Ann Surg. 2002;235:217–25.

12. Akiyoshi T. Technical feasibility of laparoscopic extended surgery beyond total mesorectal excision for primary or recurrent rectal cancer. World J Gastroenterol. 2016;22:718–26.
13. Akiyoshi T, Nagasaki T, Ueno M. Laparoscopic total pelvic exenteration for locally recurrent rectal cancer. Ann Surg Oncol. 2015;22:3896.
14. Nakamura H, Uehara K, Arimoto A, et al. The feasibility of laparoscopic extended pelvic surgery for rectal cancer. Surg Today. 2016;46:950–6.
15. Bretagnol F, Dedieu A, Zappa M, et al. T4 colorectal cancer: is laparoscopic resection contraindicated? Color Dis. 2011;13:138–43.
16. Martinez-Perez A, Carra MC, Brunetti F, et al. Pathologic outcomes of laparoscopic vs open mesorectal excision for rectal cancer: a systematic review and meta-analysis. JAMA Surg. 2017;152:e165665.
17. van der Pas MH, Haglind E, Cuesta MA, et al. Laparoscopic versus open surgery for rectal cancer (COLOR II): short-term outcomes of a randomised, phase 3 trial. Lancet Oncol. 2013;14:210–8.
18. Guillou PJ, Quirke P, Thorpe H, et al. Short-term endpoints of conventional versus laparoscopic-assisted surgery in patients with colorectal cancer (MRC CLASICC trial): multicentre, randomised controlled trial. Lancet (London, England). 2005;365:1718–26.
19. Veldkamp R, Kuhry E, Hop WC, et al. Laparoscopic surgery versus open surgery for colon cancer: short-term outcomes of a randomised trial. Lancet Oncol. 2005;6:477–84.
20. Clancy C, O'Leary DP, Burke JP, et al. A meta-analysis to determine the oncological implications of conversion in laparoscopic colorectal cancer surgery. Color Dis. 2015;17:482–90.
21. Jayne DG, Guillou PJ, Thorpe H, et al. Randomized trial of laparoscopic-assisted resection of colorectal carcinoma: 3-year results of the UK MRC CLASICC trial group. J Clin Oncol Off J Am Soc Clin Oncol. 2007;25:3061–8.
22. Fleshman J, Branda M, Sargent DJ, et al. Effect of laparoscopic-assisted resection vs open resection of stage II or III rectal cancer on pathologic outcomes: the ACOSOG Z6051 randomized clinical trial. JAMA. 2015;314:1346–55.
23. Colombo PE, Bertrand MM, Alline M, et al. Robotic versus laparoscopic total mesorectal excision (TME) for sphincter-saving surgery: is there any difference in the transanal TME rectal approach?: a single-center series of 120 consecutive patients. Ann Surg Oncol. 2016;23:1594–600.
24. Shin US, Nancy You Y, Nguyen AT, et al. Oncologic outcomes of extended robotic resection for rectal cancer. Ann Surg Oncol. 2016;23(7):2249–57.
25. Malakorn S, Sammour T, Pisters LL, Chang GJ. Robotic total pelvic exenteration. Dis Colon Rectum. 2017;60:555.
26. D'Annibale A, Pernazza G, Monsellato I, et al. Total mesorectal excision: a comparison of oncological and functional outcomes between robotic and laparoscopic surgery for rectal cancer. Surg Endosc. 2013;27:1887–95.
27. Mills JT, Burris MB, Warburton DJ, et al. Positioning injuries associated with robotic assisted urological surgery. J Urol. 2013;190:580–4.
28. Malakorn S, Sammour T, Bednarski B, et al. Three different approaches to the inferior mesenteric artery during robotic D3 lymphadenectomy for rectal cancer. Ann Surg Oncol. 2017;24:1923.
29. Ibrahim AE, Sarhane KA, Pederson JC, et al. Robotic harvest of the rectus abdominis muscle: principles and clinical applications. Semin Plast Surg. 2014;28:26–31.
30. Beyond TME Collaborative. Surgical and survival outcomes following pelvic exenteration for locally advanced primary rectal cancer: results from an international collaboration. Ann Surg. 2017;269(2):315–21.

Tsuyoshi Konishi

Oncological Rationale

Oncological outcomes of surgical treatment for rectal cancer have been dramatically improved during the past decades. With improved curability of tumors in the central pelvis by neoadjuvant therapy and total mesorectal excision (TME), attention has shifted to the lateral pelvic compartment (Fig. 30.1) [1]. In western countries, lateral pelvic lymph nodes have not been indicated for surgical resection in rectal cancer, because lateral nodal disease has been generally considered to be distant metastasis and that lateral local recurrence can be prevented by neoadjuvant therapy [2]. However, a recent study of 366 patients who were treated with neoadjuvant chemoradiotherapy and TME demonstrated that 83% of local recurrences developed in the lateral compartment and 27% of patients with enlarged lateral lymph nodes (>5 mm in diameter) before treatment developed local recurrence [3].

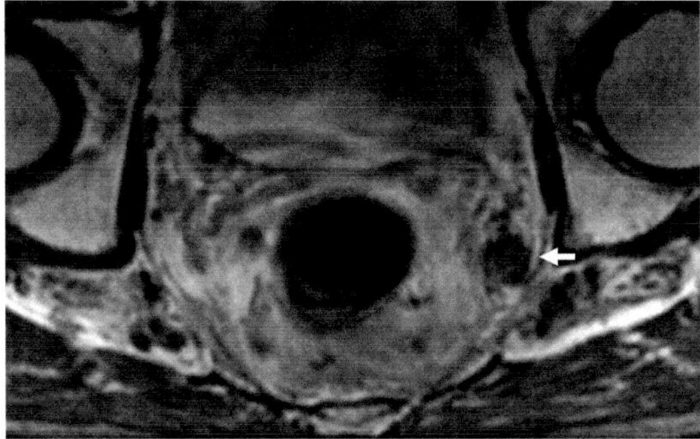

Fig. 30.1 T2-weighted axial image of a metastatic lateral pelvic lymph node. An enlarged metastatic lymph node (white arrow) is observed in the left obturator area. The patient underwent chemoradiation followed by LPLND which revealed pathological metastasis in the lateral pelvic lymph node

In the east, mainly Japan, lateral nodal disease has been treated as a regional disease. According to Japanese studies, rectal cancer above the peritoneal reflection or T1 or T2 rectal cancers rarely metastasize to the lateral compartment, whereas T3 or T4 rectal cancers that extend below the peritoneal reflection have reported incidence of lateral pelvic lymph node metastasis of 15–20% (Table 30.1) [4–7]. Even before the era of modern neoadjuvant chemoradiotherapy and adjuvant chemotherapy, lateral pelvic lymph node dissection (LPLND) alone achieved 40–50% 5-year overall survival rates in patients with histologically positive lateral nodal metastasis, which is historically better survival than with stage IV disease [2, 4, 8].

Electronic supplementary material The online version of this chapter (https://doi.org/10.1007/978-3-030-18740-8_30) contains supplementary material, which is available to authorized users.

T. Konishi (✉)
Department of Gastroenterological Surgery,
Colorectal Division, Cancer Institute Hospital
of the Japanese Foundation for Cancer Research,
Tokyo, Japan
e-mail: tkonishi-tky@umin.ac.jp

Table 30.1 Incidence of lateral pelvic lymph node metastasis without chemoradiation in rectal cancer

Author	Year	Tumor	N	LPLN metastasis
Ueno M	2005	T3-4 extraperitoneal rectal cancer	237	17.3%
Ueno H	2007	T2-4 extraperitoneal rectal cancer	244	16.8%
Kobayashi H	2009	T3-4 extraperitoneal rectal cancer	540	18.1%
Akiyoshi T	2012	T3-4 extraperitoneal rectal cancer	3832	14.6%

An important clinical question is whether we should intensify local treatment for patients with residual lateral nodes after chemoradiotherapy. The estimated incidence of lateral nodal metastasis varies among the previous reports from 5% to 20% after modern neoadjuvant chemoradiotherapy, which irradiates the lateral compartment [3, 9–11]. These findings suggest that TME alone with modern neoadjuvant therapy may decrease, but never eliminate, lateral nodal metastasis. Although patients with lateral nodal metastasis have poorer outcomes than those without disease [3, 12, 13], studies have demonstrated that 42–48% of patients with lateral nodal recurrence did not have distant metastasis [3, 10, 14], suggesting that these patients could have "regional" disease and could be cured with intensified local treatment. Supporting this argument, a recent retrospective study from Japan that combined neoadjuvant chemoradiotherapy and selective LPLND reported excellent outcomes with 2.7% local recurrence and 84% relapse-free survival at 3 years in patients with clinically enlarged lateral nodes [15]. These data challenge the western concept that lateral nodal disease is never curable with resection and supports the hypothesis that lateral nodal disease may be regional and can be cured by combining surgical resection with chemoradiotherapy.

Outcomes of Laparoscopic Lateral Pelvic Lymph Node Dissection

Short-Term Outcomes

Short-term outcomes of laparoscopic (including robotic) LPLND have been reported mainly from Asian countries since 2011 (Table 30.2) [16–23].

Although all the studies were retrospective case series, the median estimated blood loss and rates of conversion were low. The largest multicenter case-matched study from Japan comparing laparoscopic and open LPLND reported longer operative times, less blood loss, less blood transfusions, similar grade III–IV complications, and no mortality in the laparoscopic group [23]. These outcomes indicate technical safety and feasibility of laparoscopic LPLND.

The operative field of LPLND, particularly the distal internal iliac area where metastasis is commonly found, is located deep within the pelvis. For this condition, a laparoscopic approach has the advantage of providing better surgical views compared to an open approach (Fig. 30.2). Magnified high-resolution images and reduced bleeding due to pneumoperitoneum also contribute to clear identification of anatomy and enable meticulous dissection with the laparoscopic approach.

Long-Term Oncological Outcomes

Evidence regarding long-term oncologic outcomes for this procedure are relatively limited. A case series of 107 patients that underwent laparoscopic LPLND after neoadjuvant chemoradiotherapy at a single center reported 95.8% 3-year overall survival, 84.7% 3-year relapse-free survival, and 3.2% 3-year local recurrence [16]. Considering that these patients all had cT3 or T4 extraperitoneal low rectal cancers with clinically positive lateral nodes, these data support the oncologic rationale to perform this procedure. A retrospective multicenter case-matched study from Japan that compared laparoscopic and open LPLND reported 93.9% 3-year overall survival,

Table 30.2 Series of laparoscopic lateral pelvic lymph node dissection for rectal cancer

Author	Year	N	Neoadjuvant chemoradiotherapy	Operation time, min	Blood loss, mL	Number of harvested lateral pelvic lymph nodes	Conversion	Overall morbidity
Yamaguchi T	2017	118	24%	474	213	10	17%	41%
Ogura A	2016	107	100%	461	115	25[d]	0%	34%
Base SU	2014	21[a]	86%	396	200	7	0%	29%
Furuhata T	2014	18	0%	604	380	17	0%	17%
Liu T	2011	68	N/A	271	150	23[d]	N/A	7%
Park JS	2011	16[b]	56%	310	188	9	0%	31%
Liang TJ	2011	34	100%	58[c]	44[c]	6	N/A	21%
Konishi T	2011	14	100%	413	25	23[d]	0%	36%

N/A not available

[a]Including 11 robotic surgeries

[b]Including 2 robotic surgeries

[c]For unilateral lateral pelvic lymph node dissection

[d]Total retrieved lymph nodes

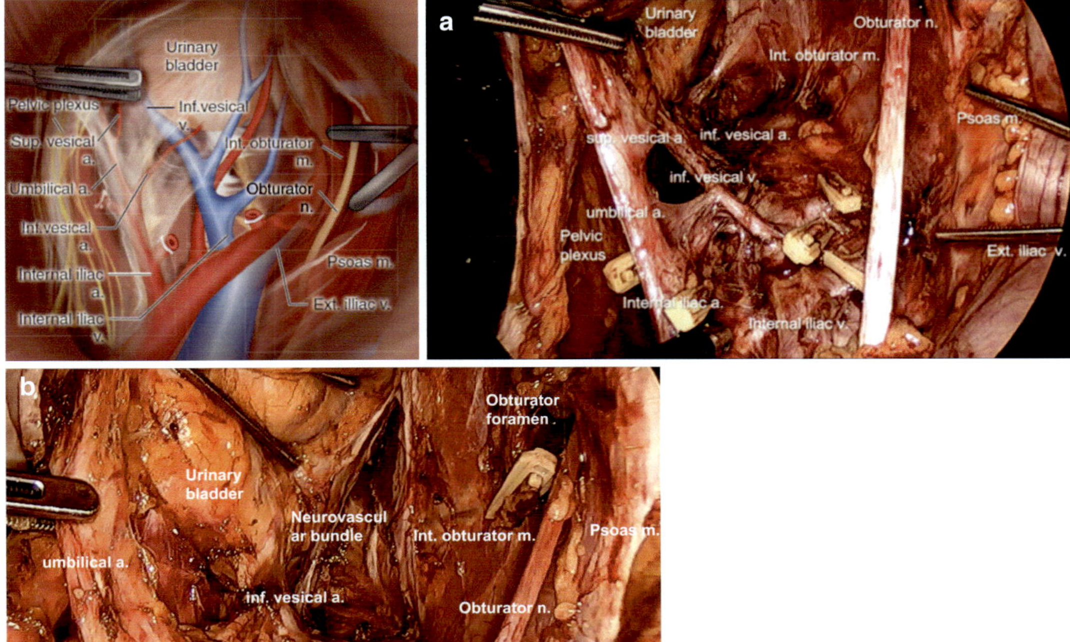

Fig. 30.2 Illustration showing preservation of the superior and inferior vesical vessels and autonomic nerves. Paired intraoperative views (**a**, distant view; **b**, closeup view) after right-sided laparoscopic LPLND, preserving the superior and inferior vesical vessels and autonomic nerves. The area around the inferior vesical vessels is the most common site for metastasis from rectal cancer

93.9% 3-year local recurrence-free survival, and 80.3% 3-year relapse-free survival in the laparoscopic group, which were all similar to or better than the open group [23].

Anatomy of Lateral Pelvic Areas

Areas to Be Dissected

Studies from Japan reported that lateral nodal metastases from rectal cancer mainly occur in the obturator and internal iliac areas and that these areas are "regional" and can be cured by resection [5, 6]. In contrast, lateral nodes in the external and common iliac areas are rarely involved with disease and are more often associated with distant metastasis. As such, obturator and internal iliac areas are two important areas to be dissected with LPLND, while the other areas can be spared unless there are suspicious grossly enlarged nodes.

Anatomic Landmarks

There are numerous anatomic structures in the obturator and internal iliac areas which are unfamiliar to GI surgeons. To simplify understanding, one should consider that the main lateral pelvic compartments, i.e., obturator and internal iliac areas, are surrounded by three planes: (1) lateral plane, psoas muscle, and internal obturator muscle; (2) internal plane, hypogastric nerve and pelvic plexus and urinary bladder; and (3) dorsal plane, internal iliac vessels, and lumbosacral nerve trunk. Another plane divides the area into obturator (lateral) and internal iliac (medial) areas: the vesicohypogastric fascia, which is comprised of the internal iliac artery, vesical branches (umbilical artery and superior and inferior vesical arteries), and urinary bladder. The proximal (cranial) border of the lateral pelvic area is usually at the bifurcation of the internal and external iliac veins.

Dissection exposing these anatomic landmarks along these planes results in complete dissection of the obturator and internal iliac lymph nodes. Importantly, metastatic nodes should be dissected en bloc without exposing or grasping the metastatic tissues. Piece-meal dissection of the nodes should be avoided as it may lead to bleeding, spillage of cancer cells, and possibly recurrence [17]. Dissection using anatomic planes enables en bloc removal of target tissues.

Preservation of Structures

The ureter, hypogastric nerve, pelvic plexus, and obturator nerve are preserved unless they are involved in cancer. A nerve-preserving technique is important to preserve postoperative urinary and sexual function [24, 25]. Careful use of electrocautery or energy devices is needed as these structures are sensitive to thermal and electric injury.

Obturator artery and vein can be resected to facilitate obturator lymph node dissection. In fact, resection of the obturator vessels does not cause dysfunction of any type after surgery. The umbilical artery and superior/inferior vesical vessels can also be resected if they are involved by metastasis. The inferior vesical vessels are often involved or abutted by metastatic nodes as this location is the most common site for metastasis [5]. For this condition, the obturator and internal iliac areas are dissected en bloc using the three planes and without the vesicohypogastric fascia (Fig. 30.3).

Preoperative Imaging Studies

Anatomic variation is common for the internal iliac vessels and their branches, particularly for the veins. Careful evaluation of preoperative contrast-enhanced computed tomography (CT) or magnetic resonance imaging (MRI) is needed for mapping the origins of the superior gluteal artery, umbilical artery, superior/inferior vesical vessels, and obturator vessels from the main trunk of the internal iliac artery and vein. The inferior vesical artery/vein should be carefully identified and evaluated for invasion. It is important to determine from preoperative imaging whether the vessels are to be resected or preserved

Fig. 30.3 Dissection planes for LPLND. (**a**) The obturator and internal iliac areas are surrounded by three planes, which are marked by the yellow dashed lines. (**b**) The vesicohypogastric fascia, which includes the internal iliac artery, vesical branches, and urinary bladder, divides the lateral area into obturator and internal iliac areas

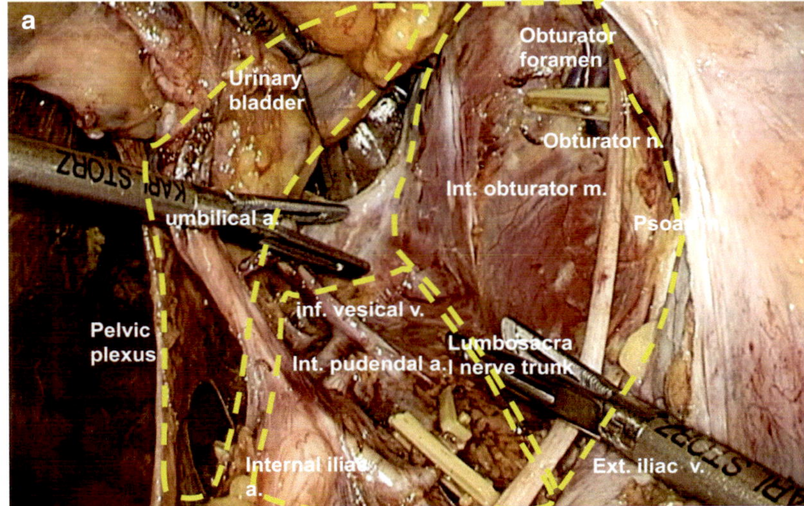

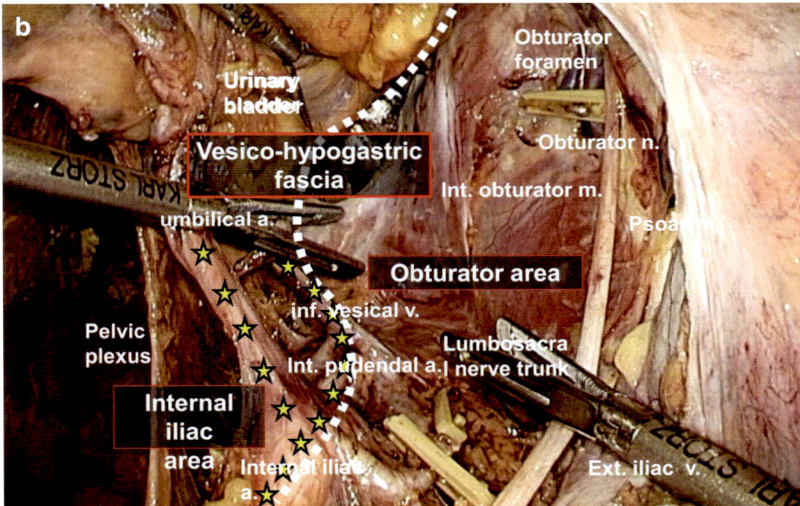

according to the location of metastatic lymph nodes. If invaded or abutted by metastatic nodes, the vessel branches must be incorporated into the resection.

Technical Details

Patient Positioning and Port Placement

LPLND is initiated after completion of TME. Patient positioning is the same as used in TME. Typically, the patient is placed in Trendelenburg position so that the small bowel, colon, and omentum are moved out of the pelvic surgical field by gravity. The degree of Trendelenburg position should facilitate appropriate exposure but should be as minimal as possible given the prolonged operating time expected for LPLND.

Port placement can also be the same as used in TME with no need for additional ports. Typical port placement is described in Fig. 30.4. We typically place a 12-mm camera port at the umbilicus, 12-mm port at the right lower abdomen, and three 5-mm ports at the right middle, left lower, and left middle abdomen. At least one 12-mm

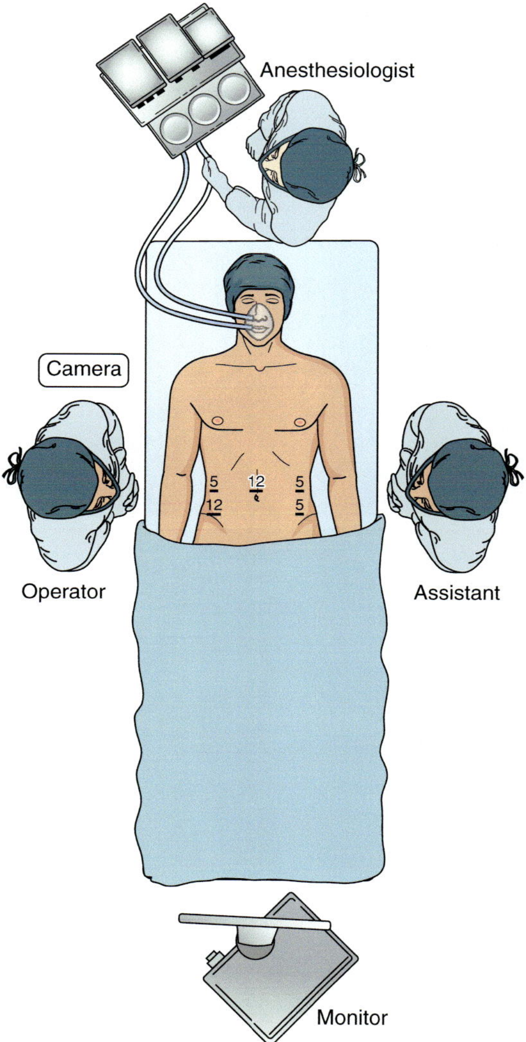

Fig. 30.4 Trocar/port and surgeon positions for LPLND

port for quick insertion of gauze is used in the case of bleeding.

For the left-side dissection, the surgeon operates from the right side of the patient. For the right-side dissection, the surgeon starts from the left side of the patient to facilitate exposing the external iliac vein, psoas muscle, internal obturator muscles, and obturator canal. The surgeon then moves the position to the right side of the patient for the remainder of the procedure.

Step-by-Step Procedure
(Video 30.1)

Isolation of the Ureter and Pelvic Plexus

The ureter is identified, taped, and isolated distally. The hypogastric nerve and pelvic plexus are also mobilized together with the ureter in the same plane, which is covered with the same connective tissue (i.e., prehypogastric nerve fascia). Isolation of the pelvic plexus is stopped before entry into the neurovascular bundle to avoid injury. Careful dissection is needed at this point, particularly avoiding thermal injury to the nerves. After isolation, the ureter may be retracted toward the midline using an umbilical tape so that the ureter and nerve are mobilized away from the internal iliac lymph nodes.

Obturator Lymph Node Dissection

Identifying Internal Border of the External Iliac Vein
The purpose of identifying the external iliac vein is to detect the psoas muscle just behind the vessel. Dissection of the external iliac lymph nodes on the surface of the vein is not performed unless there is presence of grossly enlarged nodes. This is an uncommon place for metastasis from rectal cancer, and the dissection often causes postoperative edema in the lower extremities.

At the distal end of the external iliac vein, there is a lymphatic chain from the inguinal nodes to the obturator nodes. This distal end should be ligated with a clip to avoid lymphorrhea and lymphocele after surgery.

Dissection Along Psoas and Internal Obturator Muscles
Once the psoas muscle is identified behind the external iliac vein, the dissection is continued to expose the surface of the psoas muscle followed by the internal obturator muscle. There is an

avascular plane between the obturator lymph node and fascia of the muscle. Tiny perforating veins in this layer can be dissected with electrocautery.

Identification of the Obturator Nerve and Vessels at the Obturator Canal

Dissection is continued to expose the surface of the internal obturator muscle; and the obturator nerve, artery, and vein are easily identified at the entry point to the obturator canal. The obturator nerve is preserved and the obturator vessels are ligated at this entry point.

Exposing Internal Obturator Muscle to the Tendinous Arch of the Levator Muscle

Dissection is continued on the surface of the internal obturator muscle down to the tendinous arch where the levator muscle attaches to the internal obturator muscle. Dissection is continued to expose the surface of the levator muscle and the space that communicates with the TME space. Although communication with the TME space is not needed, it avoids postoperative lymphocele in the lateral area as the discharge is drained to the TME space through the communication. This is the end of the lateral border dissection of the obturator area.

Dissection Along the Umbilical Artery and Bladder (Vesicohypogastric Fascia)

Dissection now moves to the internal border of the obturator area. The first step is to identify the umbilical artery. Obturator lymph nodes are retracted laterally, and this countertraction will expose the clear embryonic plane between the adipose tissue of the obturator lymph nodes and the adipose tissue of the bladder and vesical vessels. This layer is called the "vesicohypogastric fascia" and is typically avascular. Dissection continues following this layer, exposing the umbilical artery followed by the superior and inferior vesical vessels and the surface of the bladder. Finally, the dissection reaches the levator which was previously exposed. This is the most distal end of the obturator area.

Isolation of Obturator Nerve

Once the obturator nerve is identified at the obturator canal, the nerve is exposed and isolated from distal to proximal, detaching the obturator lymph nodes. The obturator nerve is to be isolated to the bifurcation of the internal and external iliac veins. At this point, the nerve runs behind the vessels. Importantly, electrocautery is to be avoided around the obturator nerve as it might stimulate the nerve and create unintended leg motion which could be dangerous, as well as creating potential for thermal injury to the nerve with resultant postoperative obturator nerve palsy.

Ligation of Proximal End of the Obturator Lymph Nodes

After isolating the obturator nerve, the adipose tissue of the obturator lymph nodes is ligated at the bifurcation of the internal and external iliac veins. This lymphatic chain is to be ligated using a clip to avoid postoperative lymphorrhea or lymphocele. This is the proximal end of the obturator lymph node dissection.

Exposing Internal Iliac Vessels and Lumbosacral Nerve Trunk

The dissection continues by exposing the internal iliac artery and vein lateral to the vesicohypogastric fascia. It is critical at this point to keep the plane exactly on the surface of internal iliac artery and vein so that the branch vessels (e.g., obturator artery/vein) can be identified and ligated at the root. Dissection follows exposing the surface of the lumbosacral nerve trunk. The surface of the lumbosacral nerve trunk is usually covered with thin connective tissue, and dissection of obturator lymph nodes can be performed preserving this connective tissue. If this connective tissue is taken with the nodes, the surface of the nerve is exposed, and patients may complain of lower extremity pain due to sciatic neuralgia.

Identification of Inferior Vesical Vessels and Infra-piriformis Muscle Foramen

Dissection of the dorsal plane of the obturator area culminates with identification of the inferior vesical vessels which are the last branches from the main trunk of the internal iliac vessels, followed by the infra-piriformis muscle foramen at which the main trunk of the internal iliac vessels exit the pelvis as the internal pudendal vessels. Dissection around the inferior vesical vessels and infra-piriformis muscle foramen is critical as this area is the most frequent site for metastasis. If metastatic lymph nodes abut the inferior vesical vessels or internal pudendal vessels, then resection of the vessels is required. At the infra-piriformis muscle foramen, dissection reaches the distal obturator area which was previously dissected, and thus the dissection of the obturator area is finished.

Internal Iliac Lymph Node Dissection

Preservation of Hypogastric Nerve and Pelvic Plexus

As described at the beginning of the procedure, the hypogastric nerve and pelvic plexus are separated together with the ureter from the piriformis muscle. The S4 pelvic splanchnic nerve sometimes runs adjacent to the inferior vesical vessels, which distally combine and form the neurovascular bundle at the entry point to the bladder. Dissection and isolation of the pelvic plexus can stop before the S4 pelvic splanchnic nerve is reached to avoid injury to neurovascular bundle.

Dissection of Internal Iliac Lymph Nodes

Adipose tissue on the surface of the main trunk of the internal iliac vessels internal to the vesicohypogastric fascia is dissected, exposing the surface of these vessels. The volume of adipose tissue in this area is relatively small, and the inferior vesical vessels should be exposed to ensure complete removal of the lymphatic tissue in this area.

Final Check and Drain Placement

The harvested lymph node tissues are removed from the abdomen in a plastic bag. It is important that targeted enlarged lymph nodes are also har-vested with the specimen, since metastatic nodes may adhere to the inferior vesical vessels or neurovascular bundle and are occasionally left in situ. If this is the case, combined resection of inferior vesical vessels or neurovascular bundle is needed. Finally, a drainage catheter is placed in the TME space.

Combined Resection of Vessels and Nerves

Metastatic lateral nodes often involve or abut vesical branches of the internal iliac vessels. Particularly, the inferior vesical artery and vein are the most commonly involved as this is the most frequent metastatic site. Sometimes, the main trunk of the internal iliac artery/vein or pelvic nerve plexus is involved by large metastatic nodes. In either case, involved vessels and nerves must be resected. Typical variations of LPLND are described in Fig. 30.5. When the enlarged node involves the inferior vesical vessels, these vessels are resected preserving the main trunk of the internal iliac vessels and autonomic nerves. The vesical vessels are ligated at the root from the internal iliac vessels and distally at the entry point to the bladder. The umbilical artery can also be ligated to make the procedure easier. Dissection follows the lateral, internal, and dorsal planes, and en bloc dissection of the obturator and internal iliac lymph nodes is performed (Fig. 30.6).

When the metastatic nodes involve the main trunk of the internal iliac artery, it is ligated distal to the superior gluteal artery and distally at the entry point to the infra-piriformis foramen. In this case, the dorsal dissection plane follows the surface of internal iliac vein. When the main trunk of the internal iliac vein is involved, dissection requires tremendous technical skill. Proximal ligation is similar to the artery, but the distal portion of the internal iliac vein often has multiple perforating branches to the pelvic wall. These must be carefully ligated to avoid bleeding. In this case, the dorsal dissection plane follows the lumbosacral nerve trunk.

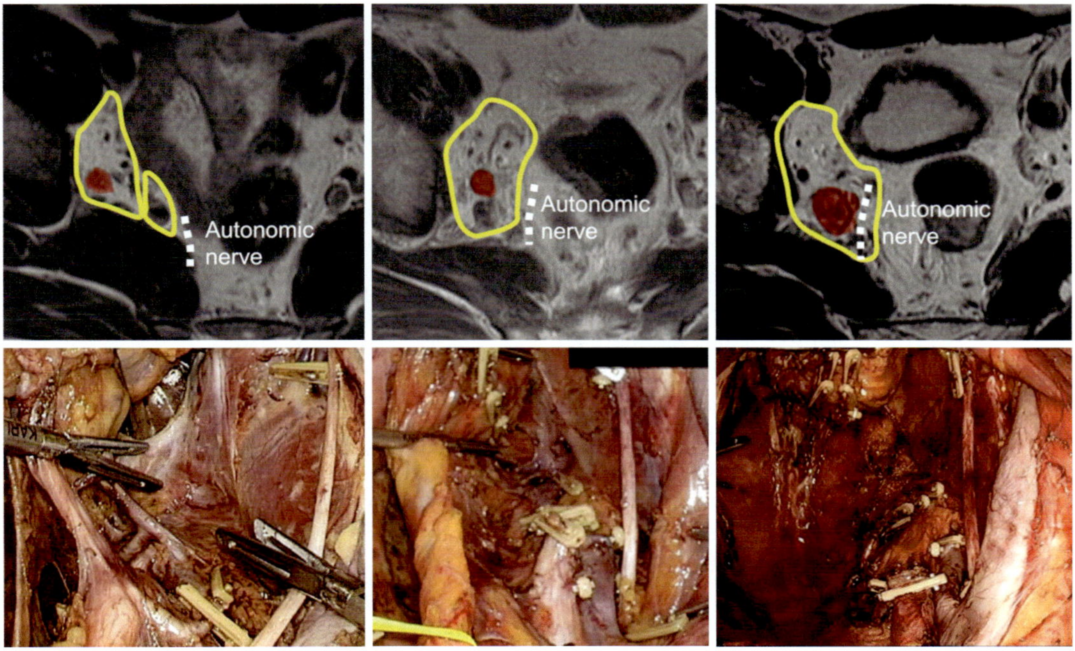

Fig. 30.5 Typical variations of LPLND. Left: an enlarged obturator lymph node did not invade or abut the inferior vesical vessels. Obturator and internal iliac areas were dissected separately while preserving all the vesical branch vessels and autonomic nerves. Middle: an enlarged internal iliac node invades the inferior vesical vessels. Obturator and internal iliac areas were dissected en bloc resecting all vesical branch vessels but preserving the autonomic nerves. Right: a large metastatic node invades the inferior vesical vessels, main trunk of the internal iliac artery and vein, and abuts the autonomic nerves. Obturator and internal iliac areas were dissected en bloc with combined resection of the internal iliac artery and vein with the vesical branch vessels and autonomic nerves. The lumbosacral nerve trunk is exposed after resecting the internal iliac vessels

Fig. 30.6 Surgical view after left-sided laparoscopic LPLND preserving autonomic nerves and main trunk of the internal iliac vessels but resecting the vesical branch vessels (umbilical artery and superior and inferior vesical vessels)

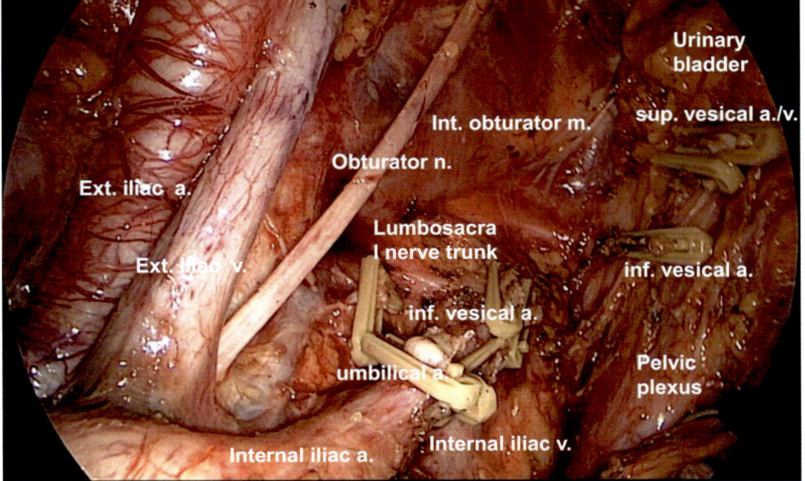

Conclusions

LPLND is an important component of the armamentarium for colorectal surgeons who practice in tertiary referral centers with specific focus on the multidisciplinary management of rectal cancer. A minimally invasive approach provides more advanced knowledge of pelvic anatomy particularly outside of what is known for TME. Standardization of this procedure through a minimally invasive approach may facilitate the dissection technique and provide optimal functional and oncological outcomes. However, before this technique is implemented into clinical practice, formal training with courses and cadaveric dissections is needed to abbreviate the learning curve and decrease the risk of intraoperative complications/injuries in the early adoption phase. As refinement of precise indications for the procedure evolves, selection of ideal candidates will further optimize outcomes.

References

1. Kusters M, Bosman SJ, Van Zoggel DM, et al. Local recurrence in the lateral lymph node compartment: improved outcomes with induction chemotherapy combined with multimodality treatment. Ann Surg Oncol. 2016;23:1883–9.
2. Konishi T, Watanabe T, Nagawa H, et al. Preoperative chemoradiation and extended pelvic lymphadenectomy for rectal cancer: two distinct principles. World J Gastrointest Surg. 2010;2:95–100.
3. Kim TH, Jeong SY, Choi DH, et al. Lateral lymph node metastasis is a major cause of locoregional recurrence in rectal cancer treated with preoperative chemoradiotherapy and curative resection. Ann Surg Oncol. 2008;15:729–37.
4. Akiyoshi T, Watanabe T, Miyata S, et al. Results of a Japanese nationwide multi-institutional study on lateral pelvic lymph node metastasis in low rectal cancer: is it regional or distant disease? Ann Surg. 2012;255:1129–34.
5. Kobayashi H, Mochizuki H, Kato T, et al. Outcomes of surgery alone for lower rectal cancer with and without pelvic sidewall dissection. Dis Colon Rectum. 2009;52:567–76.
6. Ueno H, Mochizuki H, Hashiguchi Y, et al. Potential prognostic benefit of lateral pelvic node dissection for rectal cancer located below the peritoneal reflection. Ann Surg. 2007;245:80–7.
7. Ueno M, Oya M, Azekura K, et al. Incidence and prognostic significance of lateral lymph node metastasis in patients with advanced low rectal cancer. Br J Surg. 2005;92:756–63.
8. Sugihara K, Kobayashi H, Kato T, et al. Indication and benefit of pelvic sidewall dissection for rectal cancer. Dis Colon Rectum. 2006;49:1663–72.
9. Ishihara S, Kawai K, Tanaka T, et al. Oncological outcomes of lateral pelvic lymph node metastasis in rectal cancer treated with preoperative chemoradiotherapy. Dis Colon Rectum. 2017;60:469–76.
10. Kim MJ, Kim TH, Kim DY, et al. Can chemoradiation allow for omission of lateral pelvic node dissection for locally advanced rectal cancer? J Surg Oncol. 2015;111:459–64.
11. Kim TG, Park W, Choi DH, et al. Factors associated with lateral pelvic recurrence after curative resection following neoadjuvant chemoradiotherapy in rectal cancer patients. Int J Color Dis. 2014;29:193–200.
12. Kusters M, Slater A, Muirhead R, et al. What to do with lateral nodal disease in low locally advanced rectal cancer? A call for further reflection and research. Dis Colon Rectum. 2017;60:577–85.
13. Shihab OC, Taylor F, Bees N, et al. Relevance of magnetic resonance imaging-detected pelvic sidewall lymph node involvement in rectal cancer. Br J Surg. 2011;98:1798–804.
14. Kim MJ, Chan Park S, Kim TH, et al. Is lateral pelvic node dissection necessary after preoperative chemoradiotherapy for rectal cancer patients with initially suspected lateral pelvic node? Surgery. 2016;160:366–76.
15. Akiyoshi T, Ueno M, Matsueda K, et al. Selective lateral pelvic lymph node dissection in patients with advanced low rectal cancer treated with preoperative chemoradiotherapy based on pretreatment imaging. Ann Surg Oncol. 2014;21:189–96.
16. Ogura A, Akiyoshi T, Nagasaki T, et al. Feasibility of laparoscopic total mesorectal excision with extended lateral pelvic lymph node dissection for advanced lower rectal cancer after preoperative chemoradiotherapy. World J Surg. 2017;41:868–75.
17. Liang JT. Technical feasibility of laparoscopic lateral pelvic lymph node dissection for patients with low rectal cancer after concurrent chemoradiation therapy. Ann Surg Oncol. 2011;18:153–9.
18. Konishi T, Kuroyanagi H, Oya M, et al. Multimedia article. Lateral lymph node dissection with preoperative chemoradiation for locally advanced lower rectal cancer through a laparoscopic approach. Surg Endosc. 2011;25:2358–9.
19. Park JS, Choi GS, Lim KH, et al. Laparoscopic extended lateral pelvic node dissection following total mesorectal excision for advanced rectal cancer: initial clinical experience. Surg Endosc. 2011;25:3322–9.
20. Liu T, Zhang C, Yu P, et al. Laparoscopic radical correction combined with extensive lymphadenectomy and pelvic autonomic nerve preservation for mid-to-low rectal cancer. Clin Colorectal Cancer. 2011;10:183–7.
21. Bae SU, Saklani AP, Hur H, et al. Robotic and laparoscopic pelvic lymph node dissection for rectal cancer:

short-term outcomes of 21 consecutive series. Ann Surg Treat Res. 2014;86:76–82.

22. Furuhata T, Okita K, Nishidate T, et al. Clinical feasibility of laparoscopic lateral pelvic lymph node dissection following total mesorectal excision for advanced rectal cancer. Surg Today. 2015;45:310–4.

23. Yamaguchi T, Konishi T, Kinugasa Y, et al. Laparoscopic versus open lateral lymph node dissection for locally advanced low rectal cancer: a subgroup analysis of a large multicenter cohort study in Japan. Dis Colon Rectum. 2017;60:954–64.

24. Akasu T, Sugihara K, Moriya Y. Male urinary and sexual functions after mesorectal excision alone or in combination with extended lateral pelvic lymph node dissection for rectal cancer. Ann Surg Oncol. 2009;16:2779–86.

25. Saito S, Fujita S, Mizusawa J, et al. Male sexual dysfunction after rectal cancer surgery: results of a randomized trial comparing mesorectal excision with and without lateral lymph node dissection for patients with lower rectal cancer: Japan Clinical Oncology Group Study JCOG0212. Eur J Surg Oncol. 2016;42:1851–8.

Jin-Tung Liang

Introduction

Lateral pelvic lymph node dissection (LPLND) for treatment of advanced low rectal cancer has been predominantly performed in Japan because of technical difficulties and higher incidence of surgical morbidities (e.g., genitourinary dysfunction) [1, 2]. In our institution patients with advanced low rectal cancer and synchronous clinically positive lateral pelvic nodes have been treated with preoperative concurrent chemoradiation therapy (CCRT) followed by total mesorectal excision (TME) [3–5]. However, patients who have persistent enlargement of nodes even after CCRT have selectively undergone LPLND. Although LPLND has been performed by open laparotomy, the minimally invasive approach has been rarely reported [6]. In this chapter, we present our approach to LPLND after CCRT.

Electronic supplementary material The online version of this chapter (https://doi.org/10.1007/978-3-030-18740-8_31) contains supplementary material, which is available to authorized users.

J.-T. Liang (⊠)
Department of Surgery, National Taiwan University
Hospital, Taipei City, Taiwan
e-mail: jintung@ntu.edu.tw

Indications for Lateral Pelvic Lymph Node Dissection

In our institution, LPLND has been reserved for advanced rectal cancer patients with clinically suspicious lymph node metastasis in the lateral pelvic side wall. T3 or T4 rectal cancers below the pelvic peritoneal reflection with presence of suspicious metastatic lateral pelvic lymph nodes, as detected by transrectal ultrasonography, magnetic resonance imaging, computed tomography, or positron emission tomography, were candidates for this surgical procedure. Candidate patients received preoperative CCRT protocol, which includes radiation therapy (4500 cGy during 5 weeks) and FOLFOX (5-fluorouracil, leucovorin, and oxaliplatin) with or without the addition of targeted agents, administered biweekly for six cycles. After completion of CCRT, diagnostic imaging studies were performed, and if they revealed persistence of positive lateral pelvic lymph nodes, the patients were managed by LPLND and TME at 6 weeks after completion of CCRT. Choice of unilateral or bilateral LPLND was dependent on the location of nodal involvement.

Laparoscopic Lateral Pelvic Lymph Node Dissection

Five abdominal ports (5/12-mm) are used: para-umbilical port for establishment of pneumo-peritoneum and insertion of a camera; two ports at the anterior axillary line over the right lower quadrant as working ports; and two other ports in mirror locations to the working port in the left lower quadrant as assistant ports. We perform LPLND in the period between complete mobilization of the rectum and perineal dissection or reconstruction of bowel continuity [5].

LPLND over the left pelvic side wall is performed first because it can be started immediately after mobilization of the rectosigmoid colon without changing operator position (Fig. 31.1a–g). We initiate clearance of lymphatic tissues by skeletonizing the common iliac vessels. The obturator fossa is then entered at the bifurcation of the internal and external iliac vessels. The lymphatic chains intermingled with adipose tissues within the obturator fossa and paravesical fossa are removed en bloc. During the dissection process, the obturator nerve and the pelvic plexus medial to the internal iliac vessels are carefully preserved. After completion of left-sided LPLND, the surgeon shifts to the left side of the patient and uses the left abdominal ports as the working ports and the right-sided ports as the assistant ports to perform right-sided LPLND (Fig. 31.2a–h).

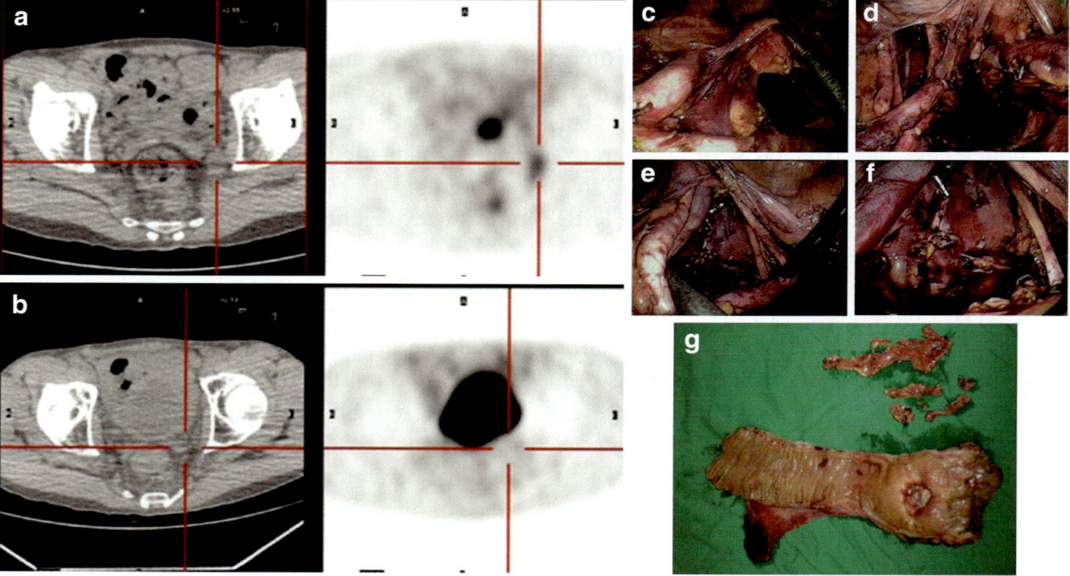

Fig. 31.1 (**a**) Positron emission tomography/computed tomography (PET/CT) scan shows suspected metastatic lymph nodes over the left obturator fossa of the pelvis before CCRT in a 71-year-old male patient with low rectal cancer. (**b**) After CCRT, PET/CT shows attenuated but persistent silhouette of suspicious lymph nodes at the same anatomic location. (**c**) The patient underwent laparoscopic lateral pelvic lymph node dissection, which started from stripping of lymphatic tissues at the left common iliac artery and vein. (**d**) The obturator fossa was explored and the lymphatic chains were cleared. (**e**) Clearance of lymph nodes over the left lateral pelvis was completed and the obturator nerve was preserved. (**f**) A closer view showing en bloc removal of lympho-adipose tissues over the left obturator fossa and paravesical fossa. (**g**) Surgical specimen showing that the patient had undergone abdominoperineal resection with cleared lympho-adipose tissues from the lateral left pelvis

Fig. 31.2 (**a**) Before CCRT, coronal view of computed tomography imaging shows an enlarged lymph node (arrow) over the right lateral pelvis in a 54-year-old male patient with low rectal cancer. (**b**) Axial view spotlighting the encasement of the iliac vein by the metastatic node (arrow). (**c**) PET/CT identified the metastatic lymph node in the right pelvis. (**d**) After CCRT, the suspected metastatic node (arrow) was identified but had altered density on CT imaging. (**e**) The metastatic lymph node was dissected from the involved iliac vein by blunt dissection. (**f**) Closer laparoscopic view of the metastatic lymph node (arrow) after CCRT. (**g**) The lympho-adipose tissues of the right lateral pelvic station were removed en bloc with preservation of the obturator nerve (arrow). (**h**) Surgical specimen showing scarred rectal cancer (arrow) around the anal dentate line with a positive lateral pelvic lymph node (arrow)

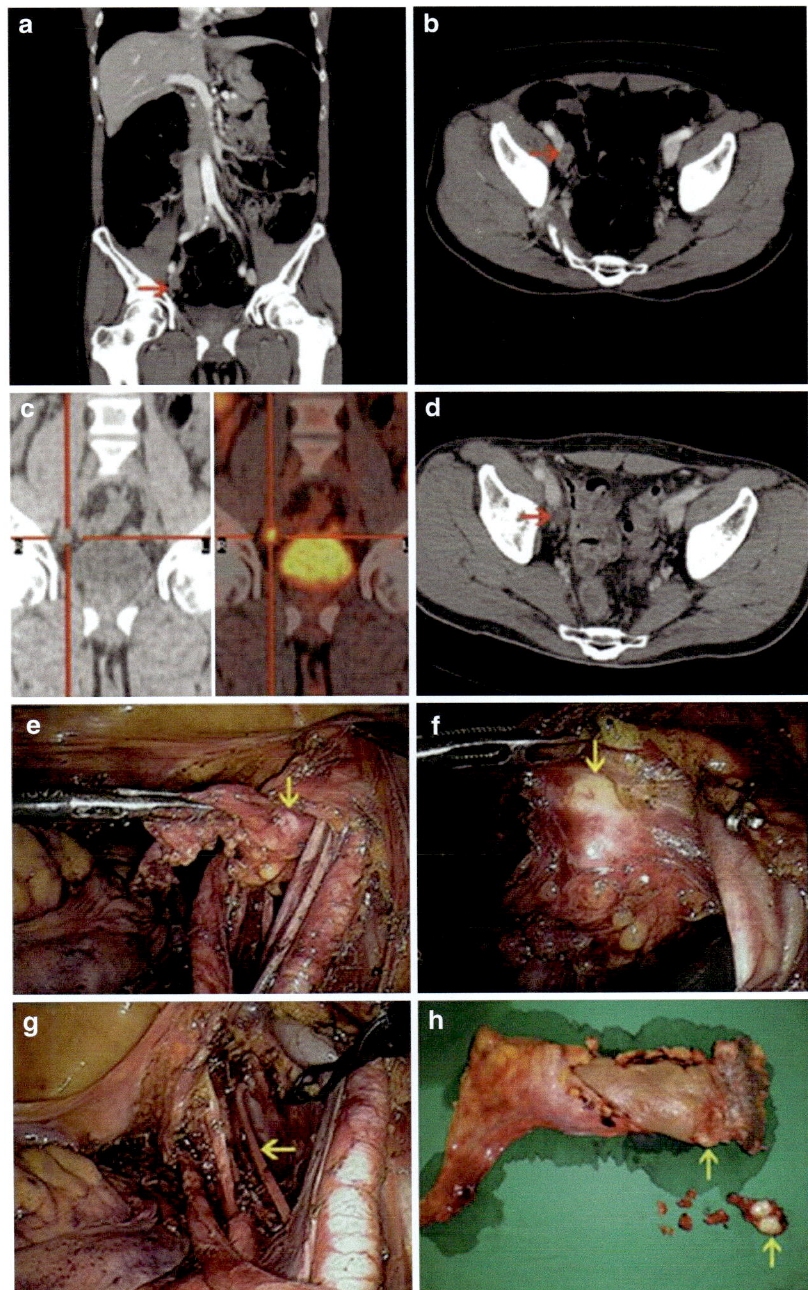

Robotic Lateral Pelvic Lymph Node Dissection (Video 31.1)

We have adopted the robotic approach to perform LPLND, especially for patients with obesity or patients with narrow or deep pelvic cavities. The surgical anatomy and extent of dissection for LPLND are shown in Fig. 31.3a, b.

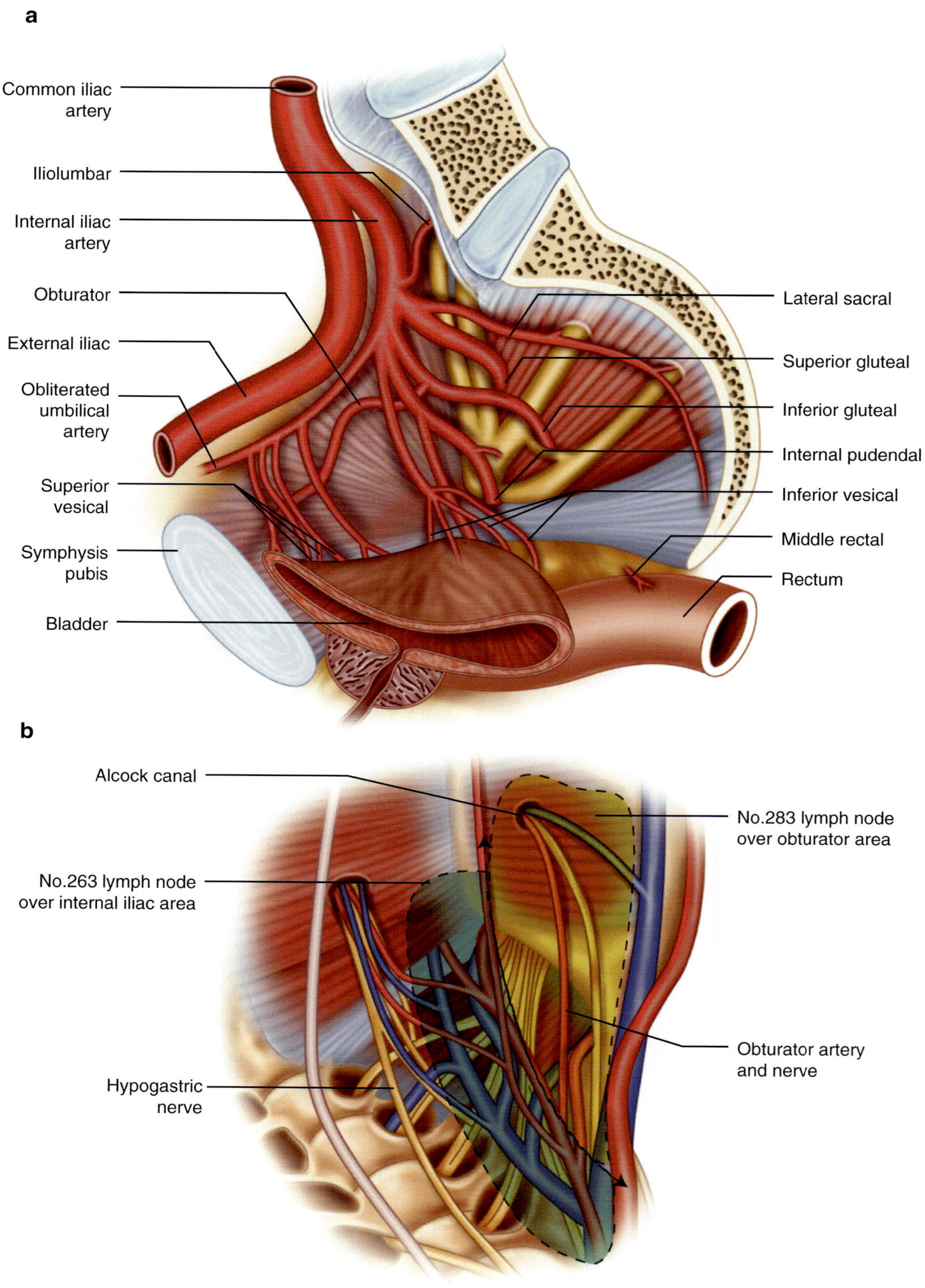

Fig. 31.3 (**a**) Surgical anatomy of right pelvic side wall. (**b**) Lateral lymph node dissection includes en bloc resection of lympho-adipose tissues over the obturator fossa

Patient Positioning and Operating Room Setup

Patients are placed in modified lithotomy position with hips straightened and knees flexed (Fig. 31.4c). We adhere to the universal port placement guidelines provided by Intuitive Surgical (Sunnyvale, CA) for trocar positioning for left lower side abdominal procedures (Fig. 31.4a, b), shifting all trocars to the right or left side depending on the location of the positive nodes and habitus of the patient. The camera port is placed at different locations for right-sided and left-sided LPLND as depicted in Fig. 31.4a, b.

After establishing pneumoperitoneum at 12 mmHg, the first 8-mm robotic trocar is placed near the umbilicus along the right para-rectus line. For left- and right-sided procedures, the trocars are placed in an oblique fashion. The other three 8-mm robotic trocars are inserted under visualization: one port over the right iliac fossa and two trocars in the left superior hemi-abdomen, one that is slightly on the left side of the supraumbilical area and another one in the left hypochondriac space. The 12-mm assistant trocar is positioned in the right or left flank depending on the location of the surgical procedure (Fig. 31.4a, b).

Robotic Lymph Node Dissection

Similar to laparoscopic LPLND, we initiate clearance of lymphatic tissues by dissection of the common iliac vessels. The obturator fossa is entered at the bifurcation of the internal and external iliac vessels. The lymphatic chains along with adipose tissues within the obturator fossa and paravesical fossa are dissected with en bloc removal. When bilateral LPLND is necessary, we alternate inserting the camera between ports as shown in Fig. 31.4a, b; and the patient is tilted down on the side opposite of the target location to facilitate better approach to the lateral pelvic lymph nodes.

Operative Considerations

We forewarn that this operation is so technically demanding that it cannot be performed by every surgeon; and every patient cannot undergo this operation. We have performed LPLND based on personal experience of over 500 laparoscopic rectal cancer operations, and we have limited recruitment to patients with mean body mass index of no more than 26.4 kg/m^2.

Stepwise Surgical Technique with the Xi Platform

1. Five or six abdominal ports are used, which includes one camera port, three robotic ports, and one or two assistant ports, depending on the need for unilateral or bilateral LPLND. The patient is tilted 15 ° either right or left side down, depending on the location of the positive nodes.
2. For left-sided dissection, the robotic cart is docked at the left hip position.
3. With traction and countertraction using instruments in robotic arms 1 and 2 and assistant port(s), we expose the root of the inferior mesenteric artery and excise the lymph nodes in this area while carefully preserving the autonomic nerves.
4. We preserve the left colic artery to maintain adequate blood supply.
5. We identify the distal end of the inferior mesenteric vein, where the superior rectal artery is transected with a laparoscopic linear stapler.
6. The pre-sacral lymph nodes overlying the sacral promontory are excised.
7. The pre-sacral region includes the triangle between the medial borders of the common iliac arteries and the line connecting the bifurcations of the internal and external iliac arteries.
8. Lymph nodes in the area of the proximal common iliac vessels are dissected.
9. Lymph nodes and lymphatic tissues are resected from the aortic bifurcation to the bifurcation of the internal and external iliac arteries.
10. Lateral lymph nodes outside the pelvic plexus around the external iliac artery, internal iliac artery, and obturator space are excised. The ureter is identified to avoid iatrogenic injury.

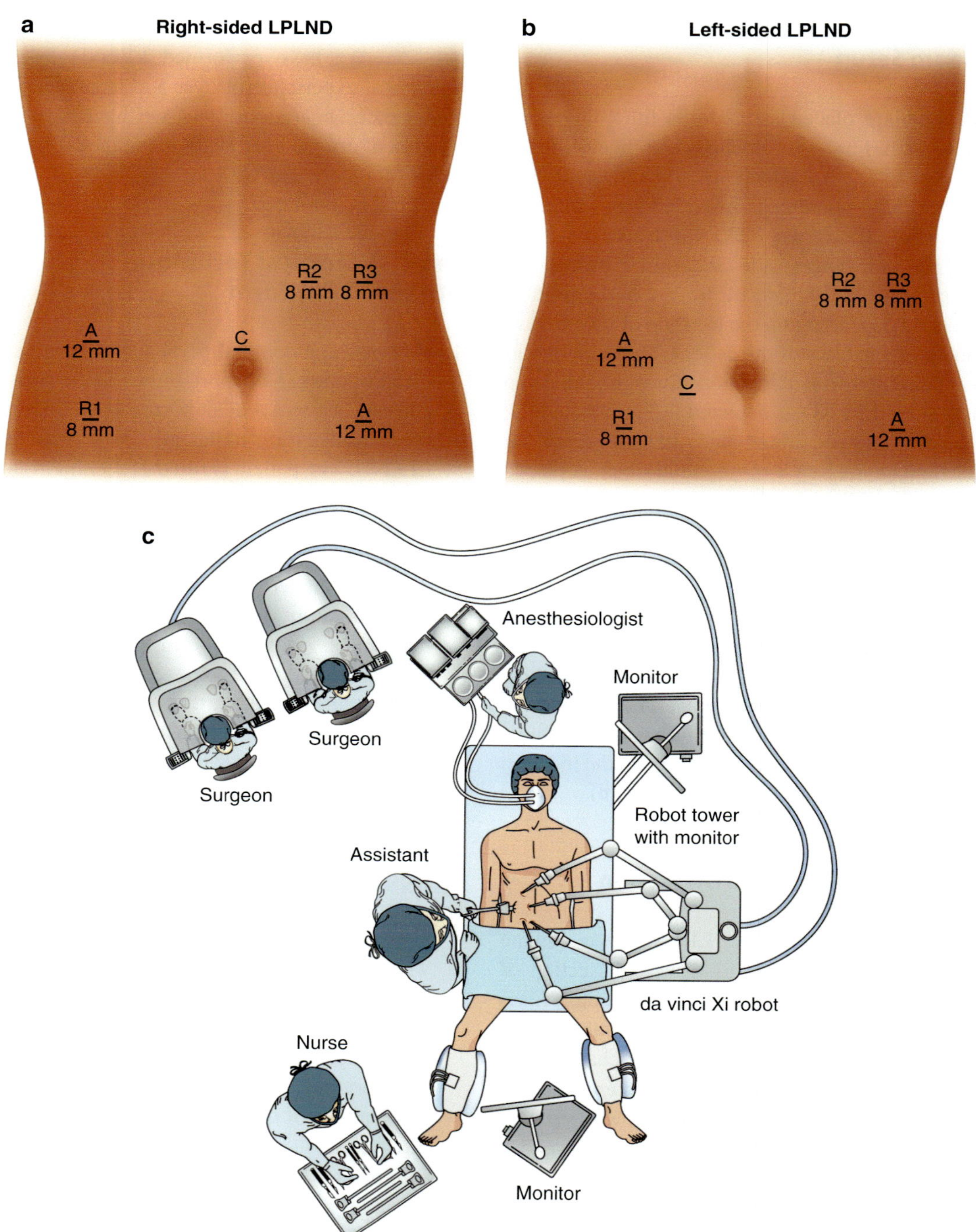

Fig. 31.4 (**a**, **b**) Trocar/port placement for robotic lateral pelvic lymph node dissection. (**c**) Patient positioning and robotic setup for lateral pelvic lymph node dissection

11. The robotic arm 3 and assistant gently push the ureter toward the superior lateral side to expose the external iliac artery, internal iliac artery, and obturator fossa.

12. The obturator fossa is entered at the bifurcation of the internal and external iliac vessels. The lymphatic and adipose tissues within the obturator fossa are removed en bloc.

13. During dissection the obturator nerve and vessels are identified medial to the external iliac artery and lateral to the superior vesicle artery.

14. Obturator lymph nodes are resected, while the obturator nerve is preserved and the obturator artery and vein are ligated.

15. At completion of pelvic lymph node dissection, the external iliac vessels, internal iliac vessels, obturator nerve, and pelvic plexus remain intact.

Conclusions

We have named this surgical procedure the "Japanese spirits" because both colorectal surgeons and patients in Japan "worship" the efficacy of this procedure. In contrast, Western surgeons contend that lateral nodal involvement of rectal cancer is an indicator of poor prognosis and that lymphadenectomy does not improve overall survival [7–18]. However, we believe that surgical removal of involved lymph nodes can provide the only chance for cure in these patients. Importantly, the treatment of rectal cancer requires multimodal and individualized therapy. Therefore, a surgical procedure alone is not appropriate for all patients. We believe that robotic approach for LPLND should be the first option for patients, since it can help provide complete cancer clearance using a minimally invasive approach [19–20].

References

1. Akasu T, Moriya Y. Abdominopelvic lymphadenectomy with autonomic nerve preservation for carcinoma of the rectum: Japanese experience. In: Wanebo HJ, editor. Surgery for Gastroinestinal cancer: a multidisciplinary approach. Philadelphia: Lippicott-Raven; 1997. p. 667–80.

2. Ueno M, Oya M, Azekura K, et al. Incidence and prognostic significance of lateral lymph node metastasis in patients with advanced low rectal cancer. Br J Surg. 2005;92:756–63.

3. Liang JT, Lee PH. Laparoscopic pelvic autonomic nerve-preserving surgery for patients with lower rectal cancer after chemoradiation therapy. Ann Surg Oncol. 2007;14:1285–7.

4. Liang JT, Huang KC, Lee PH, et al. Oncologic results of laparoscopic D3 lymphadenectomy for male sigmoid and upper rectal cancer with clinically positive lymph nodes. Ann Surg Oncol. 2007;14:1980–90.

5. Liang JT, Lee PH. Laparoscopic abdominoanal pull-through procedure for male patients with lower rectal cancer after chemoradiation therapy. Dis Colon Rectum. 2006;49:259–60.

6. Uyama I, Sugioka A, Matsui H, et al. Laparoscopic lateral node dissection with autonomic nerve preservation for advanced lower rectal cancer. J Am Coll Surg. 2001;193:579–84.

7. Ueno H, Mochizuki H, Hashiguchi Y, et al. Prognostic determinants of patients with lateral nodal involvement by rectal cancer. Ann Surg. 2001;234:190–7.

8. Kusters M, Beets GL, van de Velde CJ, et al. A comparison between the treatment of low rectal cancer in Japan and the Netherlands, focusing on the patterns of local recurrence. Ann Surg. 2009;249:229–35.

9. Yano H, Moran BJ. The incidence of lateral pelvic side-wall nodal involvement in low rectal cancer may be similar in Japan and the West. Br J Surg. 2008;95:33–49.

10. Georgiou P, Tan E, Gouvas N, et al. Extended lymphadenectomy versus conventional surgery for rectal cancer: a meta-analysis. Lancet Oncol. 2009;10:1053–62.

11. Moriya Y. Importance of lymphatic spread. In: Soreide O, Norstein J, editors. Rectal cancer surgery: optimisation standardisation documentation. Berlin: Springer; 1997. p. 153–64.

12. Takahashi T, Ueno M, Azekura K, Ota H. The lymphtic soread of rectal cancer and the effect of dissection: Japanese contribution and experience. In: Soreide O, Norstein J, editors. Rectal cancer surgery: optimisation standardisation documentation. Berlin: Springer; 1997. p. 165–80.

13. Kim JC, Takahashi K, Yu CS, et al. Comparative outcome between chemoradiotherapy and lateral pelvic lymph node dissection following total mesorectal excision in rectal cancer. Ann Surg. 2007;246:754–62.

14. Watanabe T, Tsurita G, Muto T, et al. Extended lymphadenectomy and preoperative radiotherapy for lower rectal cancers. Surgery. 2002;132:27–33.

15. Wichmann MW, Müller C, Meyer G, et al. Effect of preoperative radiochemotherapy on lymph node retrieval after resection of rectal cancer. Arch Surg. 2002;137:206–10.

16. Kim YW, Kim NK, Min BS, et al. The prognostic impact of the number of lymph nodes retrieved after neoadjuvant chemoradiotherapy with mesorectal excision for rectal cancer. J Surg Oncol. 2009;100:1–7.
17. Wanebo HJ, Turk PS. Abdominosacral resection for recurrent rectal cancer. In: Beuer JJ, Gorfine SR, Kreel 1, Gelernt IM, Rubin P, editors. Colorectal surgery illustrated: a focused approach. St. Louis: Mosby Year Book; 1993. p. 248.
18. Bernstein TE, Endreseth BH, Romundstad P, et al. Circumferential resection margin as a prognostic factor in rectal cancer. Br J Surg. 2009;96:1348–57.
19. Liang JT. Technical feasibility of laparoscopic lateral pelvic lymph node dissection for patients with low rectal cancer after concurrent chemoradiation therapy. Ann Surg Oncol. 2011;18:153–9.
20. Chen TC, Liang JT. Robotic lateral pelvic lymph node dissection for distal rectal cancer. Dis Colon Rectum. 2016;59:351–2.

Transanal Endoscopic Microsurgery

John R. Konen and Peter A. Cataldo

Introduction

No discussion regarding the utility of transanal endoscopic microsurgery (TEM) can begin without first discussing the cohort of techniques used to gain access to the rectum. Specifically, local excision (LE) techniques were initially developed for management of lesions in the distal rectum. These procedures allowed for the removal of disease while avoiding the morbidity and mortality of a larger operation such as total mesorectal excision (TME), which can carry operative morbidity and mortality rates of 33% and 2%, respectively [1].

LE approaches can be divided into techniques appropriate for the lower third, middle third, or upper third of the rectum. Traditional transanal excision (TAE) was promoted by Parks et al. in the 1950s for lesions within the lower third of the rectum [2]. While this technique has been successful in resecting lesions less than 10 cm from the anal verge, its use has also been restricted by poor visibility and limited reach by conventional tools. The trans-sphincteric approach developed by Mason was useful for lesions of the middle third of the rectum; however, this utility was balanced with the myriad functional consequences including fecal incontinence, rectal fistulas, and wound infections resulting in fibrosis of the sphincter mechanism [3, 4]. Lesions in the upper third of the rectum were traditionally approached by a low anterior resection (LAR) or abdominoperineal resection (APR); however, Kraske developed the less invasive trans-sacral approach for tumors in the mid to upper third of the rectum [5]. This technique was largely abandoned due to its high rates of morbidity and mortality. Among these three LE techniques, the trans-sacral and trans-sphincteric approaches have the distinct advantage of sampling perirectal lymph nodes, while the transanal techniques cannot.

Transanal endoscopic microsurgery (TEM) was borne out of these prior LE limitations by Gerhard Buess in the early 1980s in Tubingen, Germany. It is a unique form of transanal surgery that incorporates use of specialized equipment including an operating proctoscope, gas insufflation, and magnified stereoscopic vision for improved visualization. Lesions of the rectum extending up to 20 cm from the anal verge are potentially amenable to resection via a TEM setup, allowing much greater versatility compared to the multitude of traditional LE techniques described above.

Electronic supplementary material The online version of this chapter (https://doi.org/10.1007/978-3-030-18740-8_32) contains supplementary material, which is available to authorized users.

J. R. Konen (✉) · P. A. Cataldo
Department of Surgery, University of Vermont Medical Center, Burlington, VT, USA
e-mail: John.Konen@uvmhealth.org; Peter.Cataldo@uvmhealth.org

© Springer Nature Switzerland AG 2020
J. Kim, J. Garcia-Aguilar (eds.), *Minimally Invasive Surgical Techniques for Cancers of the Gastrointestinal Tract*, https://doi.org/10.1007/978-3-030-18740-8_32

Indications

TEM has been described in the application of many different disease processes and can be broadly classified into two categories: benign and malignant lesions.

Benign Lesions

Arguably the most common usage of TEM is for rectal polyps deemed unresectable by endoscopy. TEM in this manner spares the patient a larger, more morbid operation. Polyps closer to the rectosigmoid junction may preclude use of TEM due to the curvature of the sacrum, preventing passage of the rigid operating proctoscope. Conversely, very distal lesions about 3–4 cm from the anal verge make it challenging to maintain a seal around the proctoscope with resultant loss in pneumorectum and collapse of the operative field. Other described uses of TEM include repair of upper rectal-vaginal fistulas or extrasphincteric fistulas, pelvic abscess drainage, resection of neuroendocrine tumors, GISTs, and excision of extra-rectal masses, among others [6–8].

Malignant Lesions

Surgical therapy for rectal cancer includes both LE and radical approaches. Traditional radical operations include TME, which incorporates the lymph node basin of the specimen, and can be performed as either open or laparoscopic anterior resection (LAR) or by APR with colostomy.

LE approaches for rectal cancer have been controversial, and arguments both supporting and refuting their use abound in the literature. The central tenet surrounding surgical approach to rectal cancer is to maximize oncologic results while minimizing the impact of treatment on quality of life. Radical approaches described above are the standard of care for most stage I–III rectal cancers, and advantages include disease-free survival rates of 90% or higher and low local recurrence rates of 0–7.2% for T1-T2 disease [9,

10]. Radical resections, however, carry perioperative mortality rates of 1–2% and morbidities approaching 30% with anastomotic leak, sepsis, and perineal and/or wound complications [1, 11]. Other major disadvantages include diminished quality of life with postoperative urinary, sexual, and bowel dysfunction and temporary or permanent stoma.

Given these compelling complications, much interest over the past three decades has been devoted to LE as an alternative to radical resection. Advantages of LE include less invasive operation that avoids the major morbidities of radical resection, preserving normal anorectal and sexual function, as well as less postoperative pain, shorter length of stay, and faster return to normal activity levels. Extensive literature review reveals that when comparing LE techniques to radical excision, 5-year local recurrence rates tend to be higher for both T1 (8.2–23%) and T2 adenocarcinomas (13–37%) undergoing LE when compared to radical surgery for T1-T2 disease (0–7.2%) [10, 12, 13]. However, there has not been a significant difference in disease-free survival when compared to radical surgery (55–93% for LE vs 77–97% for radical excision) [9]. This is thought to be due to the retrospective nature of the studies and limited follow-up, as some have shown a survival benefit favoring radical excision beyond 5 years; therefore, those undergoing LE for cure should be committed to long-term follow-up [14]. In a recent study, however, O'Neill et al. demonstrated local recurrence and survival rates comparable to TME in favorable T1 N0 lesions and select T2 N0 lesions that underwent neoadjuvant chemoradiotherapy [15]. The study was limited by its single-center and retrospective analysis. LE has evolved over the past several decades, and many of these studies aggregate LE to include traditional TAE as well as TEM. The newer technology of TEM affords the surgeon improved visualization allowing for precise dissection. In fact, one study comparing TAE to TEM found that TEM had significantly less chance of tumor fragmentation (94% vs 65%), significantly more negative margins (90% vs 71%), and significantly less recurrence with TEM vs traditional TAE [16], and other studies have shown similar results [17, 18]. Another study even found a lower recurrence rate for TEM vs TAE (6% vs 29%) and identified margin status as an independent predictor of local recurrence and disease-free survival [19]. These studies highlight that despite heterogeneity in LE techniques, TEM is clearly the preferred approach for LE of rectal cancer – purportedly due to the improved dexterity and visualization in TEM.

When considering local excision, several factors must be considered. It is important to know that lymph node metastasis is directly related to tumor depth and has been reported to be 0–12% in T1 tumors, 12–28% in T2 tumors, and 36–67% in T3/T4 tumors [20–22]. It is presently not known whether LE results in locoregional control failure, which may be secondary to the inability of LE and TEM to sample the lymph node basin. As such, if LE is pursued, the surgeon must rely on preoperative staging to guide treatment decisions, and several principles regarding decision-making should be addressed. First, MRI does not accurately differentiate tumor depth. For example, in one study, MRI was able to accurately identify 100% of "favorable prognosis" tumors regardless of location within the rectum, but "favorable" was defined as T1 N0, T2 N0, or T3 <1 mm N0, which is a grouping of disease types that is not helpful in selecting patients who are appropriate for LE [23]. In fact, in this study, MRI was poor at distinguishing T1 from T2 tumors – a task that is crucial to select patients for LE. In a recent meta-analysis, the overall sensitivity and specificity of MRI for T category were 87% and 75%, respectively, and were found to be more accurate for circumferential resection margin (CRM, or predicted distance to the mesorectal fascia) involvement than for T category. Endorectal ultrasound (EUS) is better in studies assessing its ability to differentiate T stage for rectal cancer. In a recent meta-analysis, the sensitivity and specificity of EUS to determine T1 stage were 87.8% and 98.3% for T1 lesions and 80.5% and 95.6% for T2 lesions, respectively [24]. However, the sensitivity was higher for advanced (T3 or greater) disease. Thus, the surgeon must be aware of the risk of incorrect clinical staging.

Second, 12–28% of T2 lesions will have local lymph node metastasis. Imaging modalities (EUS, MRI) routinely miss 50% of nodes that contain metastasis, many of which are less than 5 mm in diameter [25, 26]. Thus, roughly 10% of patients with T2 disease will have unidentified metastatic lymph nodes making them T2N+ and are compared retrospectively to patients who have undergone radical excision who are pT2 N0. Thus, there will be a proportion of LE patients who are stage III, thus unfairly biasing oncologic results toward radical resection. However, new data suggests that using criteria such as indistinct borders and mottled or heterogeneous appearance of nodes, in addition to size, should be considered when staging lymph nodes with imaging, thus minimizing the proportion of understaged patients [27].

Fortunately, several components of tumor biology can provide clues as to the presence of local metastatic nodes, such as poor histopathologic features (lymphovascular/perineural invasion, submucosal invasion to sm_3 level, tumor budding at the leading edge, mucinous component), response to neoadjuvant chemoradiation, and location within the rectum. Additionally, poor surgical outcomes such as fragmented tumor resection or positive margins also increase the risk of recurrence [16, 28]. Those who have normal histologic features and an adequate response to neoadjuvant chemoradiation may be more appropriate candidates for LE of residual tumor via TEM. Lezoche et al. staged patients with T1 N0 or T2 N0 lesions, where T1 patients underwent TEM alone and T2 patients received neoadjuvant therapy and then underwent TEM. The T2 patients had a local recurrence of 5% and disease-free survival of 93% after median 97-month follow-up. Eighteen percent of T2 lesions had pathologic complete response (ypCR) [29]. Regarding location, several studies have demonstrated 22–34% rate of local node metastasis for T1 cancers in the lower third of the rectum, compared to 8% in the left colon and 3% in the right colon, suggesting distal rectal cancers may not be appropriate for local resection alone [30].

It is clear that decision-making for rectal cancer is increasingly complex. The authors suggest the following treatment algorithm: TEM for rectal cancer should be offered to patients with T1 N0 disease with favorable histologic features. If final pathology reveals no adverse features and adequate resection margins, then TEM alone is adequate. If final pathology identifies adverse histopathologic features or a positive margin, then that patient should undergo adjuvant chemoradiation or be offered radical resection. For T2 N0 lesions (where the tumor invades into but not beyond the muscularis propria), the algorithm is considerably more controversial. Standard of care is radical excision; however, promising results following pCR suggests there is a role for TEM [31]. These patients can be treated with LE when combined with neoadjuvant chemoradiation. If they develop a significant response, TEM for residual tumor resection is appropriate; or alternatively, if a complete response is detected by imaging, then a "watch and wait" protocol may also be appropriate, as TEM following neoadjuvant chemoradiation is associated with prolonged healing times, patient discomfort, and anorectal dysfunction. However, if they have minimal response, then a radical resection is indicated. Finally, TEM may be offered as a palliative procedure for patients with locally advanced lesions as a less aggressive approach in patients who are poor operative candidates.

Preoperative Preparation

Workup and Lesion Preparation

It cannot be stressed enough that appropriate patient selection is key in utilizing TEM in the treatment of rectal cancer. All patients being considered for TEM must undergo adequate staging workup. This begins with digital rectal exam assessing for location and mobility of the mass. A full colonoscopy with biopsy and EUS are essential to assess for the size, depth, and synchronicity of tumors. MRI may also be helpful in staging despite its limitation in distinguishing early-stage rectal lesions. TEM requires that the patient be positioned such that the tumor is oriented directly down toward the operating table, so rigid proc-

toscopy is necessary to obtain lesion position on the rectal wall (anterior, posterior and right, left, or lateral), as well as exact distance from anal verge, as flexible endoscopy is unreliable. TEM should only be offered for lesions below 15 cm from the dentate line. Lesions >15 cm from the anal verge and close to the dentate line may be limited by the bony confines of the pelvis and loss of pneumorectum, respectively. In general, TEM has much less utility for upper rectal tumors, as these patients tend to do very well with LAR. Contraindications to TEM include uncorrected coagulopathy, rectal varices, anal stenosis or node-positive carcinoma detected in workup (if TEM performed for curative intent). If a polypectomy site is the target lesion with TEM, timing of surgery becomes increasingly important. If excision proceeds too late, the site may be impossible to identify. Conversely, if surgery takes place too soon, the anatomy may be distorted by inflammation making appropriate resection difficult. Delicate tattoo of the lesion circumferentially with India ink preserves planes and visualization of the lesion at time of surgery.

Patient Consultation and Consent

A full discussion with the patient regarding the risks and benefits of TEM is necessary, specifically the opportunity to avoid major morbidities of a radical approach but with the caveat that they may require further surgical therapy depending on the final pathologic result. If TEM is performed for malignancy, it must be stressed that postoperative follow-up will be required. Risks include, but are not limited to, incontinence, bleeding, perforation, rectovaginal fistula, stoma creation, incomplete resection, and inability to perform resection. Due to the size of the proctoscope (4 cm) and long duration of the cases, incontinence is a concern. Fortunately, incontinence that develops postoperatively is usually short-term and resolves in a majority of patients. Studies examining quality of life measures and continence pre- and postsurgery were unchanged [32, 33]. Full-thickness resection of the rectal wall could result in inadvertent intraperitoneal entry, which is most common in lesions on the anterior rectal wall, since the upper two-thirds of the anterior rectum in intraperitoneal. If there is considerable concern for intraperitoneal entry and need for conversion to formal laparotomy is anticipated, this should be discussed at the time of consent. If the lesion is in the upper rectum, a more detailed discussion with the patient should occur regarding possible unresectability and should focus on whether they would desire a formal resection at the same time or at a later procedure. A full bowel preparation is recommended, along with systemic antibiotics.

TEM/TEO Equipment and Operative Setup

TEM equipment is supplied by Richard Wolf GMBH (Knittlingen, Germany), while transanal endoscopic operation (TEO) equipment is provided by Karl Storz GMBH, (Tütlingen, Germany). We will discuss the Wolf equipment, which includes all necessary components to perform the operation.

Operative Instruments/Proctoscope

Improved visualization in TEM is due to maintenance of pneumorectum and high-resolution stereoscopes. The proctoscope is 4 cm in diameter and comes in three lengths: 12, 13.7, and 20 cm (Fig. 32.1). The 12 and 20 cm shafts have oblique edges for mid and upper lesions, respectively, while the 13.7 cm shaft has a flat edge for distal lesions extending into the anus. The entire scope is mounted on an articulated arm known as the Martin arm, which is attached to the operating table and allows for precise, hands-free positioning of the proctoscope. The proctoscope has two types of detachable faceplates: a viewing plate with a window and bellows insufflation for positioning and an operating plate that contains four ports (one for the stereoscope and three for the operating instruments) (Fig. 32.1). The instrument ports are capped with a soft silicone airtight valve, which permits rapid exchange of the long

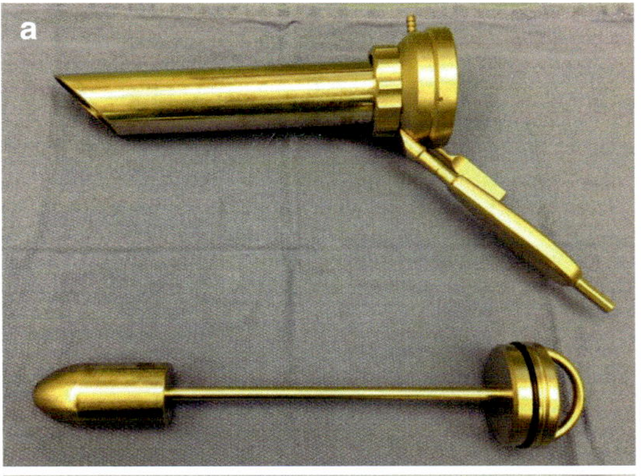
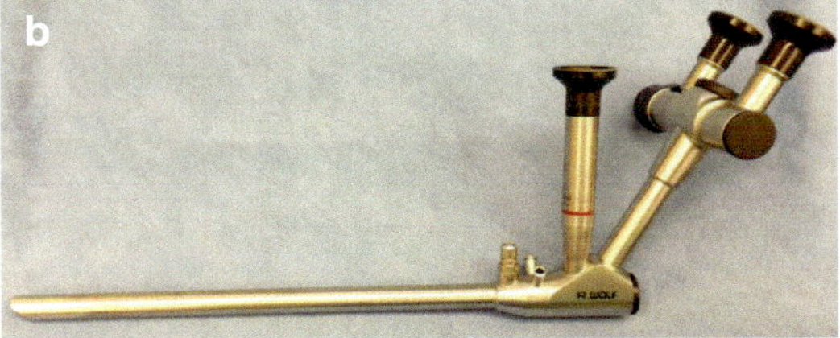
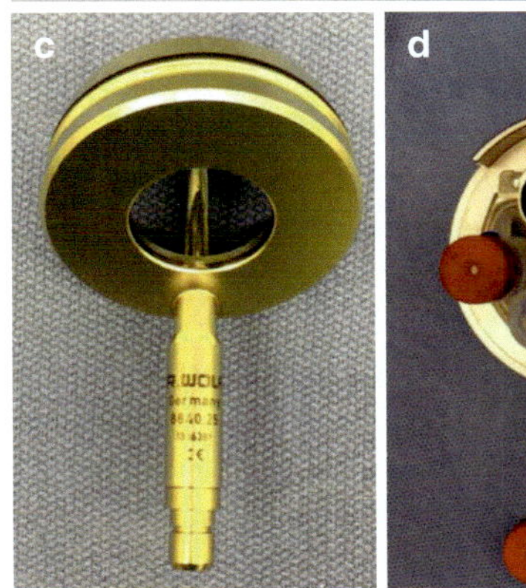
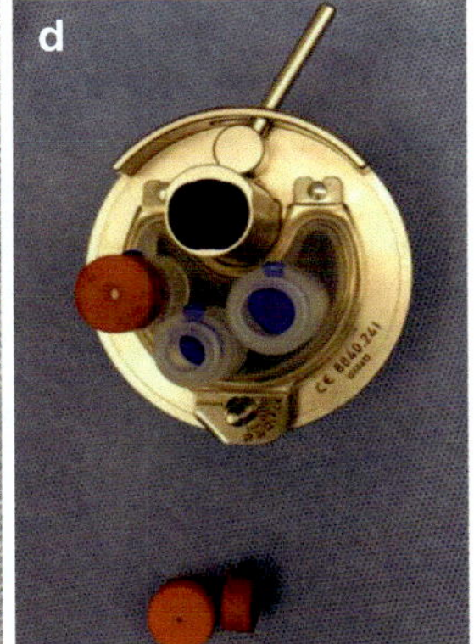

Fig. 32.1 Richard Wolf TEM rectoscope. (**a**) 12 cm proctoscope with obturator for atraumatic insertion. There are two other 4 cm shaft sizes: 13.7 cm flat-edged for distal lesions and 20 cm oblique (not shown). (**b**) Stereoscope with binocular optic and laparoscopic camera attachment. It also contains ports for CO_2 insufflation, intrarectal pressure monitor, light source, and irrigation. (**c**) The viewing faceplate depicted can be used with hand bellows (not shown) to properly position the proctoscope. The viewing faceplate is exchanged for the operating faceplace (**d**) and contains four ports: one for the stereoscope (top) and three for operative instruments. Shown at the bottom are the soft silicone caps that permit passage of instruments

operative instruments while minimizing changes in pneumorectum. The stereoscope is 10 mm in diameter and contains a binocular optic. It provides up to a 6× magnification, 50-degree downward viewing angle, and 75-degree lateral field of view (Fig. 32.1). The stereoscope also contains a 40-degree downward scope that is attached to a laparoscopic camera allowing the operation to be viewed on a video monitor. The stereoscope itself has ports for CO_2 insufflation, intrarectal pressure monitor, light cord, and a water jet to clean the lens. The instruments are 5 mm in diameter, consisting of electrocautery knife, cautery/suction tube, graspers, injection needle, needle holders, scissors, and a clip applier (Fig. 32.2). Each dissecting instrument should be well lubricated along the shaft with mineral oil prior to beginning the case, as it will decrease friction and wear on the silicone caps, which could cause loss of pneumorectum. Of note, the forceps are designed to hold tissue at the tip, while the area near the fulcrum is ridged and can grip a suture needle being passed through tissue. The needle holders have straight and angled options. The clip applier is unique to TEM and "silver bbs" are placed at the beginning and end of a working running suture, since intra-luminal knot tying is challenging during TEM.

Insufflator Unit/Other Necessary Machines

The insufflator supplies CO_2 via a port on the stereoscope and is stored in a cart/tower within the operating room. An electrocoagulation machine is also kept on the cart, along with a light source, irrigation pump with irrigation reservoir, and TEM roller pump for suction (a conventional suction machine would collapse pneumorectum). A pedal can activate irrigation (which is driven by the CO_2 pressure), and another pedal is used for coagulation (Fig. 32.3).

Operative Setup

Patient positioning is paramount to appropriate surgical setup. The surgeon should have identified the lesion location within the rectum preoperatively, but after the patient is anesthetized, the location can be re-confirmed with digital

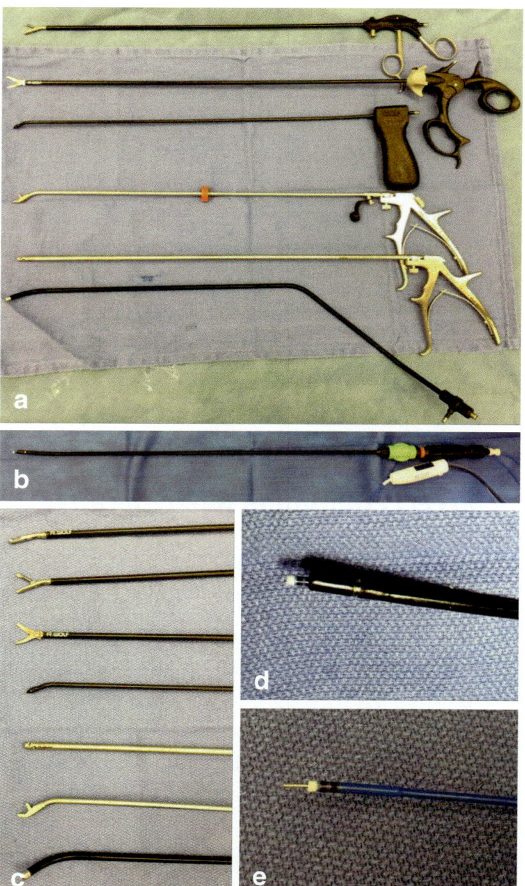

Fig. 32.2 TEM operating instruments. (**a**) From *top* to *bottom*: straight monopolar grasping forceps, scissors, articulated monopolar knife with ergonomic pistol grip, needle holder, clip applier, and suction tube. (**b**) Erbe HybridKnife® in rod handle for elevation of the submucosal plane using the high-pressure waterjet. (**c**) Enlargement of instrument heads from *top to bottom*: grasping forceps (closed, open), scissors, articulated monopolar knife, clip applier, needle holder, and suction tube. (**d**) Enlargement of Erbe HybridKnife® instrument in rod and (**e**) alone with knife tip deployed. All black instruments are insulated so they can be attached to cautery. Articulated instruments allow for greater range of motion within the operating proctoscope

rectal exam or rigid proctoscopy. The patient should then be positioned so that the lesion is oriented toward the floor (Table 32.1). A modified lithotomy position will be used for posterior rectal lesions, while a prone position will be used for anterior lesions. Patients will be positioned in left or right lateral decubitis for

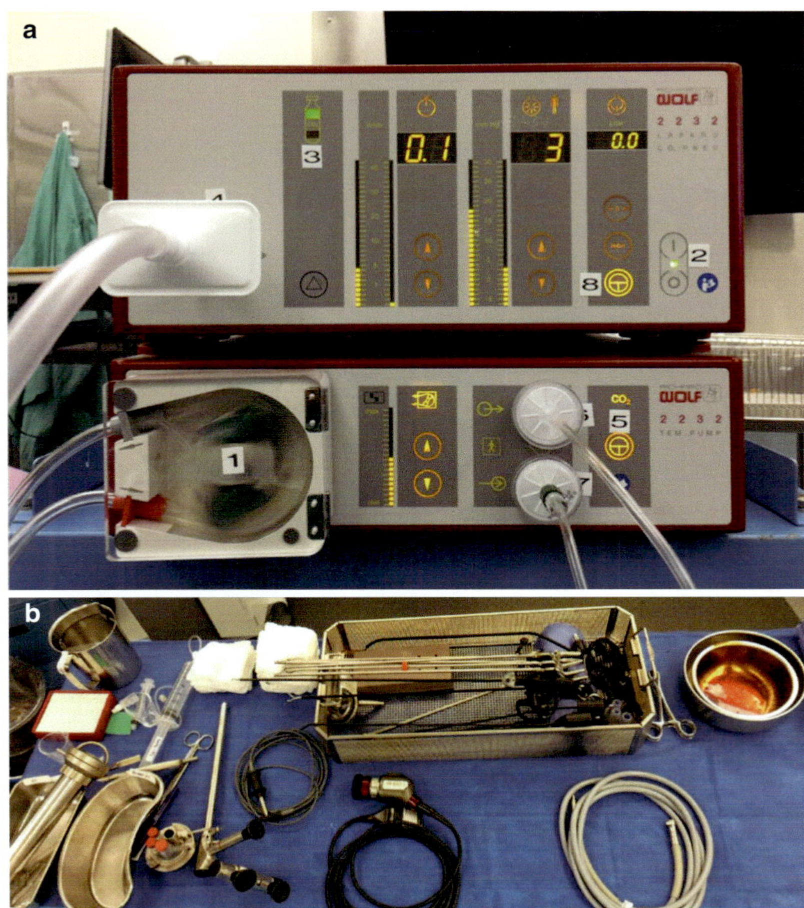

Fig. 32.3 Insufflation machine and table setup. (**a**) Richard Wolff insufflation machine, which displays flow, patient pressure, and total liters of CO_2 pumped. The lower console contains the suction device on a roller pump (1). (**b**) Operative table setup with the proctoscope, faceplates, stereoscope, laparoscopic cables, and camera, as well as the instruments

lateral lesions (Fig. 32.4). For tumors that are circumferential or near circumferential, the patient may need to be repositioned during the procedure; however, the majority of lesions can be resected without repositioning. The patient's legs should be adjusted out so that the surgeon has appropriate range of motion of the instruments. After patient positioning, the patient is draped and the Martin arm is attached to the table. The anus should be gently dilated with 2–3 fingers and the proctoscope should then be inserted. Positioning should be adjusted to properly view the lesion with the windowed faceplate (which comes with a hand bellows and can be used similar to a proctoscope) and then clamped to the Martin arm (Fig. 32.5). Ideally, the lesion will be at between the 4- and 6-o'clock positions in the viewing field. The viewing faceplate can then be exchanged for the operating faceplate, and the stereoscope and appropriate tubing and cords can be connected (Fig. 32.5). For distal lesions, the use of the viewing faceplate and hand bellows are often unnecessary, as positioning the proctoscope is simple and can be done with the operating faceplate attached.

Table 32.1 Patient positioning options in TEM

Lesion location	Patient operative position
Anterior rectum	Prone jackknife
Left lateral rectum	Left side down
Right lateral rectum	Right side down
Posterior rectum	Modified lithotomy

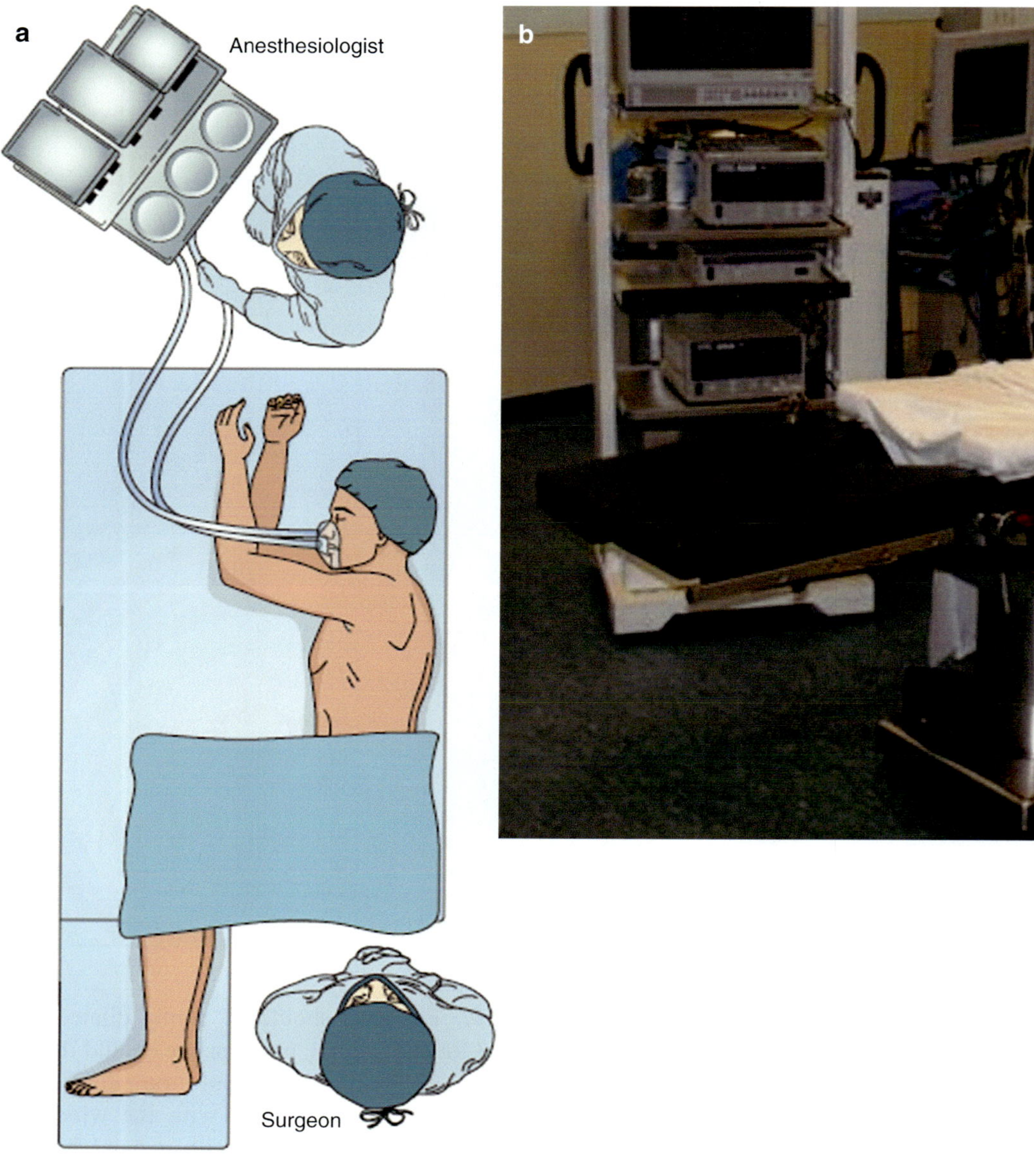

Fig. 32.4 Right lateral decubitus patient positioning. (**a**) This position would be used for a rectal lesion in the right lateral rectal wall. Note the use of foam to properly posi-tion patient's hips and knees at 90 degrees and secure them to the table with tape. A single split-leg section (**b**) can be used to support both legs

Operative Technique and Tips

Video 32.1

Once the setup is complete, excision of the lesion can begin (Table 32.2). For benign lesions and partial-thickness lesions, the injection needle is passed through the port, and local anesthesia with epinephrine should be infiltrated underneath the lesion. A solution of 1% lidocaine with 1:100,000 dilution of epinephrine is recom-

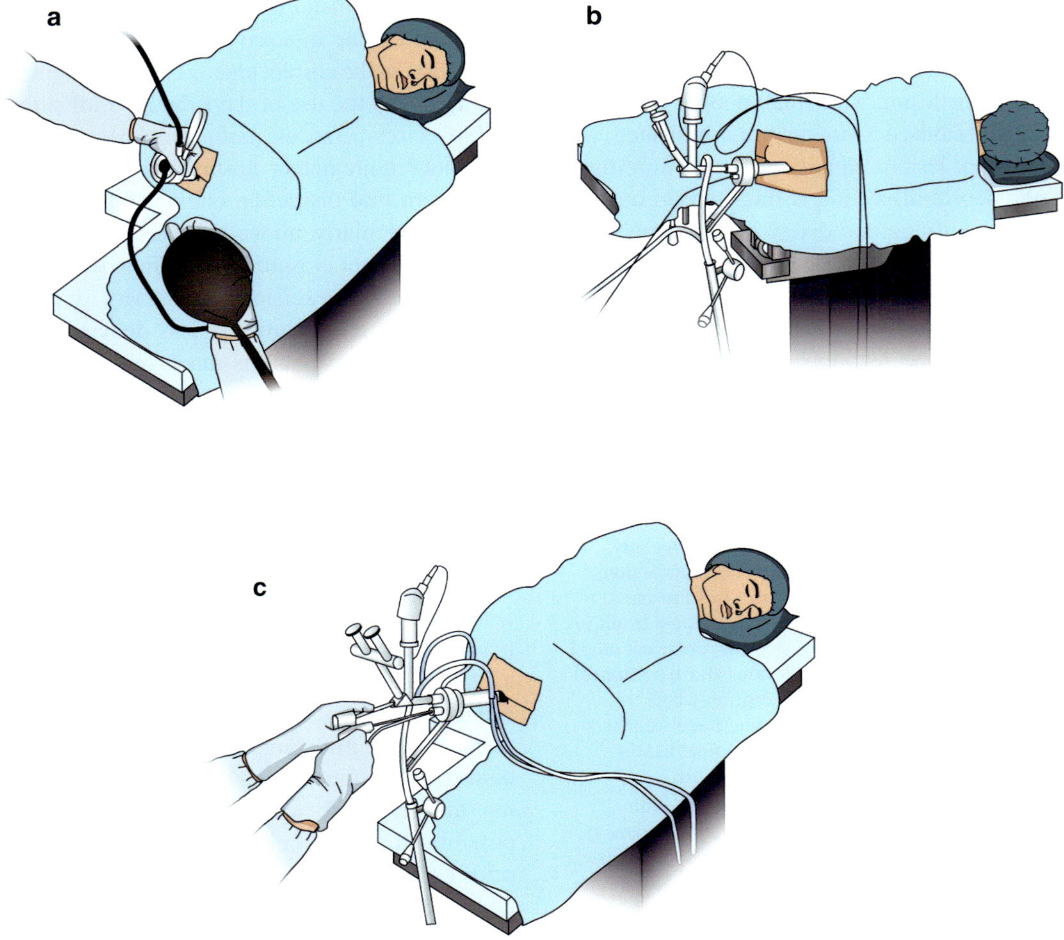

Fig. 32.5 TEM operative setup. (**a**) The viewing face-place and hand bellows are used to properly position the rectoscope for adequate view of the lesion, and then secure it to the Martin arm. (**b**) Completed setup with proctoscope secured, stereoscope/camera attached, and suction instrument inserted and (**c**) with dissection instruments at the beginning of lesion excision

mended. The importance of this step is critical, both for hemostasis and elevation of the lesion to aid in dissection and separation of the mucosa from the underlying muscular wall. Alternatively, the Erbe HybridKnife® (Erbe USA, Marietta, GA) can be used to elevate the lesions scheduled for submucosal excision (Fig. 32.2). The waterjet is a high-pressure foot-controlled pump that injects fluid via a blunt tip needle. A combination of saline, methylene blue, and lidocaine is used. This results in significant spatial separation of the mucosa and inner muscular rectal wall. The methylene blue creates blue submucosal fluid which contrasts with the white muscular layer, making identification of the correct dissection plane obvious and simple. The electrocautery knife is then used to mark circumferentially around the lesion with small dots of cautery. For benign lesions, a 5 mm margin is indicated, while malignant lesions should have a 10 mm margin. Submucosal dissection is then carried out, carefully identifying and dissecting the proper plane (Fig. 32.6). The specimen is carefully retracted superiorly to aid in exposure. Forceful elevation of the specimen will result in tearing of the tissue and should be avoided. The dissection should

continue from distal to proximal. The submucosal space can be injected as needed to facilitate dissection in the correct plane. This step is greatly facilitated by the use of the Erbe HybridKnife®. In most circumstances, partial-thickness excision does not require defect closure. However, if there is concern that dissection entered full-thickness plane, particularly above the peritoneal reflection, then defect closure is recommended.

Full-thickness excisions (mandatory for malignant lesions) are technically less demanding, as the full-thickness plane is much more forgiving than the submucosal plane. For full-thickness excision, a local anesthetic with 1:200,000 dilution epinephrine is injected into the muscular layer and into the perirectal fat for postoperative pain control and, most importantly, intraoperative hemostasis. Appropriate margins are then marked circumferentially with electrocautery. Dissection again proceeds distal to proximal. The full-thickness plane is entered with needle-knife electrocautery (alternative energy sources are rarely needed and generally only add expense and complexity) at the midpoint, distal to the lesion. The dissection continues around the perimeter, following the previously cautery-marked margins. If possible, the entire circumference is dissected prior to beginning the deep dissection. Once the perimeter is complete, the lesion is elevated with a grasper, and deep dissection is initiated. If desired, particularly for posterior lesions, a large portion of mesorectal fat (potentially containing

Table 32.2 Resection options in TEM

Resection options	Description	Indication
Partial-thickness excision	Removes rectal wall down to the inner circular muscular layer	Benign lesions only, namely, larger lesions where full-thickness excision would result in stenosis; proximal rectal lesions above peritoneal reflection where intraperitoneal entry or rectovaginal fistula would result
Full-thickness excision	Removes all layers of rectal wall with or without removal of subjacent perirectal fat	Large polyps with suspected malignancy; malignant T1 N0 and favorable T2 N0 lesions

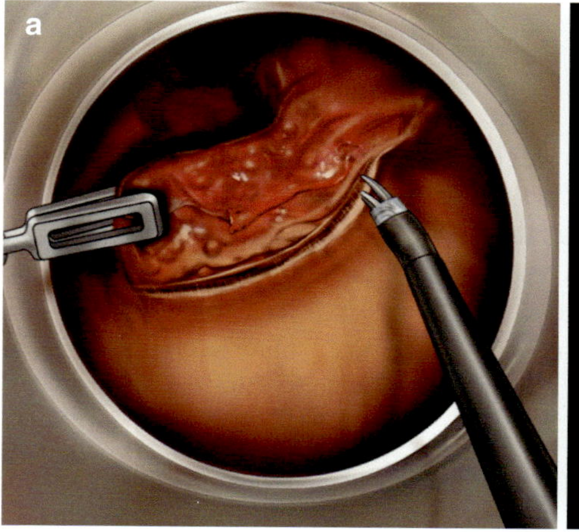
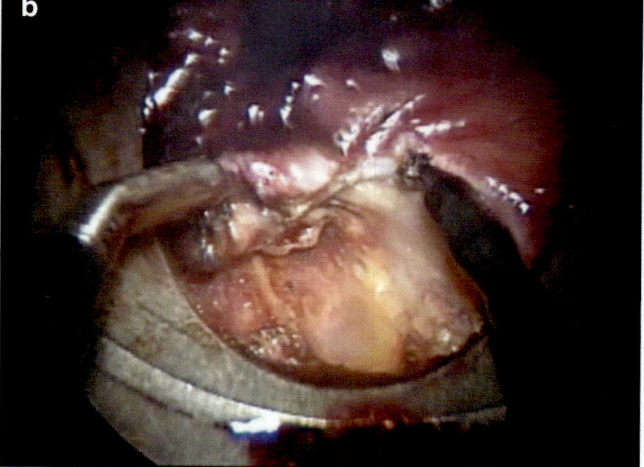

Fig. 32.6 (**a**) Illustration showing submucosal dissection with the Erbe HybridKnife®. (**b**) Paired intraoperative image demonstrating grasping tissues in the left hand while dissecting with the HybridKnife® in the right hand

regional lymph nodes) can be excised en bloc with the specimen. This portion of the procedure is quite simple, but it is important to remain vigilant regarding hemostasis, as the mesorectum can contain large vessels. During any TEM dissection, as for most surgical dissections, traction/countertraction is essential. In TEM, the surgeon only has one hand to create traction (the other hand is performing the procedure), so countertraction must be created by the pneumorectum and by appropriate positioning of the proctoscope. Proper positioning of the proctoscope (i.e., keeping the lesion in the lower half of the visual field) facilitates instrument handling and specimen manipulation. The proctoscope may have to be repositioned several times as dissection of the lesion or closure of the defect progresses. Once the lesion has been excised, the defect should be closed. Defects inferior to the peritoneal reflection do not necessarily require closure, as they will heal by secondary intention. However, our recommendation is that nearly all defects be sutured closed for two reasons: (1) proximal defects near the peritoneal reflection can secondarily penetrate into the peritoneum, resulting in significant intraperitoneal sepsis, and (2) closing the majority of full-thickness defects improves a surgeon's operative technique in the event that a full-thickness defect above the peritoneal reflection requires closure. There are two situations in which defects should be left open: (1) TEM following chemoradiation. These defects will nearly always break down if closed. (2) Defects adjacent to the dentate line, where sutures in this zone are particularly painful and wounds are at risk for disruption due to the fixed anatomy of the anus, leading to tension on the suture line. Anterior distal rectal defects are closed in females to minimize risk of anovaginal fistula.

When suturing, the suction instrument is removed from the proctoscope to leave more room for the other instruments. A grasper and needle holder are used to complete the closure. A clip or "bb" is placed 10–12 cm from the needle on a 2-0 polydioxanone (PDS) suture. The gasket is backloaded onto the needle driver, the suture is grasped 1 cm from the needle, and the instrument is passed into the proctoscope. The needle is then loaded on the needle holder and suturing can begin. All defects are closed transversely to prevent stenosis.

Small defects are closed right to left, suturing from distal to proximal. Once the defect is closed, a second bb is placed on the suture, ensuring that the suture is tight enough to close the defect, but not tight enough to strangulate the tissue. For longer areas of resection, the defect is bisected with a single suture (with a "bb" at the beginning and the end of the stitch) in order to approximate proximal and distal portions of the rectal wall. The remainder of the defect is then closed from lateral to medial on either side of the bisected suture. It is often helpful to decrease extraluminal pressure on the TEM unit to 8–10 mmHg to take tension off the suture line during closure. If the suture line is slack, the end of the suture can be grasped and gently pulled on to tighten it, and another "bb" can be applied to make it taut.

Once the specimen is resected, it can be marked at the inferior border with a stitch. The specimen should be removed from the proctoscope by opening the faceplate. The lesion should be immediately pinned to a flat surface such as corkboard to ensure that the specimen does not shrink and can be properly evaluated by the pathologist (Fig. 32.7).

Pitfalls and Complications

Above all, patient positioning is one of the most important steps and cannot be overemphasized. If after TEM setup has been completed and the surgeon identifies the lesion to be in a suboptimal position (i.e., not oriented toward the floor), it is far better to reposition the patient than to proceed with TEM. With partial-thickness excision, "button-holing" the lesion can occur, which happens when dissection is too superficial and can result in incomplete resection. Conversely, during partial-thickness resection, dissection can enter the muscularis propria and result in full-thickness excision. To correct this, the plane can be reentered, or the lesion can be excised as a full thickness. Peritoneal entry is another consequence of full-thickness excisions of intraperitoneal rectal lesions and is not considered a complication. It can be planned or inadvertent and will be immediately noticeable by collapse of the operative field as the pneumorectum is lost into the peritoneal space. It is essential that these defects be closed accurately

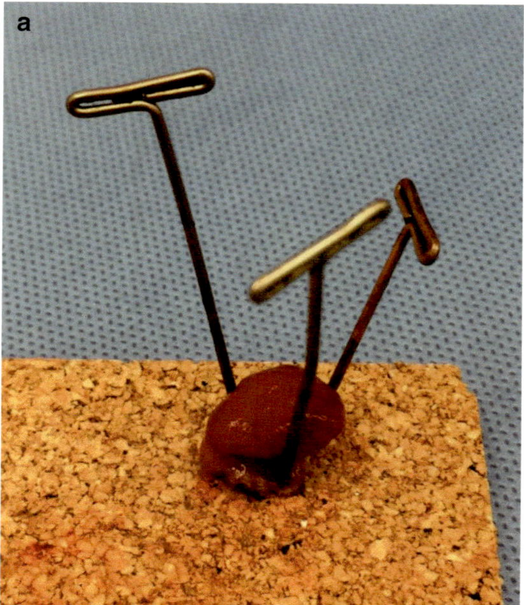

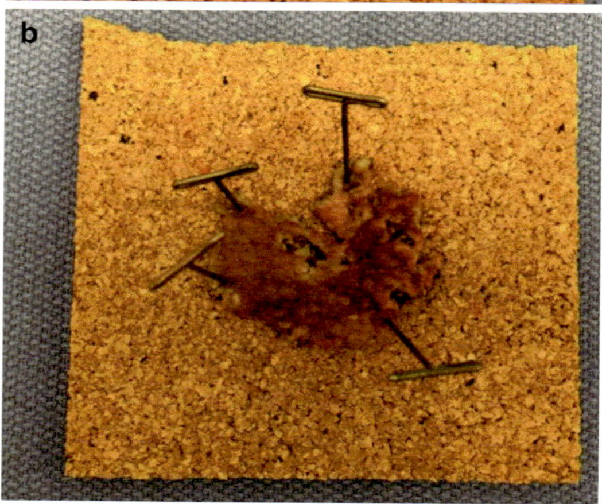

Fig. 32.7 Specimen orientation. (**a**) Immediately after resection is complete, a polypoid rectal lesion is removed through the faceplate and pinned by the operative team with T-pins to a piece of corkboard. This is essential, so the lesion does not shrink and so the anatomical margins can be assessed. (**b**) A larger lesion

and completely. A separate peritoneal and rectal wall closure is ideal but can be difficult to complete. Conversion to laparotomy may be needed if the repair cannot occur via TEM, with the conversion rate ranging from 2.6% to 4.3% in two large studies [34, 35]. If there is concern with the durability of closure, the patient may be kept for observation overnight and a water-soluble contrast enema can be ordered the following day. Bleeding is another potential complication; however, it is rarely clinically significant [36]. Suture line dehiscence may also occur and is generally cited between 0% and 15% [37]. The majority of patients can be treated conservatively with the expectation that the defect will slowly close over time. In rare circumstances, a diverting stoma may be required. Peritonitis will obviously necessitate laparotomy.

Postoperative Care and Follow-Up

TEM is generally performed as an outpatient surgery. If there are no concerns surrounding wound closure or intraperitoneal entry as discussed above, then the patient can be discharged home the day of surgery after successful voiding. Patients should begin a stool softener and a fiber supplement immediately after surgery to keep their stools loose for the first two postoperative weeks with the goal to avoid a large, hard bowel movement that could disrupt suture lines.

In general, patients undergoing TEM for malignancy should have routine surveillance at 3-month intervals for the first 24 months, which includes history and physical exam, and flexible sigmoidoscopy with CEA levels at 6, 18, and 24 months. One should examine luminal changes over time, as the local tissue can be distorted from resection. A full colonoscopy should be obtained at the 12-month mark, and CT of the abdomen and pelvis should be performed on a yearly basis.

Recurrence rates for pT1 cancers range from 0% to 12.5% and occasionally as high as 25%; however, the higher rates are from older studies and likely reflect early problems with appropriate patient selection, inferior staging technology, and a steeper learning curve [38, 39]. It has been demonstrated in a large prospective study that pT1 tumors with favorable histology have a recurrence rate around 6% [40]. In fact, a recent study by O'Neill et al. at the University of Vermont demonstrated recurrence rate of 6.7% for both T1 and T2 disease after TEM with a median follow-up of 4.6 years [15]. Overall survival rates between TEM and radical surgery have been comparable, both in excess of 90% in properly selected and matched patients [41, 42]. It is important to note that patients who undergo

TEM prior to a necessary radical resection do not have adversely affected outcomes, as demonstrated by Borschitz et al., where a subset of patients with unfavorable pT1 lesions subsequently underwent immediate radical surgery and had a local recurrence rate of 6% and a 10-year cancer-free survival of 93%, which are comparable to undergoing radical resection alone or TEM resection for favorable pT1 disease [40]. These findings were replicated in a study from 21 regional centers in the UK [43]. Collectively, completion radical surgery does not appear to alter the oncologic outcome. There has nonetheless been attention drawn as to whether TEM would adversely affect the specimen quality and tissue planes in a subsequent radical resection. A UK database identified 36 such scenarios and found that the majority ($n = 23$, 64%) had a "good"-quality resection specimen and had a significantly improved 5-year disease-free survival compared to patients with an "inferior" specimen (100% vs 51%) [44]. However, radical resection following TEM can be associated with higher perioperative complication rates and can convert patients originally amenable to LAR to APR with permanent colostomy.

Conclusions

Since its inception in the early 1980s, TEM has greatly expanded its breadth of treatment capabilities for transanal surgery – from benign, endoscopically unresectable polyps to neoplasms, complex fistulas, and abscesses, just to name a few. Its ability to provide high-resolution optics and precise endoscopic instruments allows for more complete and oncologically desirable outcomes, all the while sparing a patient the morbidities and potential poor quality of life outcomes of a larger resection. As its popularity increases, a growing body of outcomes studies demonstrates its superiority to traditional transanal techniques. Although there is no single consensus regarding its role in rectal cancer, it is becoming clear that it can, in select patients, offer similar local recurrence and survival outcomes as radical operations. In carefully selected patients with early T1 lesions, and some T2 lesions with concomitant neoadjuvant chemoradiotherapy,

TEM offers a prominent alternative to these traditional radical approaches. Future studies will be needed to examine its role in locally advanced lesions, whether a "watch and wait" approach following complete clinical response to chemoradiotherapy is appropriate or if resection of residual tumor via TEM is necessary.

References

1. Law WL, Chu KW. Anterior resection for rectal cancer with mesorectal excision: a prospective evaluation of 622 patients. Ann Surg. 2004;240:260–8.
2. Parks AG. Transanal technique in low rectal anastomosis. Proc R Soc Med. 1972;65:975–6.
3. Mason AY. Surgical access to the rectum – a trans-sphincteric exposure. Proc R Soc Med. 1970;63(Suppl):91–4.
4. Graham RA, Garnsey L, Jessup JM. Local excision of rectal carcinoma. Am J Surg. 1990;160:306–12.
5. Kraske P, Perry EG, Hinrichs B. A new translation of professor Dr P. Kraske's Zur Exstirpation Hochsitzender Mastdarmkrebse 1885. Aust N Z J Surg. 1989;59:421–4.
6. Steele RJC, Hershman MJ, Mortensen NJ, et al. Transanal endoscopic microsurgery – initial experience from three centres in the United Kingdom. Br J Surg. 1996;83:207–10.
7. Kinoshita T, Kanehira E, Omura T, et al. Transanal endoscopic microsurgery in the treatment of rectal carcinoid tumor. Surg Endosc. 2007;21:970–4.
8. Serra-Aracil X, Mora-Lopez L, Alcantara-Moral M, et al. Atypical indications for transanal endoscopic microsurgery to avoid major surgery. Tech Coloproctol. 2014;18:157–64.
9. Althumairi AA, Gearhart SL. Local excision for early rectal cancer: transanal endoscopic microsurgery and beyond. J Gastrointest Oncol. 2015;6:296–306.
10. You YN, Baxter NN, Stewart A, et al. Is the increasing rate of local excision for stage I rectal cancer in the United States justified?: a nationwide cohort study from the National Cancer Database. Ann Surg. 2007;245:726–33.
11. Vennix S, Pelzers L, Bouvy N, et al. Laparoscopic versus open total mesorectal excision for rectal cancer. Cochrane Libr. 2014;15:CD005200.
12. Garcia-Aguilar J, Mellgren A, Sirivongs P, et al. Local excision of rectal cancer without adjuvant therapy: a word of caution. Ann Surg. 2000;231:345–51.
13. Bentrem DJ, Okabe S, Wong WD, et al. T1 adenocarcinoma of the rectum: transanal excision or radical surgery? Ann Surg. 2005;242:472–7.
14. Nash GM, Weiser MR, Guillem JG, et al. Long-term survival after transanal excision of T1 rectal cancer. Dis Colon Rectum. 2009;52:577–82.
15. O'Neill CH, Platz J, Moore JS, et al. Transanal endoscopic microsurgery for early rectal cancer: a single-center experience. Dis Colon Rectum. 2017;60:152–60.

16. Moore JS, Cataldo PA, Osler T, et al. Transanal endoscopic microsurgery is more effective than traditional transanal excision for resection of rectal masses. Dis Colon Rectum. 2008;51:1026–31.
17. Lin GL, Qiu HZ, Meng WC, et al. Local resection for early rectal tumours: comparative study of transanal endoscopic microsurgery (TEM) versus posterior trans-sphincteric approach (Mason's operation). Asian J Surg. 2006;29:227–32.
18. De Graaf EJR, Burger JWA, Van Ijsseldijk ALA, et al. Transanal endoscopic microsurgery is superior to transanal excision of rectal adenomas. Color Dis. 2011;13:762–7.
19. Christoforidis D, Cho HM, Dixon MR, et al. Transanal endoscopic microsurgery versus conventional transanal excision for patients with early rectal cancer. Ann Surg. 2009;249:776–82.
20. Zenni GC, Abraham K, Harford FJ, et al. Characteristics of rectal carcinomas that predict the presence of lymph node metastases: implications for patient selection for local therapy. J Surg Oncol. 1998;67:99–103.
21. Brodsky JT, Richard GK, Cohen AM, et al. Variables correlated with the risk of lymph node metastasis in early rectal cancer. Cancer. 1992;69:322–6.
22. Madbouly KM, Remzi FH, Erkek BH, et al. Recurrence after transanal excision of T1 rectal cancer: should we be concerned? Dis Colon Rectum. 2005;48:711–21.
23. Brown G, Davies S, Williams GT, et al. Effectiveness of preoperative staging in rectal cancer: digital rectal examination, endoluminal ultrasound or magnetic resonance imaging? Br J Cancer. 2004;91:23–9.
24. Puli SR, Bechtold ML, Reddy JB, et al. How good is endoscopic ultrasound in differentiating various T stages of rectal cancer? Meta-analysis and systematic review. Ann Surg Oncol. 2009;16:254–65.
25. Kotanagi H, Fukuoka T, Shibata Y, et al. The size of regional lymph nodes does not correlate with the presence or absence of metastasis in lymph nodes in rectal cancer. J Surg Oncol. 1993;54:252–4.
26. Andreola S, Leo E, Belli F, et al. Manual dissection of adenocarcinoma of the lower third of the rectum specimens for detection of lymph node metastases smaller than 5 mm. Cancer. 1996;77:607–12.
27. Kim JH, Beets GL, Kim MJ, et al. High-resolution MR imaging for nodal staging in rectal cancer: are there any criteria in addition to the size? Eur J Radiol. 2004;52:78–83.
28. Quirke P, Dixon MF, Durdey P, et al. Local recurrence of rectal adenocarcinoma due to inadequate surgical resection: histopathological study of lateral tumour spread and surgical excision. Lancet. 1986;328:996–9.
29. Lezoche G, Guerrieri M, Baldarelli M, et al. Transanal endoscopic microsurgery for 135 patients with small nonadvanced low rectal cancer (iT1–iT2, iN0): short- and long-term results. Surg Endosc. 2011;25:1222–9.
30. Nascimbeni R, Burgart LJ, Nivatvongs S, et al. Risk of lymph node metastasis in T1 carcinoma of the colon and rectum. Dis Colon Rectum. 2002;45:200–6.
31. Garcia-Aguilar J, Shi Q, Thomas CR Jr, et al. A phase II trial of neoadjuvant chemoradiation and local excision for T2N0 rectal cancer: preliminary results of the ACOSOG Z6041 trial. Ann Surg Oncol. 2012;19:384–91.
32. Gracia Solanas JA, Ramírez Rodríguez JM, Aguilella Diago V, et al. A prospective study about functional and anatomic consequences of transanal endoscopic microsurgery. Rev Esp Enferm Dig. 2006;98:234–40.
33. Cataldo PA, O'Brien S, Osler T. Transanal endoscopic microsurgery: a prospective evaluation of functional results. Dis Colon Rectum. 2005;48:1366–71.
34. Salm R, Lampe H, Bustos A, et al. Experience with TEM in Germany. Endosc Surg Allied Technol. 1994;2:251–4.
35. Barendse RM, Dijkgraaf MG, Rolf UR, et al. Colorectal surgeons' learning curve of transanal endoscopic microsurgery. Surg Endosc. 2013;27:3591–602.
36. Floyd ND, Saclarides TJ. Transanal endoscopic microsurgical resection of pT1 rectal tumors. Dis Colon Rectum. 2006;49:164–8.
37. Schäfer H, Baldus SE, Hölscher AH. Giant adenomas of the rectum: complete resection by transanal endoscopic microsurgery (TEM). Int J Color Dis. 2006;21:533.
38. Saclarides TJ. TEM/local excision: indications, techniques, outcomes, and the future. J Surg Oncol. 2007;96:644–50.
39. Sengupta S, Tjandra JJ. Local excision of rectal cancer. Dis Colon Rectum. 2001;44:1345–61.
40. Borschitz T, Heintz A, Junginger T. The influence of histopathologic criteria on the long-term prognosis of locally excised pT1 rectal carcinomas: results of local excision (transanal endoscopic microsurgery) and immediate reoperation. Dis Colon Rectum. 2006;49:1492–506.
41. Lezoche G, Baldarelli M, Paganini AM, et al. A prospective randomized study with a 5-year minimum follow-up evaluation of transanal endoscopic microsurgery versus laparoscopic total mesorectal excision after neoadjuvant therapy. Surg Endosc. 2008;22:352–8.
42. Lee W, Lee D, Choi S, et al. Transanal endoscopic microsurgery and radical surgery for T1 and T2 rectal cancer. Surg Endosc. 2003;17:1283–7.
43. Bach SP, Hill J, Monson JRT, et al. A predictive model for local recurrence after transanal endoscopic microsurgery for rectal cancer. Br J Surg. 2009;96:280–90.
44. Hompes R, McDonald R, Buskens C, et al. Completion surgery following transanal endoscopic microsurgery: assessment of quality and short-and long-term outcome. Color Dis. 2013;15:e576–81.

The Approach to Transanal Total Mesorectal Excision

F. Borja de Lacy and Antonio M. Lacy

Introduction

The gold standard treatment for curative locally advanced rectal cancer is radical resection with a complete mesorectal excision. Combined with neoadjuvant chemoradiation therapy, total mesorectal excision (TME) has been demonstrated to reduce tumor recurrence, as the complete removal of the mesorectum limits the radial spread of cancer cells [1]. The TME technique has evolved from open to minimally invasive approaches, including laparoscopic and robotic. The superiority of one approach over another is still under debate.

Due to the difficulty of working in the low pelvis, especially in male and obese patients, which may increase the risk of incomplete mesorectal excisions or positive margins, the transanal TME (TaTME) technique has emerged as a valid alternative to the previous approaches. TaTME allows for potential increased quality of the TME, especially in mid and low rectal tumors. This has been shown in recent studies and meta-analyses [2, 3]. The real long-term oncological benefits of

TaTME are still under investigation, but the enormous potential of TaTME have opened the door to global use [4, 5].

TaTME can be technically challenging; thus structured training and standardization of the technique are necessary for its appropriate implementation [6]. In this chapter, we present a detailed description on how to approach TaTME, based on our experience from more than 400 cases.

Operative Setup

Patient Preparation

According to current guidelines, all patients with rectal cancer suitable for radical resection should undergo thorough preoperative staging that includes complete study of the colon (colonoscopy or virtual colonoscopy in cases of obstructive tumors), thoracic and abdominopelvic computed tomography, pelvic magnetic resonance imaging, and serological analysis of carcinoembryonic antigen. In patients whose tumor is not palpable by digital rectal examination, a rigid proctoscopy should be performed to measure its distance from the anal verge or anorectal junction. After appropriate staging, surgeons, medical and radiation oncologists, radiologists, and pathologists should discuss each case assessing the benefits of multidisciplinary treatment.

Electronic supplementary material The online version of this chapter (https://doi.org/10.1007/978-3-030-18740-8_33) contains supplementary material, which is available to authorized users.

F. B. de Lacy (✉) · A. M. Lacy
Gastrointestinal Surgery Department, Hospital Clinic, University of Barcelona, Barcelona, Spain
e-mail: bdelacy@aischannel.com;
amlacy@aischannel.com

© Springer Nature Switzerland AG 2020
J. Kim, J. Garcia-Aguilar (eds.), *Minimally Invasive Surgical Techniques for Cancers of the Gastrointestinal Tract*, https://doi.org/10.1007/978-3-030-18740-8_33

Once surgery is indicated, it is recommended that the patient meets an enterostomal nurse, for appropriate physical and mental education. The day before surgery, our routine practice is to perform mechanical bowel preparation, together with the administration of oral antibiotics and one dose of subcutaneous unfractionated heparin for thromboprophylaxis. Before the induction of anesthesia, intravenous antibiotic prophylaxis is given with cefazolin and metronidazole. Intermittent pneumatic compression devices are placed, and the patient is set in modified lithotomy (Lloyd-Davies) position.

Operative Room Preparation

TaTME can be performed by a one-team or a two-team approach ("Cecil approach"). The one-team approach should start with the abdominal phase of the procedure, finishing the dissection just before entering the peritoneal reflection. Then the surgical team should move to the transanal phase. The reason is that performing the transanal portion of the procedure first can cause pneumoretroperitoneum that may challenge the abdominal dissection.

If personnel are available, we strongly recommend the two-team approach. Working simultaneously allows for shorter operative time and better traction and counter-traction to facilitate the resection. Both teams should have different monitors and insufflator systems. The procedure starts with occlusion of the distal sigmoid by the abdominal team until the transanal team completes the intraluminal rectal purse-string. Until both fields are connected, the pressure should be higher in the transanal field to avoid pneumoretroperitoneum and to facilitate rectal distention.

Abdominal Phase

The abdominal approach can be determined by surgeon preference, although we favor a conventional laparoscopic medial-to-lateral colonic mobilization. The operative table is tilted in Trendelenburg position with slight patient's right

side down (Fig. 33.1). A 12-mm trocar is inserted at the umbilicus for the camera; a 5-mm trocar is inserted in the right flank, a 5-mm trocar in the right lower quadrant, and a 5-mm trocar in the left lower quadrant. Additional trocars can be added, generally in the epi- or hypogastrium for further retraction (Fig. 33.2).

The left colon should be mobilized with high ligation of the inferior mesenteric artery (preserving the pelvic nerve plexuses) and division of the inferior mesenteric vein at the lower border of the pancreas. The splenic flexure is typically mobilized to provide enough colonic length and limit anastomotic tension. Then the caudal dissection follows, as described in the traditional abdominal TME technique, while the transanal team progresses in the opposite direction. Once both teams are connected ("Rendezvous"), the abdominal team helps with traction and counter-traction and facilitates transanal dissection. At this point, the insufflation pressures of both fields are equalized, usually at 15 mmHg.

Transanal Phase

Video 33.1

The transanal approach depends on the height of the tumor and whether the transanal endoscopic platform can be inserted while ensuring a safe distal resection margin. Three-dimensional cameras and insufflators with continuous flow and smoke evacuation have further optimized the safety and quality of transanal resection.

Mid and Low Rectal Tumors Except 2–3 cm Above the Dentate Line

The transanal phase begins with rectal irrigation and placement of an anal retractor (Lonestar, CooperSurgical, Trumbull, CT, USA) to visualize the dentate line. After correct anal dilatation (Fig. 33.3), the endoscopic platform is introduced. We have considerable experience with the flexible Gelpoint Path (Applied Medical, Rancho Santa Margarita, CA, USA), which requires a shorter learning curve and provides better maneu-

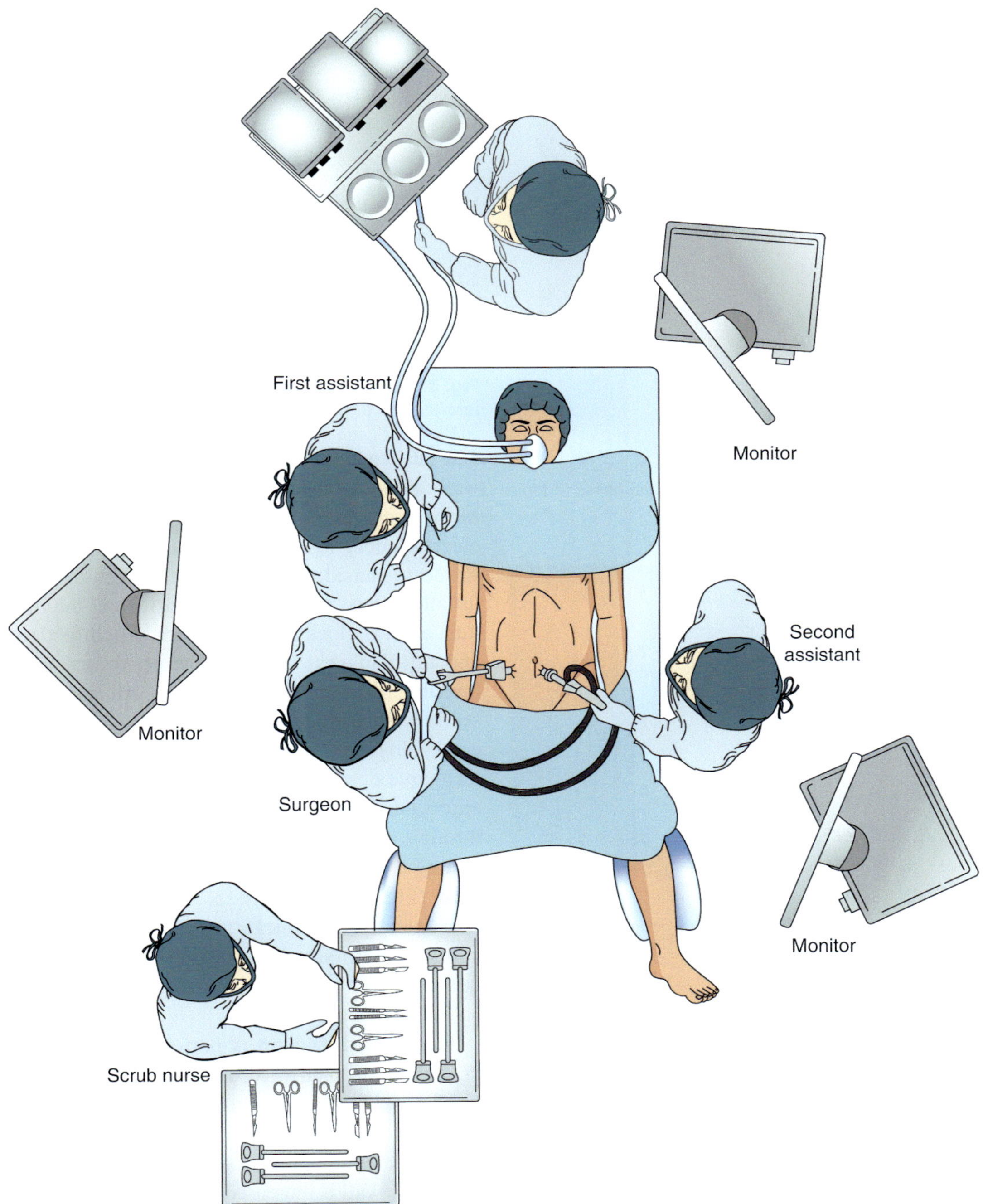

Fig. 33.1 Theater organization for abdominal phase of laparoscopic low anterior resection

verability. Three trocars are inserted in an inverted triangle (Fig. 33.4), with the camera placed at the 6-o'clock position. The abdominal team then occludes the distal sigmoid, and the pneumorec-tum is established at a pressure of 15 mmHg. The distal edge of the tumor is located, and, at the desired distance, a purse-string suture with a 26-mm needle and a size 0 polydioxanone suture

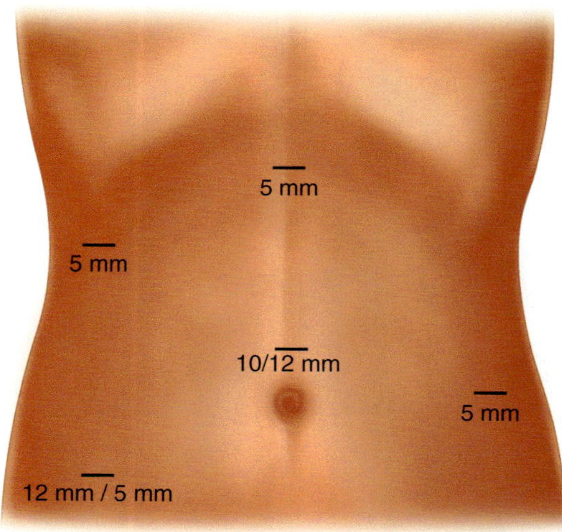

Fig. 33.2 Trocar positions for abdominal phase of laparoscopic low anterior resection

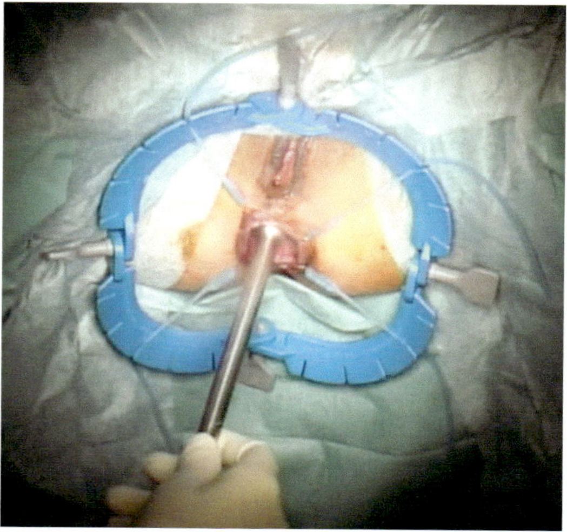

Fig. 33.3 Intraoperative image showing anal dilatation following placement of the Lonestar retractor

is made to close the rectal lumen (Fig. 33.5), with small equal bites at the same rectal level. The purse-string stitching is a crucial step of the procedure, as its tightness is imperative to prevent translocation of liquid stool and cancer cells during the dissection, which may increase the risk of pelvic abscess and locoregional recurrence.

The closed rectal stump is flooded with cytocidal solution to eliminate potential tumor cells,

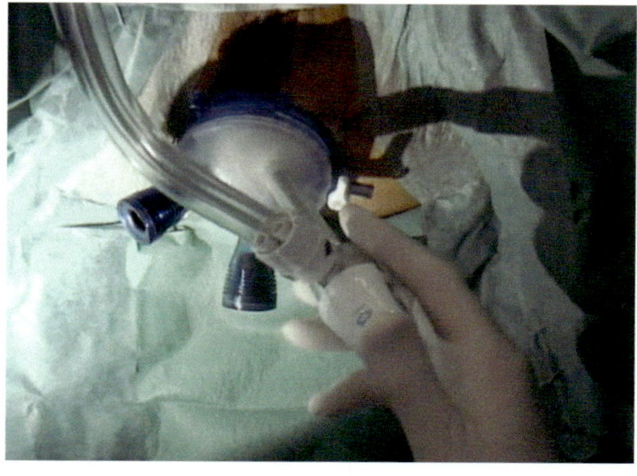

Fig. 33.4 The Gelpoint endoscopic platform has been inserted into the anal canal

and subsequently, the transection of the rectal wall starts under endoscopic visualization. This rectal transection or rectotomy is carried out with electrocautery in a circumferential fashion from inside to outside (Fig. 33.6). The rectotomy is usually started on the anterior surface of the rectum, at 12-o'clock in counterclockwise direction, and full-thickness dissection is performed until reaching the avascular TME plane. An acute dissection is carried out cranially, following the embryologically defined principles of the TME technique described by Heald [7]. The transanal approach seems to offer a more natural dissection through the "Holy plane," recognizing and dissecting inside Denonvilliers' and Waldeyer's fascias (Fig. 33.7). This is the plane where intraoperative complications (hemorrhage, autonomic nerve injury, prostate dissection, and urethral injury) can be minimized while producing optimal TME specimens.

Cephalad dissection is performed with electrocautery. Bipolar forceps can be used to control small vessels. Due to increased low pelvic space inherent to the transanal dissection, enhanced by cranial rectal retraction, the risk of damaging the pelvic sidewall is increased compared to abdominal TME. The improved visualization by laparoscopic instruments may help the surgeon identify the correct lateral planes and avoid dissecting laterally to the endopelvic fascia.

Although not the routine practice of all surgical units, we favor circumferential dissection,

Fig. 33.5 Endoscopic suturing was performed to create purse-string closure of the rectal lumen

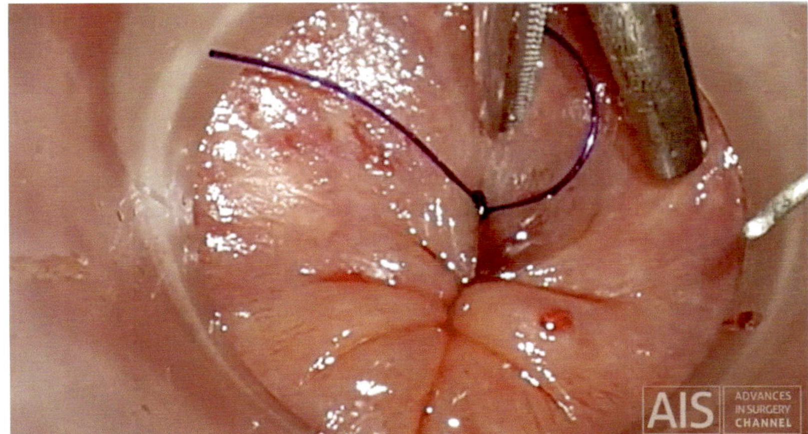

Fig. 33.6 Intraoperative image showing rectotomy that is performed with electrocautery in a circumferential fashion from inside to outside. The assistant is holding the purse-string suture

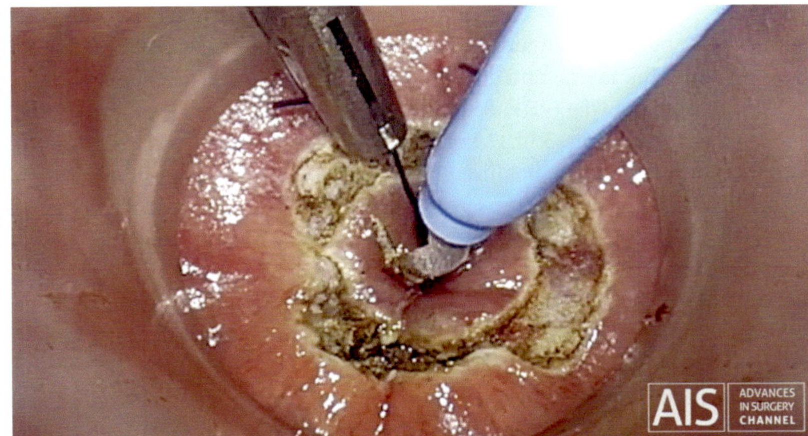

Fig. 33.7 Intraoperative image showing dissection through the "holy plane," recognizing and dissecting inside Denonvilliers' and Waldeyer's fascias

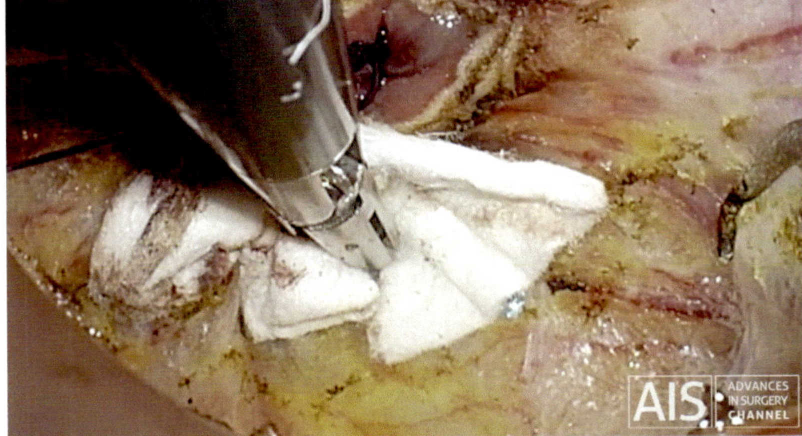

trying to maintain symmetry. Our platform allows pelvic insufflation to help to find the mesorectal innermost correct plane. It is always easier to find the TME plane at the anterior and posterior sides, so connecting them may help if any doubt arises while dissecting the lateral boundaries.

TaTME carries potential pitfalls and new complications, such as urethral or pelvic sidewall injuries. As always, the surgeon must master anatomy and the relationships with neighboring structures: Denonvilliers' fascia, prostate, seminal vesicles, urethra, and vagina anteriorly; neurovascular bundles laterally; and Waldeyer's fascia and presacral vessels posteriorly. The surgeon must remember that dissecting too posteriorly, outside Waldeyer's fascia, might lead to hemorrhage but also dangerous confusion when coming along the lateral and anterior sides.

Upon reaching the "Rendezvous" with the abdominal team (Fig. 33.8), both teams work together until the rectum is ultimately released.

Low Rectal Tumors up to 2–3 cm Above the Dentate Line

When the tumor is located so low that limits the endoscopic platform insertion, an intersphincteric dissection with conventional open instruments might be the first step. As suggested by Rullier et al. [8], a standard coloanal anastomosis may be performed in supra-anal tumors (>1 cm from the anal ring), a partial intersphincteric resection in juxta-anal tumors (<1 cm from the anal ring), and a total intersphincteric resection in intra-anal tumors, meaning that the internal anal sphincter is invaded. Once there is enough tissue to close the lumen, the purse-string suture with a size 0 polydioxanone suture is placed. Afterwards, the endoscopic platform can be inserted, and the dissection can be continued with laparoscopic instruments.

High Rectal Tumors

When the tumor is located in the high rectum (10–15 cm from the anal verge), a partial mesorectal excision with transection of the mesorectum at least 5 cm below the distal edge of the tumor can be made. After the endoscopic platform is inserted, 5 cm are measured distally to the tumor and the rectal lumen is closed. Then, the rectum and mesorectum are transected perpendicularly until reaching the proper TME plane. Dissecting inside the mesorectum carries a higher risk of bleeding, which can be limited using sealing devices. Whether the transanal approach has a clear benefit in patients with high rectal tumors is still under debate, although advantages such as shorter operative times and lower conversion rates have been suggested.

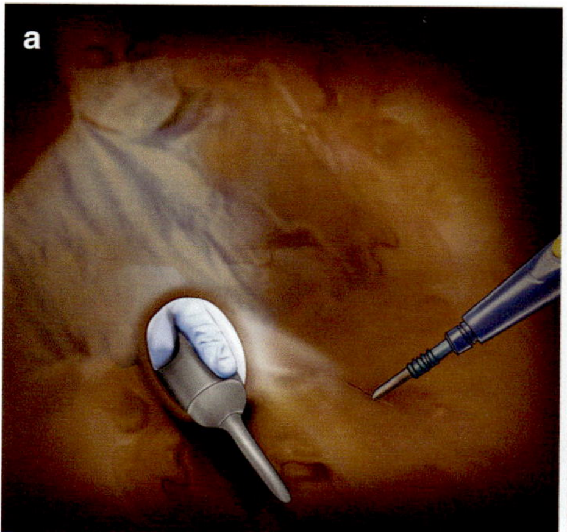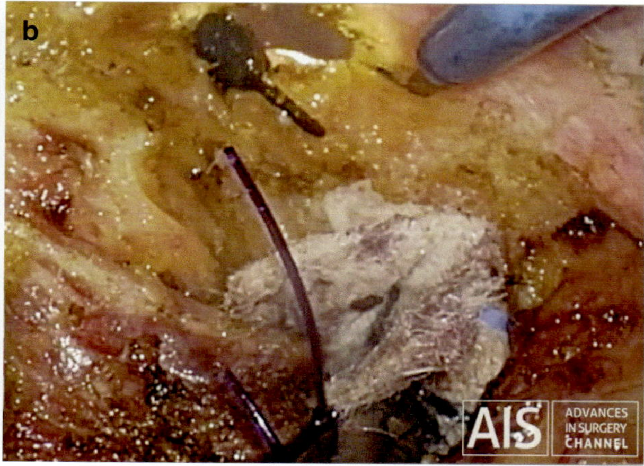

Fig. 33.8 (**a**) Illustration showing the "rendezvous" point where the abdominal team meets the transanal team. (**b**) Paired intraoperative image showing when transanal dissection reaches the abdomen and electrocautery from the abdomen meets electrocautery from the perineum

Specimen Extraction

The specimen may be extracted through the transanal or transabdominal routes. It is worth noting that transanal extraction provides greater integrity of the abdominal wall, decreasing the risk of surgical site infections and incisional hernias and improving postoperative pain and cosmesis. However, transanal extraction can be performed only when the size of the tumor, the mesorectum, and the pelvis allows it. Splenic flexure mobilization is recommended if transanal extraction is planned, to avoid excessive vascular tension during the specimen retrieval. In case of a single-stapled double-purse-string anastomosis, the purse-string on the opened distal rectal cuff should be performed before transanal extraction, preventing mucosal retraction that may increase the difficulty of specimen extraction. In case of a hand-sewn coloanal anastomosis, the transanal extraction must be performed after placing the four cardinal stitches.

In case of a large tumor, bulky mesentery, or excessively narrow pelvis, we believe that a transabdominal specimen extraction is safer than the transanal route. In the majority of these cases, a Pfannenstiel incision can be created that is tailored to the specimen size.

Regardless of the specimen extraction site, we have incorporated indocyanine green fluorescence angiography for real-time intraoperative evaluation of bowel perfusion before proximal colonic transection. If available, we strongly recommend its use, as it is considered a promising tool to reduce anastomotic leak rate [9]. Bowel perfusion may also be assessed after creation of the anastomosis.

Anastomosis

When a stapled anastomosis is attempted, we favor the single-stapled, double-purse-string method. Once the specimen has been resected, the anvil is inserted into the proximal colon either to perform a side-to-end or an end-to-end anastomosis. A second purse-string, usually with a size 0 polypropylene suture, is placed in the opened distal cuff. In mid and low rectal tumors, this purse-string may be performed by hand after removing the endoscopic platform. In cases of higher tumors, suturing by hand might be extremely challenging, and its performance with the transanal platform and laparoscopic instruments is recommended. The rectal cuff purse-string is then tied around the anvil, and the stapler is connected. Our most significant experience is with regular colorectal EEA or hemorrhoidal staplers, the latter with longer spike and delivering wider doughnuts. A 10-Fr drainage catheter might facilitate the technique: inserted on the stapler spike if a regular EEA stapler is used and removed laparoscopically or on the proximal anvil for a more natural transanal extraction in cases of hemorrhoidal stapler use. Once the anvil and the pin are connected, the stapler is fired. Post-anastomosis exploration is recommended, either with direct or endoscopic view to rule out bleeding and assess for pneumoperitoneum leak through the staples.

In cases of hand-sewn coloanal anastomoses, four cardinal 2-0 polyglycolic stitches are placed in the opened rectal cuff, leaving the needles in place. After specimen extraction, the proximal colon is positioned back to the pelvis. The colonic lumen is then opened, and the four cardinal stitches are put through the desired site. Before knotting those four points, several 3-0 polyglycolic sutures are placed to complete the coloanal anastomosis. Each stitch must include a full-thickness bite of the colon.

After completion of the anastomosis, a closed-suction drain is typically left in the pelvis, and a decompressing tube is inserted transanally to decrease sphincter-resting pressure. The surgical team assesses the need for diverting ileostomy. In cases when anastomosis is not considered, always having been agreed upon preoperatively with the patient, the rectal stump may be closed and a terminal end colostomy may be performed.

Postoperative Care

The postoperative care should follow the same principles as for any standard laparoscopic low anterior resection. With increasing adoption of enhanced recovery after surgery (ERAS) programs, patients may be treated according to "fast-track" protocols. Early feeding, mobilization, and respiratory exercises are applied and the closed-suction drain is removed before the patient's discharge.

References

1. McCall JL. Total mesorectal excision: evaluating the evidence. Aust N Z J Surg. 1997;67:599–602.
2. Xu W, Xu Z, Cheng H, et al. Comparison of short-term clinical outcomes between transanal and laparoscopic total mesorectal excision for the treatment of mid and low rectal cancer: a meta-analysis. Eur J Surg Oncol. 2016;42:1841–50.
3. Ma B, Gao P, Song Y, et al. Transanal total mesorectal excision (taTME) for rectal cancer: a systematic review and meta-analysis of oncological and perioperative outcomes compared with laparoscopic total mesorectal excision. BMC Cancer. 2016;16:380.
4. Stevenson AR, Solomon MJ, Lumley JW, et al. Effect of laparoscopic-assisted resection vs open resection on pathological outcomes in rectal Cancer: the ALaCaRT randomized clinical trial. JAMA. 2015;314:1356–63.
5. Fleshman J, Branda M, Sargent DJ, et al. Effect of laparoscopic-assisted resection vs open resection of stage II or III rectal Cancer on pathologic outcomes: the ACOSOG Z6051 randomized clinical trial. JAMA. 2015;6(314):1346–55.
6. Francis N, Penna M, Mackenzie H, et al. Consensus on structured training curriculum for transanal total mesorectal excision (TaTME). Surg Endosc. 2017;31:2711–9.
7. Heald RJ, Husband EM, Ryall RD. The mesorectum in rectal cancer surgery – the clue to pelvic recurrence? Br J Surg. 1982;69:613–6.
8. Rullier E, Denost Q, Vendrely V, et al. Low rectal cancer: classification and standardization of surgery. Dis Colon Rectum. 2013;56:560–7.
9. Keller D, Ishizawa T, Cohen R, et al. Indocyanine green fluorescence imaging in colorectal surgery: overview, applications, and future directions. Lancet Gastroenterol Hepatol. 2017;2:757–66.

Craig S. Johnson and Margaret W. Johnson

Introduction

Lesions in the colon and rectum, whether malignant or benign, require surgical intervention to treat or prevent the development of cancer. A variety of new operative options for the excision of rectal lesions have emerged in recent decades. The following chapter introduces procedures used to address rectal lesions before expanding upon the latest treatment option for such cases: robotic transanal minimally invasive surgery (TAMIS). Some key points of comparison are effectiveness, patient impact, and accessibility of the technique.

Historically, treatment for colon and rectal lesions has involved the removal of the entire affected section of the colon or rectum along with the attached mesorectum and lymph nodes, a procedure called total mesorectal excision (TME). This open operation, while curative, has been associated with high morbidity and mortality rates. It can result in permanent colostomy, bowel, bladder, and sexual dysfunction [1]. These

deleterious effects prompted surgeons to explore less invasive options that could minimize the impact on patient quality of life without sacrificing oncological outcomes.

Local excision, a procedure that removes a lesion without removing the surrounding section of the colon or rectum, is a less invasive operation available for treatment of early-stage cancer patients and patients with small benign tumors [2]. This technique was first written about in the nineteenth century and has been further explored and fine-tuned in recent years [3]. Today, many patients are candidates for local excision. Colorectal cancer is the third most common cancer diagnosis [4]; and 39% of diagnoses are localized-stage disease [5]. These patients could be eligible for a minimally invasive treatment option.

As interest in natural orifice transluminal endoscopic surgery (NOTES) emerged, so did efforts to attempt transanal local excision. With this treatment option, patients benefit from the lack of an anastomosis, as well as the lack of an external wound [6–8]. Initial attempts at local excision left much to be improved. The most common transanal local excision technique, simply called transanal excision (TAE), results in good postoperative quality of life and employs widely available instruments but has substantially worse oncological outcomes than TME. Difficulty visualizing and exposing the lesion can lead to imprecise excision and inferior oncological outcomes [9, 10]. This procedure can

Electronic supplementary material The online version of this chapter (https://doi.org/10.1007/978-3-030-18740-8_34) contains supplementary material, which is available to authorized users.

C. S. Johnson (✉)
Oklahoma Surgical Hospital, Tulsa, OK, USA
e-mail: cjohnson@satulsa.com

M. W. Johnson
The University of Texas, Austin, TX, USA

© Springer Nature Switzerland AG 2020

J. Kim, J. Garcia-Aguilar (eds.), *Minimally Invasive Surgical Techniques for Cancers of the Gastrointestinal Tract*, https://doi.org/10.1007/978-3-030-18740-8_34

treat accessible tumors within the anal canal, but patients with lesions further from the verge cannot undergo TAE. This procedure can be a good option for eligible patients, as it rarely causes anal sphincter, bladder, or sexual dysfunction. TAE is the most commonly used method of local excision because of the availability of necessary instrumentation and the limited detrimental effects on quality of life [11].

Transanal endoscopic microsurgery (TEM) was introduced in 1983 but remained infrequently used due to the cost and complexity of the instruments, the technical difficulty of the procedure, and the need for additional training [9, 12]. While TEM spares patients from the high risk of morbidity associated with TME, it can still negatively impact quality of life. The rigid scope used in the procedure combined with long operative time can result in short-term reduction in anorectal function. TEM results in inferior oncological outcomes compared to major resection but superior outcomes compared to TAE [2, 13]. TEM allows for much better visualization and, consequently, better excision than TAE especially with experienced surgeons [14]. Overall, TEM does not produce better oncological outcomes or postoperative quality of life and is more challenging for surgeons to learn due to lack of instrumentation and learning opportunities.

In 2009, laparoscopic TAMIS was developed [15]. This procedure was designed as a hybrid between TEM and laparoscopy [16]. While TEM requires specialized instrumentation, laparoscopic TAMIS employs widely available laparoscopic instruments. The accessibility of the instruments is an improvement upon earlier surgeries, but many of the difficulties associated with laparoscopic TAMIS stem from these very instruments [17, 18]. Laparoscopic TAMIS can work well for tumors 8–12 cm from the anal verge [2], but it is difficult to achieve quality visualization and excision beyond this limited range. Even within this range, suturing presents a significant technical challenge [19]. It is too early to know the long-term oncological outcomes of laparoscopic TAMIS [13]. Shortly after the introduction of laparoscopic TAMIS, robotic TAMIS was developed to build upon this advancement.

Robotic TAMIS is a minimally invasive option that uses multi-use instruments without sacrificing accuracy of excision or postoperative quality of life. The feasibility of this procedure was initially shown in a cadaveric study [20]. Later studies found that the robot allowed for improved vision, control, and maneuverability and was both safe and feasible [21–23, 24]. The author has performed robotic TAMIS on lesions from 6 to 18 cm from the anal verge and have found that the robotic platform allows for high-quality excisions that would be outside of the range of both laparoscopic TAMIS and TEM. Because this procedure was developed recently, there are relatively few articles detailing patient outcomes. The following explains this procedure in depth.

Rationale for Robotic TAMIS

Robotic TAMIS allows for minimally invasive local excision of benign and early malignant rectal lesions. It can be used to treat or prevent cancer or for palliation [25]. Robotic TAMIS allows a surgeon to overcome the limitations of the laparoscopic technique concerning closure of the defect [19] and to reach a wider range of lesions, particularly more proximal ones.

Preoperative Evaluation

Colonoscopy

Colonoscopy must be performed to exclude proximal colonic lesions.

Rigid Proctoscopy

Rigid proctoscopy allows for accurate measurement of the rectal lesion in relation to the anal verge. It also gives the surgeon an opportunity to measure the size of the lesion and determine the location of disease in relation to the valves of Houston.

MRI and Endorectal Ultrasound

Magnetic resonance imaging (MRI) or endorectal ultrasound (ERUS) shows the depth of invasion into the wall of the rectum. It also allows for assessment of the perirectal lymph nodes.

Patient Selection

Indications

Indications for robotic TAMIS include:

- Patients with benign rectal lesions or early-stage malignant lesions no lower than the first valve of Houston and no higher than 15–18 cm from the anal verge
- Patients with T2 lesions treated with preoperative radiation and chemotherapy
- Patients with lesions less than the entire circumference for benign lesions below the peritoneal reflection and up to 4 cm in diameter above the peritoneal reflection

Contradictions

Contradictions for robotic TAMIS include:

- Patients with advanced rectal cancer (i.e., T3 or T4)
- Patients with node-positive disease
- Patients with symptoms of pain and obstruction secondary to the primary tumor

Special Considerations

Robotic TAMIS can be utilized as a palliative technique for patients who are symptomatic from the primary tumor and deemed unfit for major abdominal surgery. For example, robotic TAMIS may be appropriate for patients with advanced (stage IV) rectal cancer with local symptoms such as tumor-specific hemorrhage [25].

Robot, Ports, and Instrumentation

Port

The GelPOINT Path (Applied Medical, Rancho Santa Margarita, CA; USA) is a port specifically designed for transanal surgery [9]. Unlike the rigid sleeve used for TEM, the GelPOINT Path is smaller and made of flexible silicone, preventing loss of sphincter function after surgery [19]. The GelPOINT Path consists of a sleeve that is inserted and then attached to a cap (Fig. 34.1). The cap is filled with a gel through which instruments are inserted. These components provide the airtight seal necessary for insufflation and protect the anal canal from moving instrumentation.

Insufflator

In order to maintain a stable pneumoperitoneum, CO_2 insufflation must be maintained at a constant pressure of 10–15 mmHg. Conventional insufflators will not allow for a constant pressure and cause a bellowing effect of the rectum, making TAMIS virtually impossible. Currently, there are two insufflators that create constant pressure: the Airseal (Surgiquest, Orange, CT, USA) and the Smith and Nephew insufflator (Smith and Nephew, London, UK).

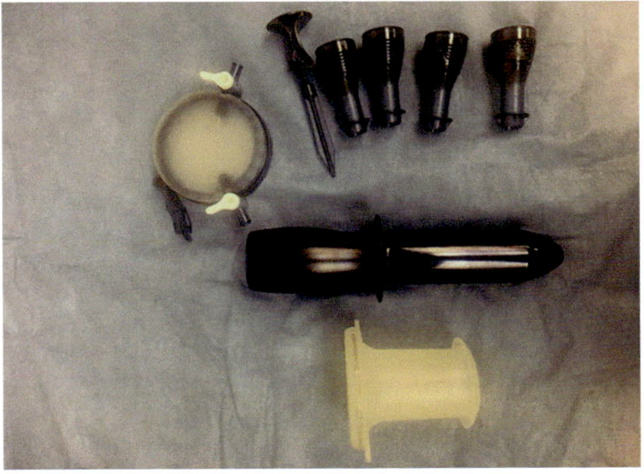

Fig. 34.1 GelPOINT Path. The preferred platform for robotic TAMIS

Robot

The da Vinci Xi robot (Intuitive Surgical, Inc., Sunnyvale, CA, USA) has many features that facilitate a TAMIS procedure. The ports can be placed only a few centimeters apart while still allowing the instruments to work in parallel. In this way, a surgeon can avoid the need to cross instruments. The arms and instruments are slimmer than previous-generation robots and can be positioned directly over the patient, allowing the robotic cart to be placed on either side of the patient (Figs. 34.2 and 34.3).

Operating Theatre and Assistants

The procedure can be carried out in a general use robotic operating room. One bedside assistant and one nurse are required. The bedside assistant is seated between the patient's legs in lithotomy position (Xi) or on the opposite side of the bedside cart in the prone position (Si). The role of the bedside assistant is to change robotic instruments during the operation, pass sutures, and provide suction. Additional responsibilities are to monitor the robotic arms for potential collisions and to make bedside adjustments as needed.

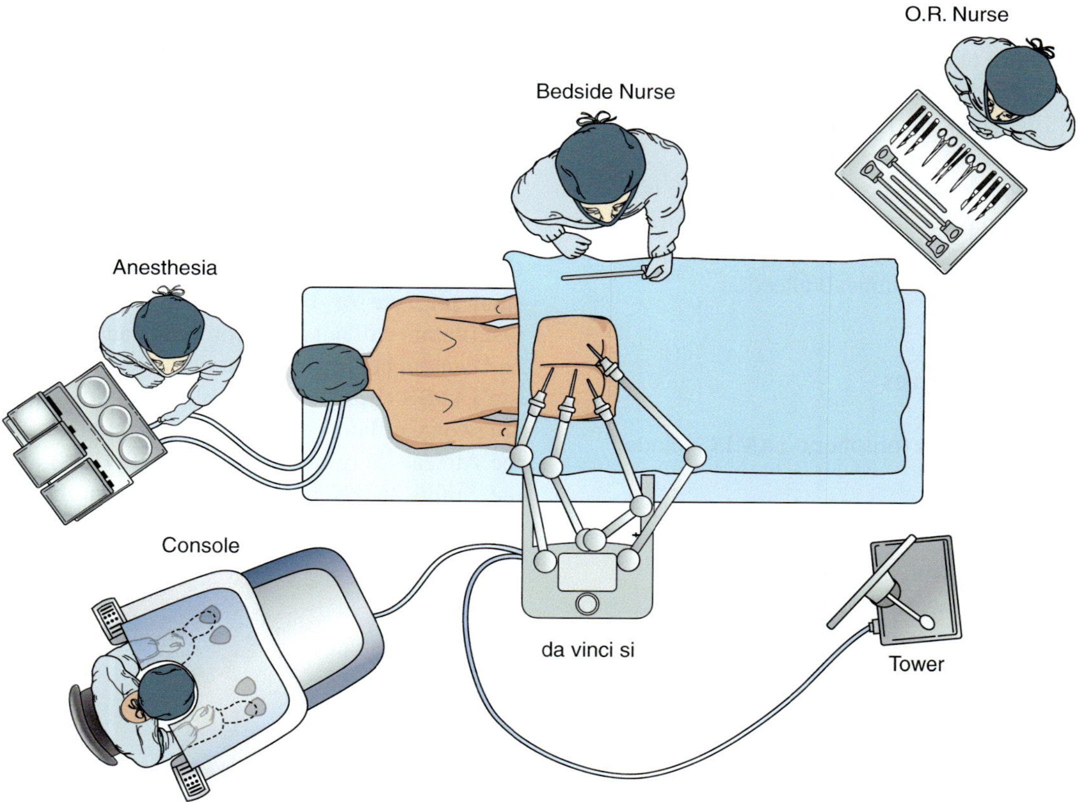

Fig. 34.2 Proper positioning of the Si in TAMIS. The port placement and instrumentation are the same as with the Xi robot. The main difference will be patient positioning. The patient should be in the prone position with the robot side docked

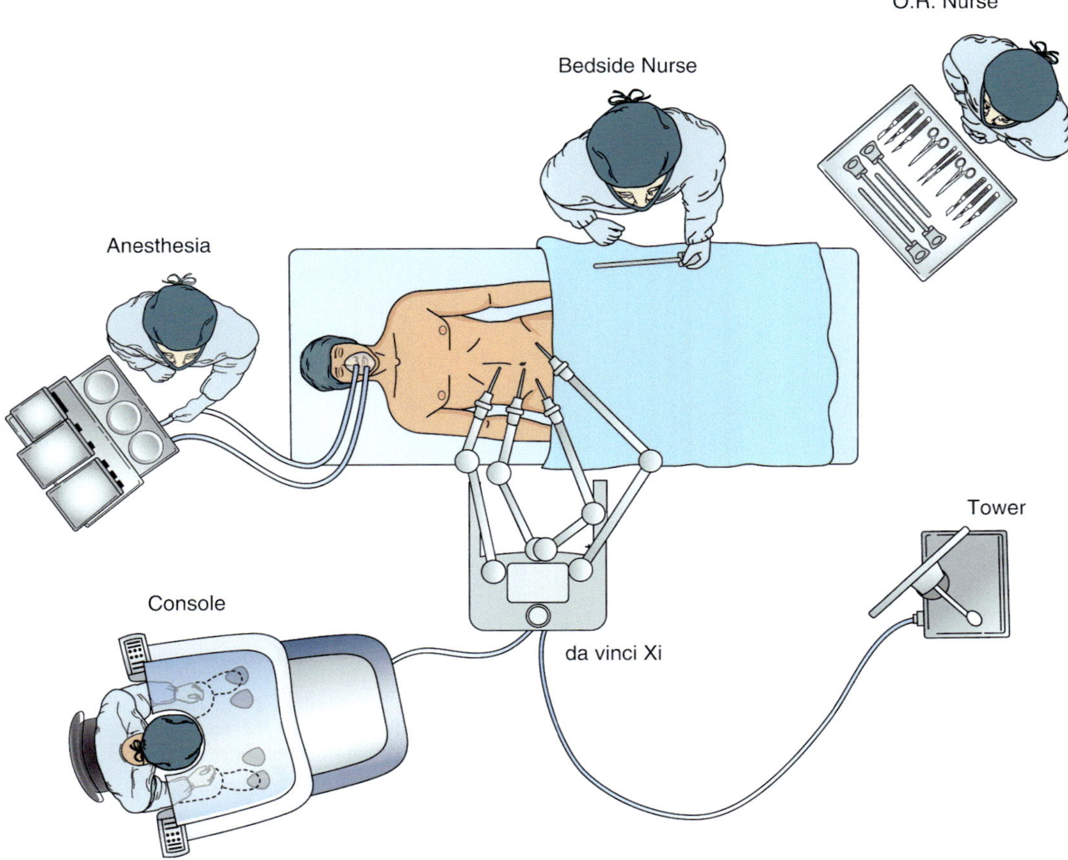

Fig. 34.3 Proper positioning of the Xi robot in TAMIS. The camera arm should be aligned with the long axis of the body with one working arm on each side. The arms are brought in as close as possible to the camera arm allowing for use of the instrument in as parallel position as possible

Patient Positioning

Modified Lloyd-Davies position is most functional for this procedure. This position allows for the anesthesiologist to have easy access to the patient's airway. This position is preferred in morbidly obese patients, as it avoids pressure on the upper torso that may impede respiration. For all patients, precautions typical for abdominal operations must be taken to prevent neurovascular injury to the lower extremities.

The vast majority of lesions can be well visualized and successfully treated in the lithotomy position. The setup of robotic TAMIS creates a seemingly paradoxical relationship between position and visualization. The prone position is best to visualize posterior lesions just above the sphincter complex but will not allow for proper visualization of anterior lesions just above the sphincter complex. Robotic TAMIS in the prone position is appropriate as long as the patient's body habitus allows for safe anesthesia. Based on tumor location and body habitus, a surgeon must choose between the prone and the supine position.

Robot Docking and Setup
(Video 34.1)

With the patient properly positioned (approximately 20° Trendelenburg) under general anesthesia with muscular blockade, prepped and

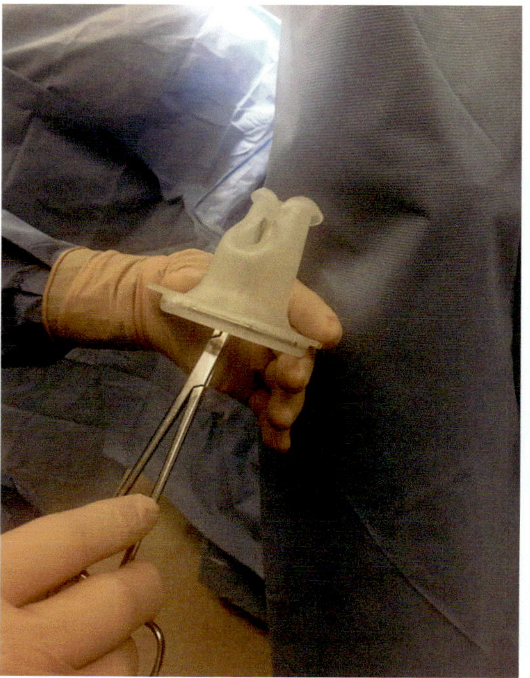

Fig. 34.4 Crimping the sleeve prior to placement in the anal canal

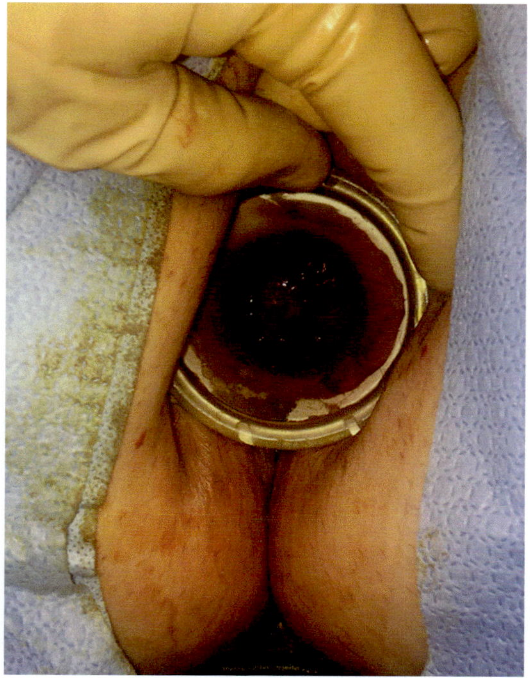

Fig. 34.5 Proper position of GelPOINT Path sleeve. Note the slight prolapse of the rectal mucosa indicating that the collar of the sleeve is above the sphincter complex and rectal ring

draped, and after a "time out," a perianal block of bupivicaine with epinephrine is given.

The GelPOINT Path anal sleeve is introduced into the anal canal. In order to insert the sleeve, the opening of the port flat is pressed and then folded into a "U" shape (Fig. 34.4), and then the folded end of the sleeve is inserted into the anus until the proximal bevel of the sleeve is above the sphincter complex (Fig. 34.5). Once the sleeve has been inserted, insert the obturator through the sleeve in order to expand the sleeve.

The anal sleeve is sutured to the perianal skin with a heavy silk suture (Fig. 34.6). The 12- and 6-o'clock positions must be unencumbered, so the sutures should be placed between the 2- to 4-o'clock and 8- to 10-o'clock positions. The GelPOINT Path cap is placed with the locking latch at the 6-o'clock position; otherwise the built-in ports could obstruct the robotic ports when placed. The insufflation port is placed at the 6-o'clock position, 5 mm from the edge of the gel cap. Insufflation should commence at 10–15 mmHg.

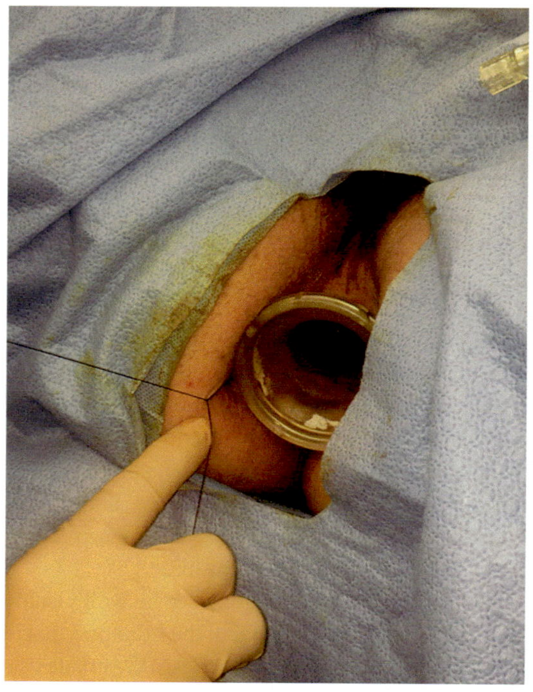

Fig. 34.6 Anchoring the GelPOINT Path sleeve

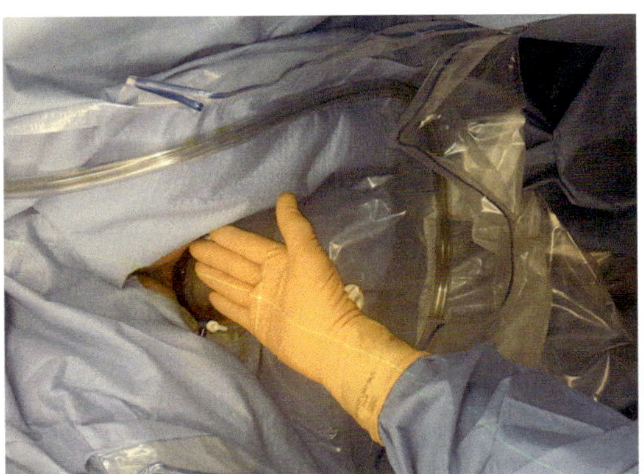

Fig. 34.7 Aligning the laser crosshairs. Place the crosshairs approximately 10 cm from the 12-o'clock position of the GelPOINT Path to align the camera arm

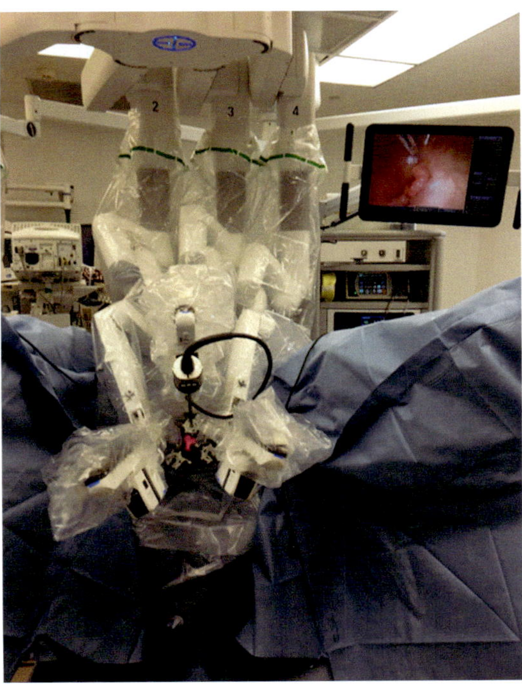

Fig. 34.8 Docked robot. Note how the arms are tucked in close allowing parallel use of the instruments

Prior to driving the Xi robotic cart to the bedside, select either the patient left or patient right setting, depending on the placement of the cart. Choose upper abdomen and deploy for docking. To position the robot, align the laser crosshairs approximately 10 cm distal to the 12-o'clock position of the gel point cap. Using the palm of the surgeon's hand as a surface to view the lasers is helpful (Fig. 34.7).

Place a robotic 8 mm port at the 12-o'clock position of the gel cap 5 mm from its edge. Place the port to a depth of midway up the port's shaft. Dock the port to one of the central robotic arms, #2 or #3. The assistant should dock the robotic ports as they are placed. Once the camera port is docked, place the camera at 30 ° up configuration. This configuration allows the camera and working arms to function with the least amount of collisions because they will be on separate planes. The camera arm must be aligned with the axis of the patient's body. Once the camera is placed, one may choose to target or not. Targeting will align the boom height at the ideal height for sterility and ensure that the working arms are in range for docking.

Place the working arm ports at the 3:15 and 8:45 positions, 5 mm from the edge of the gel cap. The depth of these two ports should be just through the gel. The gravitational center should

be visible once docked. By placing the ports in this fashion, collisions between the heads of the trocars are avoided and the robotic arms will have enough room to dock in patients who are in the lithotomy position (Figs. 34.8 and 34.9).

The instruments to be used are monopolar curved scissors or a cautery hook and needle drivers in the dominant hand and a fenestrated bipolar in the non-dominant hand. If using the scissors, place this instrument first while there remains room to pass the pointed tip of the shears safely. Then insert the other instruments into the ports.

Energy settings on the ERBE Vio electrocautery unit (ERBE Marietta, GA, USA) should initially be set on Dry Cut 1, Soft Coag 3, and Bipolar 3 with auto stop. The cautery hook produces more smoke and spray than the shears do on similar settings. The electrocautery unit can be adjusted to get the desired tissue effect with as little smoke and spray as possible.

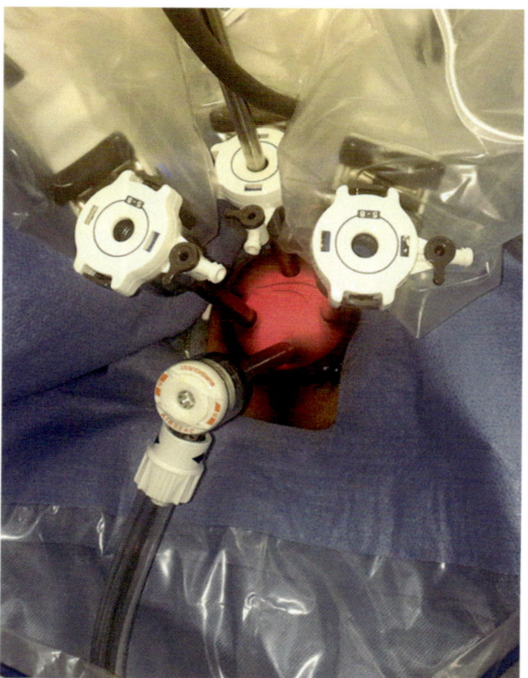

Fig. 34.9 GelPOINT Path with the trocars placed and robot docked

Visualization, Excision, and Closure

After setup and docking are complete, the surgeon goes to the console. Information gathered preoperatively can be used to locate and visualize the lesion. Advance the camera and instruments alternately, always maintaining view of the instruments while they are in motion since you cannot rely on haptic feedback for obstacles [23]. Once visualized, excision of the lesion is carried out within surgical principles, submucosal or full thickness.

There are several technical points to consider unique to the robot while working in a narrow, tight space. Keeping the shafts of the working instruments parallel and at the periphery while using the waist portions of the instruments toward each other is most efficient. Moving the arms as little as possible and in a very slow and deliberate fashion will help avoid crossing the instruments and fouling the camera.

Once the lesion has been removed, the assistant grasps it with a locking laparoscopic grasper through the assistant port. At this point, undock the

robot and remove the robotic ports, allowing the assistant to remove the gel cap with the specimen grasped. Once the specimen has been retrieved, it should be oriented and sutured to a needle board for pathologic examination. The robot is redocked according to the same guidelines followed at the beginning of the procedure. The process of undocking, retrieving the specimen, and redocking to close the defect takes 4–6 minutes.

To avoid undocking and redocking, one may choose to leave the specimen parked in the rectum during closure of the defect. There are some drawbacks to leaving the specimen parked. The lesion may get in the way during closure of the defect. It can also get "lost" in the proximal colon requiring endoscopic retrieval. Additionally, there is concern for seeding the rectal defect with neoplastic cells. Removing the specimen promptly upon excision avoids those issues and also allows for immediate inspection of margins. The potential problems associated with retrieving the specimen prior to closing the defect should be weighed against the relative minimal time it takes to go through this process.

Closure of the defect is carried out after retrieving the specimen and redocking the robot. As robotic TAMIS remains to be standardized, there is no consensus yet on whether the defect must be closed. As with TEM, the majority of authors recommend suturing the wound, but no randomized trials have proven the superiority of this technique [19, 26].

Some describe defect closure as a necessary step in any TAMIS procedure [2, 13], but others state the opposite [9]. In the largest study to address the question of closing the defect ($n = 75$), endoscopy 3 months after surgery showed that all defects that had been left open had healed. This study was the only study of TAMIS to conclude that leaving the defect open did not increase morbidity [19].

Operating robotically as opposed to laparoscopically may overcome technical difficulties that preclude defect closure. The robot allows for precise suture closure and avoids interference between instruments, even in the confined pelvic cavity [17]. Routine closure of the defect is not only possible but also preferable. It guards against avoidable complications such as those from undetected intraperitoneal microperforation [27]. We close all rectal defects in order to guard against preventable complications; and closure is mandatory if the peritoneum is entered. Some use laparoscopic assistance to inspect the abdominal contents for any potential injury and to perform a leak test if the peritoneal cavity is breeched during excision, but this is not mandatory and would depend on the circumstances [13].

Choice of suture material for closure should be re-absorbable suture lasting greater than 45 days. The type of closure can be running or interrupted. While techniques vary, we have discovered closure to be most efficient using a 3-0 V-lock (180 days) on a CV-23 needle that is 15 cm in length. Suturing should be carried out in a transverse fashion to avoid any intraluminal rectal stenosis (Fig. 34.10). Closure of the defect can be quite challenging and pushes the robot's capabilities. To work around difficulties, a surgeon can change which instrument hand is suturing, rotate the camera either to the left or right, or have the bedside assistant retract as needed.

Upon closure of the defect, the rectum is irrigated and inspected. Individual interrupted sutures can be used if a defect remains. When satisfied, undock the robot and remove the gel point path device. Rigid proctoscopy is performed for final inspection. Finally, a dry gauze dressing is applied.

Postoperative Management

Patients are admitted to the hospital for a planned overnight stay. They are started on a soft diet immediately. Activity is limited to bathroom privileges with sitting in a chair the evening of surgery. If a Foley catheter was placed at surgery, it is scheduled to be removed at midnight on the day of surgery. Having the Foley removed at midnight gives time to use urinary retention protocols by the first postoperative morning. The perianal dressing is removed on the morning of postoperative day 1. No additional bandage or care is typically required, and the vast majority of patients experience no pain. If there is discomfort, acetaminophen is recommended. The patient is discharged on postoperative day 1 with instructions to eat a soft diet, take a daily stool softener, and avoid lifting >10 lbs. for 2 weeks. We have the patient return for postoperative visit at 2 weeks. An external anal exam is done on the first postoperative visit. Postoperative endoscopy should be at 6 months to 1 year. If there was a questionable margin, endoscopy should be performed at 3 months. If the patient is doing well, the patient is allowed to return to work without restriction.

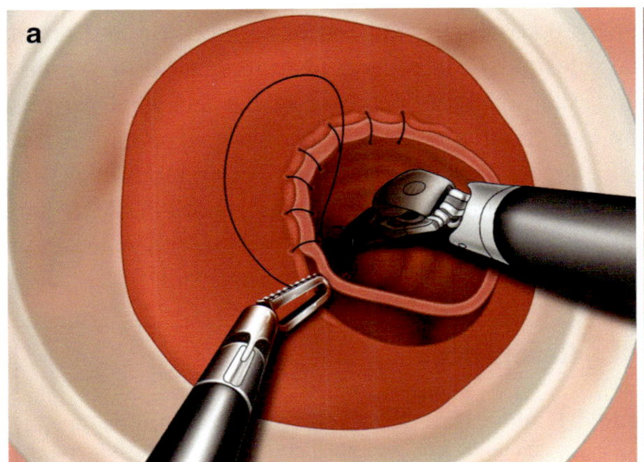

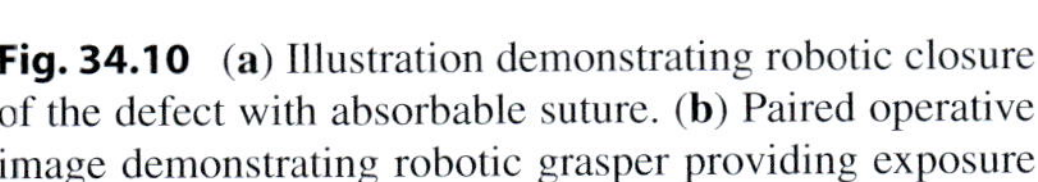

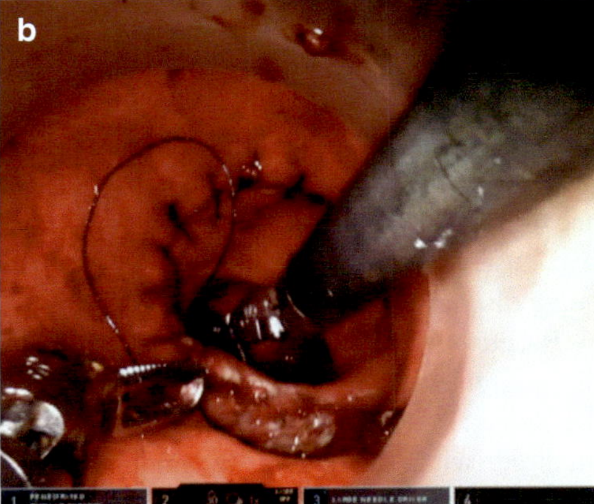

Fig. 34.10 (**a**) Illustration demonstrating robotic closure of the defect with absorbable suture. (**b**) Paired operative image demonstrating robotic grasper providing exposure and the robotic needle driver closing the rectal defect with V-Loc suture

Conversions

Conversion from robotic TAMIS is a rare occurrence in properly selected patients. Robotic assistance in rectal operations has been shown to significantly lower the conversion rate compared to purely laparoscopic operations [23, 17]. In the author's experience, cases performed according to the above protocol had no conversion, meaning that all cases that were begun robotically remained minimally invasive robotic procedures.

If a case cannot be completed robotically, the surgeon has a few options. For lesions above the peritoneal reflection, conversion from a robotic TAMIS typically results in an abdominal procedure, namely, a low anterior resection. Laparoscopic TAMIS should be the next step for lesions below the peritoneal reflection that cannot be completed robotically. It is very difficult to complete the procedure via laparoscopic TAMIS if the procedure cannot be completed robotically. Typically, lesions below the peritoneal reflection are converted to a transanal excision. It would be a rare event to convert a lesion below 8 cm to an abdominal procedure.

Complications

Urinary retention is the most common postoperative complication in robotic TAMIS. This complication is common to laparoscopic and robotic TAMIS. One study found that urinary retention was an issue for 40% of patients with hospital stays over 24 hours [14]. This complication could impede a major benefit of robotic surgery by increasing the length of hospital stay. A trial of neostigmine 0.5–1 mg IM q1h prn for a total of five doses is effective in preventing the patient being discharged with a Foley catheter.

Based on the location of the lesion, entry of the peritoneal cavity can be an expected part of the procedure. Closure of the peritoneal cavity is repaired with the suture technique described above. In a patient who has had mechanical and antibiotic bowel prep with appropriate preoperative antibiotics, no special precautions are needed postoperatively.

Postoperative rectal bleeding can occur within the first 10 days postoperatively. This complication is typically secondary to a hematoma developing in the resection bed. This bleeding can be significant and require a return to surgery; however, this bleeding usually stops with bedrest and correction of clotting abnormalities. A leak from a peritoneal entry site can occur and is treated as a postoperative anastomotic leak. Return to surgery with closure of the leak, drainage, and proximal diversion is usually required.

Postoperative infection within the closure site can occur rarely. Abscess should be drained by transanal approach, leaving the operative area open to heal secondarily. Appropriate broad-spectrum antibiotics are given for 10 days.

Rectovaginal fistula can occur on rare occasions. If acute, the typical treatment is repair of the fistula if possible and proximal diversion. Rectal stenosis can also occur with transanal excision. This can be due to technical difficulty in properly closing the defect but is usually secondary to postoperative infection. Proctoplasty versus low anterior resection may be required to correct this complication. Finally, there has been no report of urethral injury with robotic TAMIS.

Conclusion

Robotic TAMIS appears to be a safe and feasible approach for excision of some colon and rectal lesions. The robotic instrumentation may assist with overcoming some of the technical barriers of traditional TAMIS using laparoscopic instruments. Further studies are required to fully assess the long-term outcomes of robotic TAMIS and how they relate to other available procedures.

References

1. Althumairi AA, Gearhart SL. Local excision for early rectal cancer: transanal endoscopic microsurgery and beyond. J Gastrointest Oncol. 2015;6:296–306.
2. Hakiman H, Michael M, Fleshman JW. Replacing transanal excision with transanal endoscopic microsurgery and/or transanal minimally invasive sur-

gery for early rectal cancer. Clin Colon Rectal Surg. 2015;28:38–42.

3. Classic articles in colonic and rectal surgery. Jacques Lisfranc 1790–1847. Observation on a cancerous condition of the rectum treated by excision. Dis Colon Rectum. 1983;26:694–5.

4. Colorectal cancer facts & figures 2014–2016. Atlanta: American Cancer Society; 2014. https://www.cancer.org/research/cancer-facts-statistics/all-cancer-facts-figures/cancer-facts-figures-2014.html.

5. Colorectal cancer facts & figures 2017–2019. Atlanta: American Cancer Society; 2017. https://www.cancer.org/research/cancer-facts-statistics/all-cancer-facts-figures/cancer-facts-figures-2017.html.

6. Willingham FF, Brugge WR. Taking NOTES: translumenal flexible endoscopy and endoscopic surgery. Curr Opin Gastroenterol. 2007;23:550–5.

7. Flora ED, Wilson TG, Martin IJ, et al. A review of natural orifice translumenal endoscopic surgery (NOTES) for intra-abdominal surgery experimental models, techniques, and applicability to the clinical setting. Ann Surg. 2008;247:583–602.

8. Nakamura T, Mitomi H, Ihara A, et al. Risk factors for wound infection after surgery for colorectal cancer. World J Surg. 2008;32:1138–41.

9. Noura S, Ohue M, Miyoshi N, et al. Transanal minimally invasive surgery (TAMIS) with a GelPOINT® Path for lower rectal cancer as an alternative to transanal endoscopic microsurgery (TEM). Mol Clin Oncol. 2016;5:148–52.

10. Endreseth BH, Myrvold HE, Romundstad P, et al. Transanal excision vs. major surgery for T1 rectal cancer. Dis Colon Rectum. 2005;48:1380–8.

11. Garcia-Aguilar J, Mellgren A, Sirivongs P, et al. Local excision of rectal cancer without adjuvant therapy: a word of caution. Ann Surg. 2000;231:345–51.

12. Buess G, Kipfmuller K, Ibald R, et al. Clinical results of transanal endoscopic microsurgery. Surg Endosc. 1988;2:245–50.

13. Gill S, Stetler JL, Patel A, et al. Transanal minimally invasive surgery (TAMIS)- standardizing a reproducible procedure. J Gastrointest Surg. 2015;19:1528–36.

14. McLemore EC, Weston LA, Coker AM, et al. Transanal minimally invasive surgery for benign and malignant rectal neoplasia. Am J Surg. 2014;208:372–81.

15. Atallah S, Albert M, Larach S. Transanal minimally invasive surgery: a giant leap forward. Surg Endosc. 2010;24:2200–5.

16. Martin-Perez B, Andrade-Ribeiro GD, Hunter L, et al. A systematic review of transanal minimally invasive surgery (TAMIS) from 2010 to 2013. Tech Coloproctol. 2014;18:775–88.

17. Ortiz-Oshiro E, Sánchez-Egido I, Moreno-Sierra J, et al. Robotic assistance may reduce conversion to open in rectal carcinoma laparoscopic surgery: systematic review and meta-analysis. Int J Med Robot. 2012;8:360–70.

18. Jiménez Rodríguez RM, Díaz Pavón JM, de La Portilla de Juan F, et al. Prospective randomised study: robotic-assisted versus conventional laparoscopic surgery in colorectal cancer resection. Cir Esp. 2011;89:432–8.

19. Hahnloser D, Cantero R, Salgado G, et al. Transanal minimal invasive surgery for rectal lesions: should the defect be closed? Color Dis. 2015;17:397–402.

20. Hompes R, Rauh SM, Hagen ME, et al. Preclinical cadaveric study of transanal endoscopic da Vinci® surgery. Br J Surg. 2012;99:1144–8.

21. Atallah S, Quinteros F, Martin-Perez B, et al. Robotic transanal surgery for local excision of rectal neoplasms. J Robotic Surg. 2014;8:193–4.

22. Zimmern A, Prasad L, Desouza A, et al. Robotic colon and rectal surgery: a series of 131 cases. World J Surg. 2010;34:1954–8.

23. Mirnezami AH, Mirnezami R, Venkatasubramaniam AK, et al. Robotic colorectal surgery: hype or new hope? A systematic review of robotics in colorectal surgery. Color Dis. 2010;12:1084–93.

24. Hompes R, Rauh SM, Ris F, et al. Robotic transanal minimally invasive surgery for local excision of rectal neoplasms. Br J Surg. 2014;101:578–81.

25. Sumrien H, Dadnam C, Hewitt J, et al. Feasibility of transanal minimally invasive surgery (TAMIS) for rectal tumours and its impact on quality of life – the bristol series. Anticancer Res. 2016;36:2005–9.

26. Ramirez JM, Aguilella V, Arribas D, et al. Transanal full-thickness excision of rectal tumours: should the defect be sutured? a randomized controlled trial. Color Dis. 2002;4:51–5.

27. Clermonts SH, Zimmerman DD. Closure of the rectal defect after transanal minimally invasive surgery: a word of caution. Color Dis. 2015;17:642–3.

Index